HAND REHABILITATION

A Quick Reference Guide and Review

HAND REHABILITATION

A Quick Reference Guide and Review

SUSAN WEISS, OTR/L, CHT
Chief Executive Officer,
Exploring Hand Therapy Company, Inc.
St. Petersburg, Florida

NANCY FALKENSTEIN, OTR/L, CHT CEES
President,
Exploring Hand Therapy Company, Inc.
St. Petersburg, Florida

SECOND EDITION

with **400** *illustrations*

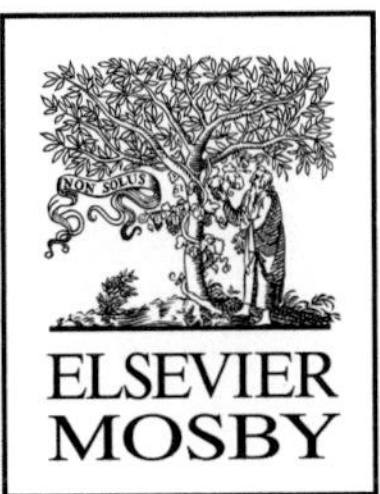

ELSEVIER
MOSBY

11830 Westline Industrial Drive
St. Louis, Missouri 63146

HAND REHABILITATION: A QUICK REFERENCE
GUIDE AND REVIEW,
SECOND EDITION

We are aware of the many techniques available to treat particular pathologies and realize this book may present debatable material. We have made every effort to verify the answers to the questions. References are provided to clarify controversial points. The material presents the technique, view, statement, or opinion of the authors and contributors, which is helpful and interesting to other practitioners. We have made every effort to ensure that the therapeutic modalities recommended are in accordance with accepted standards and the appendix material is current at the time of this publication. It is the practitioner's responsibility to evaluate the appropriateness of a particular opinion in clinical situations and to consider new developments.

One of the uses of this text is to help readers review for certification and/or examinations related to the upper extremity. This book has not been endorsed by and is not affiliated with any organization that licenses or certifies in hand rehabilitation. The authors have not been assisted in the development or publication of this text by any licensing or certifying organization.

Previous edition copyrighted 1999

ISBN-13: 978-0-323-02610-9
ISBN-10: 0-323-02610-9

Publishing Director: Linda Duncan
Managing Editor: Kathy Falk
Developmental Editor: Melissa Kuster Deutsch
Editorial Assistant: Colin Odell
Publishing Services Manager: Linda McKinley
Senior Project Manager: Jennifer Furey
Design manager: Gail Morey Hudson

Printed in the United States of America

Last digit is the print number: 9 8 7 6 5 4 3

Dedications

To my husband David, for his unconditional support of this project and for losing me for hours on end to edit and re-edit this second edition. Mom and Dad, thanks again for listening to me say how I stayed up late night after night working tediously on each chapter. To Jake my darling little boy for standing next to mommy's computer every day saying "I love you mommy," and inspiring me to continue. To Brandon and Justin for allowing me to work in the background with the light on, so I could sit with them while they watched a movie or TV. Finally, I dedicate this book to my dearly loved and missed brother Jason, in loving memory and tears.

SW

To my precious gifts from God . . . my children David and Danielle. I love you both "to the moon and back" . . . thank you for your unconditional love and support. To the love of my life, Mike Guerra, who has given me love, perspective, and friendship. Mike, you have helped make me whole, when I didn't know I wasn't. To my mother, who has given me my "drive" and for her unconditional dedication to me and all her children.

NF

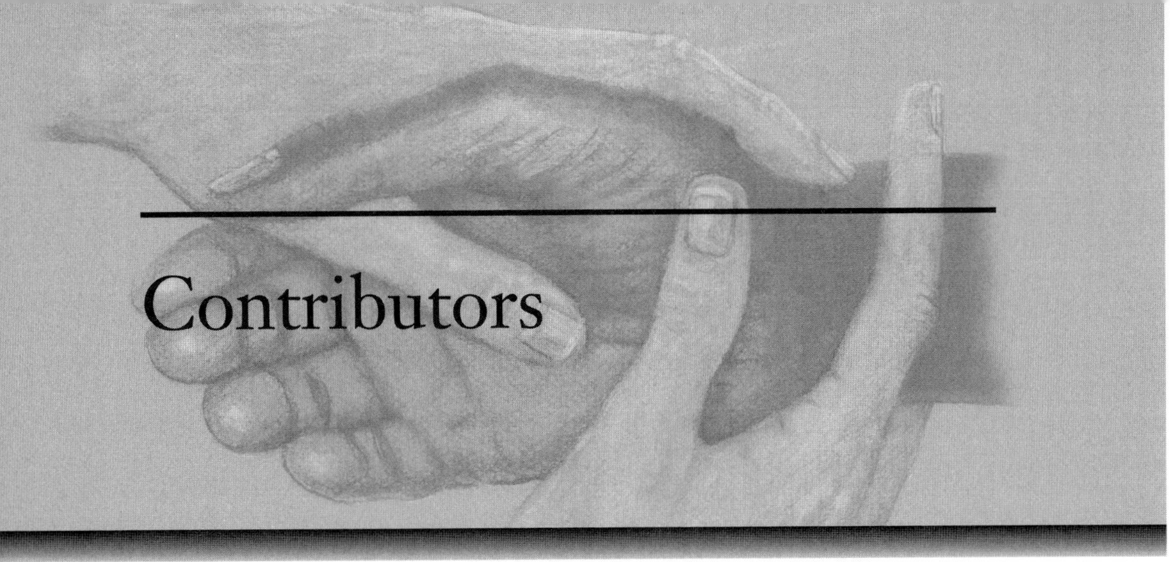

Contributors

Susan Weiss and Nancy Falkenstein developed and contributed to all chapters. Contributors are listed in alphabetical order.

Contributed topics are italicized.

Randall D. Alley, BSc, CP, FAAOP
ISPO, ABC, Chair Upper Limb Prosthetic Society
Innovative Neurotronics, Inc.
Thousand Oaks, California
Congenital Anomalies/Amputations/Prosthetics

Jacqueline Alton
St. Petersburg, Florida
Wounds/Infection

Bambi L. Anderson, OTR/L
Clinical Specialist, Upper Extremity Prosthetics
Otto Bock Health Care
Minneapolis, Minnesota
Congenital Anomalies/Amputations/Prosthetics

Karen Baker, PT, Cert. MDT
Physical Therapist
Outpatient Physical Therapy
Tampa Bay Orthopaedic Specialists
St. Petersburg, Florida
Hodge Podge of Treatment Techniques

Brigitte Borsh-Zimmer, OTR/L, CHT
Clinical Manager
Occupational Therapy—Hand Therapy Clinic
Mease Countryside Hospital
Safety Harbor, Florida
Cumulative Trauma and Differential Diagnosis

Roxanne C. Bottum, OTR/L, CHT
Director of Hand Therapy
Occupational Therapy
All Florida Orthopaedic Associates
St. Petersburg, Florida
Cumulative Trauma and Differential Diagnosis

Dale G. Bramlet, MD
Clinical Associate Professor
University of South Florida
Tampa, Florida
Director of Hand Surgery
Orthopaedic Surgery
Bayfront Medical Center
St. Petersburg, Florida
Fractures

George H. Canizares, MD
Orthopaedic Surgeon
All Florida Orthopaedic Association
St. Petersburg, Florida
Sports Injuries of the Upper Extremity

Philip A. Davidson, MD
Assistant Clinical Professor
Surgery, Division—Orthopedics
University of South Florida College of Medicine
Tampa, Florida
Tampa Bay Orthopaedic Specialists
St. Petersburg, Florida
Elbow, Shoulder

A. Lee Dellon, MD
Professor of Plastic Surgery, Professor of Neurosurgery
Johns Hopkins University
Baltimore, Maryland
Professor of Plastic Surgery, Neurosurgery, and Anatomy
University of Arizona
Tucson, Arizona
Neuroanatomy and Sensory Reeducation

Lloyd Allen Deneau, BS, CPT
Director of Physical Therapy
Physical Therapy
Commonwealth Rehabilitation
Largo, Florida
Shoulder

Karen Dhanens, OTR/L, CHT
Occupational Therapy
Trinity Medical Center
Rock Island, Illinois
Anatomy Extravaganza

Jon J. Ehrich, DO, MD
Board-Certified Physiatrist
Diplomate, American Board of Physical Medicine and Rehabilitation
Palm Beach Gardens, Florida
Complex Regional Pain Syndrome/Reflex Sympathetic Dystrophy

Leonard Elbaum, EdD, PT
Associate Professor
Department of Physical Therapy, School of Health
Florida International University
Miami, Florida
Principal
Elbaum & Associates
Research, Education, and Consultation in Physical Rehabilitation
Miami, Florida
Modalities

Georgianna Gacula Fres, OTR/L
Occupational Therapist
Hand Therapy
All Florida Orthopedic Associates
St. Petersburg, Florida
Hand Enthusiasts Vendor and Website List

Antonio J. Gayoso, MD
Plastic Surgery
All Florida Orthopaedics Associates
St. Petersburg, Florida
Flaps/Grafts/Thermal Conditions

Casey Hoover, OTR/L
Staff Occupational Therapist
Hand Therapy
All Florida Orthopaedic Associates
St. Petersburg, Florida
Evaluation, Hand Enthusiasts Vendor and Website List, Nutrition

Heather Hoyt, OTR/L
Upper Extremity Clinical Specialist
Professional Services
Otto Bock Health Care
Minneapolis, Minnesota
Congenital Anomalies/Amputations/Prosthetics

Eric P. Keefer, MD
Chief Resident
Department of Orthopedic Surgery
Lenox Hill Hospital
New York, New York
Biomechanics and Tendon Transfers

Jodi Jones Knauf, OTR, PAC
Physician Assistant
All Florida Orthopaedics
St. Petersburg, Florida
Drugs Commonly Encountered in Hand Therapy

Constance Kurash, OTR/L, CHT
Independent Contractor
Lee Memorial Health Systems
Fort Meyers, Florida
Intrinsic Mechanism

Paul C. LaStayo, PhD, PT, CHT
Associate Professor
Physical Therapy
University of Utah
Salt Lake City, Utah
Wrist

Kathryn L. Lowenstein, OTR/L
Arthritis Center
Palm Harbor, Florida
Arthritis

Mitchell B. Lowenstein, MD
Fellow of the American College of Rheumatology and Internal Medicine
Arthritis Center
Palm Harbor, Florida
Arthritis

Anne M. Lucado, MS, PT, CHT
Staff Physical Therapist
The Hand Center
Wake Forest University Baptist Medical Center
Winston Salem, North Carolina
Tendons

Amy Mills, OTR/L, CHT
Occupational Therapist
All Florida Orthopaedic Associates
St. Petersburg, Florida
Hand Enthusiasts Vendor and Website List, Nutrition

Patrick C. Prigge, CP
Upper Extremity Manager
Professional Services
Otto Bock Health Care
Minneapolis, Minnesota
Congenital Anomalies/Amputations/Prosthetics

Jorge Rodriguez, MD
Private Practice
St. Petersburg, Florida
Elbow

Julie A. Schick, CP, OTR/L
Clinical Specialist, Upper Extremity Prosthetics
Professional Services
Otto Bock Health Care
Minneapolis, Minnesota
Congenital Anomalies/Amputations/Prosthetics

Douglas R. Shier, PhD
Professor
Department of Mathematical Sciences
Clemson University
Clemson, South Carolina
Research and Statistics

Stephen D. Simonich, MD
Tampa Bay Orthopaedic Specialists
St. Petersburg, Florida
Sports Injuries of the Upper Extremity

Gerald E. Stark, Jr., BSME, CP, FAAOP
Guest Lecturer
Physical Medicine
Prosthetic-Orthotic Center
Chicago, Illinois
Vice President of Education and Technical Support
The Fillauer Companies, Inc.
Chattanooga, Tennessee
Congenital Anomalies/Amputations/Prosthetics

Charlene Stennett, OTR/L, CHT
Director of Hand Therapy
Miami Hand Center
Miami, Florida
Fractures

Shawn Swanson, BS, OTR/L
Occupational Therapist
Clinical Specialist, Upper Extremity Prosthetics
Professional Services
Otto Bock Health Care
Minneapolis, Minnesota
Congenital Anomalies/Amputations/Prosthetics

Paul Van Lede, OT, MS
Orfit Industries
Wijnegam, Belgium
Splinting

Wayne B. Whittle, BS, PT
Owner
Next Step Rehabilitation
St. Petersburg, Florida
Elbow

S. Steven Yang, MD, MPH
Assistant Adjunct
Division Hand Surgery
Department of Orthopedic Surgery
Lenox Hill Hospital
New York, New York
Biomechanics and Tendon Transfers

Contributors to the first edition:
Patricia Anderson
Brett Bolhofner
Arlicia Brown
Phyllis J. Bruni
Barbara A. Carmen
Lisa Rementer Choe
Kate Cooper
Gail P. Counts
Lawrence Gnage
Daniel Greenwald
Barbara G. Henry
Jeri Lynn Houck
Jennifer J. Jones King
John J. O'Brien, Jr.
Scott Raub
John M. Rayhack
Lori Long Root
Sharon Root Spiegel

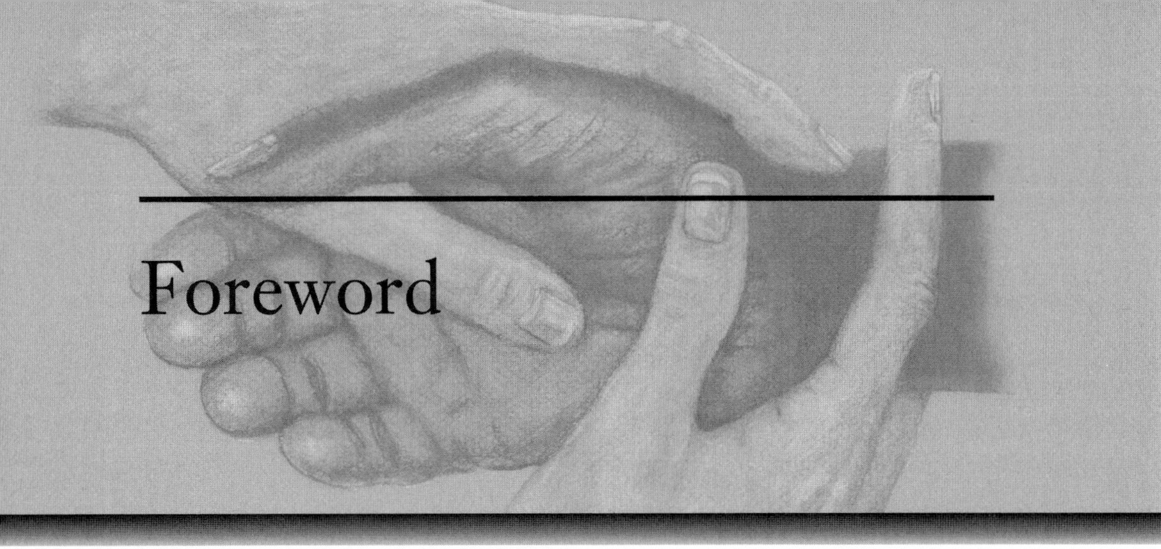

Foreword

In this expanded second edition of Hand Rehabilitation: A Quick Reference Guide and Review, Susan Weiss and Nancy Falkenstein give us a unique approach to critical thinking in hand therapy. In addition to questions relating to specific diagnoses, other areas of clinical practice are included such as anatomy, signs and symptoms, terminology, treatment decisions, use of modalities, and splinting. Unlike many texts that give us sequential information about one subject, this book requires consideration of a wide array of hand therapy information. The question format with multiple choice answers requires the reader to connect theory to real clinical circumstances. With each question being supported by specific references, the reader can conveniently pursue further study of any unfamiliar question or answer.

This text is vital for those preparing for the hand therapy certification examination or for those thinking of beginning practice in hand therapy. For those who have already been practicing in the specialty, it is an excellent review. Wrap your brain around this book . . . your clinical reasoning skills will be better for it!

Judy C. Colditz, OTR/L, CHT, FAOTA
HandLab
Raleigh, North Carolina

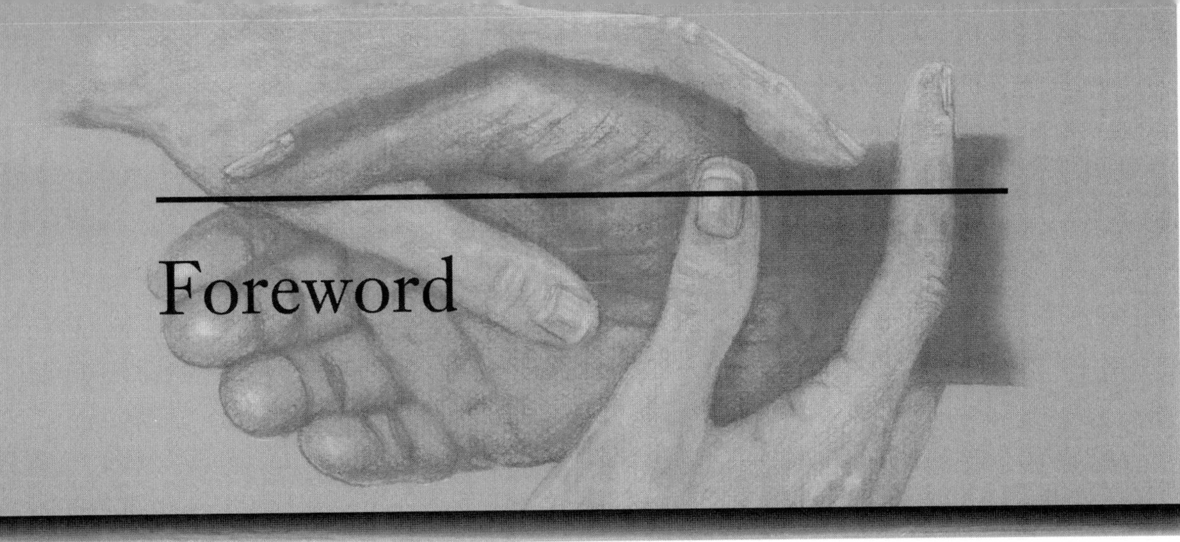

Foreword

The term "Purple Book" echoed through the cell phones and e-mails as the must-read book for future CHTs. Not until my partner, Christa Baggott, challenged me to complete a chapter (just before she passed the CHT examination), did I realize the "Purple Book" was the very same book my Florida Hand Society friends, Susan and Nancy, had published 4 years earlier. I erroneously assumed *Hand Rehabilitation: A Quick Reference Guide and Review* was primarily for pre-CHTs.

I took the challenge lightly at first, then seriously. Each question seemed to trigger those cerebral neurons to pull, gather, and blend latent and recent therapeutic knowledge, techniques, and experiences into accessible thoughts. From the commanding voice of my mentor, Dr. William Burkhalter, to a flash of a familiar photo from a landmark article, from a famous quote of Dr. Brands to the texture of a stiff brawny hand, all re-collected then recollected. Self-examination does that.

The manuscript of this second edition follows the previously proven test format of the first "Purple Book," only it is enriched with almost twice the content. Do you know how Eqawa, Jean Duchene, Andre Thomas, Masse, Wartenberg, and Froment's signs are related? Now describe each one. Like a teen lost in an interactive video game, you will anticipate each topic for the thrill of conquering an upcoming difficult question. Bonuses in the form of Clinical Gems weave a string of pearls that connect one chapter to the next. Right or wrong, there will be a continued satisfaction in settling on a final selection, each not unlike placing that final jigsaw puzzle peace, except the accomplishment is enjoyed repeatedly. Take the challenge, it's rewarding.

Have you kept up with the explosion of information? Since attaining CHT status in 1991, I had questioned the outcome of retaking the CHT examination. Well, the questions in the form of these well-planned pages fulfilled my curiosity. Seasoned therapists should take an earnest approach to this test within a text. It will not only reflect your core knowledge of hand basics, but also be the mirror of proof regarding your continuing education. Cure your curiosity.

Susan and Nancy have left personality prints throughout these pages. If you subscribe to their Exploring Hand Therapy newsletter, you are well aware of the wide appeal in the consistency of their casual and concise writing style that also permeates this edition. This appeal is so wide that their first edition spurred quite a competition at the silent auction of the International Federation of Society of Hand Therapists meeting in Scotland this year. Their newly trademarked and timely motto "Treatment to Go" follows their style. This edition, in my opinion is "Knowledge to Go." Go. Get addicted to the "Purple Book."

Nelson Vazquez, OTR/L, CHT
Co-Owner, H.A.N.D.S Rehab
Miami, Florida

Foreword to the First Edition

No doubt Socrates is smiling. In *Hand Rehabilitation: A Quick Reference Guide and Review*, Nancy Falkenstein and Susan Weiss use a mostly Socratic method—question and answer format—to teach a wide range of topics on hand therapy. In so doing, the authors demonstrate their wealth of knowledge on hand therapy and their skills in teaching hand therapy. They also reveal their creativity and sense of fun.

In this long-awaited book, health professionals and students interested in hand therapy will finally have the opportunity to test and enhance their knowledge with a series of structured questions and comprehensive answers. While other disciplines have long enjoyed this format, hand rehabilitation has been without—until now. However, Falkenstein and Weiss go well beyond the basics of question and answer. Each answer includes a well-developed rationale with references in order to bring the reader to a higher level in his or her grasp of the information. With this approach, the authors bring the reader face to face with hand therapy's core literature.

Hand Rehabilitation: A Quick Reference Guide and Review offers a great deal of information and enjoyment for students and health professionals of all levels of expertise. Falkenstein and Weiss have walked the difficult path of incorporating the breadth of hand therapy wisdom—from the basic core concepts (that always seem to need review) to the most esoteric topics. I was thrilled to finally have a name for a sign that I commonly find in my patients but have never seen referenced—despite many years of reading. Who among us is familiar with Linburg's sign? This is the anatomic interconnection between the flexor pollicis longus and the index finger flexor digitorum profundus that causes the index distal interphalangeal joint to flex when the thumb interphalangeal joint flexes and vice versa. This is only one example of the answers to career-long questions that I found in this text.

The authors have carefully sifted through the huge range of hand therapy topics and selected strategic chapters, including evaluation; flaps, grafts, and thermal conditions; wounds and infection; Dupuytren's disease and tumors; fractures; arthritis; reflex sympathetic dystrophy; tendons; splinting; congenital anomalies, amputations, prosthetics; modalities; cumulative trauma; joint mobilization and other treatment techniques; and several chapters on anatomy. This book covers all commonly seen pathologies, as well as some rarer hand pathologies. It also includes topics usually omitted from texts on hand therapy, and a resource list of vendors offering hand therapy products. I commend Falkenstein and Weiss for including a nutritional quick reference—a topic so critical to excellent outcomes and so often ignored. In keeping with the up-to-date nature of this text, the authors have also included a list of hand therapy–related Internet websites. With such a wellspring of information, no therapist should ever want for references or resources.

I predict *Hand Rehabilitation: A Quick Reference Guide and Review* will be the number one publication sought by therapists studying for the Hand Certification exam. All health professionals and students interested in hand rehabilitation will find this to be a one-of-a-kind, quick reference text that provides a comprehensive overview. It is well thought out, creatively designed, and packed with the resources we all need as hand rehabilitation professionals. I cannot thank the authors enough for providing the hand therapy community with this book.

Karen Schultz-Johnson, MS, OTR, FAOTA, CHT
Director, Rocky Mountain Hand Therapy
President, UE Tech

Foreword to the First Edition

Those in the upper extremity rehabilitation world know that it takes a Herculean effort to understand and keep up with massive amounts of information. We are now inundated with books, journals, and web pages. Continuing education and society meetings fill your calendar. So why would I agree to support yet another book on the hand and upper extremity? The reason is simple. This book amplifies and defines the areas of the upper extremity you need to bone up on and reviews the areas you are competent in. This aptitude assessment is easily evaluated with this book. As well, this book is another nice clinical resource that uses a creative and unique format (thank you Nancy Falkenstein and Susan Weiss) to present hand and upper extremity information.

At first glance this is a book of test questions and answers on the upper extremity. Although this conjures up images of hours spent reading preparatory books for standardized tests such as the SAT or GRE, **there is much more to this book**. "Clinical Gems" permeate each chapter and provide easy-to-remember pearls of wisdom regarding various anatomic regions of the upper extremity, specific pathologic states, splinting, modalities, occupational considerations, and research. Answers to the questions are clearly and concisely stated and supplemented with informative illustrations. Quick referencing is made easy through a detailed index at the front of the book. The slide rule helps suppress the desire to check the correct answer before formulating it yourself.

Obviously, the structure of this book is designed to aid readers preparing for exams on the upper extremity. There is no other book on the upper extremity available that meets this need, and it serves that purpose extremely well. I hope, however, that readers use it for more than just preparing for "the test." The format of this book lends itself to self-assessment, which all too often stops once we leave the confines of professional schooling. The exercise of testing yourself is akin to looking at your professional image in the mirror. Is there substance to what you see or is it simply superficial and without state-of-the-art content? This book is the tool for such an assessment. Certainly when areas of weakness are identified, definitive books and specialized journals are essential for in-depth discussion.

I'll never forget how failing a test in school served as a well-defined signal that I had areas of study that needed significant attention. This type of critique should not be limited to your professional education. I encourage all upper extremity rehabilitation professionals to take advantage of this opportunity to assess your level of competence and better define your areas of need. After doing this, read, attend meetings, "surf the net," question mentors and colleagues, and encourage questions from students. Then combine these academic experiences with the art of treating patients. Good luck and fear not the "test" as it is the test that crystallizes and better defines opportunities for growth.

Paul LaStayo, MPT, CHT

Northern Arizona University, Department of Biology and
DeRosa Physical Therapy, P.C.
Flagstaff, Arizona

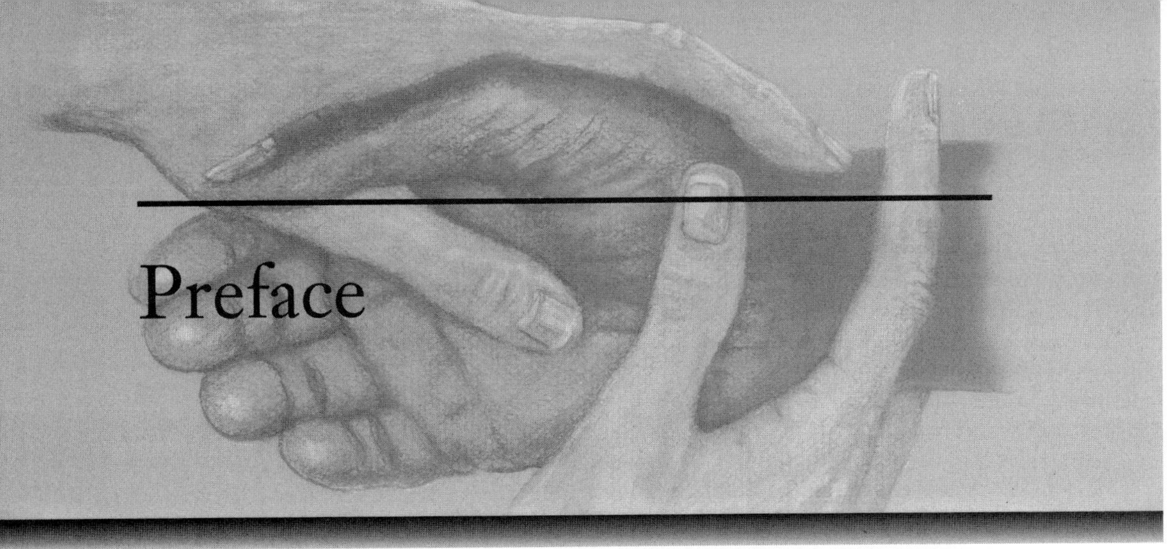

Preface

The art and science of asking questions is the source of all knowledge.—Adolf Berle

The question-and-answer format of the second edition of *Hand Rehabilitation: A Quick Reference Guide and Review* provides readers with the unique opportunity to answer questions and the inspiration to ask more. We have written this book to challenge readers to learn and develop a better understanding of the exciting art of hand rehabilitation. We hope that this book will become a premier resource for many individuals in the health sciences, including hand specialists, certified hand therapists, occupational and physical therapists and students, occupational therapy and physical therapy assistants in hand rehabilitation settings, medical and nursing students, physicians, physician assistants, operating room technicians, and orthopedic technicians. This book can be used in a classroom setting or by practitioners who work with or would like to work with patients who have hand or upper extremity disorders. In addition, of course, it is an excellent resource and study guide for professionals preparing for specialty examinations such as the Certified Hand Therapy examination, the Board-Certified Hand Surgery examination, and the Certified Orthopaedic Specialty examination. Students preparing for general registration examinations will also greatly benefit from the self-study method presented.

This book provides a comprehensive overview of hand rehabilitation through a detailed question-and-answer format that consists of multiple choice, true and false, matching, and fill-in-the-blank questions. Following the question-and-answer choices, we have provided detailed explanations of the correct answer. References, including page numbers, are cited with each question to provide the reader with a simple avenue for further study on a particular subject. In addition, many illustrations have been included to aid in the ease of learning and understanding the topics presented. This book is designed with a thorough Quick Reference Guide, found at the beginning of the book, to assist the reader in quickly finding information on any topic. A wealth of special features are provided in this book, including Clinical Gems, case studies, a slide rule to aid in self-testing, a list of drugs commonly encountered in hand rehabilitation, nutrition resources, vendors/website resources, and the addition of a bind-in CD-ROM that contains the practice questions in a quiz format, allowing the user to perform random self-tests multiple times. We have added two chapters, The Elbow and Sports Injuries of the Upper Extremity, making the book more comprehensive. In addition, we have doubled the information included in the text.

There are several different ways to use this text: (1) Readers can review questions and answer explanations as a method of learning the material. (2) The book can be used as a quick reference to access information on a particular topic or clinical problem. (3) Readers can perform self-assessments using the slide rule method, covering up the answer portion with the slide rule provided in the back of the book. (This is part of the back cover and perforated for easy removal.) Readers can take their time to come up with the correct answer and then move the slide rule down to reveal the answer. Readers may want to write their answers on a separate sheet of paper so they can test themselves more than once. (4) Case studies have been used throughout the book to show the reader how content applies to clinical practice. (5) The CD-ROM is used for random testing, allowing you to scramble the questions to test your knowledge. (6) There are four appendixes at the end of the book to use as a quick reference on various subjects.

We have included more than 200 Clinical Gems compiled by therapists, physicians, and educators. Clinical Gems range from splinting tips to mnemonics for remembering hand surgery and rehabilitation facts. The Clinical Gems provide invaluable clinical information.

This book has been developed through years of experience, preparation for specialty certification, and the desire to learn the art of exploring hand rehabilitation. Through the dedication to learning and teaching we have founded Exploring Hand Therapy, Inc. To learn more about hand therapy, please visit www.exploringhandtherapy.com and register for our comprehensive newsletter. We have devoted countless hours to preparing and writing this book. Our goal is to provide a quick reference resource that continues to fill a void in hand rehabilitation literature. We developed all of the chapters with the assistance of our contributors who have diverse professional backgrounds. We express our deep appreciation to the contributors for sharing their knowledge.

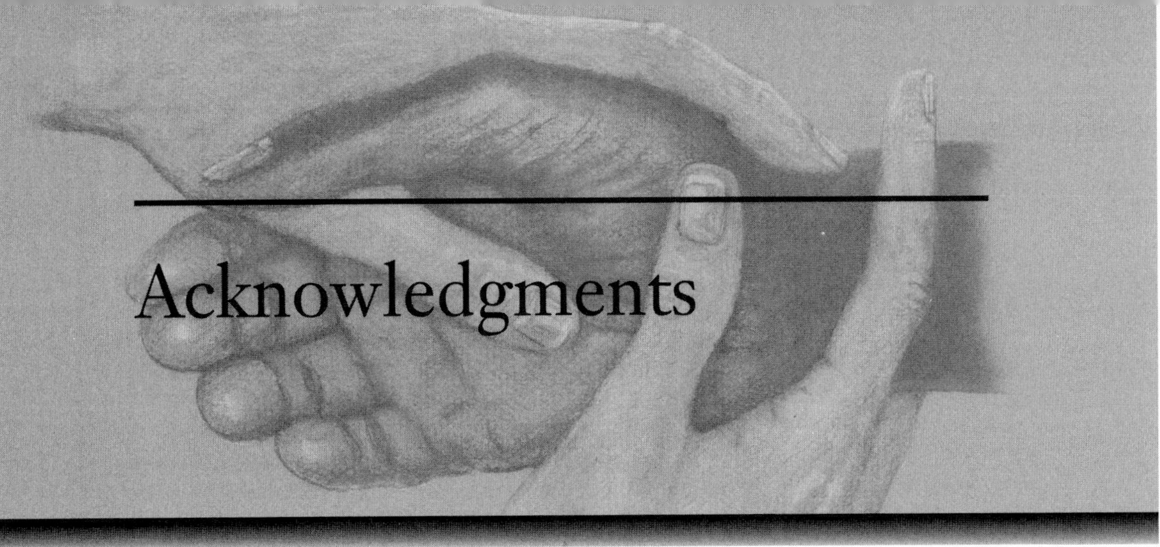

Acknowledgments

Susan expressly thanks:

- Thank you to Claudette Scott for your hard work, dedication, love you give my son Jake, and friendship. You helped make this project possible for me.
- All of our lovely contributors for their time and contributions to this work
- The Elsevier staff, including Melissa Kuster, Jennifer Furey, and Kathy Falk, for their time and patience with this project
- All Florida Orthopaedics (AFO) for allowing me to grow professionally and for providing me with a wonderful learning environment
- The doctors at AFO, including Dale Bramlet, Jorge Rodriquez, and Antonio Gayoso, for teaching me and sharing their patients with me
- My lovely friends Ali Goldenfarb, Helen Keys, Roni Murphy, and Jay Kaminsky for their friendship and love
- My friend and colleague Dermot Forde for always listening and checking up on me
- My co-author Nancy Falkenstein for being my best friend and confidant through it all, and I mean all! We did it again, girl, and my love and gratitude to you is limitless

Nancy specially recognizes:

- Mark Counts for his dedication to my sister and his family . . . we love you!
- Aunt Trish and Uncle Ron for all their direction, input, and love
- My brother Chris Falkenstein and sisters Gail Counts and Judy Bain and all my nieces and nephews
- Cassey Falkenstein and Keith Bain
- Dr. Marvin Susskind for his inspiration and his jokes
- My dear friends who have "kept me going," Nan MacDonald (Alexander), Mandy McCarty, and Nancy Brome
- Madlyn Weir, you are my spiritual inspiration, I love your singing and thanks for all your prayers
- Jayne Miller for listening to me and lending a friendly "ear"
- The contributors for their input and expertise
- All my patients present and past. . . . for without them, I would not have excelled
- My partner, co-author, and best friend, Susan Weiss. We did it again, girl! I went into this and other projects with you as a partner, and I have gained friendship, wisdom, and retrospection
- All the American military for their relentless dedication to Freedom

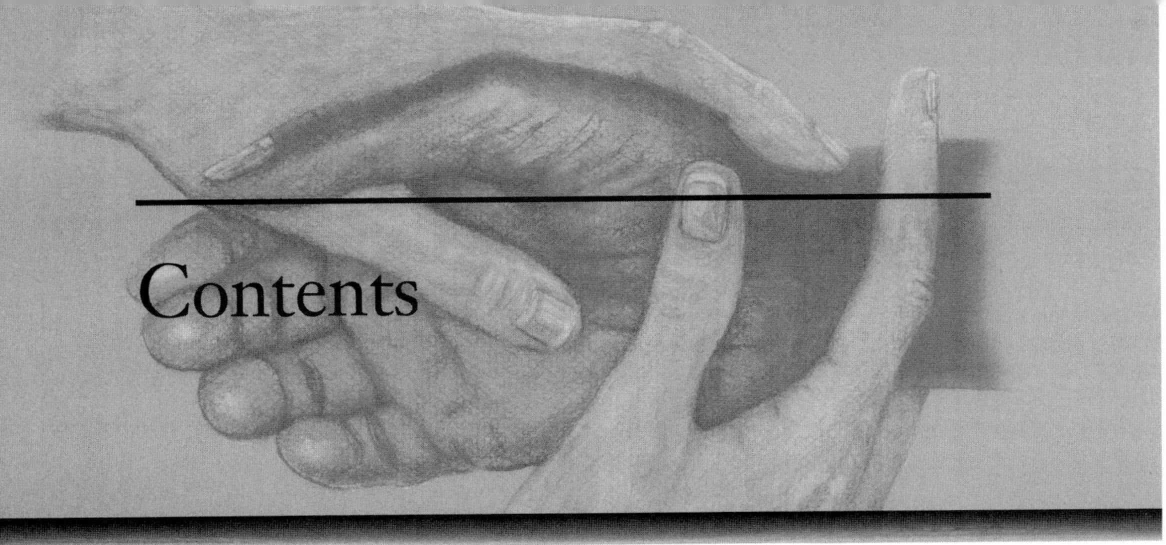

Contents

Quick Reference Guide*

*Page numbers followed by *f* indicate figures; *t*, tables; *b*, boxes.

D

G

N

O

Q

R

QUICK REFERENCE GUIDE

S

T

W

X

Y

Z

Chapter 1

Anatomy Extravaganza

1. You are treating a patient after flexor digitorum profundus repair to the ring finger. You note that he has a significant reduction of finger flexion force in the digits adjacent to the ring finger. You also recognize a flexion contracture of the ring finger. What might this patient be experiencing?

A. Lumbrical-plus phenomenon
B. Quadrigia phenomenon
C. Linburg's sign
D. Egawa's sign

When a quadrigia phenomenon occurs, the patient exhibits a flexion contracture of the involved digit and a decreased amount of flexion force in the digits next to the injured finger. The quadrigia effect can occur if the flexor digitorum profundus is advanced more than 1 cm during repair, thus resulting in limited proximal excursion of the remaining flexor digitorum profundus tendons. To prevent a quadrigia effect, one should use advancement only for the flexor pollicis longus.

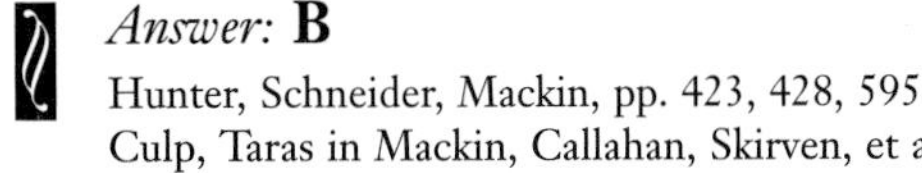

Answer: **B**
Hunter, Schneider, Mackin, pp. 423, 428, 595
Culp, Taras in Mackin, Callahan, Skirven, et al, pp. 421-426
Ejeskar, p. 63

2. Which of the following statements about Guyon's canal is false?

A. Contains the median nerve
B. Contains the ulnar nerve
C. Contains the ulnar artery
D. Borders the hook of the hamate and the pisiform

The ulnar nerve and artery are contained in Guyon's triangular canal. It is immediately ulnar to the carpal tunnel and may be a site of ulnar nerve entrapment. The borders of this canal are the hook of the hamate and the pisiform. The median nerve is in the carpal tunnel, not Guyon's canal.

Answer: **A**
Leclercq, pp. 506-507
Matloub & Yousef, pp. 201-214
Refer to Fig. 1-1

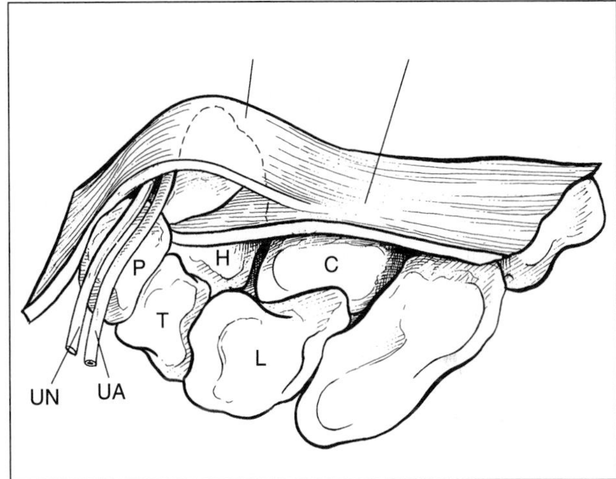

Fig. 1-1 ■ Boundaries and contents of Guyon's canal. *C*, Capitate; *H*, hamate; *L*, lunate; *P*, pisiform; *S*, scaphoid; *T*, trapezoid; *TCL*, transverse carpal ligament; *UN*, ulnar nerve; *UA*, ulnar artery; and *VCL*, carpal ligament. (From Moneim MS: Ulnar nerve compression at the wrist: ulnar tunnel syndrome, *Hand Clin* 8(2):338, 1992.)

3. Which of the following statements are true of the anatomical "snuffbox"?

A. Lunate forms the floor.
B. Abductor pollicis longus and extensor pollicis brevis tendon define the ulnar border.
C. Extensor pollicis longus tendon forms the radial border.
D. All of the above are true.
E. None of the above is true.

The anatomical snuffbox is formed by the scaphoid at the base; the abductor pollicis longus and extensor pollicis brevis define the radial border; and the extensor pollicis longus lines the ulnar border.

Answer: **E**
Mehta
Refer to Fig. 1-2

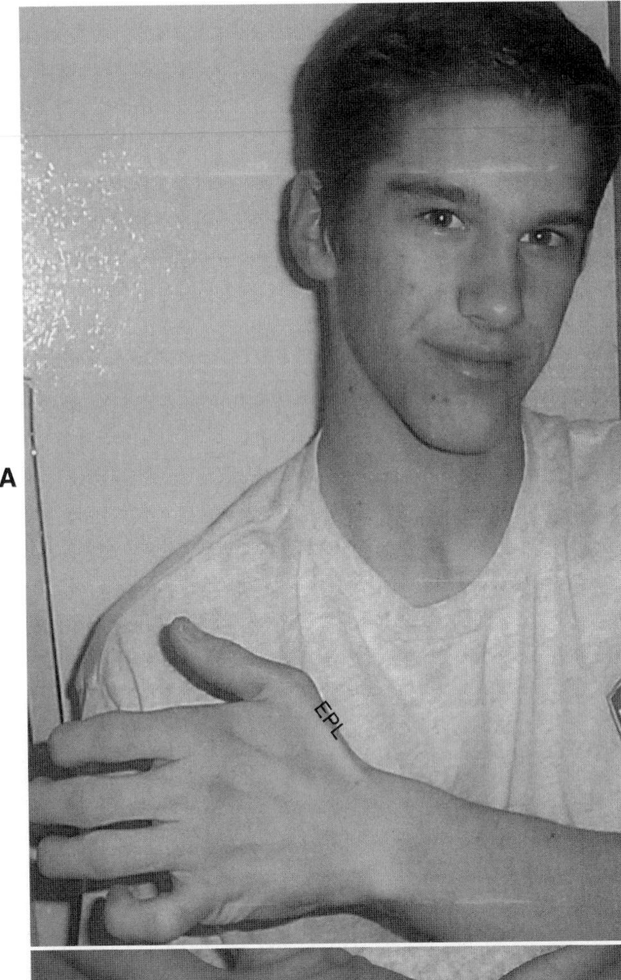

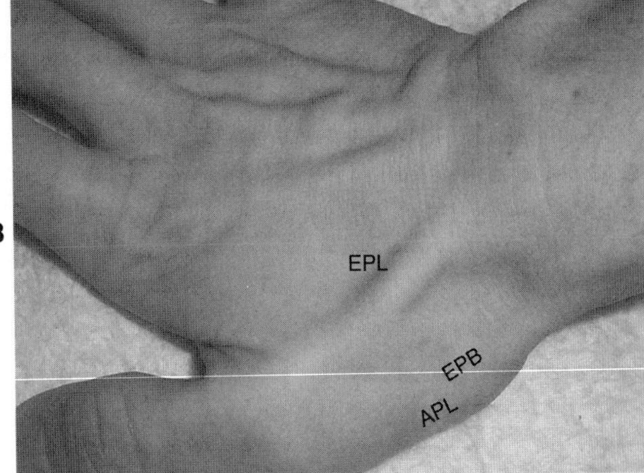

Fig. 1-2

4. Protraction—or hunching—of the shoulders is completed by which of the following muscles (pick the most complete answer)?

A. Pectoralis major and serratus anterior
B. Pectoralis major, serratus anterior, and pectoralis minor
C. Pectoralis major, serratus anterior, and anterior deltoid
D. Pectoralis major, serratus anterior, anterior deltoid, and pectoralis minor

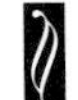

The large, strong serratus anterior as well as the pectoralis major and minor place the humerus in the "hunched shoulder" or protracted position.

Answer: **B**
Bogumill, pp. 1637-1639
Refer to Fig. 1-3

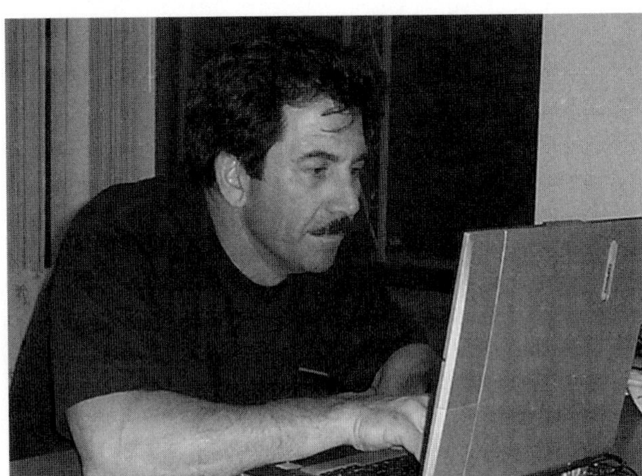

Fig. 1-3

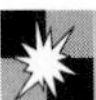

CLINICAL GEM:
If an individual works all day on a computer or is a computer enthusiast, his or her shoulder protractors are typically shortened and the retractors stretched. Stretching exercises for the protractors, strengthening exercises for the retractors, and postural reeducation are essential. Ergonomic principles for a computer workstation should be addressed.

5. Which structures run through the carpal tunnel? (Pick the most complete answer.)

A. Median nerve, flexor digitorum profundus, flexor digitorum superficialis
B. Median nerve, palmaris longus, flexor digitorum profundus, flexor digitorum superficialis
C. Median nerve, flexor pollicis longus, flexor digitorum profundus, flexor digitorum superficialis
D. Median nerve, flexor pollicis longus, palmaris longus, flexor digitorum profundus, flexor digitorum superficialis

The carpal tunnel contains ten structures: the median nerve, four flexor digitorum profundus tendons, four flexor digitorum superficialis tendons, and the flexor pollicis longus tendon. The carpal tunnel lies deep to the palmaris longus. Its borders are the pisiform, the scaphoid tubercle, the hook of the hamate, and the trapezium tubercle.

Answer: **C**
Hoppenfeld, p. 83
Refer to Fig. 1-4

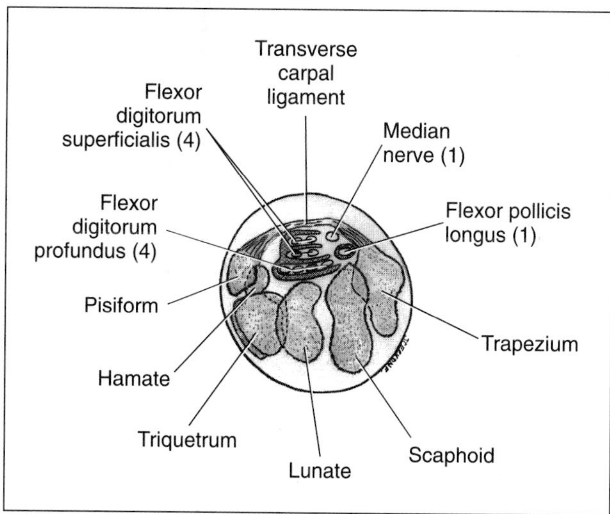

Fig. 1-4

6. What is the anatomic interconnection between the flexor pollicis longus and the index finger flexor digitorum profundus called?

A. Linburg's sign
B. Reiter's syndrome
C. Egawa's sign
D. None of the above

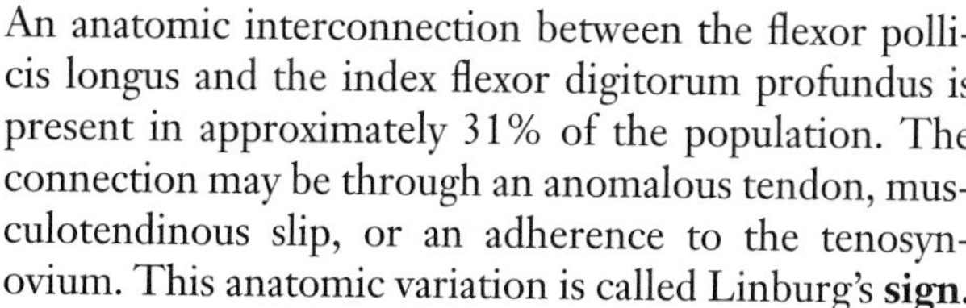

An anatomic interconnection between the flexor pollicis longus and the index flexor digitorum profundus is present in approximately 31% of the population. The connection may be through an anomalous tendon, musculotendinous slip, or an adherence to the tenosynovium. This anatomic variation is called Linburg's **sign.**

Linburg's **syndrome** can occur when this interconnection leads to pain and aggravation with activity. The discomfort is located over the radiopalmar aspect of the distal forearm and thumb.

Answer: **A**
Cooney, Linscheid, Dobyns, p. 1194
Refer to Fig. 1-5

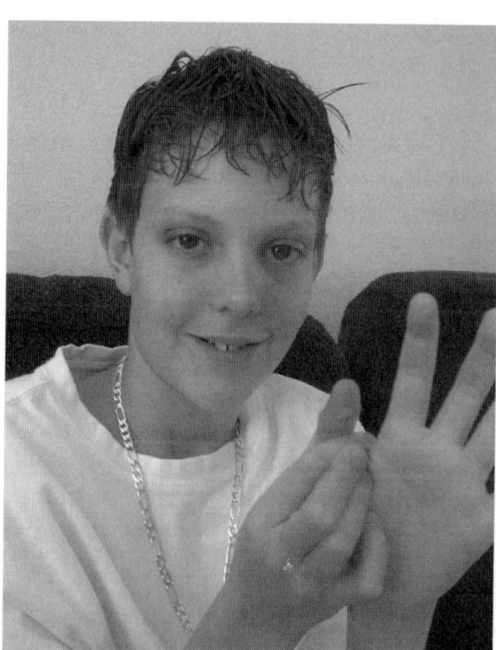

Fig. 1-5 ■ Note the flexion of the index finger when active interphalangeal (IP) thumb flexion is performed.

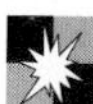

CLINICAL GEM:
To assess for Linburg's sign, have the patient actively flex the thumb interphalangeal joint. Look for involuntary motion at the index finger distal interphalangeal joint.

7. What condition is often present with Linburg's syndrome?

A. Anterior interosseus syndrome
B. Fracture of the radius
C. Trigger finger
D. Carpal tunnel syndrome

Carpal tunnel syndrome is often present with Lindburg's syndrome. Lindburg's syndrome involves tenosynovitis in the flexor pollicis longus and usually includes the flexor digitorum of the index (because of an associated anomalous interconnection). Patients complain of distal (radiopalmar) forearm and hand pain that is aggravated when distal interphalangeal (DIP) flexion of the index is blocked because the thumb is actively flexed into the palm.

Answer: **D**
Stern, pp. 467-476

8. What are the primary pathological structures that produce proximal interphalangeal joint flexion contractures?

A. Check rein ligaments
B. Collateral ligaments of the proximal interphalangeal joint
C. Lateral bands
D. Oblique retinacular ligaments

Contractures of the proximal interphalangeal joints occur after an unspecified period of time in a negative hand position (intrinsic minus). Thin fibers called *swallowtails* are extensions of the volar plate at the proximal interphalangeal joint. When these swallowtails become hypertrophied and shortened, they are termed *check rein ligaments*. Check rein ligaments can develop rapidly after edema occurs or progressively, as in Dupuytren's contracture.

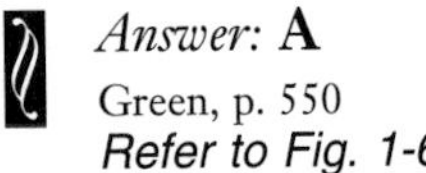

Answer: **A**
Green, p. 550
Refer to Fig. 1-6

9. Match the following dorsal wrist compartments with the tendon(s) that reside in each compartment.

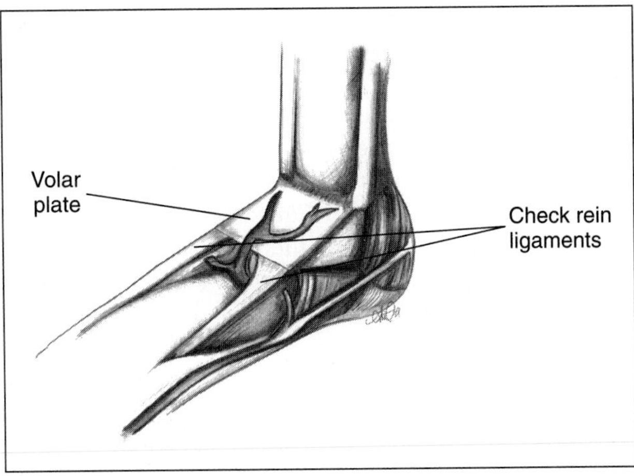

Fig. 1-6

Compartment

1. First dorsal wrist compartment
2. Second dorsal wrist compartment
3. Third dorsal wrist compartment
4. Fourth dorsal wrist compartment
5. Fifth dorsal wrist compartment
6. Sixth dorsal wrist compartment

Tendon(s)

A. Abductor pollicis longus (APL), extensor pollicis brevis (EPB)
B. Extensor digiti minimi (EDM)
C. Extensor carpi ulnaris (ECU)
D. Extensor pollicis longus (EPL)
E. Extensor digitorum (ED); extensor indicis proprius (EIP)
F. Extensor carpi radialis longus (ECRL); extensor carpi radialis brevis (ECRB)

Answers: **1, A; 2, F; 3, D; 4, E; 5, B; 6, C**
Stanley, Tribuzi, p. 9
Miller, p. 544
Refer to Fig. 1-7

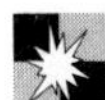

CLINICAL GEM:
To remember the dorsal compartments, one can recall the numbers 22, 12, and 11. These numbers correlate with the numbers of tendons in each of the six dorsal compartments.

Compartment	1	2	3	4	5	6
Number of tendons to recall	2	2	1	2	1	1
Tendons	EPB APL	ECRL ECRB	EPL	EDC EIP	EDM	ECU

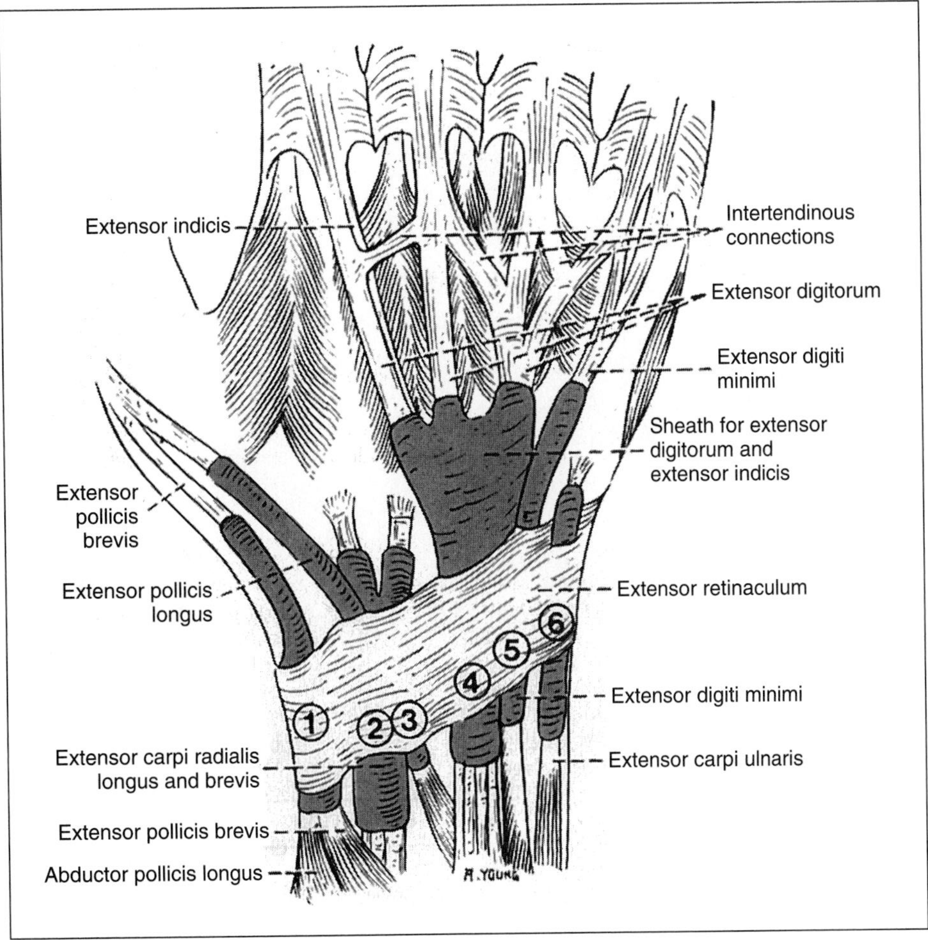

Fig. 1-7 ■ From Jenkins DB: *Linshead's functional anatomy of limbs and back*, ed 6, Philadelphia, 1991, WB Saunders.

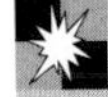
CLINICAL GEM:
To avoid confusing the fifth and sixth compartments, remember that the tendon to the fifth digit is the extensor digiti minimi (fifth digit equals fifth compartment).

10. True or false: The extensor carpi radialis brevis is the strongest wrist extensor.

The ECRB originates from the lateral epicondyle of the humerus and inserts onto the base of the third metacarpal. The ECRB has the longest extension moment arm and the largest cross-section and is the strongest and most efficient wrist extensor. The ECRL, in contrast, has the longest muscle fibers and the largest mass and therefore has a greater capacity for sustained work. The ECU has the longest moment arm for ulnar deviation. The ECU becomes a more efficient wrist extensor when the forearm is supinated.

Answer: **True**
Hunter, Mackin, Callahan, p. 523
Rosenthal in Mackin, Callahan, Skirven, et al, p. 502

11. Lateral epicondylitis is a common diagnosis in work-related injuries. Which muscle is primarily affected?

A. Extensor carpi radialis longus
B. Extensor carpi radialis brevis
C. Extensor digitorum
D. Extensor carpi ulnaris
E. Brachioradialis

The extensor carpi radialis brevis is the most commonly affected muscle in lateral epicondylitis. It causes pain with passive wrist flexion and active (and resisted) wrist

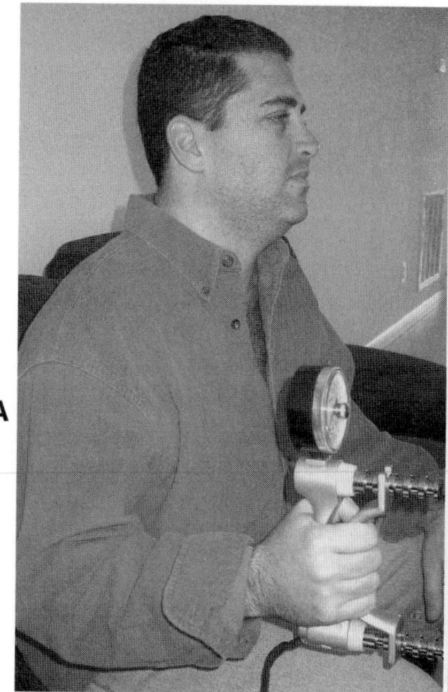

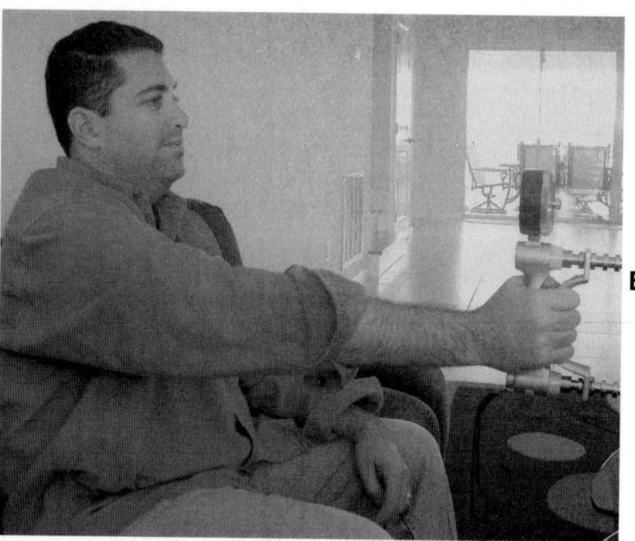

Fig. 1-8 ■ **A,** Flexed to 90 degrees for assessment. **B,** Full extension assessment.

extension. The most tender spot is located 1 to 2 cm distal to the lateral epicondyle.

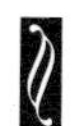

Answer: **B**

De Smet, Fabry, pp. 229-231
Nirschl, pp. 537-552

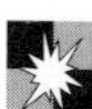

Clinical Gem:
Grip testing with the elbow flexed to 90 degrees is less painful for the patient with lateral epicondylitis versus when the grip test is performed with the elbow straight and locked. Most patients with lateral epicondylitis will benefit from education in avoiding provocative motions, such as a forceful grasp and/or lifting with elbow extended and forearm pronated. Refer to Fig. 1-8.

12. Which pulley is most commonly affected in trigger finger?

A. A1 pulley
B. A2 pulley
C. A3 pulley
D. A4 pulley
E. A5 pulley

The A1 pulley is the structure that is surgically released when trigger finger is the culprit. Although patients may complain about pain at the PIP joint level, the pathology is at the MP level at the A1 pulley. The A1 pulley can become thickened and narrow from chronic inflammation and will trap the flexor tendon.

Answer: **A**

Hunter, Mackin, Callahan, pp. 1007-1012
Lee, Nassir-Sharif, Zelouf in Mackin, Callahan, Skirven, et al, p. 939

Clinical Gem:
During trigger finger physical examination, run your finger along the flexor tendons in the palm. Often a nodule is palpable on the flexor tendon just proximal to the MCP joint.

13. Which of the following does not serve as an attachment site for the transverse carpal ligament?

A. Scaphoid
B. Trapezium
C. Hamate
D. Triquetrum
E. Pisiform

The transverse carpal ligament (TCL) attaches to the scaphoid tuberosity, the crest of the trapezium, the pisiform, and the hook of the hamate. The TCL forms the roof of the carpal canal and ranges in thickness from 1 to 3.5 mm. The TCL prevents the long flexors of the fingers from bowstringing when the wrist flexes and serves as an attachment site for thenar and hypothenar muscles.

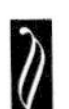

Answer: **D**

Hunter, Mackin, Callahan, pp. 905-906
Hayes, Carney, Wolf, et al, in Mackin, Callahan, Skirven, et al, p. 643

14. What is the best treatment for an acute compartment syndrome?

A. Application of ice until swelling subsides
B. Active range of motion (AROM) exercises of the affected musculature, followed first by soft tissue massage and then by application of ice pack
C. Immediate fasciotomy of all compartments involved
D. All of the above

Acute compartment syndrome may be caused by crush injury, thermal or electrical burns, snakebite, or fracture. Symptoms include pain, paresthesias, paralysis, and pulselessness. The most telling sign is pain that is out of proportion to a normal pain response and that is not alleviated by rest. Because increasing pressure in the compartment can result in necrosis—which leads to fibrosis of the muscles and other soft tissues—an immediate fasciotomy must be done after the diagnosis is reached.

Answer: **C**

Naidu, Heppenstall, pp. 13-27
Gellman, Keyur, pp. 385-389

15. True or false: A Martin-Gruber anastomosis is present in 35% to 45% of the population.

This anomaly is present in 15% to 20% of the population. The Martin-Gruber anastomosis is between the median nerve and the ulnar nerve at the forearm level. The anastomosis usually consists of median-nerve innervated motor fibers that supply the typically ulnar-innervated intrinsics. Ulnar sensory fibers also may be innervated by the median nerve when this anastomosis exists.

Answer: **False**

Kimura, p. 418
Tubiana, Thomine, Mackin, p. 277
Refer to Fig. 1-9

16. Match each muscle to the correct description:

Muscle

1. Abductor pollicis brevis
2. Extensor carpi radialis brevis
3. Extensor carpi ulnaris
4. Supinator
5. Extensor pollicis longus
6. Adductor pollicis
7. First volar interosseous
8. First dorsal interosseous

Description

A. Strong finger abductor that inserts into the base of the proximal phalanx of the index finger
B. Innervated by the median nerve and originates from the transverse carpal ligament
C. Innervated by the ulnar nerve and inserted into the ulnar side of the proximal phalanx of the thumb and the extensor expansion of the thumb
D. Inserts into the base of the third metacarpal
E. Innervated by the posterior interosseous nerve (PIN) and inserts into the base of the fifth metacarpal
F. Originates from the lateral epicondyle of the humerus and the adjacent portion of the ulna and inserts into the upper third of the radius
G. Innervated by the posterior interosseous nerve and inserts into the first distal phalanx
H. Originates from the length of the second metacarpal and adducts the index finger

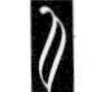

Answers: **1, B; 2, D; 3, E; 4, F; 5, G; 6, C; 7, H; 8, A**

Malick, Kasch, pp. 57-58, 66

CLINICAL GEM:
The APB is the strongest muscle of anteposition (opposition). In 1867, Duchenne called the APB muscle the *opposing phalangeal muscle of the thumb* because of its action on the tip.

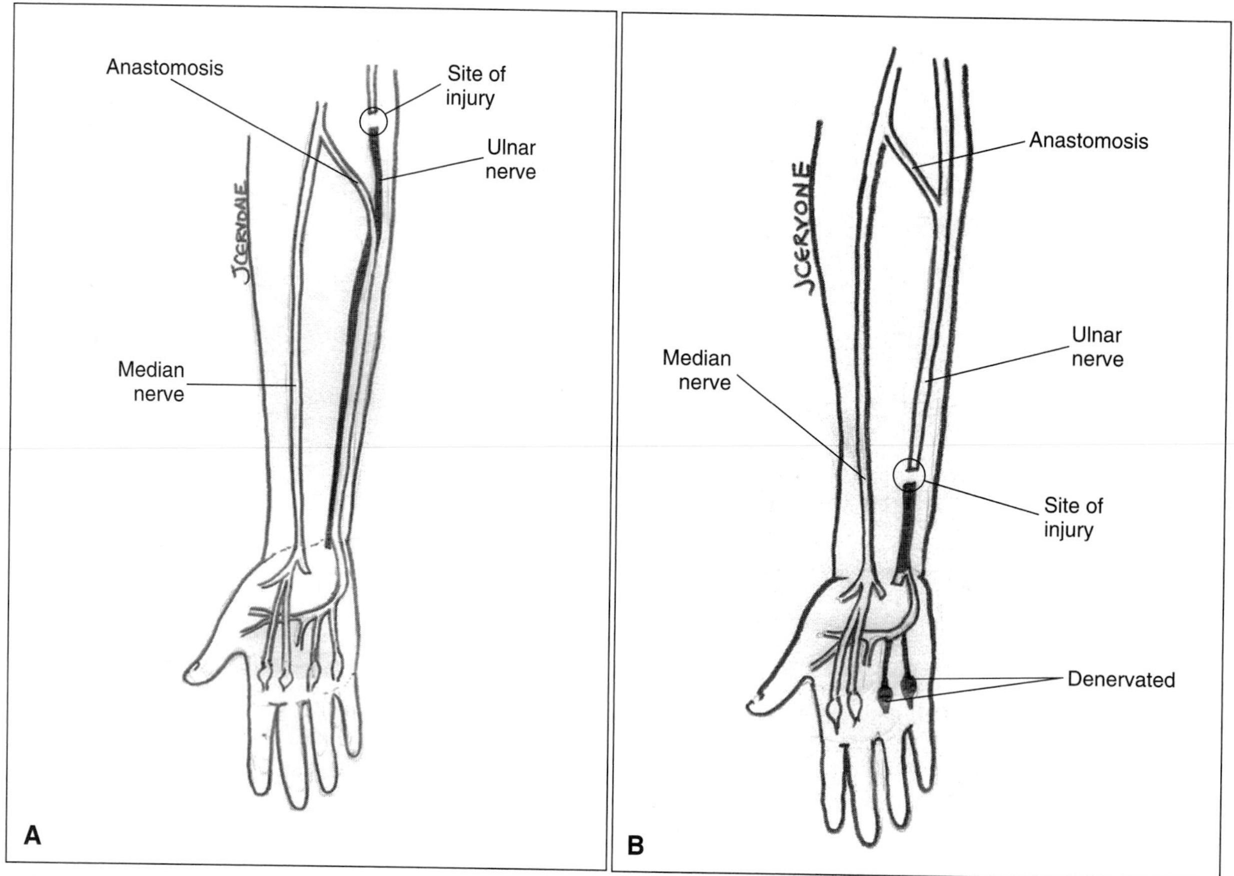

Fig. 1-9 ■ **A,** A high ulnar nerve lesion in which the anastomosis from the median to ulnar nerve occurs distal to the injury and prevents paralysis of the ulnar innervated intrinsics. **B,** A low ulnar nerve injury distal to the anastomosis, which causes paralysis of the ulnar innervated digits.

17. The elbow's main stabilizer to valgus strain is which of the following?

A. Medial epicondyle
B. Medial collateral ligament
C. Lateral epicondyle
D. Lateral collateral ligament

The medial (ulnar) collateral ligament (UCL) is the main stabilizer of the elbow joint and prevents valgus strain. The UCL originates slightly anterior and inferior to the medial epicondyle. It fans out to its attachment along the greater sigmoid fossa. It comprises anterior, posterior, and transverse bands. Damage to the UCL usually necessitates surgery.

Answer: **B**
Morrey, pp. 549-551
Refer to Fig. 1-10

18. With paralysis of the interosseous muscles, the long finger extensors are unopposed. They hyperextend the metacarpophalangeal (MCP) joints during finger extension. However, stabilization and prevention of hyperextension of the MCP joint (placing and holding the MCP in slight flexion) during extension can transfer the force from the long extensors to the PIP and DIP joints, thus resulting in extension. Which test was just described?

A. Tinels
B. Bouvier
C. Adsons
D. Finochietto-Bunnell

Bouvier is the test described and is used to determine whether the PIP joint capsule and extensor mechanism are working normally. In cases of claw hand deformity (interosseous muscle palsy), if the MCP joints are stabilized and prevented from going into hyperextension, the intrinsic muscle force is transferred distally to the PIP and DIP joints, thus aiding in reestablishing PIP and DIP extension.

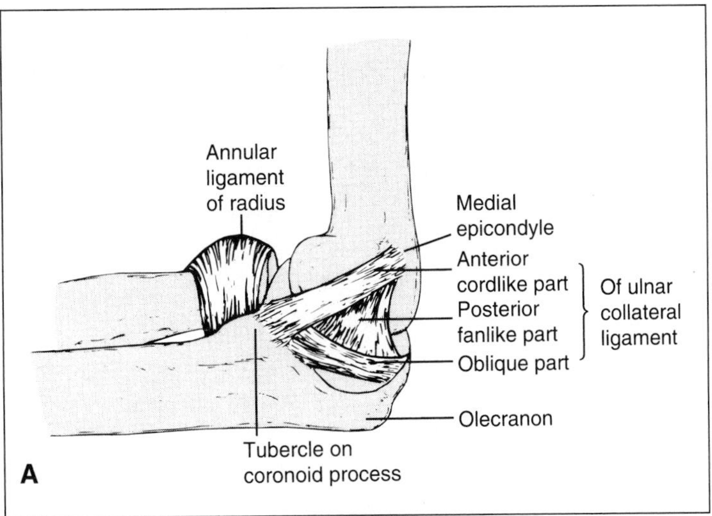

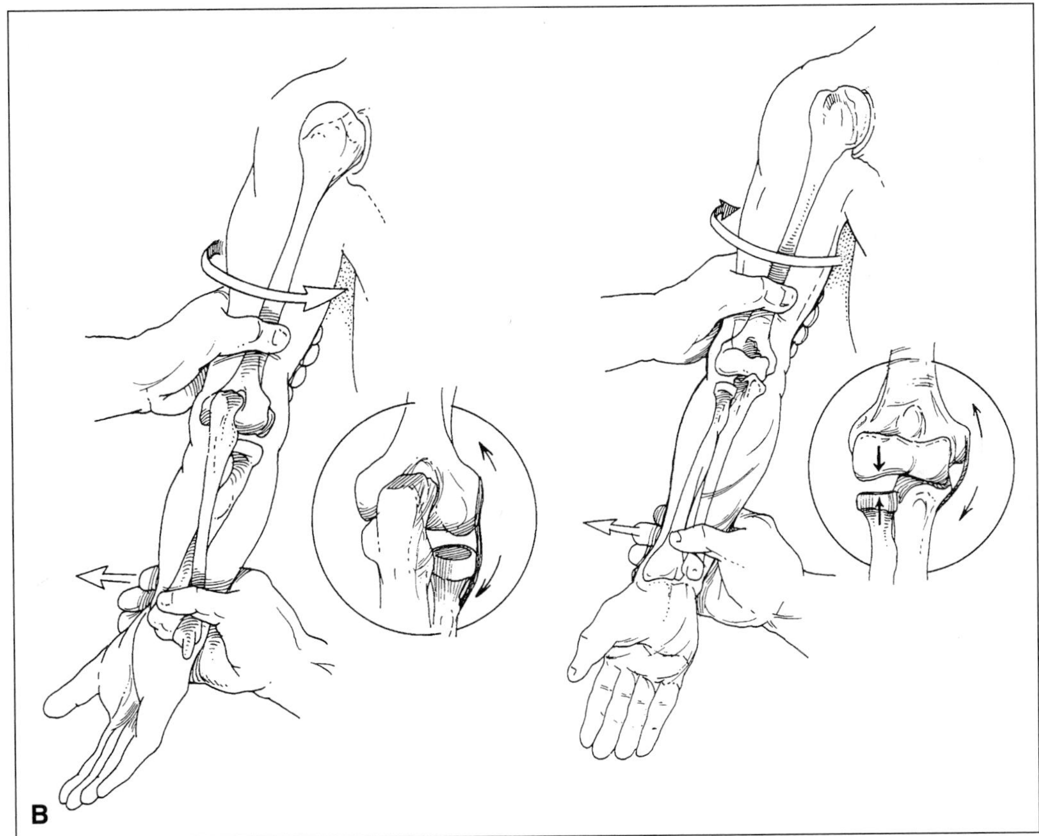

Fig. 1-10 ■ **A,** Lateral view of the bony and ligamentous anatomy of the elbow joint. **B,** *Left,* Laxity of the radial collateral ligament (varus instability of the elbow) is examined with the humerus in full internal rotation while varus stress is applied to the joint. *Right,* Laxity of the medial collateral ligament (valgus instability of the elbow) is evaluated with the humerus in full external rotation as valgus stress is applied to the joint. In both instances, rotation helps stabilize the humerus, allowing ligament laxity to be more easily appreciated. (**A,** From Mackin EJ, Callahan AD, Skirven TM, et al: *Rehabilitation of the hand and upper extremity,* ed 5, vol 1, St Louis, 2002, Mosby; **B,** from Morrey BF: *The elbow and its disorders,* ed 2, Philadelphia, 1994, WB Saunders.)

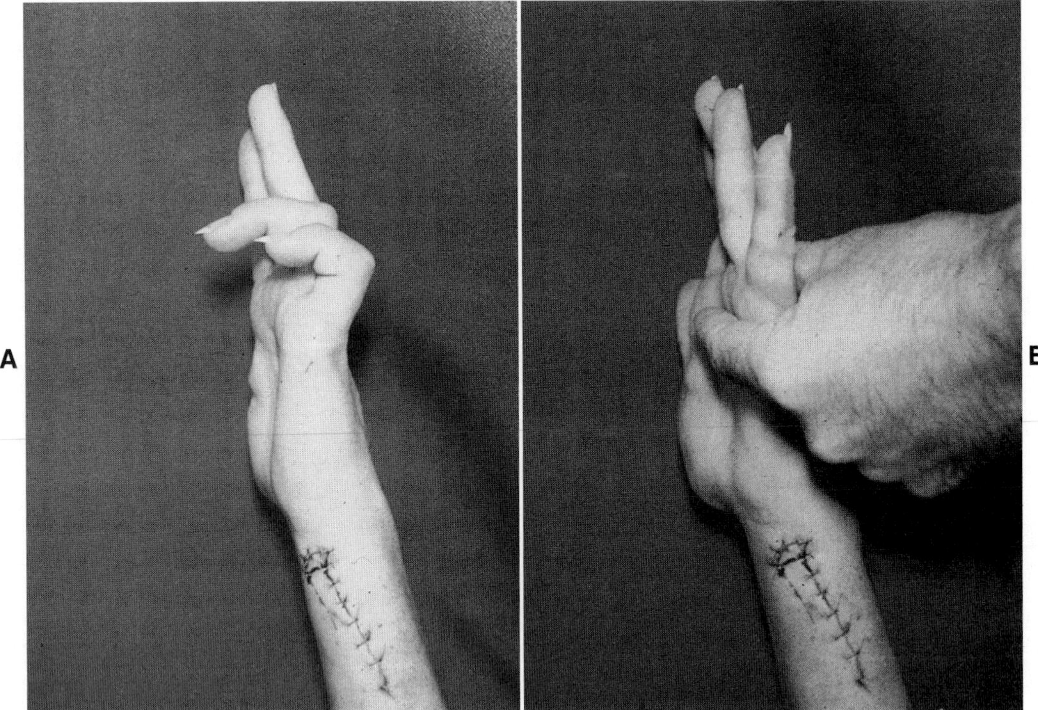

Fig. 1-11

Answer: **B**

Tubiana, Thomine, Mackin, pp. 109-110, 223

Refer to Fig. 1-11

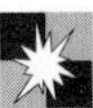
CLINICAL GEM:

When splinting, remember this principle to prevent claw hand deformity following paralysis of the interosseous muscles.

19. True or false: The most important pulleys in the flexor tendon system are A3 and A5.

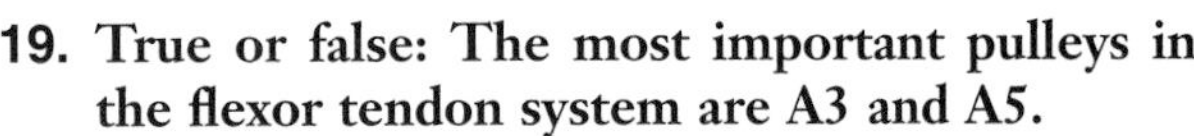

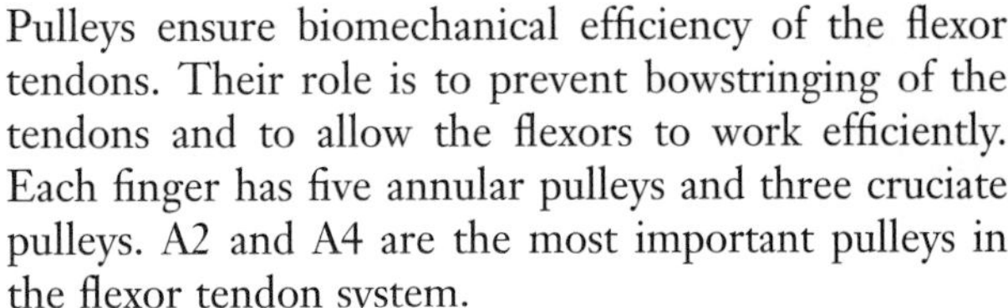
Pulleys ensure biomechanical efficiency of the flexor tendons. Their role is to prevent bowstringing of the tendons and to allow the flexors to work efficiently. Each finger has five annular pulleys and three cruciate pulleys. A2 and A4 are the most important pulleys in the flexor tendon system.

Answer: **False**

Malick, p. 43

Refer to Fig. 1-12

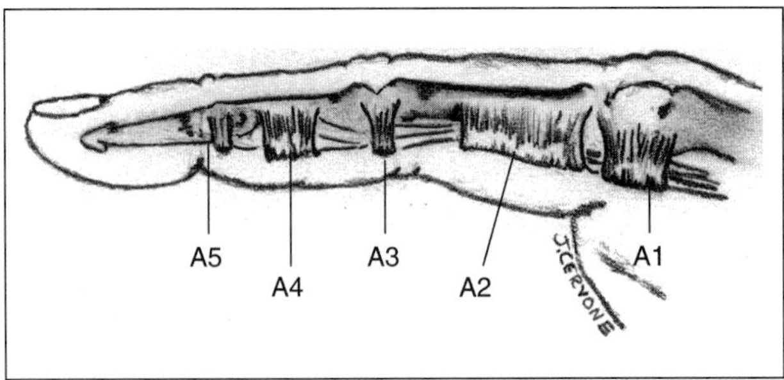

Fig. 1-12

CLINICAL GEM:

An easy way to remember the pulleys is to recall that the odd numbers for the annular pulleys correlate with finger joints:

MPJ—A1

PIPJ—A3

DIPJ—A5

20. *Wallbangers' disease* refers to persistent hard edema over the dorsum of the hand. The inexplicable edema usually occurs after a minor hand injury. This is more typically known by which of the following terms?

A. SHAFT syndrome
B. Munchausen syndrome
C. Clenched-fist syndrome
D. Secretan's syndrome

Secretan's syndrome (Wallbangers' disease) is a psychological condition that results in self-infliction of harm and exacerbation of symptoms to prolong the illness/disorder.

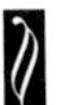

Answer: **D**
Kasdan, pp. 57-60

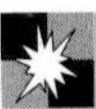

CLINICAL GEM:
Remember the S's: self-inflicted/Secretan's syndrome.

21. What is the major arterial supply to the forearm and hand?

A. Radial artery
B. Brachial artery
C. Median artery
D. Interosseous artery

The brachial artery continues from the axillary artery and travels distally along the medial arm. The median nerve is nearby. At the antecubital fossa, the brachial artery dives below the lacertus fibrosis and splits into the radial and ulnar arteries. The brachial artery is the major inflow vessel to the forearm and hand.

Answer: **B**
Spinner, p. 203
Refer to Fig. 1-13

22. How long do blood vessels require protection after surgical repair?

A. 1 to 5 days
B. 7 to 14 days
C. 14 to 21 days
D. 21 to 28 days

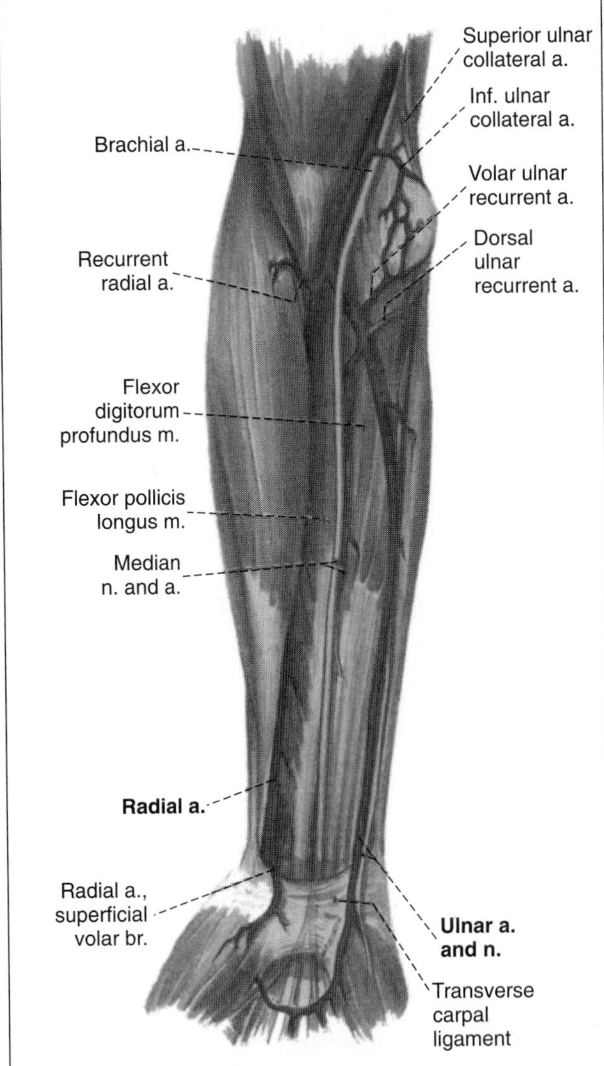

Fig. 1-13 ■ From Mackin EJ, Callahan AD, Skirven TM, et al: *Rehabilitation of the hand and upper extremity*, ed 5, vol 1, St Louis, 2002, Mosby.

Blood vessels require 1 to 2 weeks of protection. This is generally provided by the immobilization needed to protect other structures that are repaired.

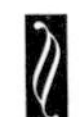

Answer: **B**
Hunter, Mackin, Callahan, p. 1059

23. What is the combined function of Cleland's and Grayson's ligaments?

A. Prevents Dupuytren's contracture
B. Stabilizes the metacarpophalangeal joint
C. Stabilizes the basal joint
D. Prevents rotary movements of the skin around the fingers

Grayson's ligament originates from the volar aspect of the flexor tendon sheath, runs volar to the neurovascular bundle, and inserts into the skin. Cleland's ligament passes dorsally to the neurovascular bundle and inserts into the skin. According to Hoppenfeld, both Grayson's and Cleland's ligaments prevent rotary movement of the skin around the fingers, thus allowing the ability to grasp objects. Grayson's ligament may contribute to a PIP joint flexion contracture in Dupuytren's disease.

Answer: **D**
Hoppenfeld, p. 65
Green, pp. 564-565
Refer to Fig. 1-14

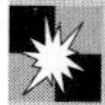

CLINICAL GEM:
Cleland's ligaments are **d**orsal to the neurovascular bundle. To remember this, recall that **"C"** for **C**leland precedes **"D"** for **d**orsal.

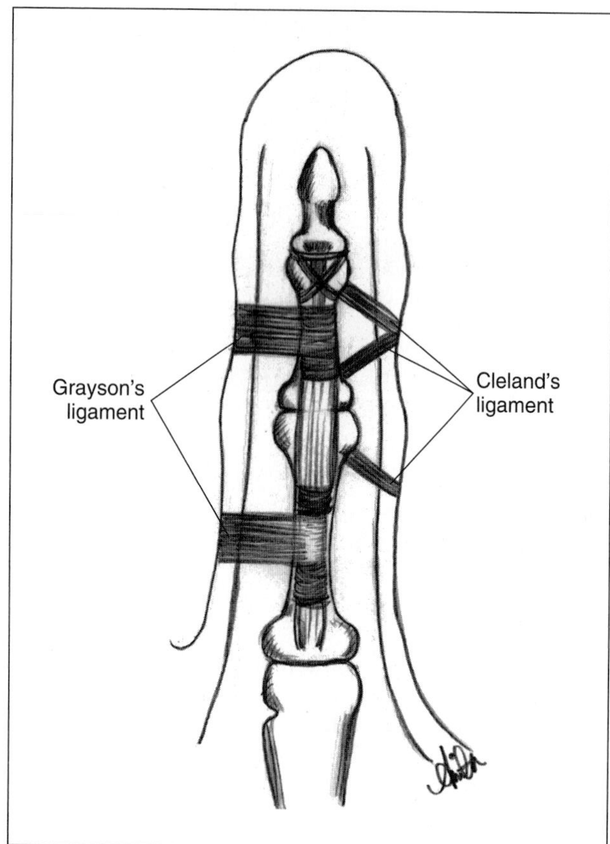

Fig. 1-14

24. Which artery provides the primary blood supply to the hand?

A. Radial artery
B. Ulnar artery
C. Persistent median artery
D. All of the above arteries supply the hand equally

The ulnar artery is larger than the radial artery and is usually the primary contributor, supplying 60% of blood to the hand. This artery supplies the superficial palmar arch in most hands, and the radial artery usually supplies the deep palmar arch. The median artery contributes to the superficial palmar arch in approximately 10% of the population. Variation in the superficial arch is greater than in the more consistent deep palmar arch. In general, arterial variations occur in up to a third of the population.

Answer: **B**
Anderson, Sec. 6-78
Refer to Fig. 1-15

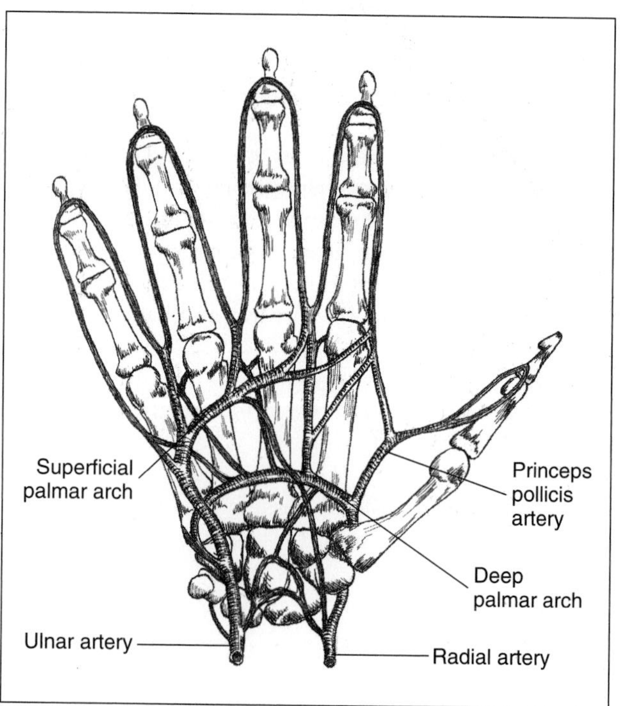

Fig. 1-15 ■ From Smith AA, Lacey SH: *Hand surgery review*, St Louis, 1996, Mosby.

25. Match each muscle with its innervation.

Muscle

1. Adductor pollicis
2. Brachioradialis
3. Extensor indicis proprius
4. Palmaris brevis
5. Abductor pollicis brevis
6. Pronator quadratus

Innervation

A. Superficial branch of ulnar nerve
B. Deep branch of ulnar nerve
C. Posterior interosseous nerve
D. Anterior interosseous nerve
E. Median nerve
F. Radial nerve

Answers: **1, B; 2, F; 3, C; 4, A; 5, E; 6, D**
Hunter, Mackin, Callahan, pp. A1-A40
Malick, pp. 57-66

26. Sensory changes, motor changes, and atrophy of the thenar musculature may indicate which of the following?

A. Syringomyelia
B. Peripheral neuritis secondary to diabetes
C. Lead intoxication
D. Charcot-Marie-Tooth disease

Individuals with diabetes may complain of sensory and motor changes and have evidence of thenar muscle atrophy. It may be confused with carpal tunnel compression of the median nerve at the wrist. In fact, carpal tunnel syndrome may coexist in persons with diabetes.

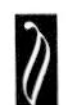

Answer: **B**
Tubiana, p. 16

27. Fingernails generally grow at what rate per month?

A. 1 to 2 mm per month
B. 2 to 3 mm per month
C. 3 to 4 mm per month
D. 4 to 5 mm per month

Two to three millimeters per month of nail growth is the expected growth rate. Thus the nail can provide a fairly accurate timetable of systemic insults, whether from toxic substances or disease.

Answer: **B**
Tubiana, Thomine, Mackin, p. 5

28. During "normal" flexing into a fist, the fingers converge and point toward what structure?

A. Hook of the hamate
B. Tubercle of the trapezium
C. Base of the first metacarpal
D. Scaphoid tubercle

The scaphoid tubercle is the point of finger convergence when a fist is made. When the digits flex into a digitopalmar grip, the more ulnar the digit, the more obliquely it deviates as it comes into the palm. Thus with each digit flexed at the MCP and PIP joints, their axes converge toward the scaphoid bone.

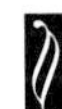

Answer: **D**
Tubiana, Thomine, Mackin, p. 6
Weinzweig, p. 13
Refer to Fig. 1-16

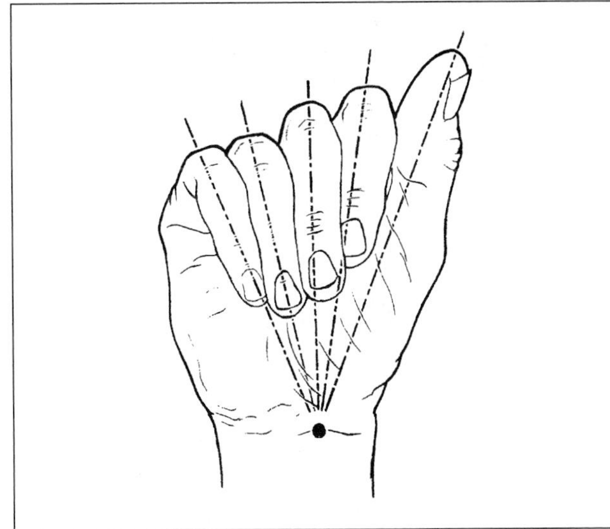

Fig. 1-16 ■ From Weinzweig J: *Hand and wrist surgery secrets,* Philadelphia, 2000, Hanley & Belfus.

29. Which structure plays a crucial role in the stability of the shoulder?

A. Teres major
B. Glenoid labrum
C. Long head of the biceps
D. Coracoacromial ligament

The stability of the glenohumeral joint is sacrificed because of its great freedom of movement. The humeral head articulates against the glenoid cavity of the scapula. The labrum is important because it gives the glenoid a deeper cavity, thus allowing for increased surface area and stability. The head of the humerus is held in the glenoid cavity by the rotator cuff muscles. The glenoid labrum is a fibrocartilaginous rim that is attached around the margin of the glenoid process.

Answer: **B**
Netter, p. 34
Refer to Fig. 1-17

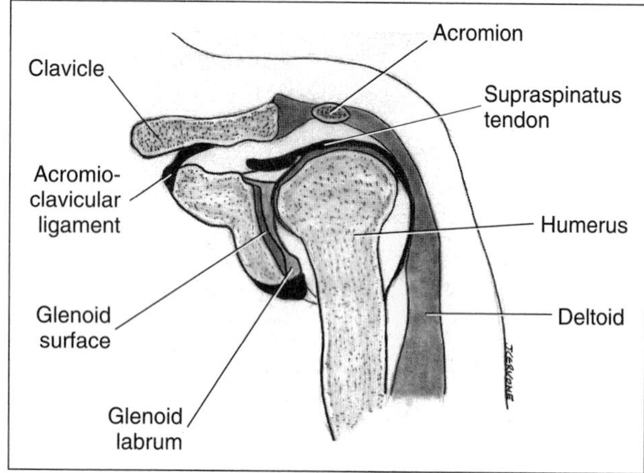

Fig. 1-17

30. Which pole of the scaphoid has a generous blood supply?

A. Distal pole
B. Waist
C. Proximal pole
D. All of the above have excellent vascularity.

The scaphoid most often receives its arterial blood supply from the radial artery through ligamentous attachments. The distal pole has a rich blood supply and tends to heal promptly, whereas the proximal pole has poor vascularity and may result in avascular necrosis or nonunion after fracture.

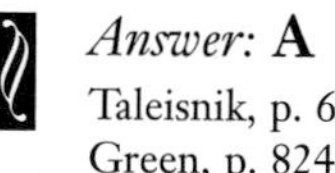

Answer: **A**
Taleisnik, p. 67
Green, p. 824

31. Which of the following statements is false with regard to the metacarpophalangeal (MCP) joint collateral ligaments?

A. With the MCP joint extended, the collateral ligaments are loose, and the portion from the metacarpal to the palmar plate is taut.
B. With the MCP joint flexed, the collateral ligaments are tight, and the portion from the metacarpal to the palmar plate is lax.
C. This structure allows for lateral movement during MCP extension and prohibits lateral movement during flexion.
D. This information is not important to consider when one splints the MCP joints.

The information in A through C is vital when splinting the MCP joints. Splinting the MCP joints in extension for prolonged periods tightens the MCP joint collateral ligaments into a shortened position.

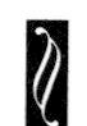

Answer: **D**
Boscheinen-Morrin, Conolly, pp. 3-5.
Refer to Fig. 1-18

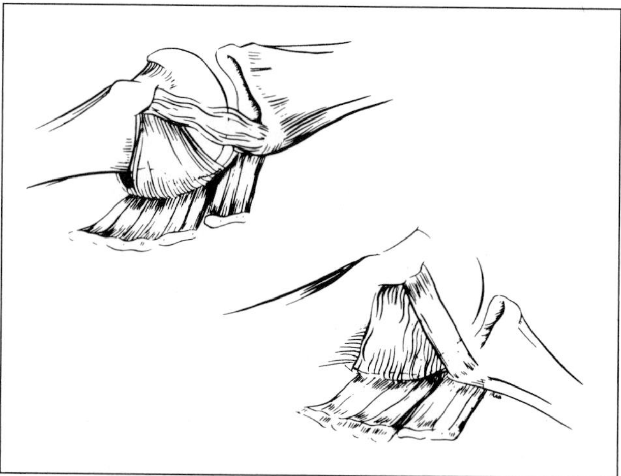

Fig. 1-18 ■ From Jupiter JB: *Flynn's Hand surgery*, ed 4, Philadelphia, 1991, Williams & Wilkins.

32. Identify the following features (1-7) of the dorsal aspect of the hand in Fig. 1-19.

A. Abductor pollicis longus (APL)
B. Juncturae tendinum
C. Dorsal tubercle of the radius/Lister's tubercle
D. Extensor pollicis longus (EPL)
E. Tendon to extensor carpi radialis longus (ECRL)
F. Extensor retinaculum
G. Extensor digitorum

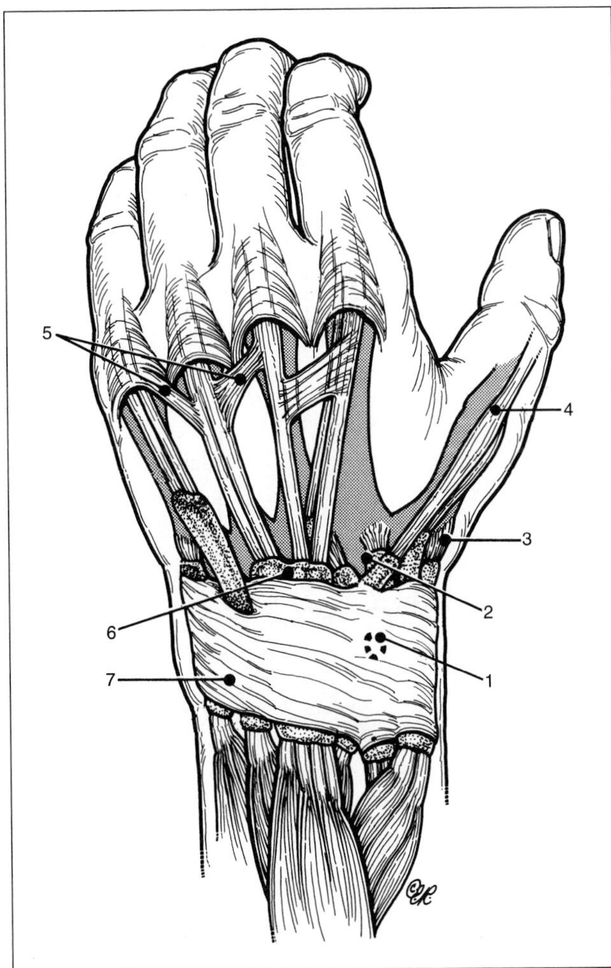

Fig. 1-19 ■ Copyright Elizabeth Roselius. Green DP, Hotchkiss RN, Pederson WC: *Green's Operative hand surgery*, ed 4, Philadelphia, 1999, Churchill Livingstone.

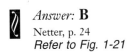

Answers: **1, C; 2, E; 3, A; 4, D; 5, B; 6, G; 7, F**
Boscheinen-Miller, Conolly, p. 44

33. Which two muscles line the medial and lateral borders of the cubital fossa?

A. Biceps medially and brachioradialis laterally
B. Brachioradialis laterally and pronator teres medially
C. Pronator teres laterally and brachioradialis medially
D. Flexor carpi ulnaris medially and biceps ulnarly

The brachioradialis forms the lateral border, and the pronator teres forms the medial border of the cubital fossa.

Answer: **B**
Hunter, Mackin, Callahan, p. 46
Mackin, Callahan, Skirven, et al, p. 29
Morrey, p. 67
Omer in Mackin, Callahan, Skirven, et al, p. 676

34. Label the creases (1-8) of the hand and wrist in Fig. 1-20 with the following terms.

A. Thenar crease
B. Proximal crease of the wrist
C. Distal crease of the wrist
D. Proximal flexor crease (proximal palmar crease)
E. Distal flexor crease (distal palmar crease)
F. Palmar digital crease
G. Proximal interphalangeal crease (middle digital crease)
H. Distal interphalangeal crease (distal digital crease)

Answers: **1, E; 2, A; 3, F; 4, B; 5, H; 6, C; 7, D; 8, G**
Chase in Mackin, Callahan, Skirven, et al, p. 64

35. Which nerve and artery pass through the quadrangular space?

A. Musculocutaneous nerve and posterior circumflex artery
B. Axillary nerve and posterior circumflex artery
C. Musculocutaneous nerve and anterior circumflex artery
D. Axillary nerve and anterior circumflex artery

The quadrangular space is bordered by the teres minor superiorly, the teres major inferiorly, the humerus laterally, and the triceps medially. The axillary nerve and posterior circumflex artery pass through this space.

Answer: **B**
Netter, p. 24
Refer to Fig. 1-21

36. Which artery passes over the floor of the anatomic snuffbox?

A. Radial artery
B. Ulnar artery
C. Median artery
D. Anterior interosseous artery

The anatomic snuffbox is a concave space made by the convergence of the extensor pollicis longus tendon with the extensor pollicis brevis and the abductor pollicis longus tendons. On the floor, the radial artery passes toward the back of the hand to the dorsal carpal branch.

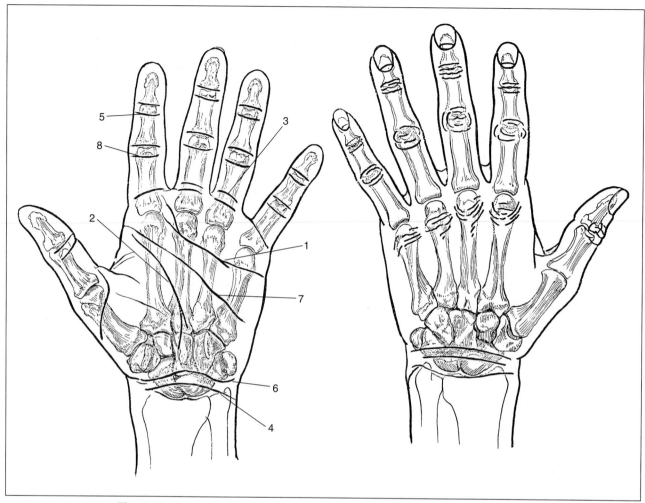

Fig. 1-20 ■ From Jupiter JB: *Flynn's Hand surgery,* ed 4, Philadelphia, 1991, Williams & Wilkins.

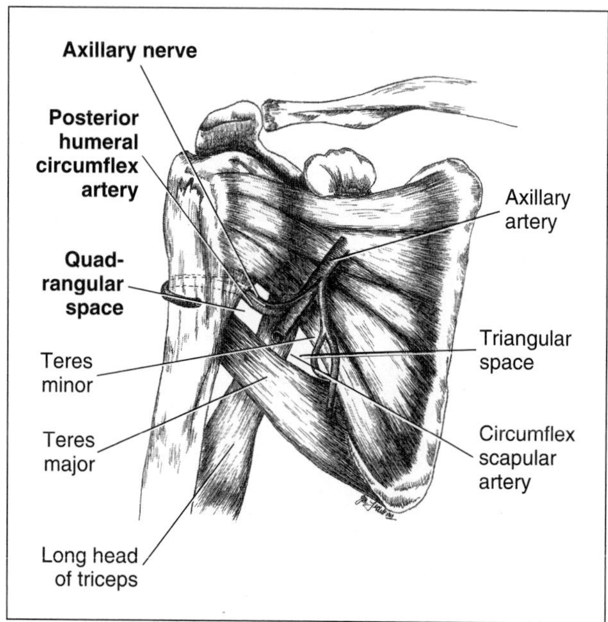

Fig. 1-21 ■ From Smith AA, Lacey SH: *Hand surgery review,* St Louis, 1996, Mosby.

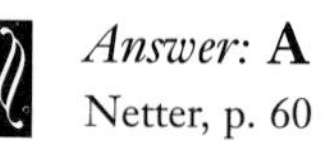

Answer: **A**
Netter, p. 60

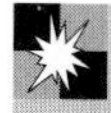

CLINICAL GEM:
Tenderness in the snuffbox may indicate a scaphoid fracture.

37. In the forearm, at the level of the elbow, which three veins make the M shape?

A. Median cubital vein, basilic vein, and lateral cutaneous vein
B. Basilic vein, cephalic vein, and median cubital vein
C. Cephalic vein, lateral cutaneous vein, and basilic vein
D. None of the above

The cephalic vein that runs on the lateral (radial) aspect of the upper extremity and the basilic vein that travels along the medial (ulnar) upper extremity form an M shape with the median cubital vein at the elbow.

Answer: **B**

Hunter, Mackin, Callahan, p. A-17
Hunter in Mackin, Callahan, Skirven, et al, p. 19
Refer to Fig. 1-22

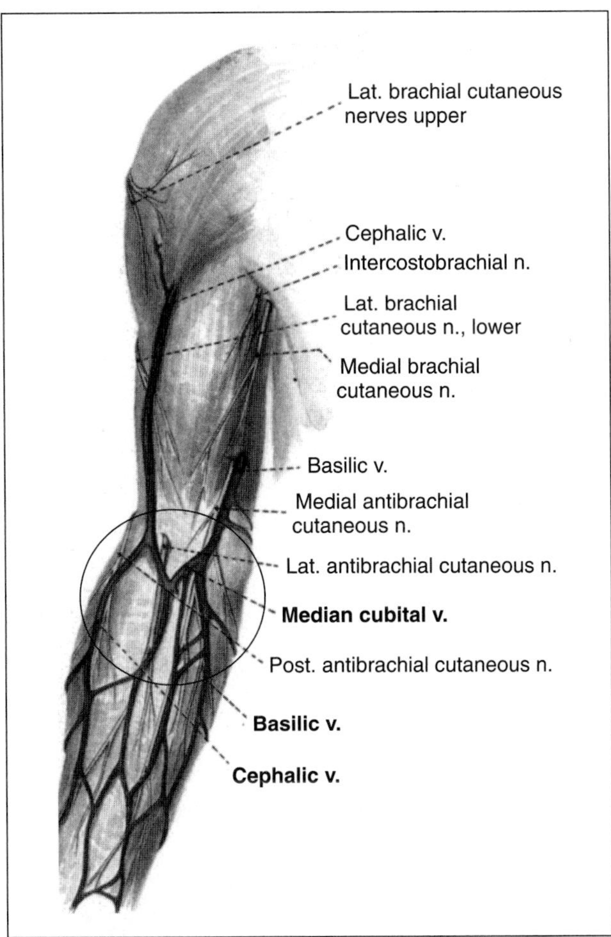

Fig. 1-22 ■ From Mackin EJ, Callahan AD, Skirven TM, et al: *Rehabilitation of the hand and upper extremity*, ed 5, vol 1, St Louis, 2002, Mosby.

38. Match the following vascular terms with the correct definitions.

Terms

1. Thrill
2. Bruit
3. Aneurysm
4. Doppler echocardiography
5. Hemangioma

Definitions

A. An adventitious sound heard on auscultation and of venous or arterial origin
B. An abnormal tremor that accompanies a vascular or cardiac murmur felt on palpation
C. Localized abnormal dilation of a blood vessel, usually an artery
D. A benign tumor of dilated blood vessels
E. A sensitive noninvasive technique for determining blood flow

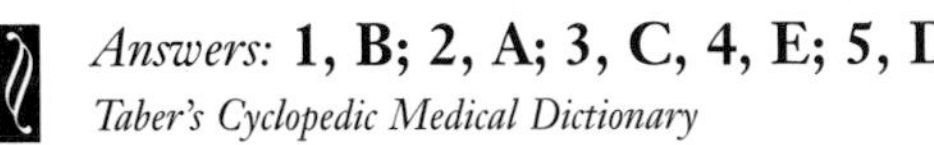

Answers: **1, B; 2, A; 3, C, 4, E; 5, D**

Taber's Cyclopedic Medical Dictionary

39. What is the space of Poirier?

A. A gap between the scaphoid and lunate bones
B. An area of avascularity in the scaphoid
C. Weakness from an absence of ligamentous support
D. T-shaped ligaments over the hamate and triquetrum

The volar wrist capsule often contains an area of weakness called the *space of Poirier.* This weakness is caused by the absence of a volar lunocapitate ligament. Some authors report that this lack of ligament support causes wrist instability.

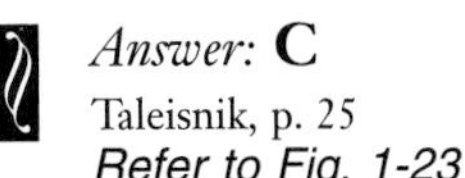

Answer: **C**

Taleisnik, p. 25
Refer to Fig. 1-23

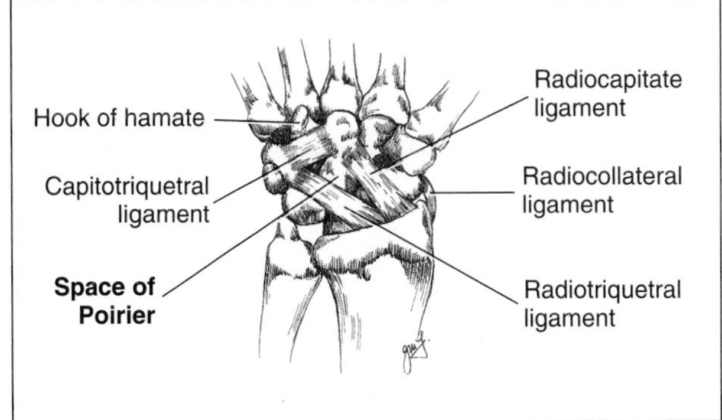

Fig. 1-23 ■ From Smith AA, Lacey SH: *Hand surgery review*, St Louis, 1996, Mosby.

40. Blood supply to the thumb comes primarily from which of the following?

A. The superficial branch of the ulnar artery
B. The deep branch of the radial artery
C. The superficial branch of the radial artery
D. The deep branch of the ulnar nerve

The deep branch of the radial artery provides the primary blood supply to the thumb.

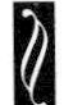

Answer: **B**

Hunter, Mackin, Callahan, pp. 34-35

41. Place the correct nerve innervation next to the muscle.

Key

1. Radial nerve = R
2. Median nerve = M
3. Ulnar nerve = U

Muscle

A. Extensor pollicis longus
B. Extensor pollicis brevis
C. Abductor pollicis longus
D. Abductor pollicis brevis
E. Adductor pollicis
F. Flexor pollicis longus
G. Flexor pollicis brevis
H. Volar interossei
I. Dorsal interossei
J. Lumbricals II and III
K. Lumbricals V and IV

Answer: **A, R; B, R; C, R; D, M; E, U; F, M; G, M & U; H, U; I, U; J, M; K, U**

Omer, Spinner, Van Beek, pp. 42-47

Refer to Table 1-1

42. Which of the following is *not* a sign of arterial insufficiency?

A. Pallor
B. Decreased temperature
C. Sluggish capillary refill
D. Cyanosis

Arterial insufficiency results in pallor (lack of color), decreased temperature, increased pain, slow capillary refill, and loss of pulse. Venous insufficiency is recognized by cyanosis (bluish discoloration of the skin caused by reduced amounts of hemoglobin in the blood) and abnormal capillary refill. Excessive elevation above the level of the heart can stress the arterial system during the acute phase and should be avoided. Elevation at the level of the heart is the recommended position. In general, slight elevation above the heart is beneficial for venous stasis, and slight lowering below the heart is helpful for arterial system management.

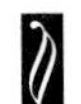

Answer: **D**

Hunter, Mackin, Callahan, pp. 1059, 1092

Pettengill in Mackin, Callahan, Skirven, et al, pp. 1413-1418

43. What is the lacertus fibrosus?

A. Part of the arcade of Frohse
B. Continuation of the arcade of Struthers
C. The ligament of Struthers
D. Synonymous with the bicipital aponeurosis

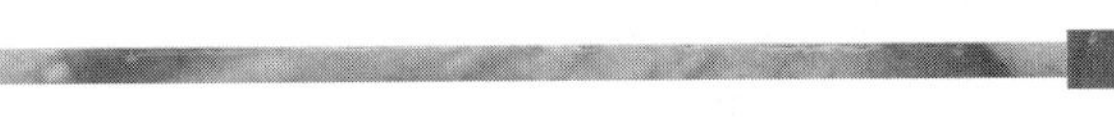

The *lacertus fibrosus* is another name for the bicipital aponeurosis. It is a fibrous band that originates from the tendon of biceps brachii. The lacertus fibrosus is tightened with pronation. Active flexion of the elbow in conjunction with pronation may contribute to compression of the median nerve at the lacertus fibrosus.

Answer: **D**

Green, pp. 1342-1343

Refer to Fig. 1-24

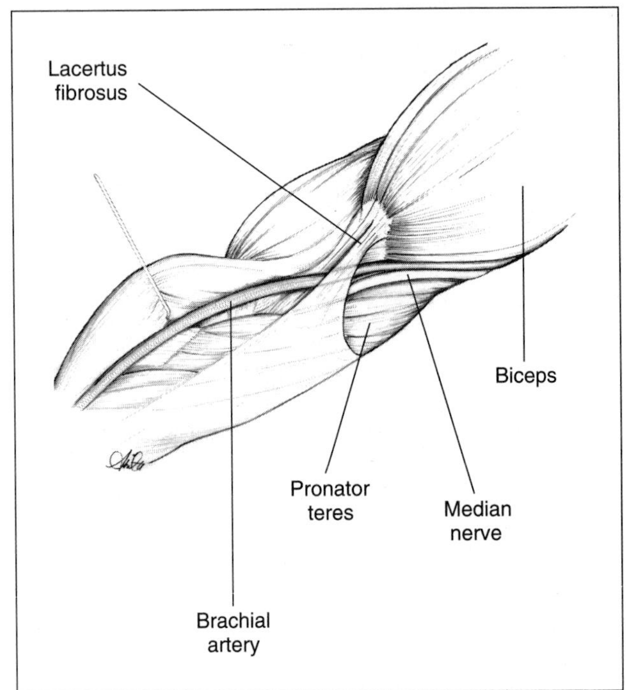

Fig. 1-24

Table 1-1

Upper Extremity: Motor and Sensory Nerve Contribution to Peripheral Nerves

Nerves	Branch	Muscle innervation	Sensory distribution
Dorsal scapular, C4-C5		Rhomboid major, rhomboid minor, levator scapulae	None
Suprascapular, C4-C6		Supraspinatus, infraspinatus	None
Nerve to subclavius, C5		Subclavius	None
Subscapular, C5-C7		Teres major	None
Long thoracic, C5-C7		Serratus anterior	None
Thoracodorsal, C6-C8		Latissimus dorsi	None
Lateral pectoral, C6		Pectoralis major, pectoralis minor	None
Medial pectoral, C7-C8		Pectoralis major, pectoralis minor	None
Axillary, C5-C6	Lateral, brachial, cutaneous	Deltoid, teres minor	Over deltoid, lateral aspect of upper arm, lateral portion of shoulder joint
Musculocutaneous, C5-C7	Lateral antebrachial cutaneous	Biceps brachii, brachialis, corocobrachialis (together with radial nerve), pronator teres	Volar radial forearm to wrist; may extend to thenar eminence
Medial brachial cutaneous (medial cord) C8-T1		None	Medial aspect of upper arm
Radial, C5-C8	Posterior interosseous Posterior, brachial, cutaneous, antebrachial, cutaneous, superficial, radial	*Triceps brachii, brachioradialis,* anconeus, *extensor carpi radialis* (*brevis* and *longus*), *extensor digitorum communis II-V,* brachialis, supinator, *extensor carpi ulnaris, extensor digiti minimi, extensor pollicis longus, extensor pollicis brevis, extensor indicis proprius*	Dorsal distal upper arm Dorsal radial forearm Dorsal *first web space* Radial dorsum of hand, wrist joint
Medial antebrachial cutaneous, C8-T1 (medial cord)	Anterior ulnar	None	Ulnar forearm
Median, C5-T1	Anterior interosseous Recurrent motor branch Palmar cutaneous	Pronator teres, pronator quadratus, *flexor carpi radialis,* palmaris longus, flexor palm and radial fingers profundus (second and third), *flexor pollicis longus, abductor pollicis brevis,* flexor pollicis brevis (superficial head), opponens pollicis, lumbricales (first and second)	*Pulp of thumb and index, proximal palm and thenar eminence,* radial
Ulnar, C8-T1	Superficial palmar	*Flexor carpi ulnaris,* flexor pollicis brevis (deep head), flexor digitorum profundus (fourth and fifth), *flexor digiti minimi brevis, opponens digiti minimi,* palmaris brevis, adductor pollicis, flexor pollicis brevis, abductor digiti, lumbricales (third and fourth), interossei	*Pulp of little finger, dorsal ulnar surface of hand,* ulnar palm, and ulnar fingers

Italics: Key muscles, most reliable sensory distribution.

From Omer GE, Spinner M, Van Beek AL: *Management of peripheral nerve problems*, ed 2, Philadelphia, 1998, Saunders.

44. Match the following terms with the correct definitions.

Terms

1. Fascia
2. Muscle
3. Sprain
4. Strain
5. Erythematous

Definitions

A. Injury to the joint with ligamentous damage
B. Injury to the muscle or musculotendinous unit
C. A fibrous membrane that covers, supports, and separates muscles
D. A type of tissue composed of contractile fibers
E. Dry, pink patches of skin that are itchy and burn

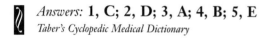

Answers: **1, C; 2, D; 3, A; 4, B; 5, E**
Taber's Cyclopedic Medical Dictionary

45. Which of the following muscles does not originate from the common flexor origin on the medial epicondyle of the humerus?

A. Pronator quadratus
B. Flexor carpi radialis
C. Flexor digitorum superficialis
D. Flexor carpi ulnaris
E. Pronator teres

Muscles originating from the common flexor origin include the pronator teres, flexor carpi radialis, flexor digitorum superficialis, palmaris longus, and flexor carpi ulnaris. Pronator quadratus is a distal forearm muscle that originates from the distal ulna.

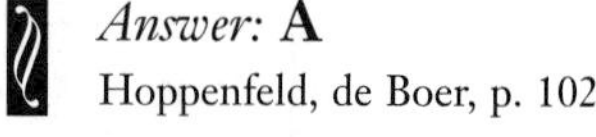

Answer: **A**
Hoppenfeld, de Boer, p. 102

46. The basilic vein and the brachial vein form which vein?

A. Axillary vein
B. Cephalic vein
C. Thoracoepigastric vein
D. Thoracodorsal vein

The basilic vein joins the brachial vein at the lower border of the teres major and goes on to form the axillary vein. The axillary vein is termed the *subclavian vein* at the first rib.

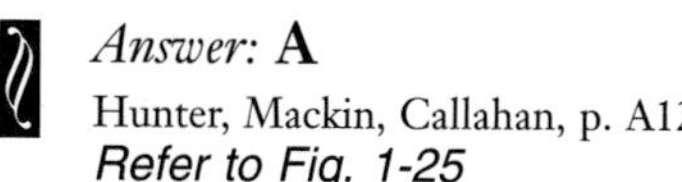

Answer: **A**
Hunter, Mackin, Callahan, p. A12
Refer to Fig. 1-25

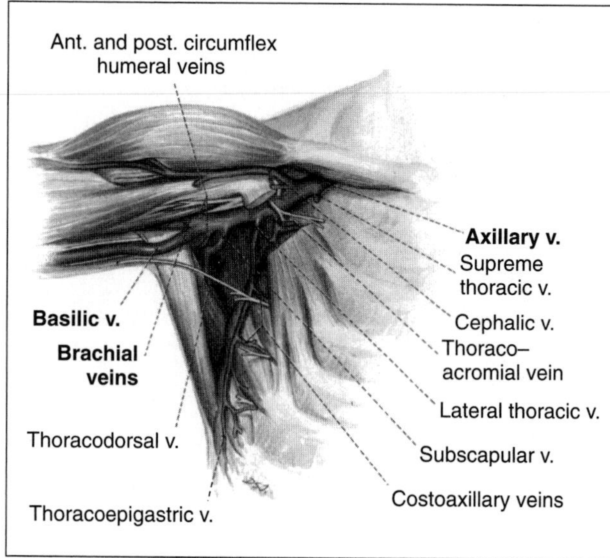

Fig. 1-25 ■ From Mackin EJ, Callahan AD, Skirven TM, et al: *Rehabilitation of the hand and upper extremity*, ed 5, vol 1, St Louis, 2002, Mosby.

47. True or false: All vein grafts should be marked and reversed when they are used in arterial reconstruction.

Both veins and arteries have been used for interposition grafts and microsurgery, but venous grafts are more readily available and appear to have the highest patency rate. All vein grafts should be marked and reversed when they are used in arterial reconstruction because even the smallest digital vessels have been shown to contain valves. Veins have valves that prevent backward circulation; therefore if veins are not reversed, blood will not flow properly.

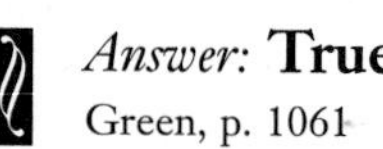

Answer: **True**
Green, p. 1061

48. Which thumb pulley is the most important?

A. A1 pulley
B. Oblique pulley
C. A2 pulley
D. Pulleys are not important in the thumb.

The oblique pulley, which is located in the mid-portion of the proximal phalanx, is the most important pulley. The pulley system in the thumb comprises the A1 pulley located at the MCP joint level, the oblique pulley at the mid-portion of the proximal phalanx, and the A2 pulley located at the IP joint. IP joint motion in the thumb will decrease if the oblique pulley is damaged.

Answer: **B**
Hunter, Mackin Callahan, p. 418
Chase in Mackin, Callahan, Skirven, et al, p. 69
Refer to Fig. 1-26

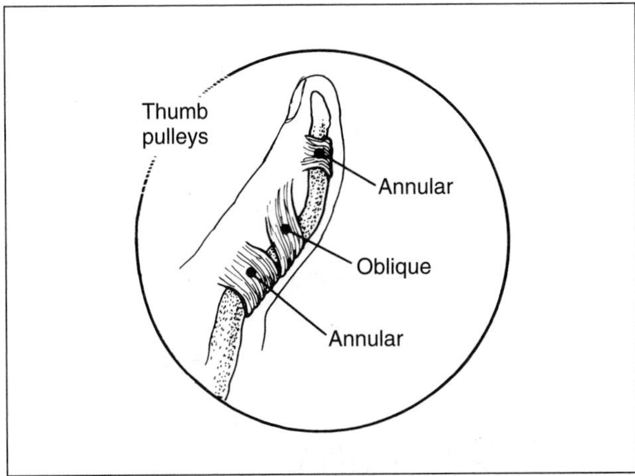

Fig. 1-26 ■ From Chase RA: *Atlas of hand surgery*, vol 2, Philadelphia, 1984, WB Saunders.

49. Which muscle's function would be affected by a lesion of the posterior interosseous nerve?

A. Brachioradialis
B. Extensor carpi radialis brevis
C. Extensor digitorum
D. All of the above

The extensor digitorum communis is affected as the deep branch of the radial nerve innervates the extensor digitorum communis, abductor pollicis longus, extensor pollicis longus, and extensor pollicis brevis.

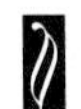
Answer: **C**
Hunter, Mackin, Callahan, p. 633

50. Lister's tubercle is a bony prominence located on which of the following?

A. Scaphoid
B. Proximal ulna
C. Distal radius
D. Distal ulna

Lister's tubercle is located on the distal radius. The extensor pollicis longus (EPL) takes a 45-degree turn around Lister's tubercle, which acts as a pulley on its course to the thumb. Rupture of the EPL is not uncommon in patients with rheumatoid arthritis. The EPL may rupture after a distal radius fracture if the tubercle is disrupted.

Answer: **C**
Hoppenfeld, p. 78

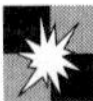
CLINICAL GEM:
The SL ligament can be palpated approximately 1 cm directly distal to Lister's turbercle on the distal radius.

51. Which structure articulates with the cupped surface of the proximal radius?

A. Trochlea
B. Coronoid
C. Capitulum
D. Medial epicondyle

The capitulum is spherical and smaller than the trochlea. The capitulum articulates with the cupped surface of the radius (radial head). The trochlea is shaped like a spool and is superior to the coronoid fossa.

Answer: **C**
Netter, p. 31
Refer to Fig. 1-27

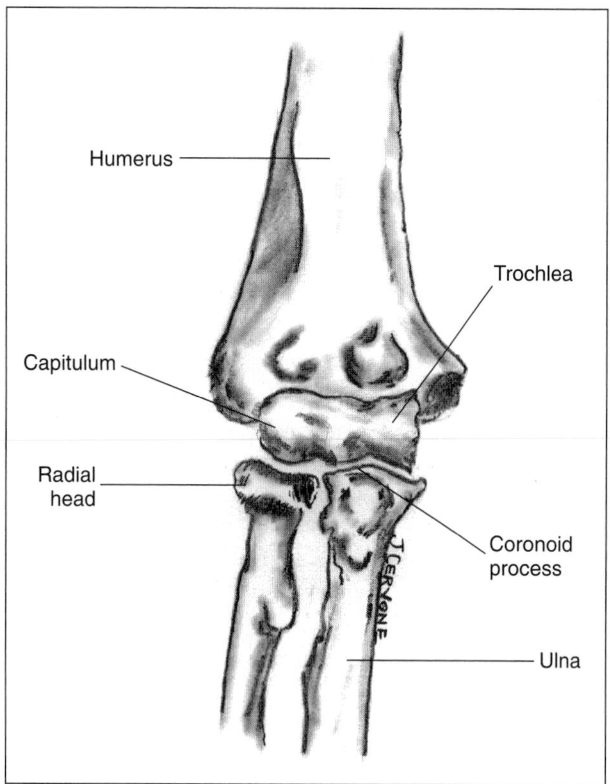

Fig. 1-27

52. Match each muscle with the correct insertion.

Muscle

1. Subscapularis
2. Pectoralis major
3. Coracobrachialis
4. Brachialis
5. Supraspinatus

Insertion

A. Bicipital groove
B. Coronoid process of ulna
C. Greater tubercle of humerus
D. Shaft of humerus
E. Lesser tubercle of humerus

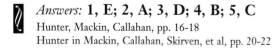

Answers: **1, E; 2, A; 3, D; 4, B; 5, C**
Hunter, Mackin, Callahan, pp. 16-18
Hunter in Mackin, Callahan, Skirven, et al, pp. 20-22

53. Which muscle is *not* included in the wad of Henry?

A. Brachioradialis
B. Supinator
C. Extensor carpi radialis brevis
D. Extensor carpi radialis longus

Hoppenfeld describes the brachioradialis, extensor carpi radialis brevis, and extensor carpi radialis longus as "the mobile wad of Henry" or "mobile wad of three." These muscles are best palpated as a unit, which is easily held and moves between the fingers. One can assess this group of muscles when the patient's forearm and wrist are in the neutral position. The supinator is not part of the wad of Henry.

Answer: **B**
Hoppenfeld, p. 47
Refer to Fig. 1-28

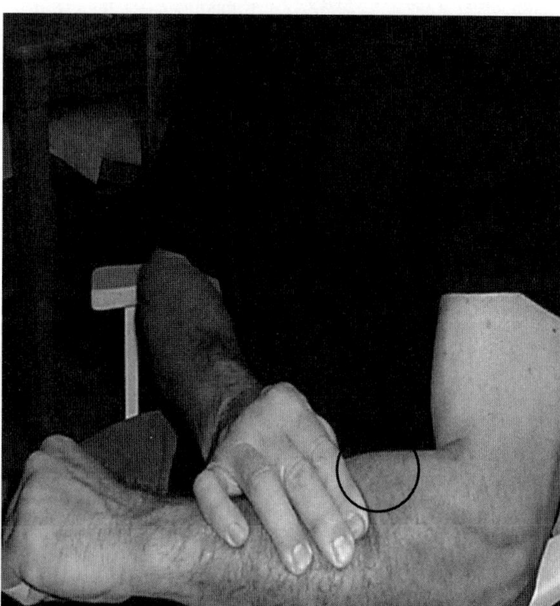

Fig. 1-28 ■ Mobile wad of Henry.

54. Match each plane with the correct definition.

Plane

1. Coronal plane
2. Frontal plane
3. Sagittal plane
4. Transverse plane

Definition

A. Another name for coronal plane
B. Divides the body into superior and inferior portions at right angles to the long axis of the body
C. Divides the body into right and left parts; called *the median plane*
D. Divides the body into front and back portions

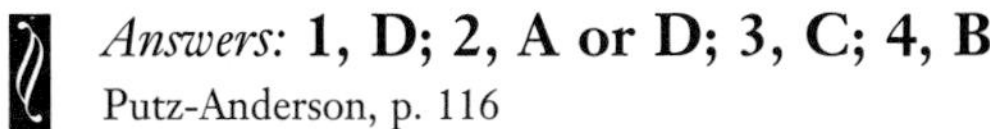

Answers: **1, D; 2, A or D; 3, C; 4, B**
Putz-Anderson, p. 116

55. Which of the following statements is false with regard to the blood supply to the hand?

A. The supply of blood to the hand depends on the venous pressure.
B. The arterial system, which brings blood into the hand, is situated on the volar aspect of the hand.
C. The venous and lymphatic system, which returns blood back into the system, is located dorsally.
D. The return flow through the veins and lymphatics normally depends on active movement of the hand and arm, which acts as a pumping mechanism.

Statement A is an incorrect or a false statement because the blood supply to the hand depends on *arterial* pressure and not *venous* pressure.

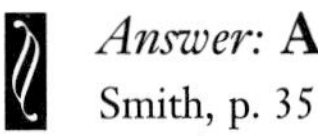

Answer: **A**
Smith, p. 35

56. *Landsmeer's ligament* is another term for which structure?

A. The oblique retinacular ligament
B. The transverse retinacular ligament
C. The triangular ligament
D. Cleland's ligament

The oblique retinacular ligament (ORL) was described by Landsmeer in 1949. This ligament coordinates the movement of the interphalangeal joints. The functional value of this ligament is controversial in normal fingers but evident in pathological conditions. The ORL is taut in DIP joint flexion; therefore if this ligament is contracted in extension, the DIP joint is not able to fully flex. When the ORL is contracted, it contributes to the boutonniere deformity.

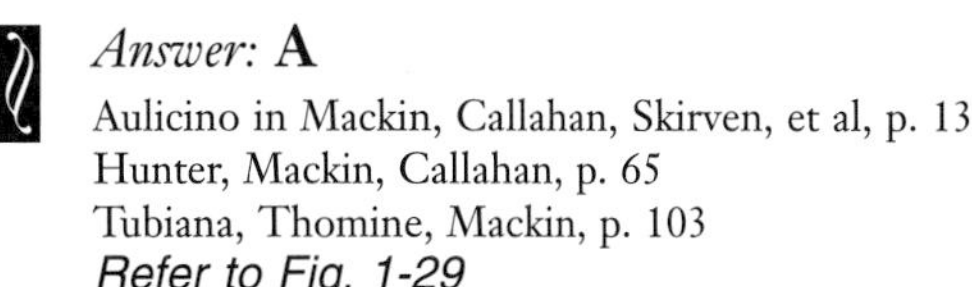

Answer: **A**
Aulicino in Mackin, Callahan, Skirven, et al, p. 133
Hunter, Mackin, Callahan, p. 65
Tubiana, Thomine, Mackin, p. 103
Refer to Fig. 1-29

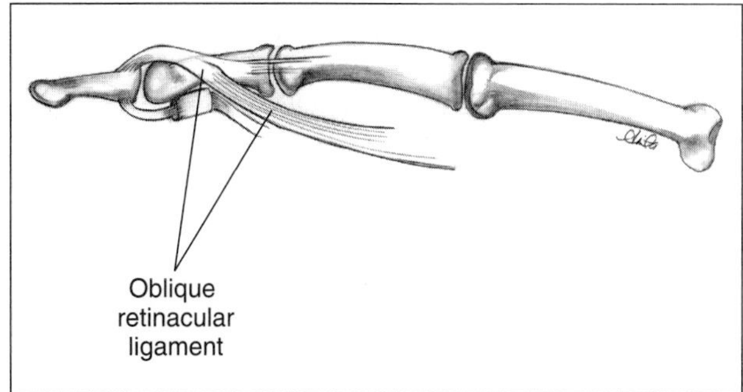

Fig. 1-29

57. True or false: A ligament attaches a muscle to a bone.

A ligament is a band or sheet of strong, fibrous, connective tissue that connects the articular ends of bones; it binds them together and facilitates or limits motion. A tendon is a fibrous, connective tissue that attaches muscle to bone.

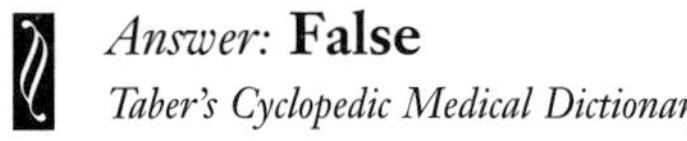

Answer: **False**
Taber's Cyclopedic Medical Dictionary

58. A fingerprint is made from which of the following?

A. Reticular dermis
B. Skin bulging
C. Papillary ridges
D. Oil in the fingertips

Fingerprints are formed from cutaneous striations that are reflective of organized papillary ridges in the underlying dermis. The reticular dermis is incorrect because it is a deeper layer that comprises collagen and elastic fibers.

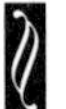

Answer: **C**

Tubiana, Thomine, Mackin, p. 131
Refer to Fig. 1-30

A

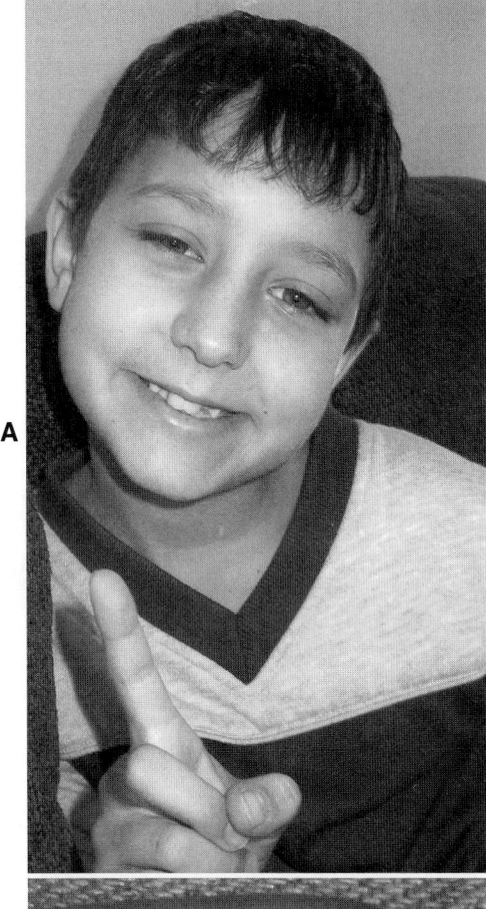

B

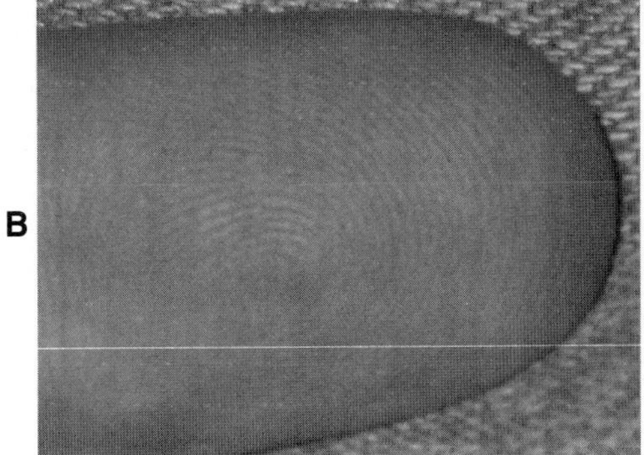

Fig. 1-30 ■ **B**, Papillary ridges.

59. Which of the following is the term for the white area at the base of the fingernail?

A. Hyponychium
B. Eponychium
C. Paronychia
D. Lunula

The lunula is the white convex area seen at the base of the nail. The hyponychium is under the nail bed. The eponychium is the embryonic structure from which the nail develops. A paronychia is an acute or chronic infection around the nail.

Answer: **D**

Tubiana, Thomine, Mackin, p. 151
Taber's Cyclopedic Medical Dictionary

60. Results of Allen's test are considered abnormal when the reflow into all or part of the hand takes longer than what amount of time?

A. 1 second
B. 3 seconds
C. 5 seconds
D. 7 seconds

7 seconds is the baseline to determine latent reflow. Slowness of more than 7 seconds indicates inadequate flow due to obstruction or anomaly. The Allen's test can also be used to assess digital flow. Testing to measure return of flow can be supplemented by laser Doppler flowmetry and pressure manometry.

Answer: **D**

Kasdan, Amadio, Bowers, p. 282
Aulicino in Mackin, Callahan, Skirven, et al, pp. 140-141
Refer to Fig. 1-31

61. Pain is present in approximately two thirds of patients with upper extremity vascular disease. Match the cause of vascular disease–related pain with the appropriate symptoms.

Cause

A. Sudden arterial occlusion
B. Vasospasm
C. Obstructive arterial problem
D. Severe arterial insufficiency

A

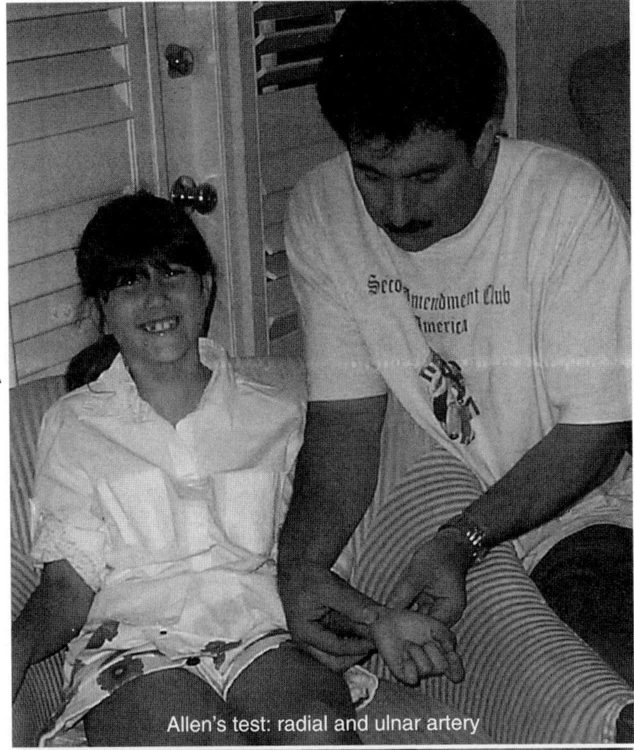

B

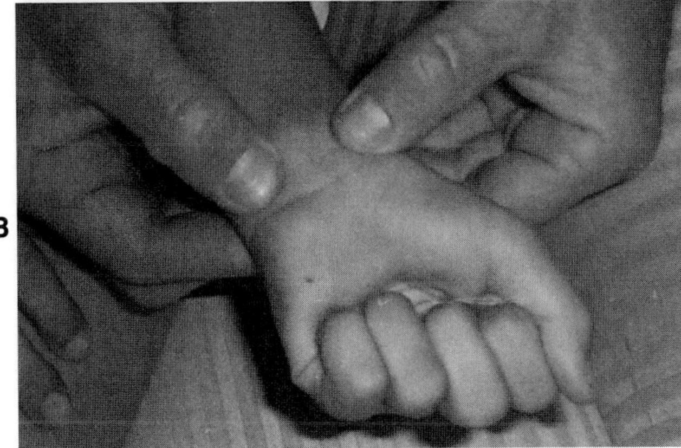

Fig. 1-31

Symptoms

1. Pain with exertion that is alleviated by rest
2. Mild paresthesias and marked pallor
3. Severe pain with sudden onset
4. Pain at rest

Answer: **A, 3; B, 2; C, 1; D, 4**

Hunter, Mackin, Callahan, pp. 961-962
Taras, Lemel, Nathan in Mackin, Callahan, Skirven, et al, pp. 882-883

62. Label Fig. 1-32.

1. Distal phalanx
2. Hyponychium
3. Nail bed
4. Eponychium
5. Nail plate

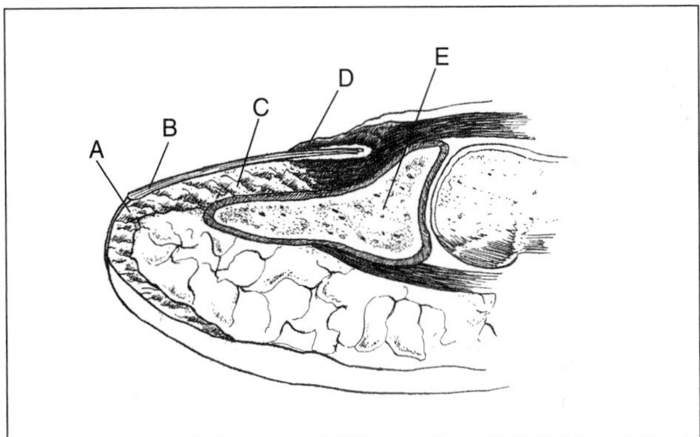

Fig. 1-32 ■ Modified from Smith AA, Lacey SH: *Hand surgery review*, St Louis, 1996, Mosby.

Answers: **1, E; 2, A; 3, C; 4, D; 5, B**

Green, p. 1283

63. The palmaris longus is absent in what percent of the population?

A. 30% to 40%
B. 5% to 8%
C. 13% to 20%
D. 75% to 85%

The palmaris longus is absent in 13% to 20% of the population. It originates from the medial epicondyle of the humerus and inserts into the palmar aponeurosis. The palmaris longus tendon is easily detected as it courses over the transverse carpal ligament. This tendon often is sacrificed when tendon transfers are performed.

Answer: **C**

Hunter, Mackin, Callahan, p. 26
Chase in Mackin, Callahan, Skirven, et al, p. 62

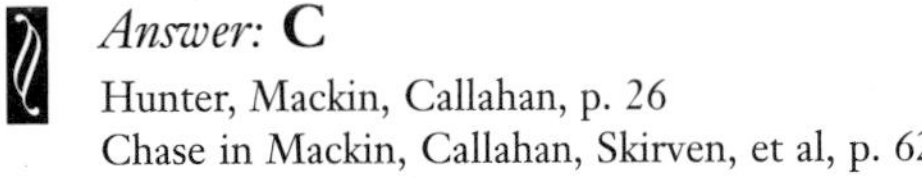

64. The fingernails of digits two and three receive their sensation from which nerve?

A. Median nerve
B. Ulnar nerve
C. Radial nerve
D. Anterior interosseous nerve

As the proper digital nerves pass toward their destination in the pad of the finger, they give off branches for the innervation of the skin on the dorsum of the fingers and matrices of the fingernails. Digital nerves for the first, second, third, and half of the fourth fingers are median nerve–innervated.

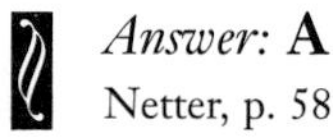
Answer: **A**
Netter, p. 58

65. The "attitude" of the hand in Fig. 1-33, *A*, depicts which of the following?

A. Position of rest
B. Lumbrical plus position
C. Intrinsic minus position
D. Intrinsic plus position

The "attitude" of the hand is an important factor to evaluate. The position of rest occurs when the metacarpophalangeal joints and the interphalangeal joints are slightly flexed and the fingers line up almost parallel to each other (Fig. 1-33, *A*). If one finger is extended (perpendicular to the others), its flexor tendon may have been damaged (Fig. 1-33, *B*).

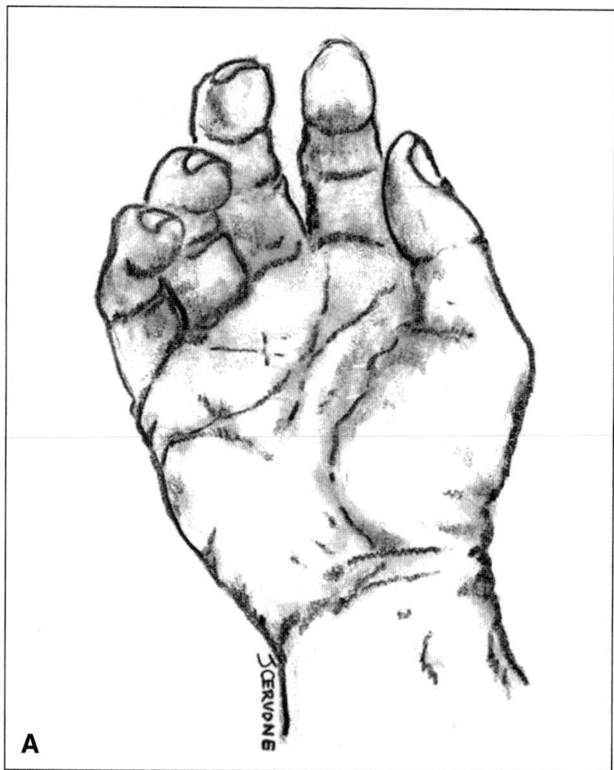

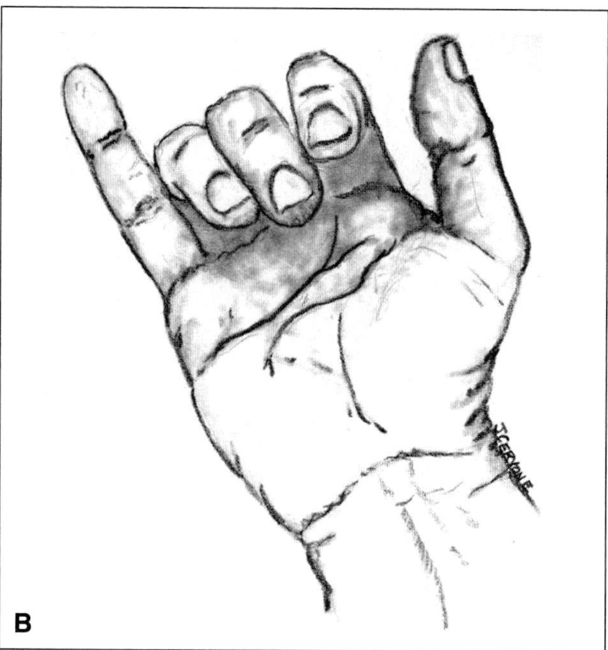

Fig. 1-33

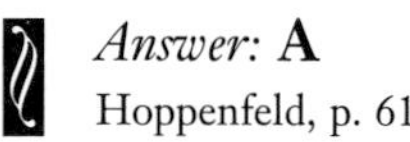
Answer: **A**
Hoppenfeld, p. 61

66. Which of the following would patients with vascular disease not experience?

A. Color changes
B. Cold intolerance
C. Stiffness in the digits after exposure to cold
D. Mild to severe pain that is relieved when the hand is warmed
E. Patients may experience all the above symptoms.

Patients with vascular disease, such as Raynaud's phenomenon, may complain of fingertips turning white then bluish, and redness may be reported when blood flow returns to the digits. Many of these patients will complain of pain when the extremity is cold. The pain is relieved when the extremity is warmed, but stiffness in the digits may follow warming of the extremity.

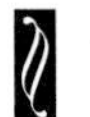

Answer: **E**

Kasdan, Amadio, Bowers, pp. 282-283
Hunter, Mackin, Callahan, p. 962

67. Ligaments about the elbow provide roughly what percent of joint stability?

A. 25%
B. 50%
C. 75%
D. 90%

Roughly half of elbow joint stability is provided by ligaments. Acute or recurrent instability can occur medially or posterolaterally. An acute tear of the medial collateral ligament is the most common isolated ligament injury of the elbow.

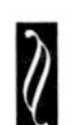

Answer: **B**

Varitimidis, pp. 66-71
Barnes, Tullos, pp. 62-67

68. Match the following muscles with their actions.

Muscle

1. Middle deltoid
2. Upper trapezius
3. Latissimus dorsi
4. Coracobrachialis
5. Pectoralis minor

Actions

A. Protraction, depression, and downward rotation of the scapula
B. Flexion and adduction of the humerus
C. Elevation and upward rotation of scapula
D. Extension, internal rotation, and adduction of the humerus
E. Abduction of humerus to 90 degrees

Answers: **1, E; 2, C; 3, D; 4, B; 5, A**

Sieg, Adams, p. 30

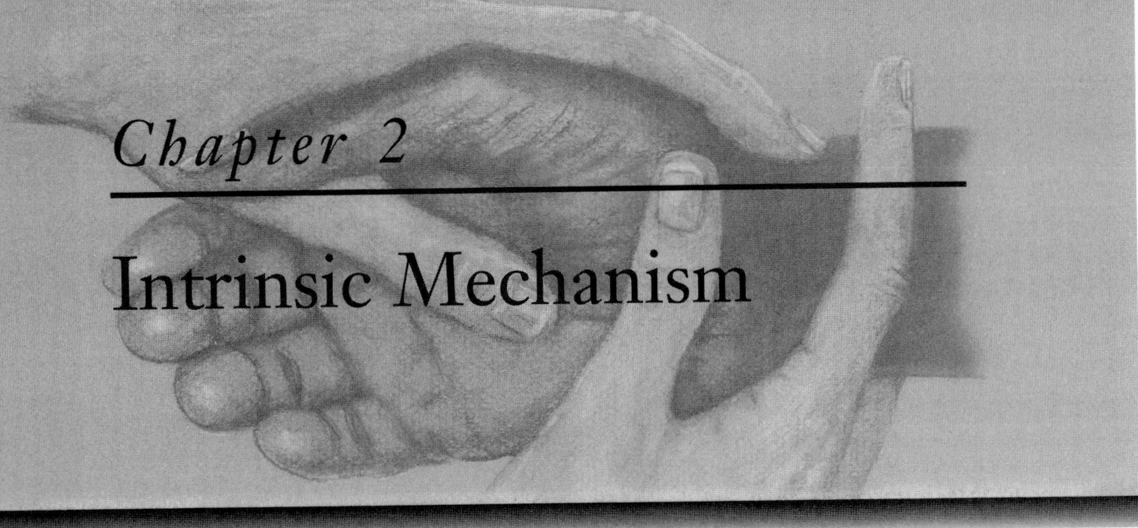

Chapter 2

Intrinsic Mechanism

1. Match the following numbers with the corresponding letters in Fig. 2-1.

1. Sagittal band
2. Triangular ligament
3. Terminal tendon
4. Lateral bands
5. Interosseous muscle
6. Lumbrical muscle
7. Long extensor tendon

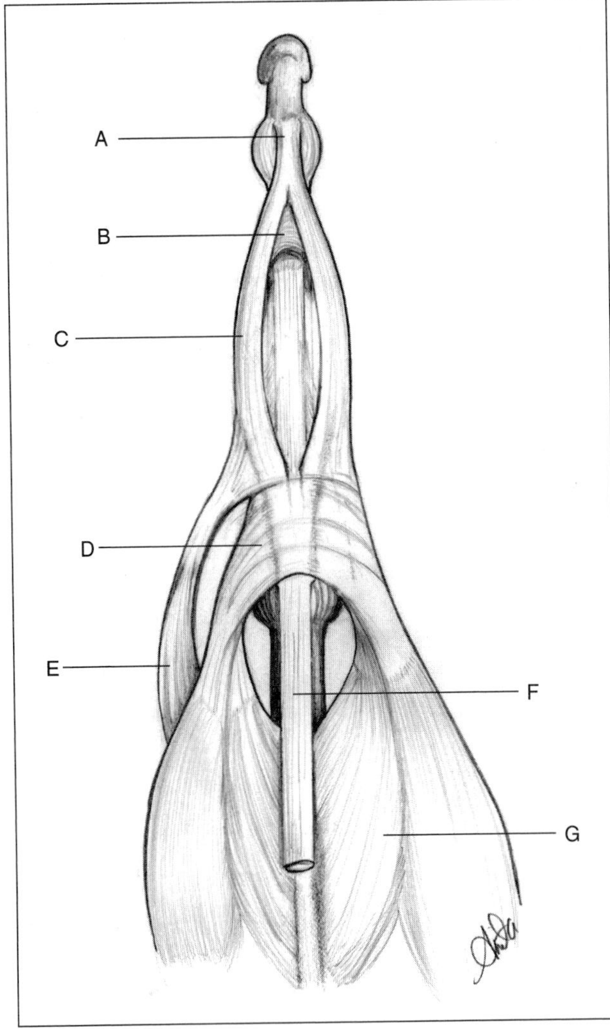

Fig. 2-1

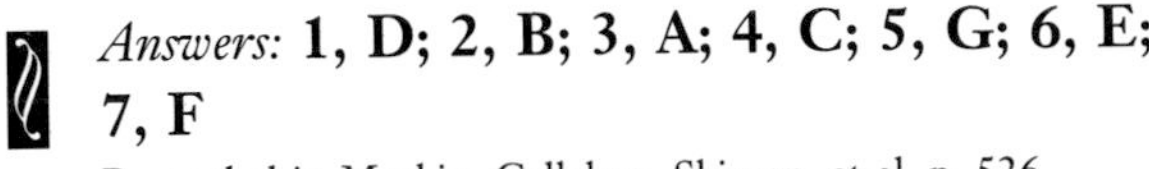

Answers: **1, D; 2, B; 3, A; 4, C; 5, G; 6, E; 7, F**

Rosenthal in Mackin, Callahan, Skirven, et al, p. 526
Hunter, Schneider, Mackin, p. 549
Mackin, Callahan Skirven et al, p. 37, 520–529

2. You are treating a patient with an ulnar nerve injury at the level of the wrist. One of your goals is to strengthen the intrinsic musculature. Which exercise is best suited for this patient?

A. Joint blocking
B. Hyperextension of the metacarpophalangeal (MCP) joints against rubber band traction
C. Pinching putty into a cone with the interphalangeal (IP) joints held in extension
D. Grip strengthening by using a hand helper with mild resistance

The lumbricals contract when the MCP joints are in flexion and the IP joints are in extension. When pinching putty into a cone by flexing the MCP joints and maintaining IP joint extension (Fig. 2-2), you are able to strengthen the lumbricals, interossei, and thumb adductors. The patient can also use a piece of thermoplastic material and push it into putty to facilitate the same muscles (Fig. 2-3). Grip strengthening would not be as effective because the IP joints flex during the exercise; therefore the patient is able to use the extrinsic flexors. Joint blocking is also incorrect because it is a nonresistive exercise for the extrinsic flexors and because hyperextension of the MCP joints facilitates the extrinsic extensors.

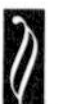

Answer: **C**

Stanley, Tribuzi, pp. 193, 199

Refer to Figs. 2-2 and 2-3

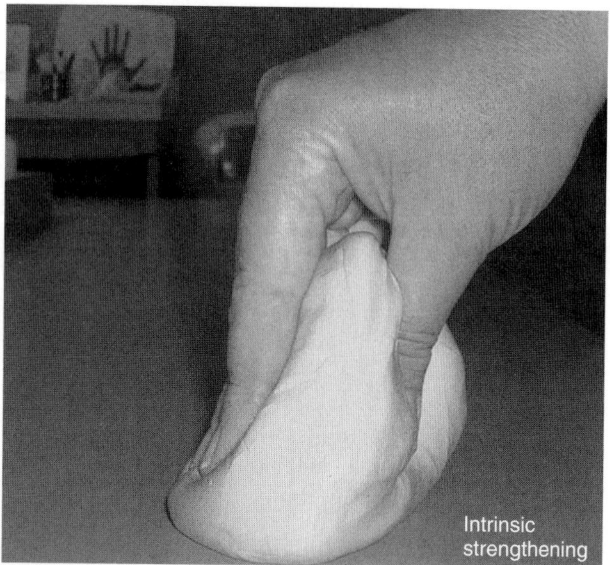

Fig. 2-2

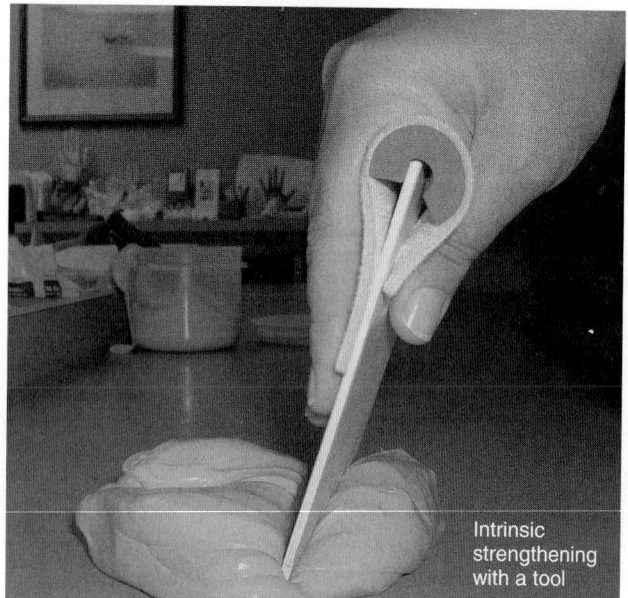

Fig. 2-3

3. A boutonnière deformity presents with which of the following?

A. MCP joint extension with IP joint flexion

B. Flexion of the proximal interphalangeal (PIP) joint with hyperextension of the distal interphalangeal (DIP) joint

C. Hyperextension of the PIP joint with flexion of the DIP joint

D. Hyperextension of the PIP joint with DIP joint flexion

A boutonnière deformity is caused by an injury to the complex extensor mechanism of the digit. The central tendon is ruptured or interrupted at the PIP joint (zone III) level, thus contributing to a loss of function of the triangular ligament. The rupture of the central slip causes proximal displacement of the extensor mechanism and a palmar subluxation of the lateral bands. The extensor force is therefore concentrated on the DIP joint, which results in hyperextension and loss of flexion at the DIP joint. The flexor digitorum superficialis is unopposed, which causes increased PIP joint flexion. As the lateral bands sublux further, the PIP joint is unable to achieve full extension actively or passively.

Answer: **B**

Rosenthal in Mackin, Callahan, Skirven, et al, p. 514
Hunter, Mackin, Callahan, p. 536
Blair, p. 610

Refer to Fig. 2-4

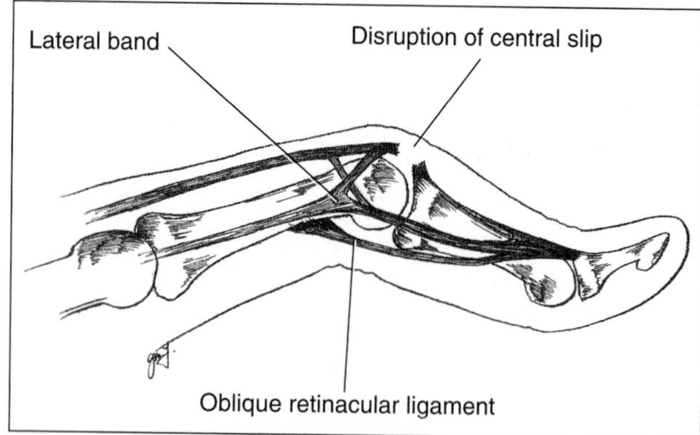

Fig. 2-4 ■ From Smith AA, Lacey SH: *Hand surgery review,* St Louis, 1996, Mosby.

4. Which exercise is most important for a patient to perform when developing a boutonnière deformity?

A. Isolated DIP joint flexion
B. Isolated PIP joint flexion
C. PIP joint extension
D. Composite digital extension

Active and passive flexion exercises of the DIP joint (Fig. 2-5) prevent oblique retinacular ligament (ORL) tightness, centralize the lateral bands, and advance the central slip. It is important to note that the most disabling element of the boutonnière deformity is the limitation of DIP joint flexion, not the lack of PIP joint motion. Patients often complain of a weak grip and an inability to grasp and manipulate small objects with the tip of the digit.

Answer: **A**
Blair, p. 614

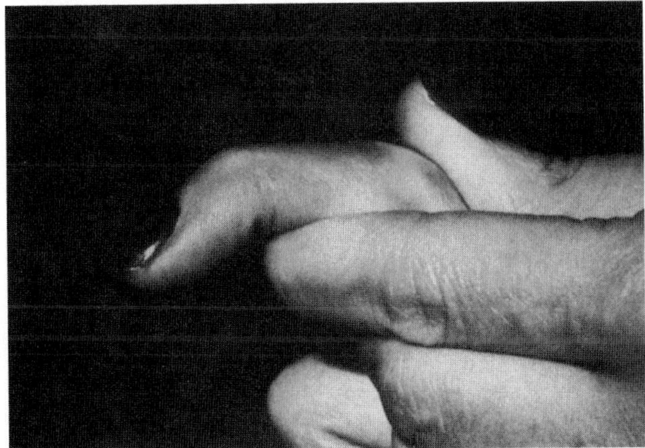

Fig. 2-5 ■ From Hunter JM, Mackin EJ, Callahan AD: *Rehabilitation of the hand: surgery and therapy*, ed 4, St Louis, 1995, Mosby.

5. You are treating a patient after a hand replantation from transmetacarpal amputation. What dysfunction often develops that can be prevented?

A. Intrinsic-plus posture
B. Boutonnière deformity
C. Intrinsic-minus posture
D. Extensor retinaculum lengthening

Hands replanted after a transmetacarpal amputation often develop an intrinsic-minus posture (claw hand). This occurs when the intrinsic muscles are injured. The distal portion becomes ischemic and causes loss of muscle function and may scar the intrinsic tendons into their canals in a lengthened position. This causes an imbalance in which the MCP joint remains extended during flexion while the IP joints move into flexion. It can be treated by splinting the MCP joints in slight flexion to help shorten the injured intrinsic tendons and by providing an outrigger for active-assistive IP extension to mimic intrinsic function 3 to 6 days postoperatively. A static anticlaw orthosis is applied around 3 to 4 weeks postoperatively.

Answer: **C**
Scheker, Hodges, pp. 473-480

6. You are treating a patient in the clinic 8 weeks after a middle phalanx fracture and observe when the PIP joint is passively flexed at 90 degrees, the DIP joint can achieve 50 degrees of flexion; however, when the PIP joint is placed at 0 degrees, the DIP can achieve only 25 degrees of flexion. This is caused by which of the following?

A. Intrinsic tightness
B. Extrinsic tightness
C. Triangular ligament tightness
D. ORL tightness
E. Extensor tendon adherence

If DIP joint flexion is more limited when the PIP joint is passively extended than when it is flexed, a tightness of the ORL results. To treat this condition, the therapist should perform ORL stretches (passive DIP joint flexion with the PIP joint held in extension) or joint-blocking exercises or apply a dynamic DIP joint flexion splint with a P2 block.

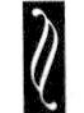

Answer: **D**
Aulicino in Mackin, Callahan, Skirven, et al, p. 133
Hunter, Mackin, Callahan, p. 65
Walters, pp. 116-123

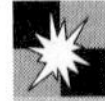

CLINICAL GEM:
P1 refers to the proximal phalanx; *P2* refers to the middle phalanx; and *P3* refers to the distal phalanx.

7. You are treating a patient who sustained a Colles fracture 4 months ago. The following is noted during the re-evaluation:

Range-of-motion assessment	Active (degrees)	Passive (degrees)
MCP	0/70	0/75
PIP	0/85	0/90
DIP	0/55	0/60

(NOTE: Wrist is at neutral during active and passive measures.)

When the fist is fully flexed in the available range of motion and the wrist is passively flexed to 25 degrees, tension is felt in the digits as they pull into extension and are unable to maintain their flexed position. What might cause this patient to experience this tension?

A. Flexor tightness distal to the wrist
B. Flexor tightness proximal to the wrist
C. Joint capsular tightness
D. Extensor tightness distal to the wrist
E. Extensor tightness proximal to the wrist

During ongoing assessments of patients, it is important to determine the origin of the limitation and treat it accordingly. Therefore one must observe the surrounding joints and their effect on range of motion. The following definitions describe various levels of tightness patients may have.

EXTENSOR TIGHTNESS PROXIMAL TO THE WRIST: To test, passively hold the digits in composite flexion while passively flexing the wrist. If the digits are pulled into extension as the wrist is passively flexed, extrinsic tightness proximal to the wrist exists. Note the position of the wrist when the extensor tension is first detected to document stiffness.

EXTENSOR TIGHTNESS DISTAL TO THE WRIST: To test, passively hold the PIP and DIP joints in flexion and passively flex the MCP joint. If the PIP and DIP joints are pulled into extension when the MCP joint is passively flexed, extensor tightness distal to the wrist exists.

FLEXOR TIGHTNESS DISTAL TO THE WRIST: To test, passively hold the PIP and DIP joints in extension and passively extend the MCP joint. If the PIP and DIP joints are pulled into flexion as the MCP joint is passively extended, flexor tightness distal to the wrist exists.

FLEXOR TIGHTNESS PROXIMAL TO THE WRIST: To test, passively maintain digits in full extension and passively extend the wrist. If flexor tension develops and the digits are pulled into flexion as the wrist is extended, extrinsic flexor tightness proximal to the wrist exists. Note the position of the wrist when the flexor tightness is first detected to document stiffness.

JOINT CAPSULAR TIGHTNESS: To test, measure active range of motion and passive range of motion. If the measurements are the same regardless of the position of the proximal and distal joints, joint capsular tightness is present.

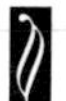

Answer: **E**
Colditz in Mackin, Callahan, Skirven, et al, p. 1032
Hunter, Mackin, Callahan, p. 1148
Walters, pp. 116-123

8. Which intrinsic muscle is the strongest?

A. Opponens pollicis
B. Flexor pollicis longus (FPL)
C. Abductor pollicis brevis (APB)
D. Adductor pollicis (AP)

The AP is the strongest of the thumb intrinsics and is stronger than the extrinsic FPL. The abductor pollicis brevis is small and is the weakest. The AP is not only used for pinching, it assists in thumb supination, provides thumb MCP stability, and assists in extending the thumb IP joint to 0 degrees of extension through the extensor mechanism. If the EPL is impaired or lost, weak IP joint extension is achieved via insertion of fibers of the AP into the lateral bands. Together with APB, IP joint extension of the thumb is achieved.

Answer: **D**
Brand, pp. 287, 291-293

9. Terminal tendon tenotomy (for treating a boutonnière deformity) restores which of the following?

A. PIP joint flexion
B. Complete PIP joint extension
C. DIP joint flexion
D. Partial DIP joint extension

A terminal tendon tenotomy is performed primarily to improve DIP joint flexion; secondarily, the PIP joint extensor deficit may show improvement. DIP joint extension is provided by the ORL through a static tenodesis effect. Patients can begin active range of motion immediately after tenotomy. If after surgery extensor deficits at the DIP joint are greater than 10 to 15 degrees, some surgeons recommend splinting the PIP and DIP joints in full extension for 10 days. The DIP joint must be monitored closely for extensor lags and appropriate splinting adjustments made.

Answer: **C**
Blair, pp. 610-614
Rosenthal in Mackin, Callahan, Skirven, et al, p. 526
Alter, Feldon, Terrono in Mackin, Callahan, Skirven, et al, p. 1551
Hunter, Mackin, Callahan, pp. 549, 1318

10. Which of the following is not a possible cause of swan-neck deformity?

A. Intrinsic tightness
B. Loss of the superficialis tendon
C. Increased force from the extensor digitorum communis
D. Landsmeer's ligament tightness

The postural collapse deformity called a *swan-neck deformity* has numerous causes. When the lateral bands displace dorsally, the imbalances of forces present as hyperextension of the PIP joint with flexion of the DIP joint. A swan-neck deformity can be caused by increased forces through the extrinsic extensor or intrinsic tendons, PIP joint instability, loss of the flexor digitorum superficialis tendon, stretching of the transverse retinacular ligament, a lax volar plate, or release of the distal extensor attachment. Answer D is incorrect because in a swan-neck deformity, the ORL (Landsmeer's ligament) lengthens.

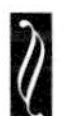
Answer: **D**
Aucilino in Mackin, Callahan, Skirven, et al, p. 133
Rosenthal in Mackin, Callahan, Skirven, et al, p. 526
Hunter, Mackin, Callahan, pp. 65, 549
Stanley, Tribuzi, pp. 405-407
Refer to Fig. 2-6

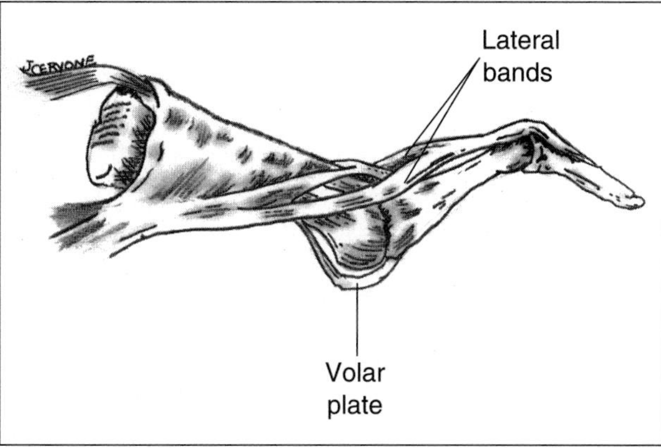

Fig. 2-6

11. In a swan-neck deformity, the lateral bands sublux volarly. True or False?

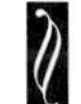

A swan-neck deformity presents with hyperextension of the PIP joint and flexion of the DIP joint. This deformity is caused by an imbalance of forces in the digit. This imbalance is summarized as follows: the transverse retinacular ligaments stretch, the triangular ligament fibers shorten, and the lateral bands sublux dorsally, causing attenuation of the PIP joint volar plate.

Answer: **False**
Rosenthal in Mackin, Callahan, Skirven, et al, p. 526
Alter, Feldon, Terrono in Mackin, Callahan, Skirven, et al, p. 1551
Hunter, Mackin, Callahan, pp. 549, 1318
Refer to Fig. 2-6

12. Which splint is most appropriate for a swan-neck deformity?

A. Silver ring to the PIP joint
B. Stack splint
C. Gutter splint to the PIP and DIP joints
D. No splint will help.

A Siris Swan-Neck Silver Ring Splint or a thermoplastic figure-of-eight splint at the PIP joint reduces or eliminates PIP joint hyperextension and decreases the imbalance of the lateral bands. It is important to understand that swan-neck deformity splints do not permanently correct the imbalance; after they are removed, the deformity will reoccur.

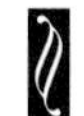
Answer: **A**
Silver Ring Splint Company Catalog
Malick, Kasch, p. 132
Refer to Fig. 2-7

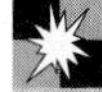
CLINICAL GEM:
Siris Silver Ring Splints are durable, attractive, and functional. Patients may choose to have gems inserted into these rings; the rings also are available in gold.

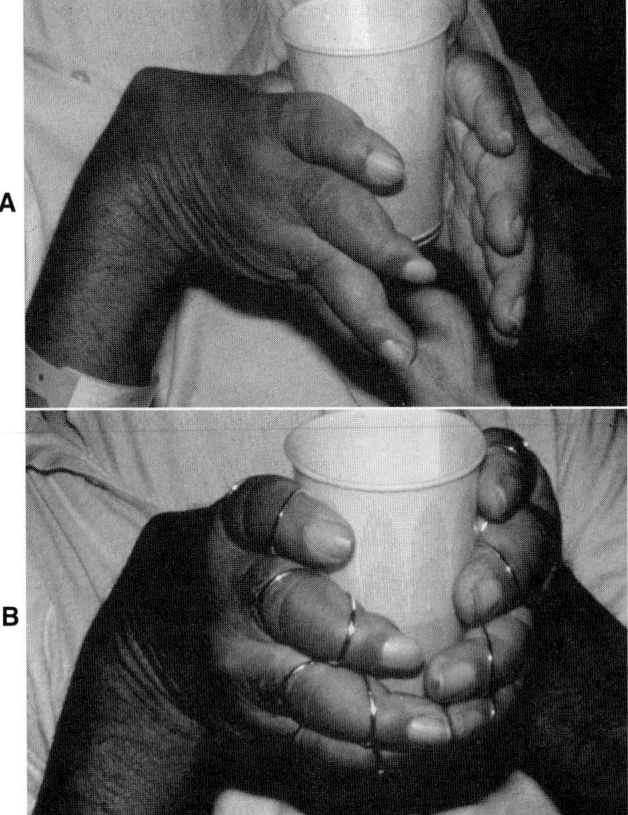

Fig. 2-7 ■ Courtesy of the Silver Ring Splint Company; Charlottesville, VA.

13. Which of the following is *not* true about the lumbricals?

A. Four of the muscles are innervated by the median nerve.
B. They insert onto the extensor assembly.
C. They link the extrinsic flexor and intrinsic extensor mechanisms.
D. They are weaker than the interossei muscles.

There are four lumbrical muscles that originate from the profundus tendon in the palm and insert on the radial side of the finger onto the dorsal apparatus. The lumbricals and the interossei flex the MCP joints and extend the IP joints. Because of its origin on the profundus, the lumbrical maintains its unique ability to modify tension between the FDP and IP extensors in all positions of the finger. The interossei are much stronger than the lumbricals. Answer A is incorrect because the two radial lumbricals are innervated by the median nerve and the ulnar two lumbricals are innervated by the deep branch of the ulnar nerve.

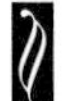

Answer: **A**

Hunter in Mackin, Callahan, Skirven, et al, p. 32
Aulicino in Mackin, Callahan, Skirven, et al, pp. 129-132
Hunter, Mackin, Callahan, pp. 65, 549
Green, Hotchkiss, Pederson, pp. 605, 606
Linscheid, p. 12

14. If a patient has intrinsic tightness, which of the following is true about the PIP joint?

A. Flexes more when the MCP joint is in flexion
B. Flexes more when the MCP joint is extended
C. Flexes the same degree regardless of the position of the MCP joint
D. Does not flex at all

When testing for intrinsic tightness, the MCP joint is held in extension while the PIP joint is passively stretched in flexion (Fig. 2-8, *A*). Next, the MCP joint is placed in flexion while the PIP joint is again passively stretched in flexion (Fig. 2-8, *B*). If the PIP joint can be passively flexed to a greater extent when the MCP joint is flexed than when it is extended, intrinsic tightness exists. If the PIP joint flexes more when the MCP joint is extended, as in answer B, extrinsic extensor tightness exists.

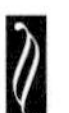

Answer: **A**

Aulicino in Mackin, Callahan, Skirven, et al, p. 133
Colditz in Mackin, Callahan, Skirven, et al, p. 1032
Hunter, Mackin, Callahan, pp. 66, 1148

15. The mallet finger can progress to which type of deformity if untreated?

A. Hyperplasia
B. Boutonnière
C. Swan-neck
D. Jersey finger

A swan-neck deformity can occur from a mallet lesion. The severity of the deformity is proportional to the stability of the palmar plate at the PIP joint. If the PIP joint palmar plate is lax, swan-neck deformity increases, and the FDP flexes the DIP joint, thus further contributing to the deformity. If the possibility of surgery is entertained, the finger can be rebalanced with tenotomy of the central tendon at the PIP joint. It also can be treated with reconstruction of the ORL by using a free tendon graft.

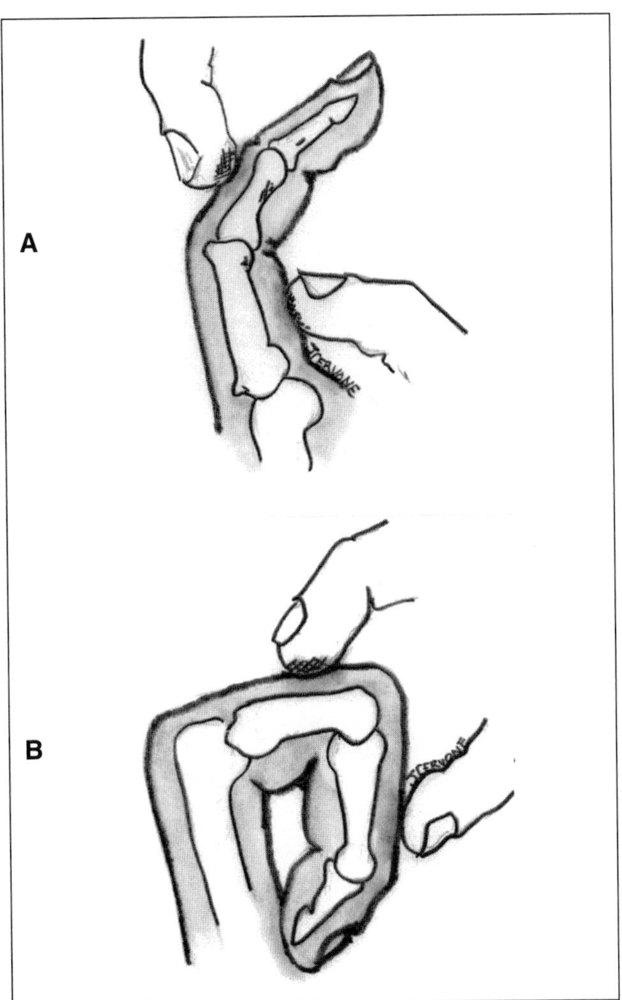

Fig. 2-8

Answer: C
Rosenthal in Mackin, Callahan, Skirven, et al, p. 521
Hunter, Mackin, Callahan, p. 544
Refer to Fig. 2-6

16. A mallet deformity with bone avulsion should be splinted for how long?

A. 4 to 6 weeks, with the DIP joint in full extension
B. 4 to 6 weeks, with the DIP joint in slight flexion
C. 6 to 8 weeks, with the DIP joint in full extension
D. 6 to 8 weeks, with the DIP joint in slight flexion

A mallet finger occurs when the extensor tendon is disrupted at the terminal tendon. The patient presents with an inability to actively extend the DIP joint. Conservative management is recommended for the patient if less than one third of the articulating surface is avulsed. The DIP joint is splinted at 0 degrees of hyperextension (the PIP joint is free) for 6 to 8 weeks (Fig. 2-9). Immobilization for 8 weeks is indicated in injuries that are more than 3 weeks old. An additional 2 weeks is indicated in a patient who loses extension quickly when the splint is weaned at 6 weeks. Studies have shown excellent results with compliant patients.

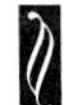
Answer: C
Malick, Kasch, p. 62
Grothe, pp. 21-24

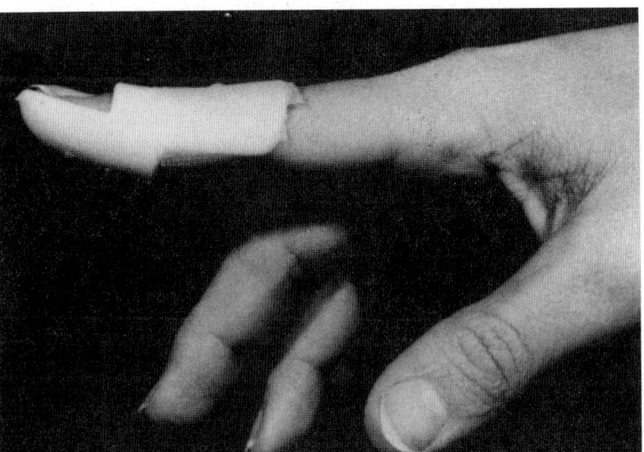

Fig. 2-9 ■ From Evans RB: Therapeutic management of extensor tendon injuries, *Hand Clin* 2:157, 1986.

17. Which of the following is not an accurate statement about the ORL?

A. If there is greater flexion of the DIP joint when the PIP joint is flexed rather than when the PIP joint is extended, there is a tightness of the ORL.
B. It originates from the volar proximal phalanx and inserts into the distal phalanx.
C. Its primary role is to extend the distal phalanx.
D. It is taut at 70 degrees of DIP joint flexion.

Extension of the distal phalanx has been postulated as a combination of the lateral bands and tenodesis of the ORL. However, most authors agree that the primary extensor of the DIP joint is from the action of the conjoined lateral bands that insert into the distal phalanx as the terminal tendon. The ORL contributes little to DIP joint extension. The ORL is considered a retaining ligament that maintains tendon centralization on the dorsum of the finger. Therefore answer C is incorrect. The ORL originates from the volar aspect of the proximal phalanx and passes obliquely dorsally and joins the lateral bands as it inserts into the distal phalanx. If this ligament is tight, DIP flexion will be limited more with

PIP extension than with PIP flexion. The ORL is taut at 70 degrees of DIP flexion.

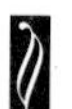

Answer: **C**

Aulicino in Mackin, Callahan, Skirven, et al, p. 133
Rosenthal in Mackin Callahan, Skirven, et al, pp. 509-510
Hunter, Mackin, Callahan, p. 65
Harris, Rutledge, pp. 713-716
Refer to Fig. 2-10

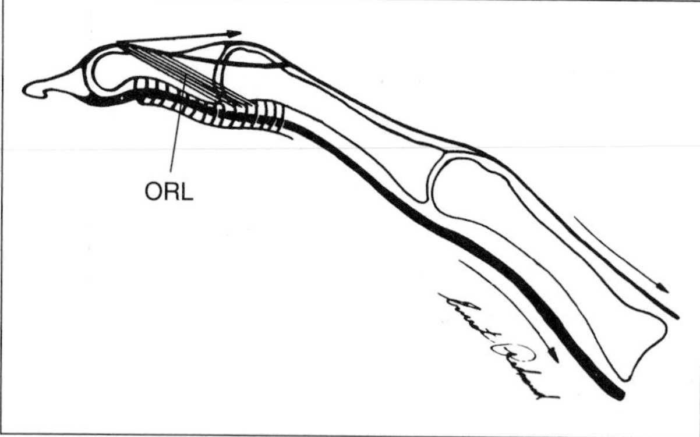

Fig. 2-10 ■ Redrawn from Tubiana R: *The hand*, Philadelphia, 1981, WB Saunders.

18. Your 29-year-old patient is demonstrating increased PIP joint flexion with the MCP joint in flexion and less PIP joint flexion with the MCP joint in extension. What exercise is best suited for this patient?

A. Graded putty exercises to allow MCP, PIP, and DIP joint flexion
B. Table top exercise, flexion of the MCP joint while maintaining IP joint extension
C. Joint blocking exercises while maintaining MCP joint extension
D. Terminal extension exercises with the palm on the table while applying pressure over the PIP joint

If PIP joint flexion is less when the MCP joint is extended than when it is flexed, it is considered a positive intrinsic tightness test. Holding the MCP joint in extension or hyperextension and passively flexing the IP joints can stretch the intrinsic muscles. Therefore joint-blocking exercises to the PIP and DIP joints with the MCP joints held in extension or hyperextension would be the best choice. This exercise needs to be repeated frequently throughout the day. A joint-blocking device or orthosis can be fabricated to assist patients with their program (Fig. 2-11). Fig. 2-12 shows the patient's active fist before performing the MCP joint blocking exercises. Fig. 2-13 shows the patient's fist immediately after 10 repetitions in the blocking splint; active motion is increased significantly.

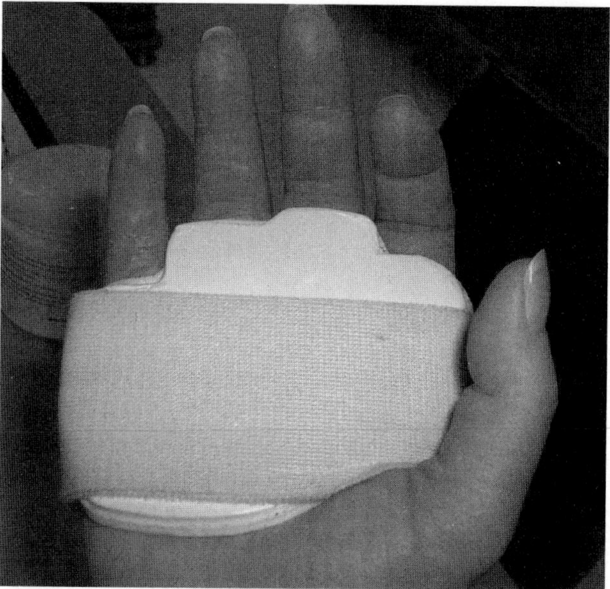

Fig. 2-11

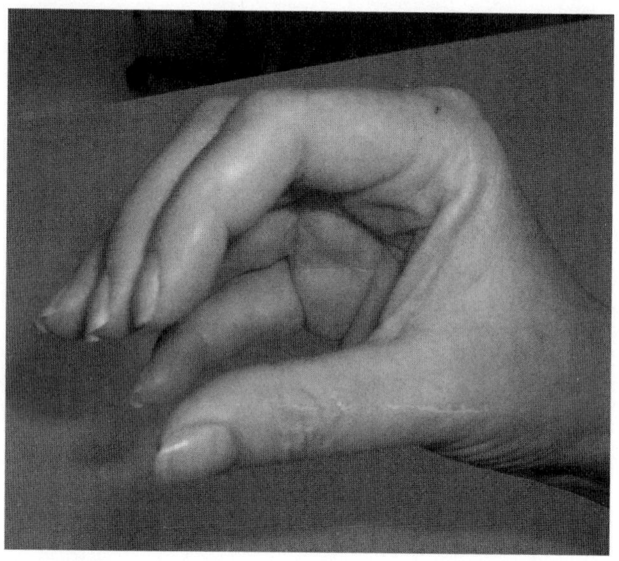

Fig. 2-12

Answer: **C**

Smith in Green, Hotchkiss, Pederson, pp. 607-608
Refer to Fig. 2-13

CLINICAL GEM:
Stretching of the lumbrical muscles can only be achieved by positioning the MCP joint in hyperextension and actively flexing the IP joint. The splint can be used to block, or one can simply be aware of the MCP joint.

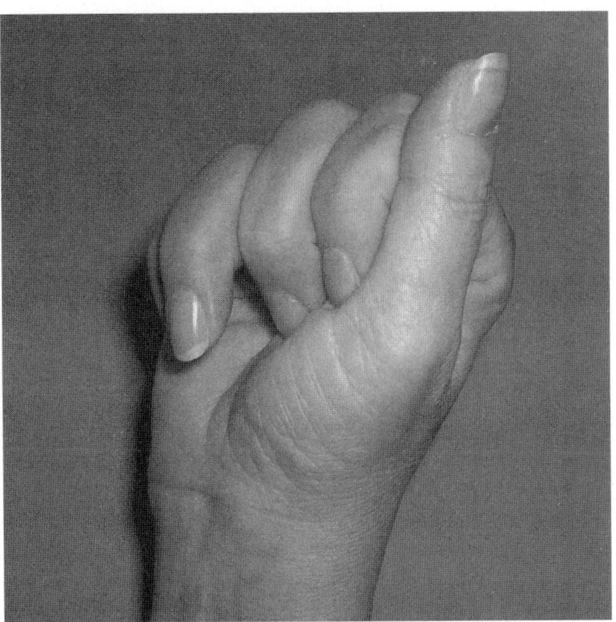

Fig. 2-13

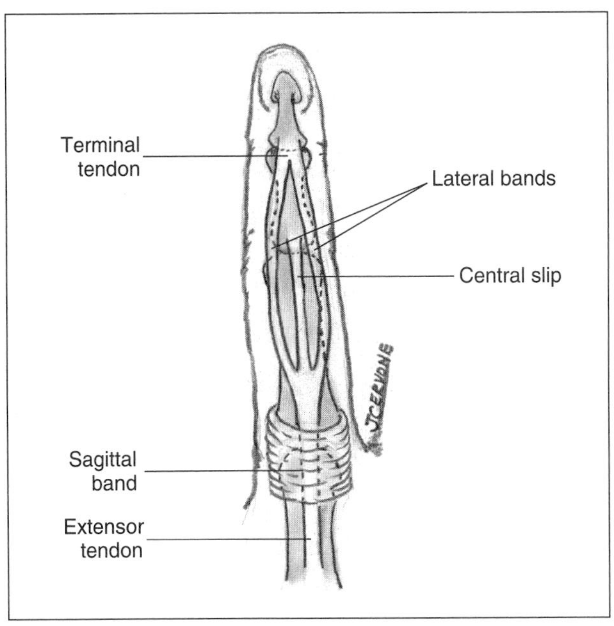

Fig. 2-14

19. Which structure(s) maintains the central position of the extensor tendon over the MCP joint?

A. Collateral ligaments
B. Shroud fibers/sagittal bands
C. Central slip
D. Lumbricals

The shroud fibers/sagittal bands stabilize the extensor tendons over the MCP joint. They arise from the extrinsic extensors and insert into the volar plate of the MCP joint. When these structures become attenuated, the patient is unable to extend the MCP joint from the flexed position. However, the patient is able to hold the finger at zero when placed there as the tendon relocates over the MCP joint. Nonoperative management involves splinting the MCP joint at zero for 3 to 4 weeks while allowing PIP joint motion. If this does not work, surgical repair is indicated.

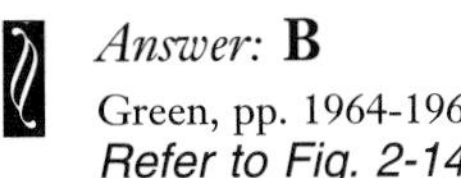

Answer: **B**
Green, pp. 1964-1965
Refer to Fig. 2-14

20. You are treating a patient 3 months after a FDP tendon graft to the ring finger. You notice that every time he attempts to make a fist the IP joints extend rather than flex. Why might this be happening?

A. Paradoxical extension
B. Quadrigia
C. The patient is not giving full effort
D. The tendon graft has ruptured

Normally, flexion of the IP joints depends on contraction of the profundus and relaxation of the lumbricals. In contrast, paradoxical extension is an abnormal phenomenon that occurs when the patient attempts to contract the profundus but instead the lumbrical is pulled proximally, thus resulting in PIP and DIP joint extension rather than flexion. Tendon laxity after a tendon graft can cause this phenomenon because the profundus contraction may have a greater effect on the lumbrical than on the graft. Paradoxical extension may also occur if the lumbrical is fibrotic or contracted and the profundus force is transmitted to the lumbrical tendon rather than the distal phalanx during muscle contraction.

Answer: **A**
Green, p. 623

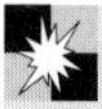

CLINICAL GEM:
The involved finger will assume an intrinsic-plus position when paradoxical extension occurs.

21. How is digital extension achieved?

A. Extrinsic tendons and sagittal bands extend the MCP joint; intrinsic musculature forming oblique fibers extend the PIP joint; and lateral bands conjoin to extend the DIP joint.
B. Extrinsic tendons extend the MCP joint and the PIP joint; lateral bands and the ORL extend the DIP joint
C. Sagittal bands extend the MCP joint; the central slip extends the PIP joint; and the ORL extends the DIP joint.
D. Lumbricals extend the MCP joint; the extensor hood extends the PIP joint; the terminal tendon extends the DIP joint.

The extensor digitorum communis, extensor indicis proprius, and extensor digiti quinti tendons combined with the encircling series of fibers of the sagittal bands extend the MCP joint and proximal phalanx. The extensor mechanism then trifurcates into the central slip and lateral bands. This mechanism is held centered by the transverse retinacular ligament and is joined by the tendons of the interossei and lumbricals. The central slip and intrinsic musculature extend the PIP joint and middle phalanx. The lateral bands conjoin to form the terminal tendon that inserts into the distal phalanx to extend the DIP joint.

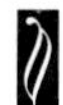

Answer: **A**
Harris, Rutledge, pp. 713-716
Smith in Green, Hotchkiss, Pederson, pp. 604-606
Martin, Collins, pp. 236-237
Refer to Fig. 2-15

22. You wish to strengthen thumb adduction for your patient. Which Baltimore Therapeutic Equipment (BTE) tool would be the best choice?

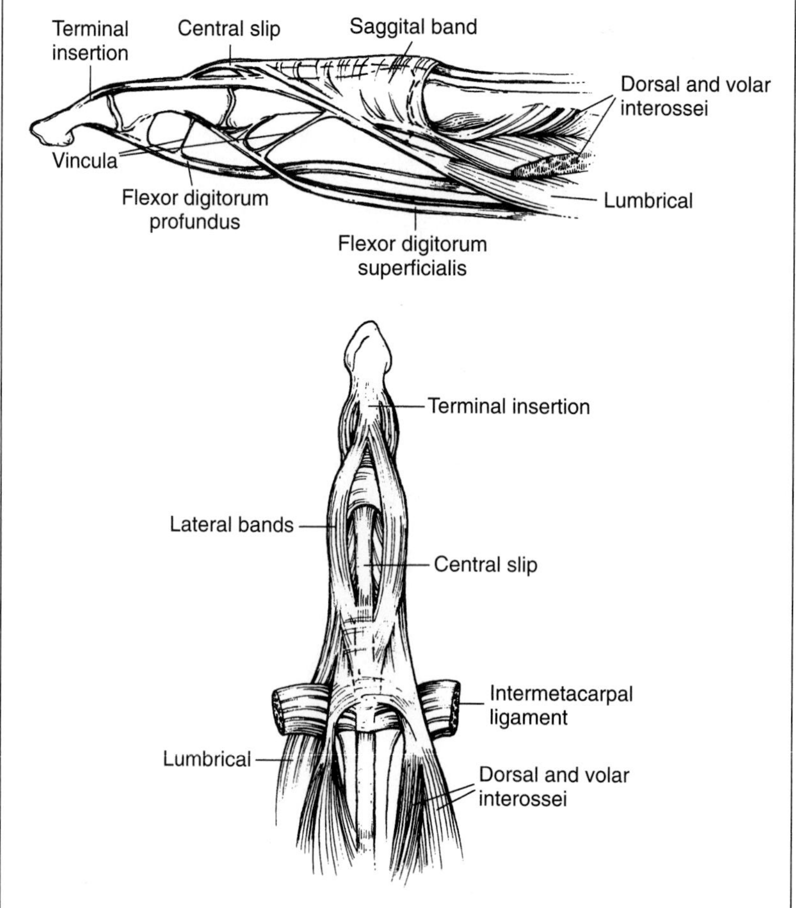

Fig. 2-15 ■ The extensor apparatus of a finger. Coordinated interactive motions between lateral forces (from interossei and lumbricals) and between central forces from the extrinsic extensor tendons allow diverse finger motion and position. (From Martin DS, Collins ED: *Manual of acute hand injuries*, St Louis, 1998, Mosby.)

A. 181—rope pull
B. 701—wrist flexion and extension
C. CPM mode
D. 202—key-shaped

Tool number 202 is key-shaped. BTE Company recommends using this attachment to simulate keys of all types for lateral pinch strengthening. Thumb adduction is strengthened in lateral pinch. The other attachments would not be appropriate choices to strengthen thumb adduction.

Answer: **D**

BTE user's guide, p. 305

23. What is the preferred method for treating a closed boutonnière deformity?

A. Immediate surgery to reconstruct the central slip
B. Splinting the PIP joint in full extension while allowing flexion of the DIP joint
C. Splinting the PIP and DIP joints in full extension while allowing MCP joint flexion
D. A PIP joint spring extension splint

A prefabricated static splint, a serial cast, or a custom-molded thermoplastic splint that provides uninterrupted PIP joint extension at 0 degrees is worn for 6 weeks to allow sufficient healing time for the central slip (Fig. 2-16). It is crucial that the splint place the PIP joint at 0 degrees, otherwise it may result in the tendon healing in an elongated position and result in a lag secondary to tendon gapping. DIP joint flexion is encouraged to stretch the ORL, realign the lateral bands, and restore muscular balance. The splint is to be worn continuously until extensor lag is no longer present. If an extensor lag develops after active motion has begun, the patient is to return to immobilization for another week. Some experienced therapists begin the patient on limited active motion at the PIP joint after 5 weeks.

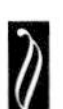

Answer: **B**

Evans in Mackin, Callahan, Skirven, et al, p. 555
Hunter, Mackin, Callahan, p. 578
Stanley, Tribuzi, pp. 375-376
Doyle in Green, Hotchkiss, Pederson, p. 1973

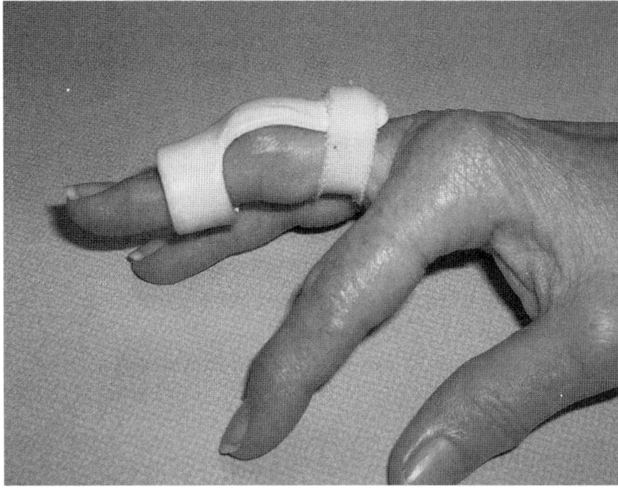

Fig. 2-16

24. A 36-year-old butcher has been referred to you after a laceration to his left index finger dorsally in zone III. His surgery included primary repair of the central slip and lateral bands with K-wire fixation 3 weeks ago. The doctor wants therapy to begin with an early motion protocol. His K-wire was removed earlier that day. How do you begin his treatment?

A. Fabricate a thermoplastic splint that maintains the PIP joint in 0 degrees of extension and begin exercises outside of the splint to the PIP joint 3 times a day; allow as much motion as possible.
B. Fabricate a thermoplastic splint that provides 0 degrees of extension for the PIP and DIP joints and begin gentle DIP joint flexion and extension exercises.
C. Begin PIP and DIP joint flexion and extension exercises immediately to decrease adhesions and fabricate a digital extension splint for night use only.
D. Fabricate a thermoplastic splint that maintains the PIP joint in 30 degrees of flexion and begin DIP and PIP joint flexion and extension exercises.

When the central slip and lateral bands are repaired the PIP joint as well as the DIP joint need to be supported in extension for 4 to 6 weeks. However, immobilization for 6 weeks can result in limited digital motion. Mobilization schedules can vary for each patient. Splinting the PIP and DIP joints in full extension for up to 6 weeks and beginning early motion exercises outside of the splint as early as 3 weeks are recommended. DIP joint flexion and extension are begun so as to glide the lateral bands and gentle active flexion of the PIP joint is initiated, to no more than 30 degrees, at 3 to 4 weeks. If no extensor lag develops at the PIP joint, motion can progress to 40 to 50 degrees and 60 to 80 degrees by the next week. The extension splint is to be worn between exercise sessions. The average thickness of the central slip just proximal to the PIP joint is only 0.5 mm; therefore, flexion exercises are to be performed with caution. Complications include elongation of the central slip because of aggressive exercises or adhesions limiting the central slip from gliding over the proximal phalanx, which will increase tension at the repair site and cause attenuation or a gap formation. Take care not to be overly aggressive. Advance according to tendon integrity.

Answer: **B**

Evans in Mackin, Callahan, Skirven, et al, pp. 554-556
Doyle in Green, Hotchkiss, Pederson, pp. 1974-1975
Hunter, Mackin, Callahan, pp. 577-578

25. True or false: The ulnar intrinsics of a patient with rheumatoid arthritis become tighter than the radial intrinsics.

The ulnar intrinsics become contracted because of a variety of dynamic and anatomic factors that occur in the rheumatoid hand, which can result in ulnar drift (Fig. 2-17, *A*). Cross intrinsic transfers can be performed by resecting the ulnar intrinsics and rerouting them to the radial side of the proximal phalanx (Fig. 2-17, *B*). These transfers can be performed in a patient exhibiting early rheumatoid arthritis or in conjunction with MCP joint arthroplasty in an attempt to rebalance the hand.

Answer: **True**

Green, pp. 617-618

26. What is the only muscle that arises from and inserts into tendon?

A. Abductor digiti minimi quinti
B. Dorsal interosseous
C. Volar interosseous
D. Lumbricals

The lumbrical muscles are the only muscles that arise and insert into tendons. They arise from the FDP tendons and insert into the extensor expansion of the extensor digitorum communis. The lumbricals are known as the "workhorses" of the hand; however, a consensus about the actual role of the lumbricals has not been reached. Jacobsen and associates have shown that the lumbricals are designed for high excursion and velocity production. Backhouse and Catton have indicated that the primary action of the lumbricals is to extend the IP joints and that they are weak flexors of the MCP joint. Brand and Hollister have indicated that the lumbricals ensure that the MCP joints flex ahead of the IP joints, thus allowing the hand to grasp a large object. The lumbricals have fascinated researchers for years and will require further research before their role is fully understood.

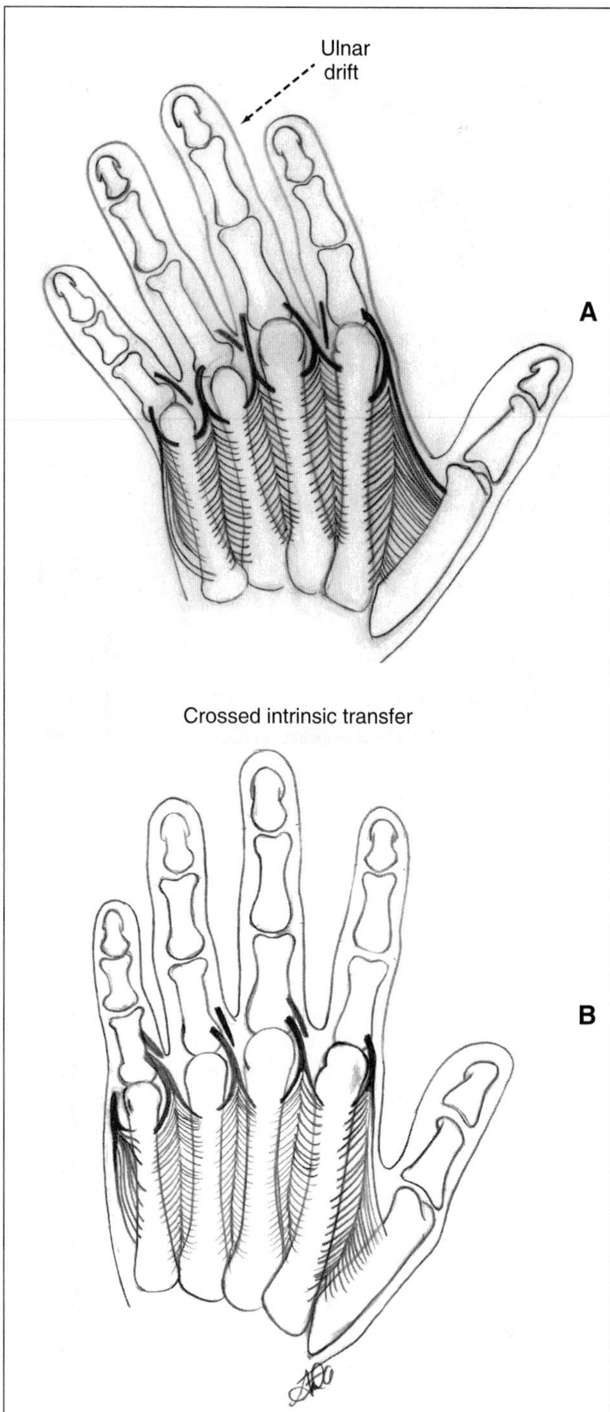

Fig. 2-17

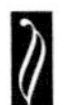

Answer: **D**

Schreuders, Stam, pp. 303-305
Brand, Hollister, p. 330
Refer to Fig. 2-18

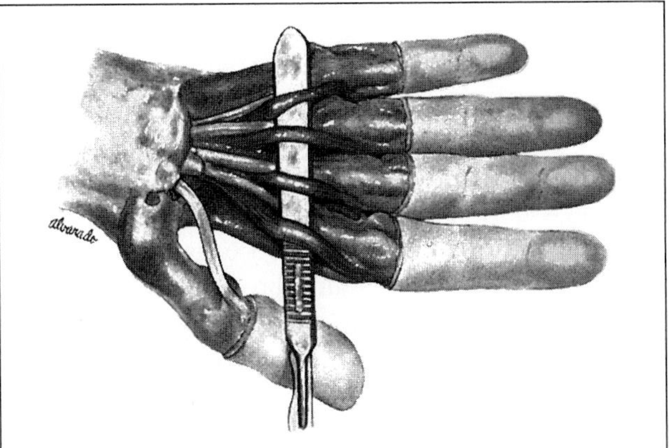

Fig. 2-18 ■ The four lumbrical muscles. (From Brand PW, Hollister A: *Clinical mechanics of the hand,* ed 2, St Louis, 1993, Mosby.)

27. A 34-year-old patient sent to you from the emergency room with a diagnosis of a sprained middle finger presents with a painful, tender, and swollen PIP joint. Active motion is decreased and the finger is held in a semiflexed position. During testing you observe a 30-degree loss of active extension of the PIP joint when the wrist and MCP joints are held in full flexion. What may develop?

A. PIP joint subluxation
B. Boutonnière deformity
C. Extensor hood inflammation
D. Collateral ligament sprain

In closed injuries, the boutonnière deformity may not be present at the time of injury. The boutonnière deformity presents with PIP joint flexion secondary to disruption of the central slip and DIP joint hyperextension caused by volar migration of the lateral bands. The deformity may take up to 20 days to develop. Early recognition may be facilitated by holding the PIP joint in full extension and testing the amount of DIP joint passive flexion. If the lateral bands have migrated volarly, DIP joint flexion will decrease.

Answer: **B**

Evans in Mackin, Callahan, Skirven, et al, p. 554
Hunter, Mackin, Callahan, p. 577
Doyle in Green, Hotchkiss, Pederson, p. 1971
Refer to Fig. 2-19

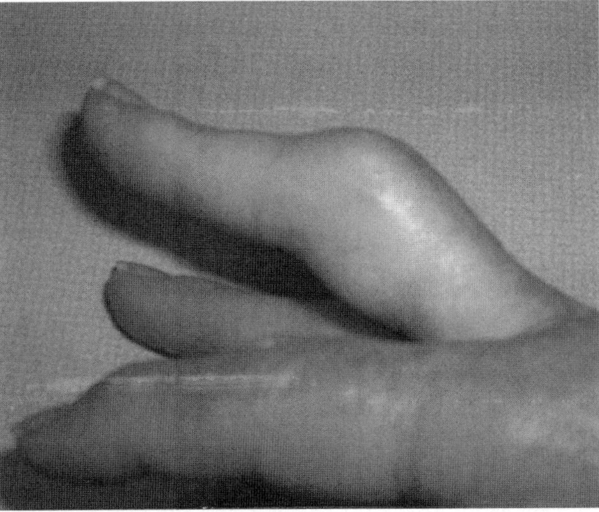

Fig. 2-19

28. What muscle is the first to recover after a lesion to the wrist in a patient with ulnar nerve paralysis?

A. Flexor pollici brevis
B. First dorsal interossei
C. Opponens digiti minimi
D. Abductor digiti minimi

In early signs of recovery after an injury to the ulnar nerve, the muscles will return in order of innervation. The first muscle to return is the abductor digiti minimi, then the two remaining hypothenar muscles, and next is the ulnar two lumbricals and the interossei. The last three muscles to return are the first dorsal interossei, the adductor pollicis, and the deep head of the flexor pollicis brevis. Contraction of the abductor digiti minimi muscle is best sought when the patient opposes the thumb to the little finger. Usually a flicker is seen before the prime-mover action is detected. As recovery proceeds, the small finger will become abducted.

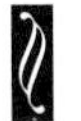

Answer: **D**

Wynn Parry, p. 89
Stanley, Tribuzi, p. 330

29. The critical corner is formed from what structures?

A. Volar plate, proper collateral ligament, and accessory collateral ligament
B. Common extensor tendon, lumbrical and interossei tendon insertions
C. Joint capsule, A2 pulley, volar plate
D. Transverse retinacular ligament, lumbrical and interossei tendon insertions

The critical corner is formed by the volar plate, proper collateral ligament, and the accessory collateral liga-

2 INTRINSIC MECHANISM

ment where they converge at the base of the middle phalanx to provide stability to the PIP joint.

Answer: **A**

Campbell, Wilson in Mackin, Callahan, Skirven, et al, p. 396
Hunter, Mackin, Callahan, p. 378

30. Which of the following statements about the PIP joint is *not* true?

A. It is a hinged joint.
B. The accessory collateral ligament folds during maximal joint flexion.
C. The lateral bands displace dorsally during flexion.
D. The volar plate is thick and prevents hyperextension.

Motion at the PIP joint occurs primarily in flexion and extension. The soft tissues and osseous structures allow this articulation to function as a hinged joint. The radial and ulnar collateral ligaments are supportive structures. The accessory collateral ligament is taut in extension and the proper collateral ligament is taut in flexion. The volar plate lies volar to the PIP joint and prevents hyperextension. Answer C is incorrect because when the PIP joint flexes, the lateral bands displace palmarly so that the moment arms of the lateral bands decrease progressively. This assists in the mechanically linked movements of the PIP and DIP joints.

Answer: **C**

Linscheid, pp. 7-8
Hunter, Mackin, Callahan, Schneider, Osterman, p. 378
Campbell, Wilson in Mackin, Callahan, Skirven, et al, pp. 396-397

31. To restore MCP flexion in a patient with intrinsic paralysis due to ulnar nerve palsy, which procedure might the surgeon select?

A. ECRL 4-tail (Brand's intrinsic transfer)
B. FDS 4-tail (modified Stiles, Bunnell transfer)
C. FDS lasso (Zancolli's lasso procedure)
D. All are appropriate surgical procedures.

All three of the above-named tendon transfer techniques are used to help restore gripping, correct claw deformity, and increase hand function after intrinsic paralysis.

THE FDS 4-TAIL (MODIFIED STILES, BUNNELL TRANSFER): The FDS tendon to the long finger is split longitudinally into four equal tails. Each slip is passed through the lumbrical canal of each finger and inserted into the radial lateral bands of the middle, ring, and small fingers and the ulnar lateral band of the index (Fig. 2-20).

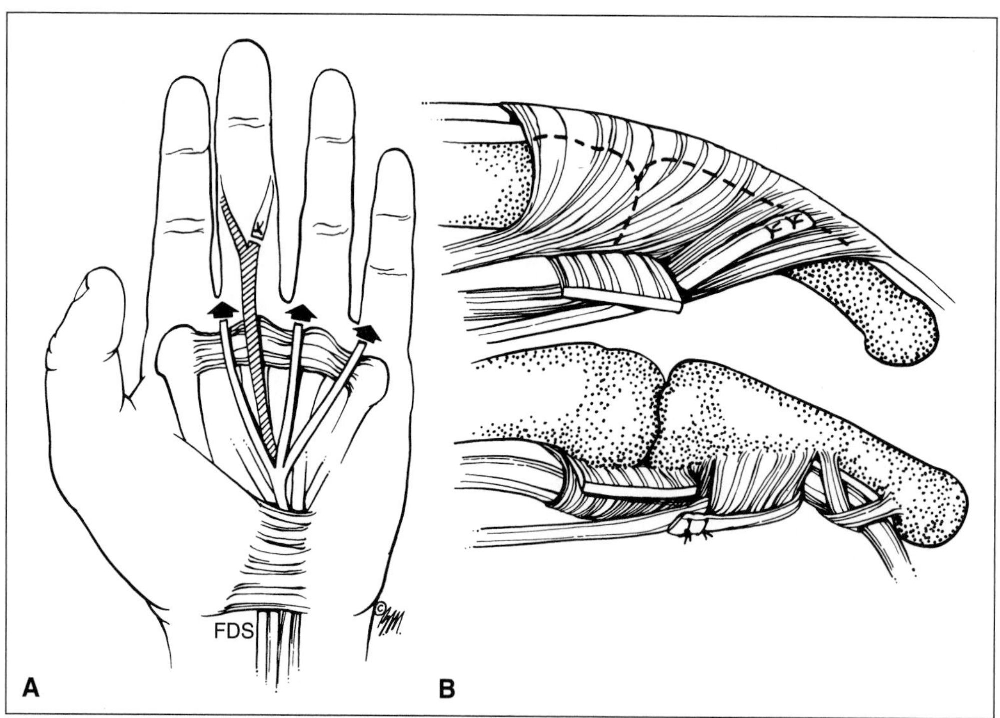

Fig. 2-20 ■ Transfer of a flexor digitorum superficialis (FDS) to control "claw finger" deformity. Half of the distal tendon of the donor superficialis tendon (long or ring) is tenodesed initially across the PIP joint to prevent hyperextension deformity of the PIP joint. The superficialis tendon is divided into two to four slips, which are passed volar to the deep transverse metacarpal ligament and through the lumbrical canals to the dorsal apparatus. The individual slips may be inserted into **(A)** the lateral band of the dorsal apparatus or **(B)** the A2 pulley of the flexor sheath. This transfer does not add power to finger flexion. (Copyright Elizabeth Roselius. From Green DP, Hotchkiss RN, Pederson WC: *Green's Operative hand surgery*, ed 4, New York, 1999, Churchill Livingstone.)

THE ECRL 4-TAIL (BRAND'S INTRINSIC TRANSFER): A free tendon graft (usually the plantaris tendon) is sutured to the distal end of the ECRL tendon and divided into four slips. With the aid of a tendon passer, the four slips are passes through the interosseous space volar to the deep transverse metacarpal ligament and are stitched to the radial lateral bands of the middle, ring, and small fingers and the ulnar lateral band of the index finger or to the radial aspect of the proximal phalanx (Fig. 2-21).

THE FDS LASSO (ZANCOLLI'S LASSO PROCEDURE): The FDS tendon is divided at the level of the proximal phalanx of each finger. The proximal stump of each tendon is pulled back, looped around the A1 pulley, and sutured on itself at the level of the MCP joint.

After surgery, the MCP joints are maintained at 60 to 70 degrees of flexion and the IP joints in full extension. The position of the wrist varies according to the type of transfer. This intrinsic-plus positioning is used to prevent recurrence of the deformity. Protective splinting may be continued for up to 12 weeks.

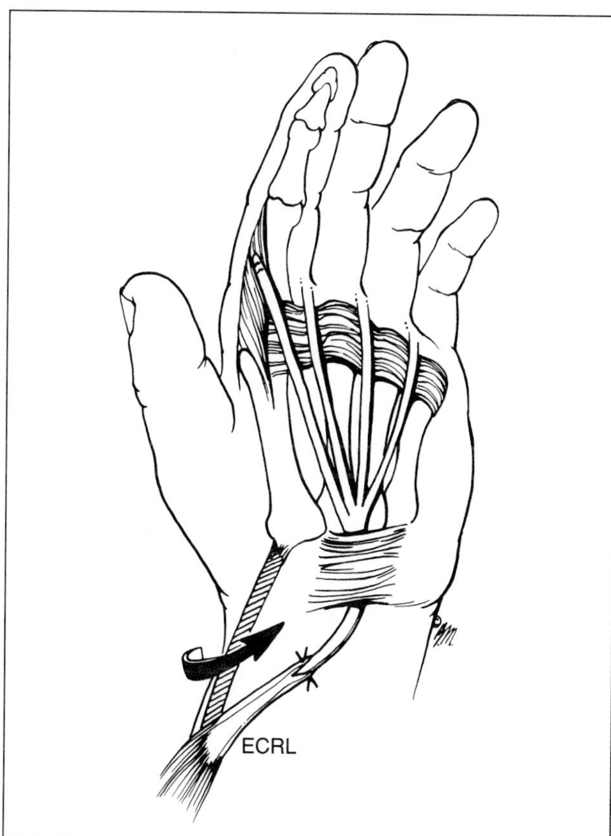

Fig. 2-21 ■ Alternative transfer of the ECRL to control "claw finger" deformity. The ECRL is passed around the radial side of the forearm and extended by a free tendon graft in two to four slips that pass through the carpal tunnel and volar to the deep transverse metacarpal ligament, through the lumbrical canals, and into the lateral band of the dorsal apparatus. This transfer adds power to finger flexion. (Copyright Elizabeth Roselius. From Green DP, Hotchkiss RN, Pederson WC: *Green's Operative hand surgery*, ed 4, New York, 1999, Churchill Livingstone.)

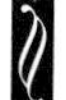

Answer: **D**

Ozkan, Ozer, Gulgonen, pp. 35-42
Toth, p. 244
Omer in Green, Hotchkiss, Pederson, pp. 1531-1533

32. Which of the following is *not* true about a claw hand deformity?

A. The muscle imbalances and deformities are progressive.
B. The patient will be unable to flex the MCP joints and extend the IP joints.
C. The patient presents with an intrinsic-plus position.
D. All are true.

In ulnar nerve injuries with intrinsic paralysis, there is loss of the hypothenar musculature, ulnar two lumbricals, interossei, and adductor pollicis muscles. The lumbricals and interossei supply balance to the flexor and extensor systems. Without these intrinsic muscles the patient will be unable to flex the MCP joints and extend the IP joints or fully flex or extend his or her digits. The digits will collapse when attempting extension, flexion, or when gripping or manipulating objects with any resistance. This imbalance usually becomes more exaggerated over time, and remodeling of the skin and joints will occur. The MCP joints will elongate and stretch into hyperextension, and the IP joints will stiffen into flexion. The extensor tendons eventually become attenuated. If the imbalance progresses into deformity, this will compromise tendon transfer surgery results. Answer C is incorrect because the claw deformity will present as the intrinsic-minus posture.

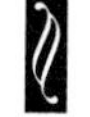

Answer: **C**

Bell-Krotoski in Mackin, Callahan, Skirven, et al, pp. 800-802
Hunter, Mackin, Callahan, pp. 730-732

33. Match each muscle to the correct description:

Muscle

1. Lumbricals
2. Opponens pollicis brevis
3. Volar interossei
4. Adductor pollicis

5. Interosssei
6. Abductor digiti minimi
7. Abductor pollicis brevis
8. Palmaris brevis
9. Opponens digiti minimi
10. First dorsal interossei

Description

A. Increases span of grasp and assists with flexion of the fifth MCP joint
B. Rotates and draws fifth metacarpal anteriorly
C. Adducts thumb to the palm, gives power for grasping, and inserts into the extensor mechanism to assist the IP joint of the thumb into 0 degrees of extension
D. Inserts on the medial or lateral aspects of the proximal phalanx into the lateral band of the extensor mechanism
E. Have a moving site of origin
F. Originates from the fascia and transverse carpal ligament and inserts on the proximal phalanx and extensor mechanism of the thumb; helps to extend the IP joint to 0 degrees of extension
G. Inserts all along the body of the first metacarpal and rotates the thumb medially
H. Assists with thumb adduction and plays a significant role for writing and typing
I. Adducts the thumb, index, ring, and small fingers
J. Wrinkles the skin on the ulnar side of the palm

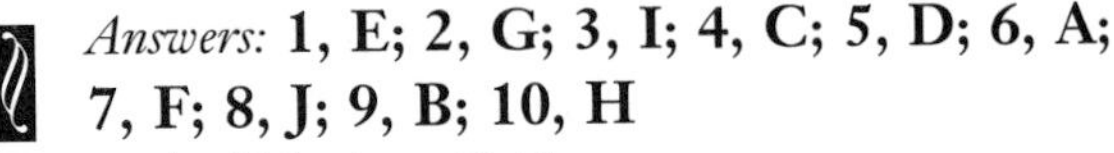

Answers: **1, E; 2, G; 3, I; 4, C; 5, D; 6, A; 7, F; 8, J; 9, B; 10, H**
Stanley, Tribuzi, pp. 20-21
Hunter, Mackin, Callahan, p. 34
Chase in Mackin, Callahan, Skirven, et al, p. 71

34. True or False: A rupture of the transverse retinacular ligament results in development of a swan-neck deformity.

The transverse retinacular ligament encircles the PIP joint. This ligament restrains dorsal displacement of the lateral bands. If the transverse retinacular ligament is injured, the lateral bands bowstring dorsally and contribute to the development of a swan-neck deformity (see Fig. 2-6). In contrast, the triangular ligament holds the lateral bands dorsally, and loss of this ligament results in the development of a boutonnière (see Fig. 2-19).

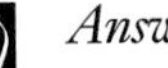

Answer: **True**
Rosenthal in Mackin, Callahan, Skirven, et al, p. 509
Hunter, Mackin, Callahan, p. 530

35. True or false: The first dorsal interossei plays an important role during lateral pinch.

The first dorsal interossei is usually considered an index finger abductor and MCP flexor. Many of its fibers have their origin on the first metacarpal shaft and therefore act on the first metacarpal serving as a weak thumb adductor. The very important role that the first dorsal interossei plays is stabilizing the first CMC joint during lateral pinch and power grip. Without the first dorsal interossei, the CMC joint would radially sublux when it is loaded in the position of lateral pinch.

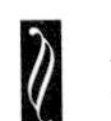

Answer: **True**
Brand, pp. 294-296

36. Match each ligamentous structure to the correct description:

Structure

A. Deep transverse metacarpal ligament
B. Proper collateral ligament
C. Accessory collateral ligament
D. Sagittal bands
E. MCP collateral ligaments
F. Triangular ligament
G. Transverse retinacular ligament
H. Transverse carpal ligament

Description

1. Taut at 25 degrees of IP flexion
2. Prevents dorsal bowstringing
3. Prevents volar shifting of the lateral bands
4. Provides the pulley mechanism for the flexor tendon sheath
5. Stabilizes the MCP volar plates
6. Contractures of this ligament prevent MCP flexion
7. Prevents dorsal shifting of the lateral bands
8. Works with the volar plate to stabilize the IP joint from lateral stresses

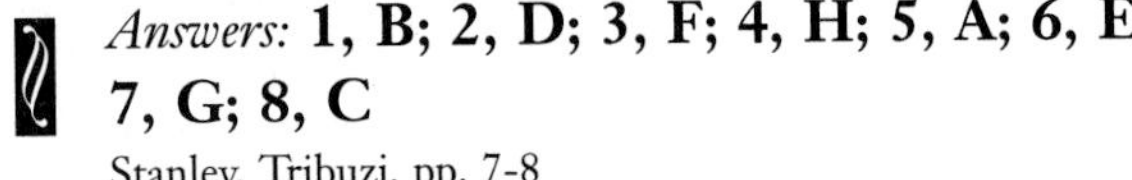

Answers: **1, B; 2, D; 3, F; 4, H; 5, A; 6, E; 7, G; 8, C**
Stanley, Tribuzi, pp. 7-8

37. True or false: Initiating active muscle contraction of the intrinsic musculature at 4 weeks is important for the treatment of a patient after a hand transplant.

The intrinsic musculature innervated distal to the level of the replantation will not be functional at this time as nerve regeneration will not have reached the intrinsic muscles at 4 weeks. An accepted concept is that nerve regeneration occurs roughly 1 mm/day or 1 inch/month in the hand. At 4 weeks, thumb and small finger opposition will not be possible. The patient will compensate by using the FPL for lateral pinch. Decreased active PIP and DIP extension will be observed because of the denervated lumbricals and interosseous muscles.

Answer: **False**
Kader, pp. 185-186

38. True or false: A sprain to the PIP joint most frequently involves injury to the ulnar collateral ligament.

A sprain to the PIP joint is common in athletics and occupational settings. This common sprain usually injures the radial collateral ligament and the volar plate. In the usual injury, the collateral ligament ruptures proximally. This event is followed by tearing of the accessory collateral ligament and then rupture of the distal volar plate.

Answer: **False**
Vicar, p. 6

39. A pseudoboutonnière deformity most commonly occurs in which finger?

A. Index
B. Ring
C. Middle
D. Small

A pseudoboutonnière deformity is a flexion deformity of the PIP joint without DIP joint hyperextension. It results from a proximal avulsion of the volar plate that develops into a flexion contracture after the patient protectively holds the finger in a flexed position over time. The volar plate heals in a proximal position. This occurs most often in the small finger. If conservative treatment with PIP joint extension splinting is to no avail, the patient may require surgical intervention to release the proximal volar plate, excise the accessory collateral ligament, and free up the lateral bands. Extension can then be maintained with a K-wire, followed by assisted range of motion (AROM) and intermittent extension splinting.

Answer: **D**
Vicar, p. 10

40. You are treating a patient after volar dislocation of the PIP joint. What structure(s) might be damaged?

A. Lateral bands
B. Superficialis tendon
C. Central slip
D. A and C are correct
E. A, B, and C are correct

Volar or anterior dislocations of the PIP joint are less common than dorsal dislocations. Volar dislocations are often complex because they are irreducible closed and may involve extensive soft tissue damage. The mechanism of injury is usually a rotary force combined with compression. It usually occurs when an extended digit is forcibly flexed at the PIP joint. This lateral stress may rupture a collateral ligament, thus allowing the head of the proximal phalanx to buttonhole between the lateral band and the central slip. The central slip can then rupture or slip around the head of the proximal phalanx and be volar to it (Fig. 2-22). If the central slip remains

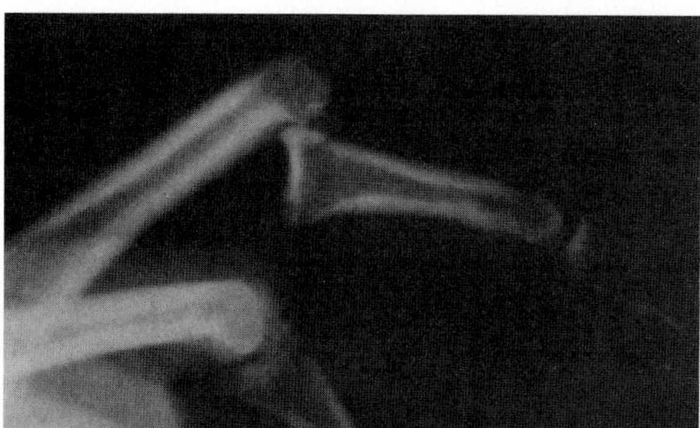

Fig. 2-22 ■ Volar dislocation of the PIP joint is a relatively uncommon injury. It should be obvious from this radiograph that the central slip must be torn for this injury to occur; therefore these patients should be treated in the same manner as those with a boutonnière injury. (From DeLee JC, Drez D, Miller MD: *DeLee & Drez's Orthopaedic sports medicine*, ed 2, Philadelphia, 2003, Saunders.)

dorsal to the head of the proximal phalanx, the lateral bands can lock under the condyle. The FDS is not injured with this injury.

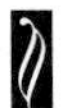

Answer: **D**

Vicar, p. 10
DeLee, Drez, Miller, pp. 1392-1393

41. Secondary defects of a hand with intrinsic paralysis include all but which of the following?

A. Flexion contractures of the PIP joints
B. Extrinsic flexor tightness
C. Anterior displacement of the lateral bands
D. Attenuation of the extensor mechanism
E. All are true.

Intrinsic paralysis can be caused from penetrating injuries, fractures, and entrapment syndromes. Most hands with paralysis of the ulnar innervated muscles will eventually develop clawing. When paralysis is progressive, the intrinsic-minus posture will be more evident. Without lumbrical or interossei activity the MCP joints are unable to flex and will hyperextend because of the unopposed pull from the EDC. The IP joints will be unable to extend; therefore the PIP joints will rest in a flexed position. Because of this positioning, the patient often develops PIP joint flexion contractures, adaptive shortening of the extrinsic finger flexors, adaptive growth of the extensor hood, and anterior displacement of the lateral bands.

Answer: **E**

Hunter, Mackin, Callahan, p. 732
Bell-Krotoski in Mackin, Callahan, Skirven, et al, pp. 802-803
Brandsma, pp. 14-17

42. How much strength do the intrinsic muscles contribute for power grasp?

A. 30%
B. 50%
C. 40%
D. 20%

The intrinsic muscles contribute half the strength of power grasp. In high ulnar nerve palsy grasp weakens by 60% to 80% secondarily to the additional loss of the ulnarly innervated fourth and fifth FDP.

Answer: **B**

Hastings, Davidson, p. 171

43. All but which of the following can cause paradoxical extension?

A. Unrepaired profundus tendon distal to the insertion of the superficialis tendon
B. Heavy adhesions on the profundus tendon distal to the lumbrical insertion
C. Gap formation of a repaired profundus tendon in zone V
D. An FDP graft that is too long

Paradoxical extension (lumbrical plus) is a phenomenon in which the FDP glides too far proximally, thus transmitting its force to the extensor mechanism via the lumbricals. The lumbricals originate from the FDP and insert onto the radial side of the MCP joint and into the central slip and lateral bands. When the patient attempts to make a fist, the MCPs flex and the IPs extend because of the increased tension on the lumbricals. Paradoxical extension can be caused by an unrepaired FDP injury distal to the lumbrical origin, flexor tendon grafts of excessive length, adhesions of the lumbricals to a repaired FDP, or heavy FDP adhesions usually occurring in zone III. Answer C is incorrect because zone V is too proximal.

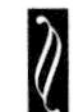

Answer: **C**

Stanley, Tribuzi, p. 38

44. True or false: A patient with median nerve palsy can continue to achieve true opposition of the thumb to each of the fingertips by using the ulnar innervated half of the flexor pollicis brevis.

With median nerve palsy, the ulnar innervated one half of the FPB can substitute for palmar abduction and allow the patient to touch the thumb to each fingertip. However, this is with a lateral approach. The thumb makes contact with the lateral aspect of the digit. Without the opponens pollicis, the thumb is unable to rotate or pronate and cannot achieve true opposition (tip to tip).

Answer: **False**

Stanley, Tribuzi, pp. 333-334

45. True or false: Surgical overcorrection of a paralytic claw hand will turn into an intrinsic-plus deformity.

Overcorrection will reverse an intrinsic-minus deformity into an intrinsic-plus deformity. The hypermobile hand will develop PIP joint hyperextension with DIP joint flexion (also known as swan-neck deformity; see Fig. 2-23). Some of the causes include an overly strong muscle transferred to the extensor apparatus, a strong tendon transfer to the A1 pulley that limits MCP extension (the patient will attempt to straighten the finger and pull too hard with the long extensor tendons), and loss of the FDS can unbalance the PIP joint and cause hyperextension.

Answer: **True**

Brand, Hollister, pp. 203-204

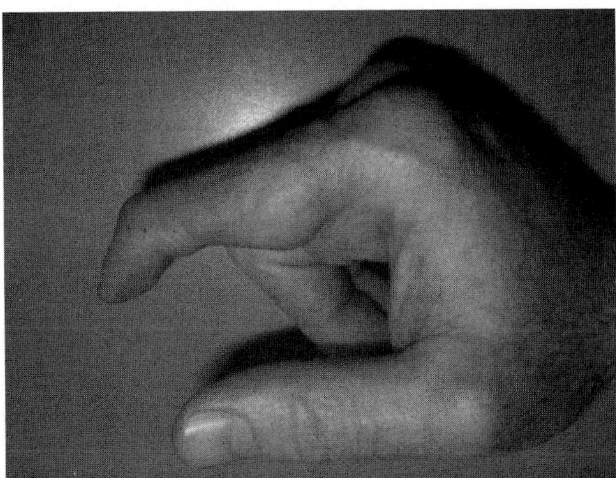

Fig. 2-23

46. Which of the following does not apply to the accessory collateral ligament at the PIP joint?

A. It is a stabilizer of the PIP joint.
B. It is taught in extension.
C. It inserts into the volar plate.
D. It is taut in flexion.

The proper collateral ligament (PCL) and accessory collateral ligament (ACL) are primary stabilizers of the PIP joint. The ACL is an anterior continuation of the joint capsule and attaches to the volar plate. In full extension, the ACL becomes taut; the PCL is taut in flexion. These ligamentous structures must be considered when splinting. Splinting the PIP joint at 0 to 15 degrees of flexion is recommended for treating collateral ligament injuries.

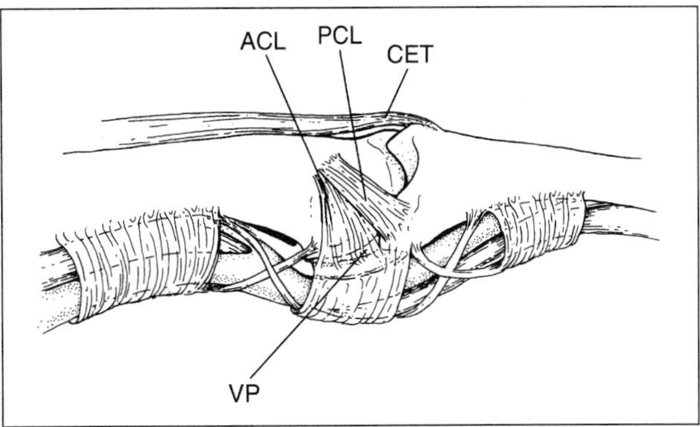

Fig. 2-24 ■ PIP joint. The major retaining ligaments of the PIP joint include the proper and accessory collateral ligaments (*PCL* and *ACL*), the volar plate (*VP*), and the dorsal capsule, with its central extensor tendon (*CET*). The VP acts as a gliding surface for the flexor tendon. (From Mackin EJ, Callahan AD, Skirven TM, et al: *Hunter, Mackin, & Callahan's Rehabilitation of the hand and upper extremity*, ed 5, St Louis, 2002, Mosby.)

Answer: **D**

Campbell, Wilson in Mackin, Callahan, Skirven, et al, p. 396
Hunter, Mackin, Callahan, p. 378
Refer to Fig. 2-24

47. The diagnosis "saddle syndrome" refers to which of the following?

A. Inflammation of the thumb carpometacarpal joint
B. Pain in the saddle-shaped joint surfaces of the upper extremity
C. Inflammation of the sagittal bands
D. Painful adhesions of the interosseous-lumbrical tendons

The interosseous and lumbrical tendons join distal to the deep transverse metacarpal ligament radial to the MCP joint of the long, ring, and small fingers. After closed injuries or repetitive microtrauma to the hand there can be painful adhesions to these structures.

The painful condition in which the interosseous-lumbrical adhesions are impinging on the deep transverse metacarpal ligament during intrinsic contraction is called *saddle syndrome* or *saddle deformity* (Fig. 2-25). The patient will experience pain with the Bunnell test (passive flexion of the IP joints while the MCP joints are supported in extension), while gripping, and during active intrinsic function.

Answer: **D**

Rosenthal in Mackin, Callahan, Skirven, et al, pp. 511-512
Hunter, Mackin, Callahan, pp. 532-534
Tan, Rothenfluh, Beredjiklian, pp. 639-643

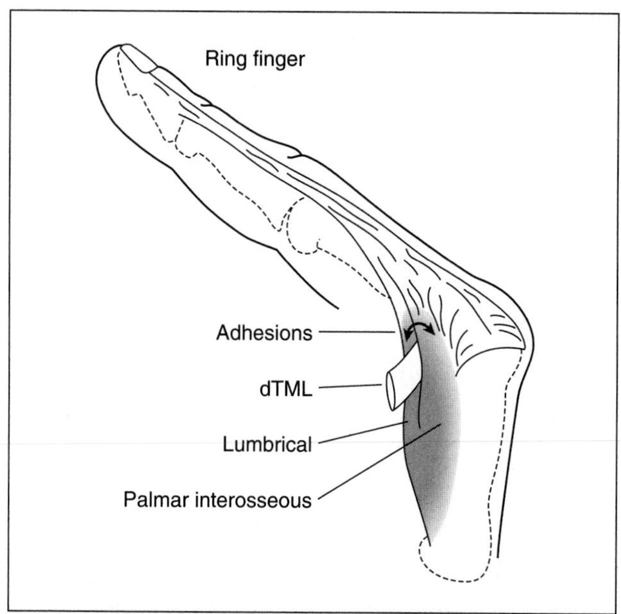

Fig. 2-25 ■ From Tan V, Rothenfluh DA, Beredjiklian PK, et al: Interosseous-lumbrical adhesions of the hand: contribution of magnetic resonance imaging to diagnosis and treatment planning, *J Hand Surg* [Am] 27(4):639-43, 2002.

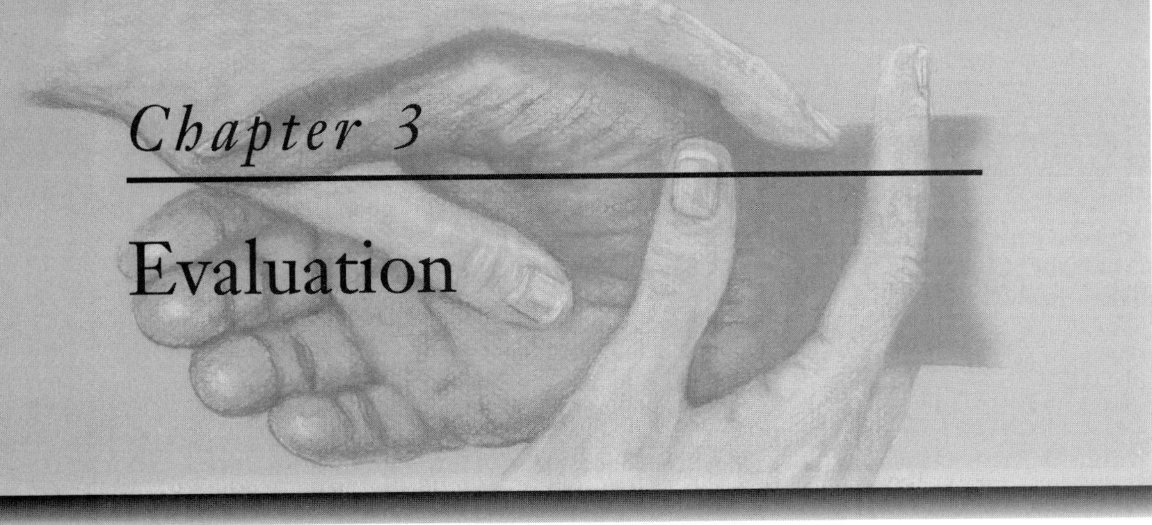

Chapter 3

Evaluation

1. Which of the following images represents a normal attitude of the hand?

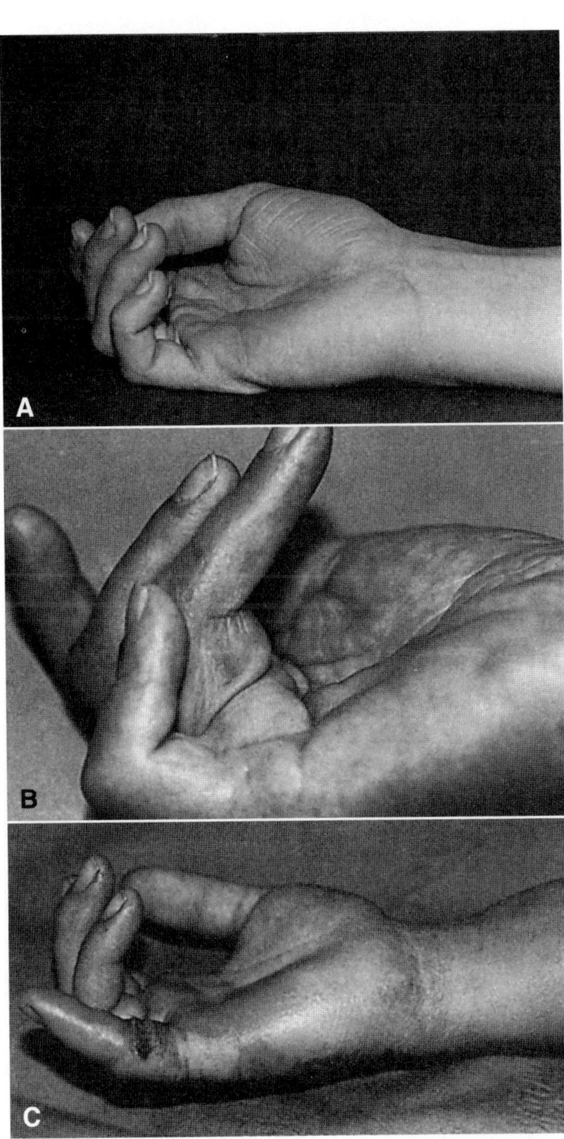

D. None of the above

Fig. 3-1 ■ **A, B,** and **C** From Mackin EJ, Callahan AD, Skirven TM, et al: *Rehabilitation of the hand and upper extremity*, ed 5, vol 1, St Louis, 2002, Mosby.

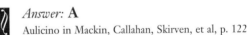

Fig. 3-1, *A*, represents the normal attitude of the hand in the resting position. Notice the fingers are progressively more flexed as one moves from the radial to the ulnar digits. In Fig. 3-1, *B*, the fingers are contracted as a result of Dupuytren's disease; therefore the normal attitude of the hand is lost. In Fig. 3-1, *C*, the normal attitude of the hand is lost because of lacerations of the flexor tendons in the fifth digit.

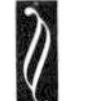

Answer: **A**
Aulicino in Mackin, Callahan, Skirven, et al, p. 122

2. You are treating a patient who injured his middle finger while playing basketball. He is unable to extend the tip of his finger. What is the most likely diagnosis?

A. Jersey finger
B. Mallet finger
C. Oblique retinacular ligament (ORL) injury
D. Crush injury to the distal interphalangeal (DIP) joint

The patient most likely has a mallet finger in which the digit presents with a "droop" of the tip of the finger at the DIP joint as a result of injury to the extensor tendon at the distal phalanx level. The treatment plan will be immobilization of the DIP joint in full extension for 6 to 8 weeks to allow the tendon to heal.

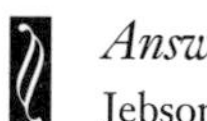

Answer: **B**

Jebson, Kasdan, p. 15

3. A right hand–dominant patient is referred to you with a diagnosis of right wrist pain. Upon evaluation you note that the onset of symptoms was approximately 1 week ago, after the patient performed excessive digging with a shovel while installing a fence. The patient has tenderness over the flexor carpi radialis (FCR) insertion and reports severe pain with passive extension. The patient has no signs of atrophy, crepitus, or loss of sensation. You consider possible FCR tendonitis. All but which of the following represent symptoms of acute tenopathy?

A. Localized pain
B. Pain with stretch to the tendon
C. Pain with resisted tendon function
D. Localized swelling
E. Crepitus

Acute tendonitis typically can present with all of the above except crepitus, which is a sign for more chronic cumulative trauma. Crepitus occurs as the tendon glides through adhesions and thickened tissues between the tendon and synovium that have developed over time. It is important to identify the stage of injury to provide appropriate treatment for the patient. For example, in this patient's case, splinting is indicated to rest the tendon and allow for inflammation to subside. In a more chronic case of tendonitis, tendon gliding may be a primary goal in treatment.

Answer: **E**

Lee, Nasser-Sharif, Zelouf in Mackin, Callahan, Skirven, et al, pp. 931-932, 943

4. A patient is referred for conservative treatment of posttraumatic DeQuervain's tenosynovitis 6 months after a motor vehicle accident (MVA). During the evaluation, you note tenderness 4 to 5 cm proximal to the radial styloid as well as at the anatomical snuffbox. The patient has a positive Finkelstein's test, negative hitchhiker's test, negative Watson's test, negative Grind test, pain with resisted wrist extension, no significant superficial tenderness on the dorsal aspect of the wrist, and no radiographic evidence of fracture. What other diagnosis may be indicated in addition to or instead of DeQuervain's?

A. Scaphoid nonunion
B. Basal joint arthritis
C. Scapholunate (SL) injury
D. Intersection syndrome
E. All of the above

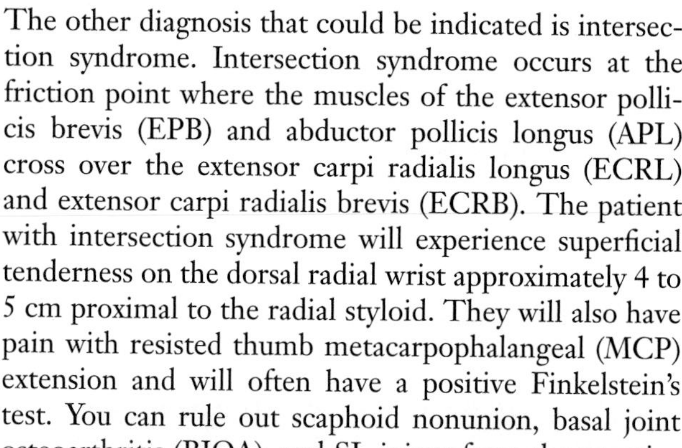

The other diagnosis that could be indicated is intersection syndrome. Intersection syndrome occurs at the friction point where the muscles of the extensor pollicis brevis (EPB) and abductor pollicis longus (APL) cross over the extensor carpi radialis longus (ECRL) and extensor carpi radialis brevis (ECRB). The patient with intersection syndrome will experience superficial tenderness on the dorsal radial wrist approximately 4 to 5 cm proximal to the radial styloid. They will also have pain with resisted thumb metacarpophalangeal (MCP) extension and will often have a positive Finkelstein's test. You can rule out scaphoid nonunion, basal joint osteoarthritis (BJOA), and SL injury from the negative tests described in the question.

Answer: **D**

Lee, Nasser-Sharif, Zelouf in Mackin, Callahan, Skirven, et al, p. 945

Skirven, Osterman in Mackin, Callahan, Skirven, et al, p. 1103

Refer to Fig. 3-2

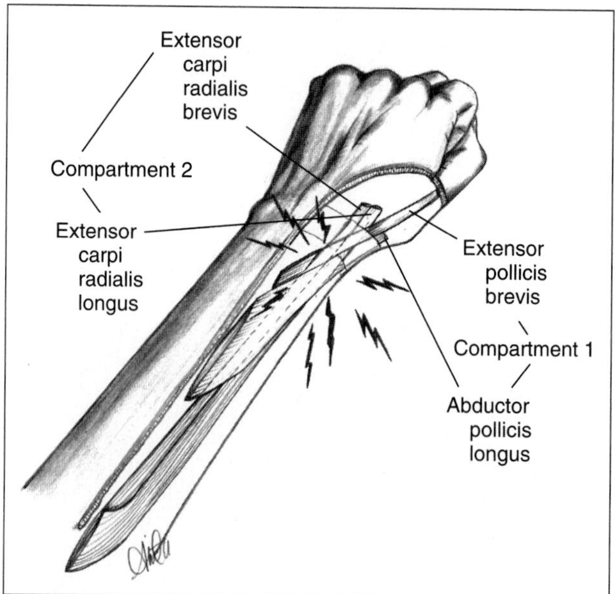

Fig. 3-2

5. A patient who is employed as a data entry technician is referred to you with a diagnosis of lateral epicondylitis. The patient has received two cortisone injections without relief and is now sent for conservative treatment. The patient describes pain throughout the lateral arm but reports the most pain in the mobile wad of Henry. Some tenderness is noted at the lateral epicondyle. Patient has pain with resisted supination and resisted middle finger extension. Which of the following is a likely differential diagnosis?

A. Radial tunnel
B. Dorsal wrist syndrome
C. Radiocapitellar joint pathology
D. ECRL tendonosis

The differential diagnosis is radial tunnel. Differentiation between the two syndromes is difficult because of the overlapping symptoms and difficulty with physical examination. Radial tunnel and lateral eipicondylitis can coexist. Radial tunnel syndrome typically presents with pain without palsy in the dorsal forearm, localized at the ECRL/ECRB/brachioradialis muscle bellies (mobile wad of Henry). Pain is worst approximately 4 to 5 cm distal to the lateral epicondyle. Patients will typically complain of deep, burning pain that is exacerbated with activities requiring forearm pronation and wrist flexion. Patients may also report resting and night pain. Resisted extension of the middle finger with the elbow extended, wrist in neutral, and the forearm pronated will elicit pain in the radial nerve distribution and the edge of the ECRB. Also, testing resisted supination with the forearm extended will elicit pain in those patients with radial nerve compression at the arcade of Frohse. The latter two tests are typically negative in patients with tennis elbow.

The following were incorrect choices. The radiocapitellar joint is not involved because of the patient's report of pain distal to the lateral epicondyle. If the ECRL were involved, the insertion of this muscle would cause the patient to complain of pain proximal to this point. Finally, the patient with dorsal wrist syndrome will have pain elicited in the SL region and resisted finger extension while the wrist is flexed (Fig. 3-3).

Answer: **A**

Hornbach, Culp in Mackin, Callahan, Skirven, et al, pp. 691-692
DeLee, Drez, Miller, p. 1328
Szabo in Green, Hotchkiss, Pederson, pp. 1433-1437

CLINICAL GEM:
Interestingly, some patients present with weakness in the extensors with a radial tunnel syndrome. This "pseudo" weakness occurs because the patient's protection from pain and is not a "true" muscle weakness.

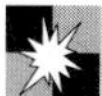

CLINICAL GEM:
Radial tunnel can occur with racquet sport injuries and manual labor workers.

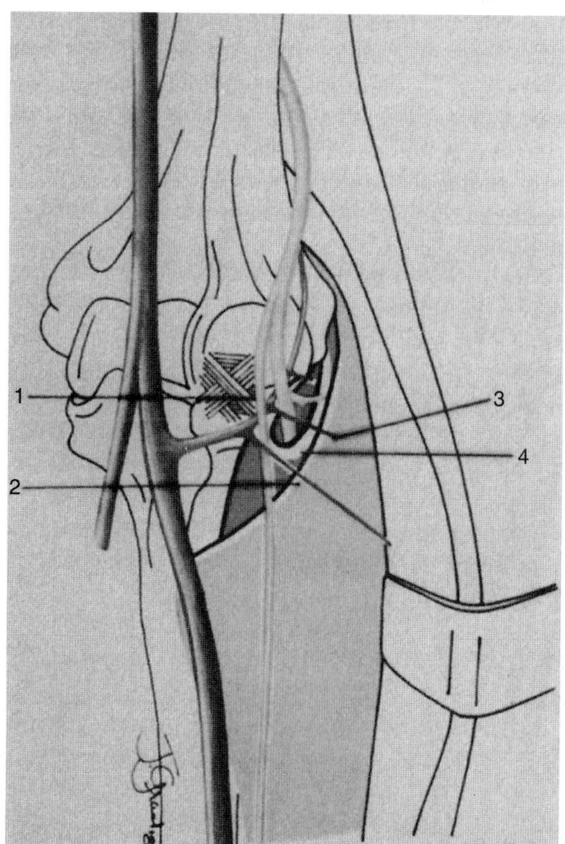

Fig. 3-3 ■ Four potentially compressive anatomic elements of the radial nerve: (1) fibrous bands overlying radial head and capsule; (2) fibrous origin of the ECRB; (3) radial recurrent arterial fan; and (4) arcade of Frohse. The distal margin of the supinator muscle has been considered a fifth site of compression. (From Moss S, Switzer H: Radial tunnel syndrome: a spectrum of clinical presentations, *J Hand Surg* 8:415, 1983.)

6. A patient is referred to therapy 6 weeks status-post intraarticular fracture of the small finger proximal interphalangeal (PIP) joint. The patient was not splinted after injury, and at the time of evaluation, the finger assumed a PIP joint flexion posture. When the patient passively flexes the DIP joint with the PIP joint in extension and then repeats with the PIP joint in flexion, you discover that greater motion exists when the PIP joint is flexed then when it is extended. What is indicated as the cause for decreased DIP joint motion?

A. ORL tightness
B. Joint contracture at the DIP joint
C. Triangular ligament tightness
D. All of the above could be indicated.

The ORL in this case has shortened secondarily to the flexed posture of the PIP joint. The ORL originates at the A2/C1 pulley area on the volar aspect of the proximal phalanx and inserts on the dorsal surface near the DIP joint. To test for ORL tightness, hold the PIP joint in extension and passively flex the DIP joint (Fig. 3-4, *A*). If flexion is less in this position than that measured with the PIP joint in flexion (Fig. 3-4, *B*), then ORL tightness is present. Joint contracture and/or triangular ligament tightness would present with limited passive DIP joint flexion regardless of the position of the PIP joint.

Answer: **A**

Aulicino in Mackin, Callahan, Skirven, et al, p. 133
Refer to Fig. 3-4

7. A patient is referred after open reduction internal fixation (ORIF) of the distal radius and ulnar styloid after sliding into home plate at a softball game. Evaluation demonstrates limited digit active range of motion (AROM) is as follows 6 months after his injury:

	MCP	PIP	DIP
Index finger	WNL	WNL	WNL
Middle finger	WNL	WNL	WNL
Ring finger	+35/88	−25/98	−15/72
Small finger	+40/90	−30/100	−15/72

NOTE: Positive (+) indicates hypertension. *WNL*, Within normal limits.

True or false: These numbers indicate a high ulnar nerve lesion is present.

Clawing of the ring and small fingers will be more dramatic in a low ulnar nerve palsy secondary to intact flexor digitorum profundus (FDP) innervation and unopposed FDP function of the ulnar innervated intrinsics. In a high ulnar nerve lesion, clawing is less noticeable secondary to the noninnervated FDP, which limits the clawing appearance at the interphalangeal (IP) joint level.

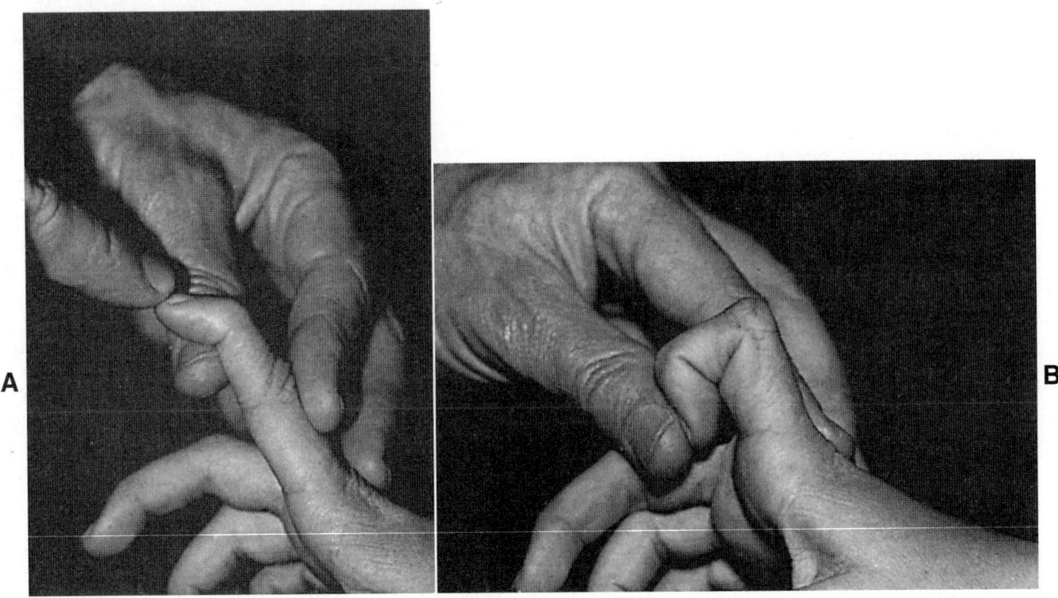

Fig. 3-4 ■ From Mackin EJ, Callahan AD, Skirven TM, et al: *Rehabilitation of the hand and upper extremity*, ed 5, vol 1, St Louis, 2002, Mosby.

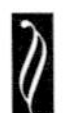

Answer: **False**

Skirven, Callahan in Mackin, Callahan, Skirven, et al, p. 605

8. Reflex testing is used to evaluate the integrity of nerve supply. The triceps reflex commonly is assessed for radial nerve function. This reflex is largely a function of what neurological level?

A. C5
B. C6
C. C7
D. C8

The radial nerve innervates the triceps. This reflex is largely a function of the C7 neurological level. To assess the triceps, place the patient's arm over your opposite arm so that it rests on your forearm. Hold the patient's arm under the medial epicondyle. Have the patient put his or her arm in a slightly flexed position, with the arm relaxed. With the narrow end of a reflex hammer, tap the triceps tendon where it crosses the olecranon fossa. You should be able to see the reflex or feel it slightly as the patient's arm jerks your supporting arm.

Answer: **C**

Hoppenfeld, p. 55

Refer to Fig. 3-5

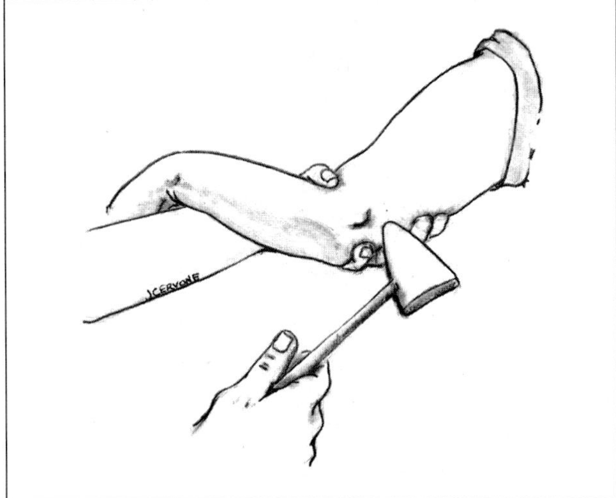

Fig. 3-5

CLINICAL GEM:
To assess C5, perform a biceps reflex test. To assess C6, perform a brachioradialis reflex test.

CLINICAL GEM:
A reflex is an involuntary response to a stimulus. Reflexes depend on intact neural pathways.

9. For optimal results during discriminative sensory reeducation, certain requirements must be met. A specific level of return in touch perception must be present for successful sensory retraining. With regards to Semmes-Weinstein monofilaments, the patient must be able to perceive which level of sensory return in order to begin discrimination testing?

A. 6.65 monofilament
B. 5.07 monofilament
C. 4.56 monofilament
D. 4.31 monofilament

A patient must have protective sensation (4.31) on the fingertips with monofilament testing before discrimination retraining can be initiated. If discriminative sensory reeducation is begun before this sensibility is obtained, the treatment will not be beneficial, and the patient may become discouraged.

Answer: **D**

Hunter, Mackin, Callahan, p. 706
Fess in Mackin, Callahan, Skirven, et al, p. 637

10. You are manual muscle testing (MMT) the triceps muscle and note that the patient can achieve full AROM only in the gravity-eliminated plane (no added resistance). The triceps should be rated:

A. Poor minus
B. Poor
C. Poor plus
D. Fair minus
E. Fair

MMT involves observing, palpating, and manually resisting muscles or groups of muscles to determine the quality and quantity of muscle contraction. Contraindications to MMT include spasticity and situations in which AROM or resistance is not allowed, such as during the healing of bone, muscle, and tendon. Several grading scales have been noted in the literature and are used in academic programs.

The following are the classifications and definitions from Trombly and Scott's grading system.

Word	Number	Definition
Zero (0)	0	No contraction palpable; no movement at joint
Trace (T)	1	Contraction/tension palpated in the muscle or tendon; no movement at joint
Poor–(P–)	2–	Part moves through only a portion of range of motion on a gravity-eliminated plane
Poor (P)	2	Part moves through full range of motion on a gravity-eliminated plane with no added resistance
Poor + (P+)	2+	Part moves through full range of motion on a gravity-eliminated plane; takes minimal resistance and then "breaks"
Fair–(F–)	3–	Part moves through less than full range of motion against gravity
Fair (F)	3	Part moves through full range of motion against gravity with no added resistance
Fair + (F+)	3+	Part moves through full range of motion against gravity with minimal resistance
Good–(G–)	4–	Part moves through full range of motion against gravity with less than moderate resistance
Good (G)	4	Part moves through full range of motion against gravity with moderate resistance
Normal (N)	5	Part moves through full range of motion against gravity with maximum resistance

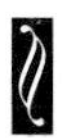

Answer: **B**

Casanova, pp. 47-52
Trombly, Scott, p. 174

11. Which is the most useful and widely known noninvasive test for evaluating the contribution of the radial and ulnar arteries to the hand?

A. Allen's test
B. Plethysmography
C. Arteriography
D. Radionuclide studies

The Allen's test is used to assess both ulnar and radial arteries of the hand. The examiner performs this test by compressing the arteries at the patient's wrist (Fig. 3-6, *A*) and asking the patient to make a fist several times to exsanguinate the blood (Fig. 3-6, *B*). Next, the patient is asked to open the hand approximately 90% while one artery is released and the refill time is noted (Fig. 3-6, *C*); the patient should not open the hand forcefully. The test is performed again with the other artery. The test is positive if there is no arterial flush in 5 to 15 seconds. This is a modification of the test originally described by Allen (see Fig. 1-31).

Answer: **A**

Green, p. 2254
Hunter, Mackin, Callahan, p. 74
Aulicino in Mackin, Callahan, Skirven, et al, p. 141

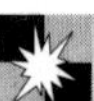

CLINICAL GEM:
A modification of Allen's test can be performed on a single digit. The steps are the same as described in the question except that the examiner occludes and releases the radial and ulnar **digital** arteries.

12. For a quick check of ulnar nerve status, which muscle would you test?

A. Abductor pollicis brevis
B. Extensor indicis proprius
C. Dorsal interossei
D. Palmaris longus

Assessment of the dorsal interossei, which abduct the digits, is a quick test for ulnar nerve function. The extensor indicis proprius is innervated by the radial nerve; the abductor pollicis brevis and palmaris longus are innervated by the median nerve.

Answer: **C**

Hoppenfeld, p. 95

CLINICAL GEM:
To remember the actions of the interossei, remember **PAD** and **DAB**. **PAD** refers to **P**almar interossei **AD**duct, and **DAB** refers to **D**orsal interossei **AB**duct.

13. When one measures the radial and ulnar deviation of the wrist, the axis of the goniometer should be placed at which of the following?

A. Scaphoid
B. Lunate
C. Triquetrum
D. Capitate
E. Distal radius

During measurement of wrist deviation, the goniometer is positioned so that the stationary arm is aligned with the forearm, the axis is at the capitate, and the moveable arm is placed along the third metacarpal. Wrist flexion and extension should be avoided during the assessment. Normal range of motion is as follows: radial deviation, 0 to 20 degrees; ulnar deviation, 0 to 30 degrees.

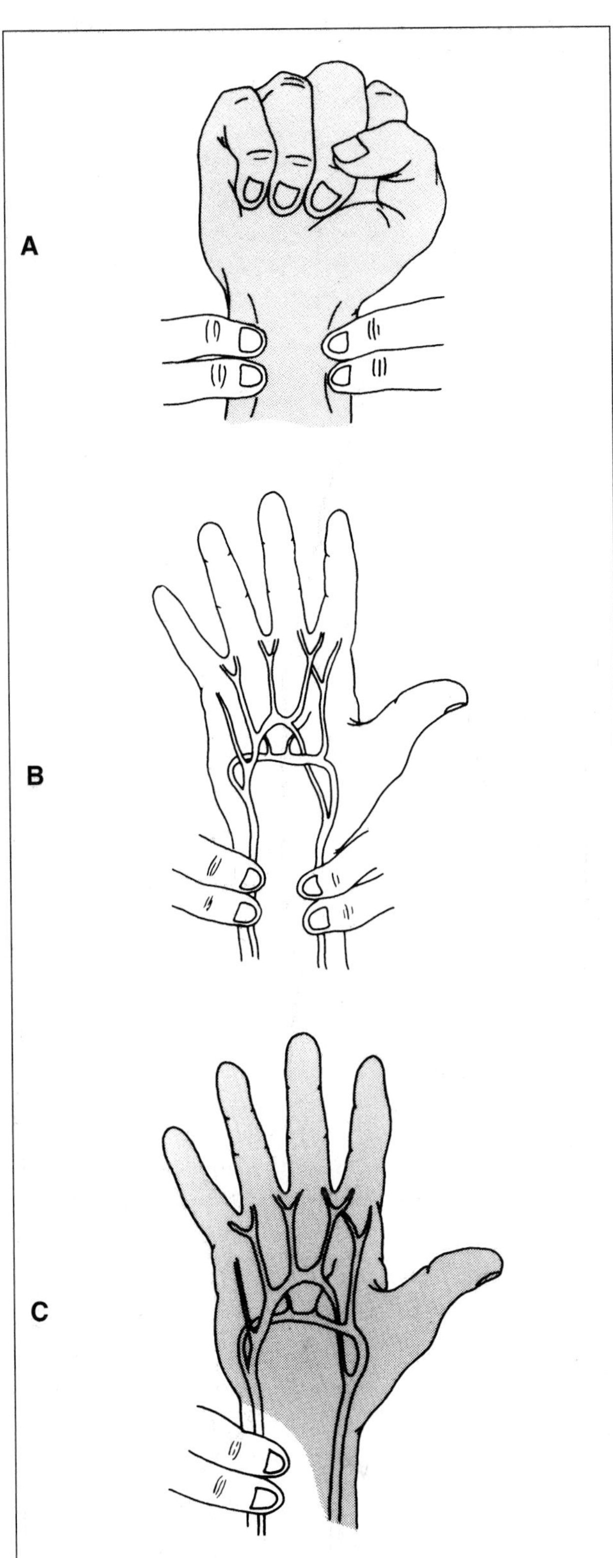

Fig. 3-6 ■ Redrawn from American Society for Surgery of the Hand: *The hand, examination and diagnosis*, Aurora, CO, 1978, The Society.

When assessing range of motion, the therapist should indicate whether active, passive, or torque range of motion is being measured. Joints typically are measured on the dorsal aspect, with the axis of the goniometer lining up with the axis of the joint. Recording any deviations in the method of assessing range of motion is imperative to allow for accurate future comparisons.

Answer: **D**

Clinical Assessment Recommendations, p. 57
Hunter, Mackin, Callahan, pp. 102-103
Cambridge in Mackin, Callahan, Skirven, et al, pp. 176-178

CLINICAL GEM:
A quick way to find the capitate is to slide your finger down the patient's middle finger until you feel a divot in the wrist. The waist of the capitate lies beneath your finger.

14. A grind test on the thumb is performed to assess which of the following?

A. Osteoarthritis
B. Tenosynovitis
C. Rheumatoid arthritis
D. Ligament weakness

The grind test is performed by applying mild axial compression and gentle rotation of the thumb. If osteoarthritis is present, this test will cause pain at the first carpometacarpal joint.

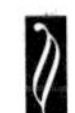

Answer: **A**

Hunter, Mackin, Callahan, p. 72
Aulicino in Mackin, Callahan, Skirven, et al, p. 138
Refer to Fig. 3-7

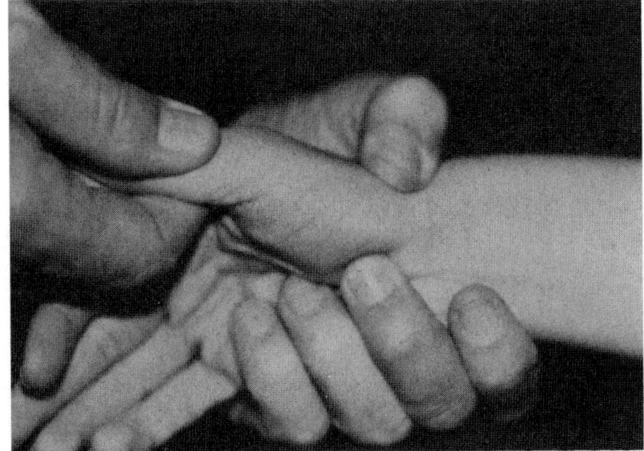

Fig. 3-7 ■ From Mackin EJ, Callahan AD, Skirven TM, et al: *Rehabilitation of the hand and upper extremity*, ed 5, vol 1, St Louis, 2002, Mosby.

15. A patient developed a chronic stiff hand after immobilization of a distal radius fracture and has attended therapy for 6 weeks. Therapy has included joint mobilization, static progressive splinting, and active/active-assisted/passive range of motion (A/AA/PROM). Reevaluation shows that PROM of the digits is 90% of the contralateral hand; however, power grip remains limited because of decreased active DIP joint flexion. The patient has limited active clawing but full passive IP joint flexion in the hook (claw) position. This patient has most likely developed which of the following?

A. Interossei tightness
B. Lumbrical tightness
C. Limited FDP glide
D. Both B and C
E. All of the above

Lumbrical tightness is present, and because of the FDP origin of the lumbricals on the FDP, limited FDP glide also occurs and affects the functional power grip of the hand. The interossei are not tight; this fact is evidenced by full passive IP joint flexion in the claw position.

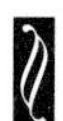

Answer: **D**
Colditz in Mackin, Callahan, Skirven, et al, p. 1044
Refer to Fig. 3-8

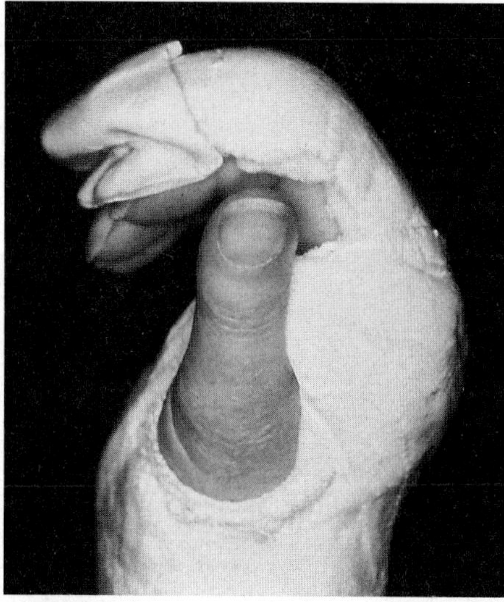

Fig. 3-8 ■ From Mackin EJ, Callahan AD, Skirven TM, et al: *Rehabilitation of the hand and upper extremity*, ed 5, vol 1, St Louis, 2002, Mosby.

CLINICAL GEM:
The casting motion to mobilize stiffness (CMMS) technique described by Judy Colditz will be useful to position the DIP joints in greater flexion and to aid in pull-through of the profundus tendons when treating patients with decreased active DIP joint flexion due to chronic stiffness (Fig. 3-8).

16. A patient is seen s/p Smith's fracture and has been progressing well in treatment. Functional range of motion (ROM) is achieved; however, the patient continues to complain of ulnar-sided wrist pain that is exacerbated with supination. The patient also experiences pain with power grip combined with supination; however, the patient's grip is pain-free when combined with pronation. Which of the following is the most likely joint dysfunction that is contributing to pain and functional loss?

A. Triangular fibrocartilage complex (TFCC) injury
B. Ulnar abutment
C. Distal radioulnar (DRU) joint volar instability
D. Posttraumatic arthritis

Volar instability at the DRU joint is likely the cause of joint dysfunction in this case. One can draw this conclusion from the mechanism of injury (volar dislocation) seen in Smith's fractures. This patient presents with pain in supination when power gripping, which is a more unusual presentation than is often seen with a typical Colles fracture and resultant TFCC injury. However, with a TFCC injury or in ulnar abutment, the ulnar structures are relatively unloaded with supination, and pain would be predominantly associated with pronated power grip. If the patient had posttraumatic arthritis the pain will occur with both supination and pronation.

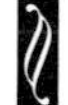

Answer: **C**
Frykman, Watkins in Mackin, Callahan, Skirven, et al, p. 1132
LaStayo in Mackin, Callahan, Skirven, et al, p. 1157

17. Match the following test to the correct description:

Test

1. Jebsen hand function test
2. Crawford small parts dexterity test
3. Rosenbusch test of finger dexterity
4. Purdue pegboard
5. Minnesota rate-of-manipulation test

Description

A. Fine-motor coordination test that uses tweezers and screwdrivers
B. Gross-motor coordination test that addresses bilateral turning and placing
C. Test that focuses on the ability to simultaneously hold, manipulate, and place small objects
D. Test that involves the manipulation of washers, small pins, and collars
E. Test that is used to assess activities-of-daily-living skills

Answers: **1, E; 2, A; 3, C; 4, D; 5, B**
Hunter, Mackin, Callahan, p. 211
Fess in Mackin, Callahan, Skirven, et al, pp. 278-279

18. To what does a coefficient of variation (COV) of 20% refer?

A. A good level of effort
B. Consistent effort
C. Inconsistent effort
D. Malingering

A COV provides a percentage of variation between trials of a test. This information can be used to assess a patient's level of effort during testing. Factors that may interfere with a patient's performance include anxiety, fear of pain or reinjury, difficulty understanding the testing procedures, and other impairments. According to an accepted standard, a COV of 15% or less means that the patient's performance is at a good level of effort; a COV of greater than 15% is considered inconsistent. The authors believe that COV results should be interpreted with caution.

Answer: **C**
Hunter, Mackin, Callahan, pp. 1739-1774
Schultz-Johnson in Mackin, Callahan, Skirven, et al, pp. 1981-2025

19. Which handle position on the Jamar dynamometer is widely accepted for testing?

A. Handle position I
B. Handle position II
C. Handle position III
D. Handle position IV
E. Handle position V

The Jamar dynamometer (Fig. 3-9) is a standardized instrument used for grip testing. It has five adjustable settings. The American Society of Hand Therapists (ASHT) recommends that the patient be seated comfortably during testing, with the shoulder adducted, the elbow flexed to 90 degrees, and the forearm and wrist in neutral positions. There is controversy regarding the optimal wrist position. Most authors report that the wrist should be positioned between 0 and 30 degrees. Extension that exceeds 30 degrees should be noted. Both the American Society of Surgery of the Hand (ASSH) and ASHT recommend testing in the second-handle position (if only one handle span is used) as well as obtaining three grip trials.

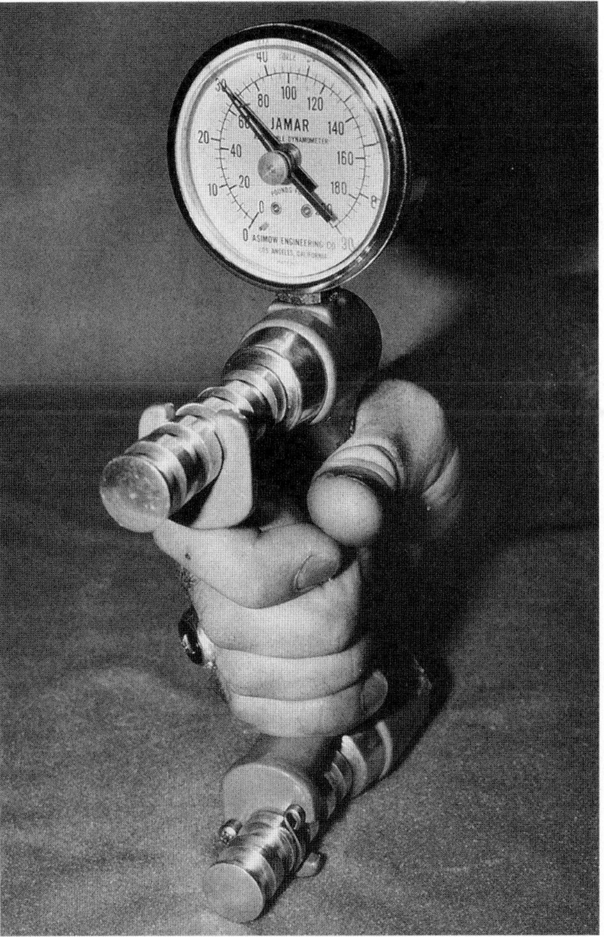

Fig. 3-9 ■ From Pedretti LW: *Occupational therapy: practice skills for physical dysfunction*, ed 4, St Louis, 1996, Mosby.

Answer: **B**

Clinical Assessment Recommendations, pp. 41-44
Aulicino in Mackin, Callahan, Skirven, et al, p. 134

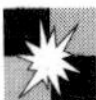

CLINICAL GEM:
Research has indicated that a 5% to 10% difference between the normal dominant hand and the normal nondominant hand usually exists.

20. A 5-year-old girl is referred to you for evaluation of her sensibility 3 months after a median nerve repair. Which test would best determine her status of sensibility?

A. Two-point discrimination (2PD)
B. Semmes-Weinstein monofilament testing
C. Moberg pick-up test
D. O'Connor tweezer dexterity test

The Moberg pick-up test is the best choice for testing a child's functional level of sensibility because a child may find other sensory tests may be confusing and therefore could easily misunderstand them. The Moberg test is a nonstandardized test that consists of picking up everyday objects and placing them in a container. One may choose to use this as a clinical tool for sensory and motor reeducation; however, if the Moberg test is used in this manner, it should not be used for testing.

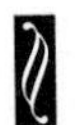

Answer: **C**

Dellon, pp. 86-104

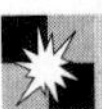

CLINICAL GEM:
When addressing tactile gnosis after a median nerve injury, the therapist should decrease sensory input to the ulnar nerve–innervated digits to ensure that object recognition is being determined by the median nerve–innervated digits. One way to ensure this is to modify a glove by cutting away the median-innervated digits (index, thumb, and long) and keeping ring and little finger glove material intact.

21. Match each Semmes-Weinstein monofilament classification with the correct filament thickness.

Classification

1. Normal
2. Diminished light touch
3. Diminished protective sensation
4. Loss of protective sensation
5. Not testable

Filament Thickness

A. 3.22
B. Greater than 6.65
C. 5.46
D. 2.44
E. 4.08

Color key to correlate with monofilament results

Green	Normal sensation	1.65-2.83
Blue	Diminished light touch	3.22-3.61
Purple	Diminished protective sensation	3.84-4.31
Red	Loss of protective sensation	4.56-6.65
Red-lined	Not testable	Greater than 6.65

Answers: **1, D; 2, A; 3, E; 4, C; 5, B**

Hunter, Mackin, Callahan, pp. 120-121
Bell-Krotoski in Mackin, Callahan, Skirven, et al, pp. 199, 204

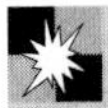

CLINICAL GEM:
When assessing with the Semmes-Weinstein monofilament (SWM) classification, remember to bowstring the monofilament at a perpendicular angle to the finger. Monofilaments 1.65 through 4.08 are applied three times per targeted area. One out of three quantifies as a correct response; larger monofilaments are applied only one time to each targeted area.

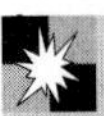

CLINICAL GEM:
Each monofilament thickness has a range of numbers that correlates with a specific color. When the Semmes-Weinstein monofilament results are completed, a hand diagram is color-coded. Color coding provides a quick reference to the person's level of sensibility. Repeat mappings should be performed to determine sensory recovery.

22. Your patient is being referred for an arthrogram to confirm which of the following suspected diagnosis?

A. TFCC tear
B. Scaphoid fracture
C. Dorsal wrist ganglion
D. All of the above are good candidates for arthrograms.

Wrist arthrography is often indicated to confirm suspected tears of the TFCC as well as other ligament tears, such as the SL or lunotriquetal ligaments. This technique is useful to detect leakage of fluids into joint spaces and diagnose tears of these ligaments. The ganglion could be confirmed by using an ultrasound imaging technique to confirm its existence, and the scaphoid fracture could be confirmed with X-ray or magnetic resonance imaging (MRI).

Answer: **A**
Jebsen, Kasdan, p. 39

23. A patient is seen 2 years after a crush injury to the middle finger (MF). The patient reports hitting the dorsal PIP joint approximately 6 months ago and feeling a "snap." The PIP joint rests in 60 degrees of flexion but is passively correctable. The patient is unable to initiate PIP joint extension with the joint in flexion. You also discover that with the MCP joint at neutral and the PIP joint placed in extension the patient can hold the digit in relative extension. Additionally, while placing the wrist and MCP joints in flexion and assessing active PIP joint extension the patient has a 15- to 20-degree lag at the PIP joint. The likely diagnosis is which of the following?

A. Lumbrical weakness
B. Central slip rupture
C. Lateral band subluxation
D. Central slip adhesion

The patient incurred a central slip rupture when the finger was struck. The central slip provides initiation of extension of the PIP joint as well as the final 15 to 20 degrees of extension. The patient's ability to hold extension when the PIP joint is placed in extension is performed by the lateral bands. The patient is unable to initiate PIP joint extension because of loss of the central slip.

Answer: **B**
Rosenthal in Mackin, Callahan, Skirven, et al, pp. 513-514
Refer to Fig. 3-10

24. A 36-year-old man presents with "balloon" edema in the right, dominant hand. You choose to test the edema using a volumeter. When this test is performed, the patient should lower his hand until the stop dowel rests at which web space?

A. Web one
B. Web two
C. Web three
D. Web four

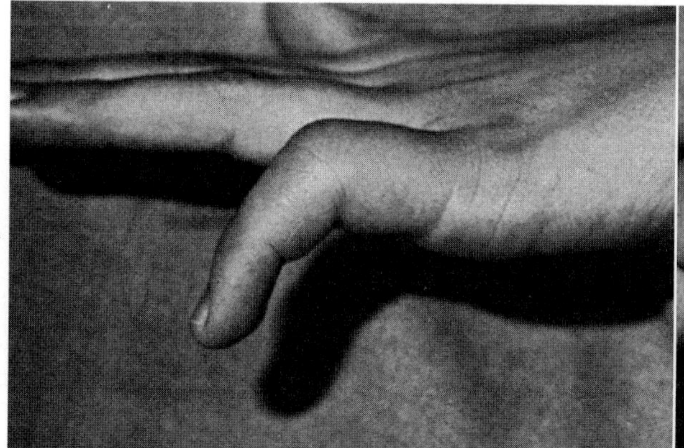

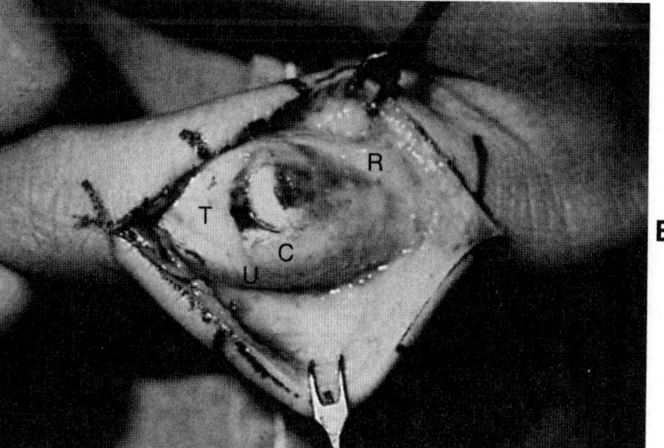

Fig. 3-10 ■ Closed rupture of extensor tendon about the PIP joint. Active and passive extension were limited. There was no resistance to flexion of distal joint. **A,** Clinical posture of injured finger. **B,** Operative findings: central tendon ruptured with herniation of head and proximal phalanx; triangular ligament was preserved. Radial lateral band is trapped beneath the condyle of the proximal phalanx. Inability to passively extend the PIP joint is indication for primary operative repair in extensor tendon injuries at this level. *C,* Central tendon; *R,* radial lateral band; *T,* triangular ligament; *U,* ulnar lateral band. (From Mackin EJ, Callahan AD, Skirven TM, et al: *Rehabilitation of the hand and upper extremity,* ed 5, vol 1, St Louis, 2002, Mosby.)

In a hand volumeter test, water is poured into the volumeter until overflow occurs and the overflow is discarded. Remove all jewelry from both upper extremities of the patient. Next, while the patient is standing, ask him to lower his hand slowly into the volumeter with his thumb facing the spout and forearm in pronation (palm facing the patient), until the third web rests on the stop dowel (the third web is between digits three and four) (Fig. 3-11). The patient's hand is removed, and water is measured in the graduated cylinder.

Answer: **C**

Hunter, Mackin, Callahan, p. 81
Villeco, Mackin, Hunter in Mackin, Callahan, Skirven, et al, p. 188

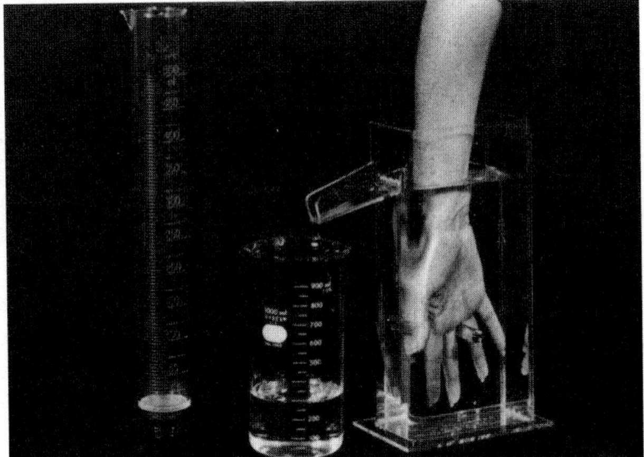

Fig. 3-11 ■ From Mackin EJ, Callahan AD, Skirven TM, et al: *Rehabilitation of the hand and upper extremity*, ed 5, vol 1, St Louis, 2002, Mosby.

Clinical Gem:
When only one or two digits are involved, circumferential measurement is more useful because the edema in an individual joint or digit may not be detected with the volumeter.

25. True or false: A neural tension test is positive if a patient feels any tingling or discomfort during the test.

A neural tension test, according to Butler, is positive when it reproduces the patient's symptoms or current complaints. One must realize that in "normal" people tension testing may cause some discomfort or numbness. Clinicians should familiarize themselves with the expected responses.

Answer: **False**

Butler, p. 162

26. True or false: A safety pin is a good tool for assessing pain perception.

A sharp/dull test is used to assess pain perception. According to Waylett-Rendall, a sterile needle should be used instead of a safety pin because denervated skin lacks calluses for protection and is more susceptible to damage. The test is performed to slight blanching to prevent puncture.

According to Moberg, Dellon, and others, pinprick (sterile needle) is not recommended because of discomfort and poor correlation with functional sensation. However, if sensibility return is absent, it may be used to determine when protective sensation is intact.

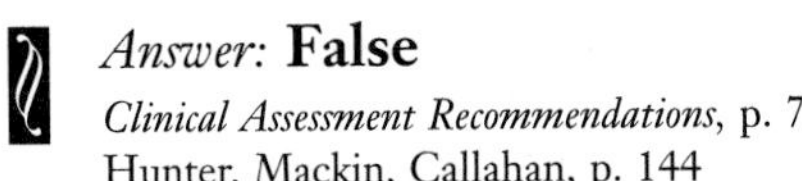

Answer: **False**

Clinical Assessment Recommendations, p. 73
Hunter, Mackin, Callahan, p. 144

27. Match each of the following tests with the correct description/names.

Tests

1. Ninhydrin test
2. Semmes-Weinstein
3. Moving two-point
4. Static two-point
5. Moberg pick-up test

Description/Names

A. Weber
B. Dellon
C. Threshold testing
D. Sudomotor function
E. Functional test for tactile gnosis

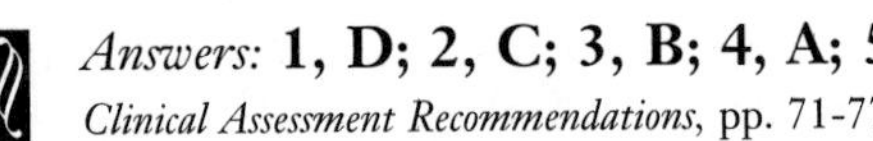

Answers: **1, D; 2, C; 3, B; 4, A; 5, E**

Clinical Assessment Recommendations, pp. 71-77

28. Which of the curves in Fig. 3-12 represents a treatable torque angle curve for a 50-degree PIP joint contracture, *A* or *B*?

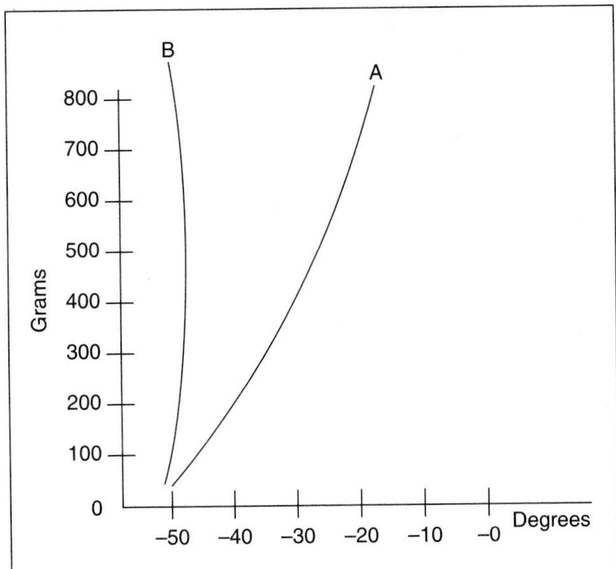

Fig. 3-12

Brand and Hollister have suggested the use of torque range of motion (TROM) to improve objectivity in measuring ROM. TROM can be performed in the clinic using a goniometer, a strain gauge, and a finger cuff. Force is applied at a right angle to the digit that is to move. One must remember to note the position of the proximal joints. A curve with a soft slope, such as curve *A*, changes rapidly with increased gram load and indicates that the joint should respond to treatment. However, if the joint is in a fixed joint contracture, the slope (curve *B*) is steep with increased loading. This may indicate that conservative treatment (e.g., splinting) may not be effective.

Answer: **A**
Hunter, Mackin, Callahan, pp. 170-174
Brand, Hollister, pp. 115-119

29. Using the Weber test, you are testing a patient with median nerve damage. The resulting score is a 12 on digits one through three. According to the normative scale, this would be rated:

A. Normal
B. Fair
C. Poor
D. Protective

The Weber two-point discrimination test assesses innervation density and can be used to determine tactile gnosis. Testing should begin with the discriminator 5 mm apart. The patient responds as to whether one or two points are perceived. Seven out of 10 correct responses must be obtained to receive a score. Categories are as follows:

Normal:	0 to 5 mm
Fair:	6 to 10 mm
Poor:	11 to 15 mm
Protective:	One point perceived
Anesthetic:	No points perceived

Answer: **C**
Clinical Assessment Recommendations, p. 79

30. A patient is referred to you with a diagnosis of wrist contusion after an MVA. The patient presents with diffuse pain throughout the wrist and forearm and multiple structures are tender on palpation. You initially address the overall pain, and the patient is now localizing pain in the central dorsal and radial dorsal zones of the wrist. Because the patient was injured when gripping a steering wheel and because of her description of pain, you suspect a possible scaphoid injury. Radiographs are retaken and unremarkable. You are now assessing for a possible SL injury. All but which of the following tests are appropriate?

A. Watson shift test
B. Clenched fist X-ray
C. SL ballottement test
D. Linsheid test

All of the above can be used to rule out SL injury except the Linsheid test. The Linsheid test is used to detect II and III carpometacarpal (CMC) injury. The Watson Shift test is performed by applying pressure to the volar prominence of the scaphoid, which can be palpated at the base of the thenar crease as the wrist is moved from ulnar deviation (UD) to radial deviation (RD) with slight wrist flexion. When the pressure is released a positive test will elicit a painful clunk as the scaphoid returns, thus reproducing the patient's symptoms. A clenched fist X-ray will load the SL ligament, and in the case of injury a Terry Thomas sign will be present with a gap between the scaphoid and the lunate. Finally, the SL ballottement test may be used to assess SL instability. This test involves grasping the scaphoid with the thumb and finger with one hand while stabilizing the lunate with the other. The scaphoid is then moved in a volar and dorsal direction on the lunate, and any pain or increased movement relative to the other side is noted.

Answer: **D**
Skirven, Osterman in Mackin, Callahan, Skirven, et al, pp. 1105-1106
Wright, Michlovitz in Mackin, Callahan, Skirven, et al, pp. 1187-1189

31. A patient is seen for evaluation with the diagnosis of cubital tunnel syndrome. The patient complains of intermittent numbness and tingling in the volar forearm and ulnar two fingers as well as burning pain proximal to shoulder. Which of the following is the appropriate upper limb tension test (ULTT)?

A. Shoulder abduction and external rotation, supination, wrist/finger/elbow extension, shoulder depression, and cervical contralateral lateral flexion
B. Shoulder abduction and external rotation, either pronation or supination, wrist/small finger extension, elbow flexion, shoulder depression, and cervical contralateral lateral flexion
C. Shoulder abduction and external rotation, pronation, wrist/small finger extension, elbow extension, shoulder depression, and cervical contralateral lateral flexion
D. Shoulder abduction and internal rotation, pronation, wrist/thumb/index flexion, elbow extension, shoulder depression, and cervical contralateral lateral flexion

Answer B is the appropriate position for ULTT for a patient with ulnar nerve symptoms. Answer A is the appropriate test for patients with median nerve symptoms, and answer D is the appropriate position for patients with radial nerve symptoms.

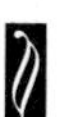
Answer: **B**
Walsh in Mackin, Callahan, Skirven, et al, p. 768

32. Total active motion (TAM) is derived by which of the following?

A. Summation of flexion minus the summation of the extension deficits
B. Summation of extension minus the summation of flexion
C. Summation of flexion and extension
D. All of the above are acceptable ways to calculate TAM

TAM is the summation of joint flexion minus the summation of joint extension deficits. For example: (MCP joint 90 degrees + PIP joint 90 degrees + DIP joint 45 degrees) – (MCP joint 0 degrees + PIP joint – 10 degrees + DIP joint – 10 degrees) = 205 degrees of TAM. Using TAM is helpful for doing comparison data and it provides useful information on the composite motion of a finger. The measurement is performed in the fisted position.

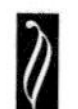
Answer: **A**
Clinical Assessment Recommendations, p. 68

33. To determine whether the biceps head is stable in the bicipital groove, which of the following should be performed?

A. Roos test
B. Wright's maneuver
C. Yergason test
D. Elbow flexion test
E. Valgus/varus test

The Yergason test (Fig. 3-13) is performed by having the patient fully flex the elbow. The examiner grasps the flexed elbow with one hand while using the other hand to hold the wrist. The patient should be instructed to resist motion while the examiner externally rotates the arm. At the same time, the examiner pulls the patient's elbow into extension. This test will determine whether the head of the biceps is stable in the bicipital groove. If the tendon is not stable, the patient may experience pain or the tendon may pop out.

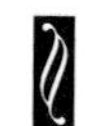
Answer: **C**
Hoppenfeld, p. 32

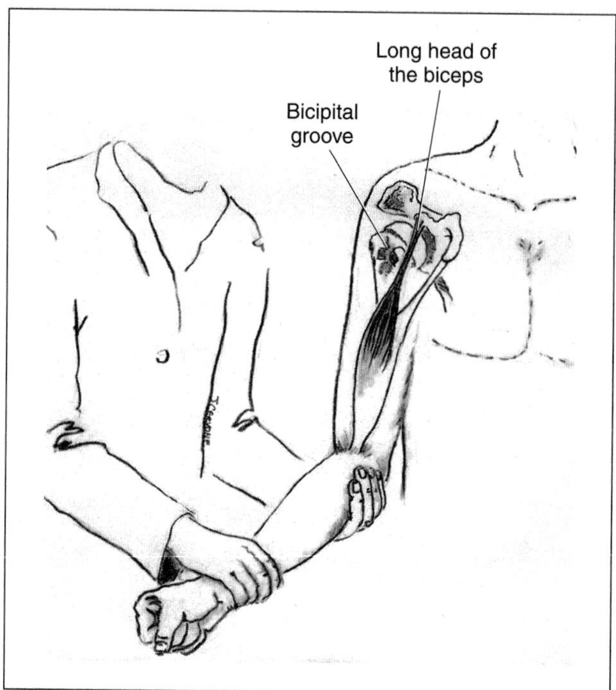

Fig. 3-13

34. What is a disadvantage of using the visual analog scale (VAS)?

A. It is a highly sensitive test.
B. It is difficult and awkward to use.
C. It has a high failure rate because patients have difficulty interpreting the instructions.
D. Examiners must have experience using the test.

The VAS is performed by drawing a 10-cm line horizontally or vertically, with the ends labeled "no pain" and "pain as bad as it could be." The patient marks the line to indicate his or her current level of pain. The test may have a high failure rate because patients may have difficulty interpreting the instructions. Completing pain assessment with supervision is recommended to ensure proper patient understanding. Answer A is an advantage of this test, but answers B and D do not apply. Other pain tests include an array of rating scales and pain questionnaires such as the McGill or Schultz pain assessment.

Answer: **C**
Clinical Assessment Recommendations, p. 100

35. True or False: The temperature of the water has no effect on the results of volumetric measurements.

According to a study by Theodore King in 1993, water temperature should be controlled. His study revealed statistical significance related to variation in temperature. Therefore cool or "tepid" water is recommended for accurate results (see Fig. 3-11).

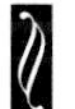

Answer: **False**
King, p. 203

36. A 40-year-old woman is referred to you for ulnar-sided wrist pain. She has no history of trauma and no radiographic signs of fracture. Upon examination, her pain is localized in the ulnar aspect of the wrist and is worse with UD, grip, and pronation. No instability is detected at end range of supination and pronation. The patient is positive for the articular disc shear test, gripping rotary impaction test (GRIT), and TFCC load test. Which of the following is the likely diagnosis?

A. Peripheral TFCC tear
B. Central disc tear
C. Lunotriquetral (LT) tear
D. Dorsal radioulnar ligament tear

The patient likely has a central disc tear of the TFCC, possibly because of early degeneration. The articular disc shear test (Fig. 3-14) is used to assess for central lesions of the TFCC. This test is performed with the patient's elbow resting on a table and the forearm in neutral. The examiner stabilizes the radius with one hand and places the thumb of the other hand dorsally over the distal ulna while placing the radial aspect of the index PIP joint over the pisotriquetral complex volarly. The examiner then squeezes the thumb and index finger together, thus creating a dorsal glide of the pisotriquetral complex on the ulnar head and shearing of the central disc.

The GRIT is a measurement of grip strength in full supination, full pronation, and neutral forearm position. The values are calculated as a ratio of supination/pronation due to the loading principle of ulnar structures

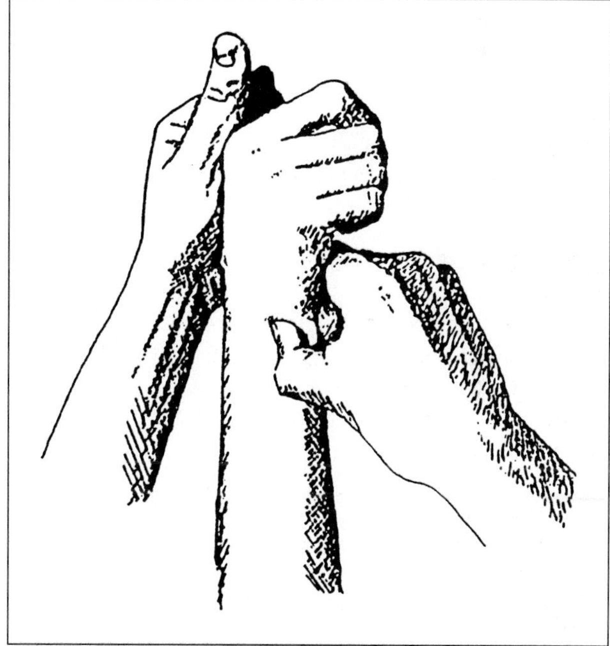

Fig. 3-14 ■ The *articular disc shear test* is a joint mobilization described by Hertling and Kessler (also known as the *ulnomeniscotriquetral dorsal glide*) and has been used as a provocative maneuver for assessing articular disc or triangular fibrocartilage pathology. The technique requires that the patient be seated or supine with the elbow resting on the tabletop and the forearm in a neutral vertical position. If the right wrist is to be inspected, the examiner's left hand stabilizes the patient's radius and hand while the examiner's right thumb is positioned dorsally over the head of the distal ulna. The examiner's radial side of the right index PIP joint is then placed over the palmar surface of the pisotriquetral complex. The examiner then squeezes the thumb and index finger together to produce a dorsal glide of the pisotriquetral complex on the distal ulnar head, thereby shearing the articular disc. A positive response to this test is a reproduction of the patient's painful symptoms and/or excessive laxity in the ulnomeniscotriquetral region. (From Hertling D, Kessler RM: *Management of common musculoskeletal disorders: physical therapy principles and methods,* Philadelphia, 1990, Lippincott.)

during grip with forearm rotation. If a patient has a GRIT ratio greater than 1.0 on the involved side and no greater than 1.0 on the un-involved side, the potential for a disc tear is high.

The standard TFCC load test (Fig. 3-15) can indicate either a peripheral or central lesion. However, the patient with a peripheral tear will likely have a history of trauma and/or instability noted at end range of supination and pronation.

Answer: **B**

Skirven, Osterman in Mackin, Callahan, Skirven, et al, p. 1108
LaStayo in Mackin, Callahan, Skirven, et al, pp. 1157, 1165-1167

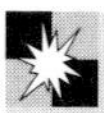

CLINICAL GEM:
Conservative management for articular disc tears that do not produce any DRU joint instability includes an ulnar gutter splint and education to avoid functional activities that require forearm pronation and gripping.

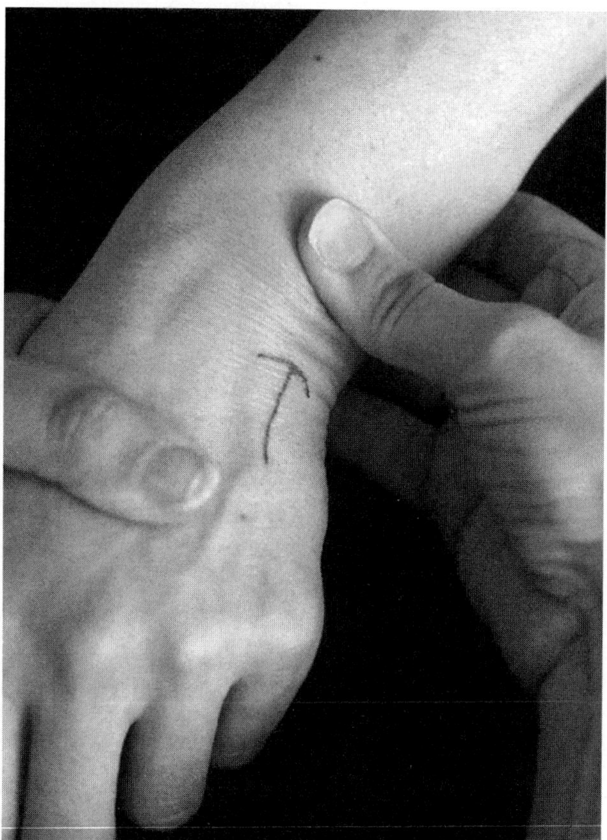

Fig. 3-15 ■ TFCC load test. Axial load, ulnar deviation, and rotation are applied to the wrist to detect a painful TFCC tear or ulnocarpal abutment. (From Mackin EJ, Callahan AD, Skirven TM, et al: *Rehabilitation of the hand and upper extremity*, ed 5, vol 1, St Louis, 2002, Mosby.)

37. The presence of axons in the process of regeneration can be detected by which of the following?

A. 256-Hz tuning fork
B. Phalen's sign
C. Iodine test
D. Tinel's sign

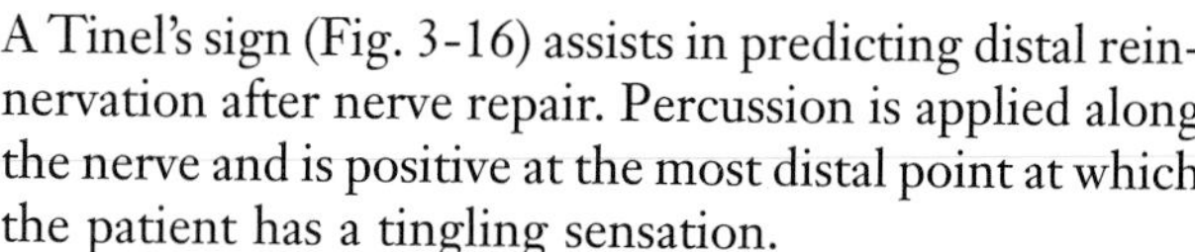

A Tinel's sign (Fig. 3-16) assists in predicting distal reinnervation after nerve repair. Percussion is applied along the nerve and is positive at the most distal point at which the patient has a tingling sensation.

A tuning fork is used for vibratory perception testing. The iodine assessment tests the sudomotor function of a nerve to assess sympathetic return. The Phalen's sign is a test performed to assist in the diagnosis of median nerve compression at the wrist.

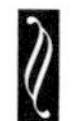

Answer: **D**

Clinical Assessment Recommendation, p. 71
Dellon, pp. 44-45

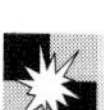

CLINICAL GEM:
Sensations during nerve regeneration may include sharp pain, shooting pain, hot and cold flashes, the sensation of water running down the arm, numbness, tingling, or no sensation at all.

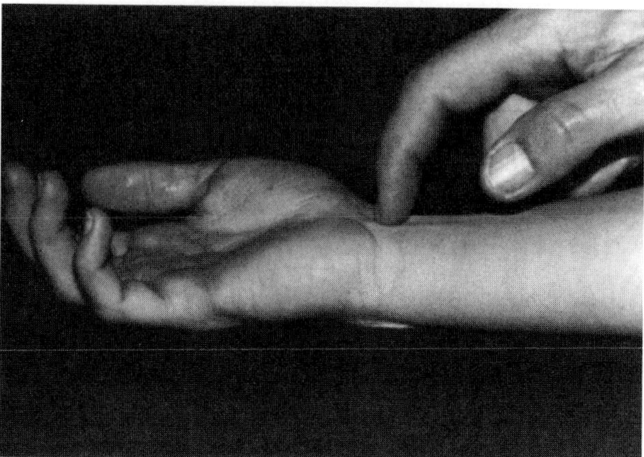

Fig. 3-16

38. A patient's primary care doctor is referred for an elbow contusion. The patient's onset of symptoms began after a blow to his flexed elbow with which he felt a pop and severe pain while playing in a football game. The patient presents with anterior pain at cubital fossa and upon MMT, 3+/5 for both supination and elbow flexion. The patient is tender at the cubital fossa and upon palpation of the biceps tendon. The patient's AROM is -20/125 (-indicates lack of full extension), and PROM is WNL but painful with elbow extension. X-rays were taken and are unremarkable; no numbness or tingling is noted. Circumferential measurements at the elbow crease are equal bilaterally. The likely diagnosis is which of the following?

A. Biceps tendon rupture
B. Partial biceps tendon tear
C. Ulnar nerve entrapment
D. Olecranon fracture

This patient likely incurred a partial biceps tendon tear because of the unexpected extension force to his elbow, pop felt, and weakness in elbow flexion and supination. In this case, the tendon is palpable and therefore not completely ruptured. No numbness or tingling indicates ulnar nerve entrapment, and an olecranon fracture would be visible by X-ray.

Answer: **B**
McAuliffe in Mackin, Callahan, Skirven, et al, p. 1208

Clinical Gem:
The bony landmarks of the elbow (i.e., medial and lateral epicondyles and the olecranon) should form an upside down triangle when the elbow is flexed and a straight line when the elbow is extended. Disruption of the triangle may indicate an elbow dislocation (Mackin, Callahan, Skirven, p. 1205).

Chapter 4

Neuroanatomy and Sensory Reeducation

1. The current approach to evaluating the success of decompression of a peripheral nerve requires which of the following?

A. Measurement of peripheral nerve function to permit staging of the degree of compression
B. Designing better questionnaires
C. Instructing therapists in telephone interview techniques
D. Alpha-, beta-, and meta-analyses

Outcome studies are in the forefront of analysis techniques to study the results of peripheral nerve decompression. Outcome is foremost determined by the initial stage of the nerve compression, and this requires preoperative measurements. Repeating these measurements after peripheral nerve surgery permits statistical analysis of results of the sensory and motor improvement by using a numerical grading scale and nonparametric statistics, thus permitting a different view of outcomes from the questionnaires. Meta-analysis is used to arrive at a conclusion from many studies of a single operation and is helped if all the patients in the studies have been staged preoperatively so that similar groups can be compared.

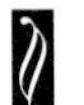
Answer: **A**
Dellon, pp. 229-240

2. A patient is evaluated for complaints of numbness in the thumb and index finger *after* a carpal tunnel decompression. Another nerve might be compressed causing the numbness. What is the compression site?

A. Deep head of the pronator teres or the lacertus fibrosis
B. Arcade of Froshe
C. Medial head of the triceps
D. Fascia between the brachioradialis and extensor carpi radialis longus

Compression of the radial sensory nerve in the distal third forearm can cause numbness in the index finger and thumb, but the numbness would occur on the **dorsal** surface of the thumb and index. The site of compression occurs where the nerve exits from subfascial to subcutaneous, between the brachioradialis and the extensor carpi radialis longus.

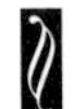
Answer: **D**
Dellon, Mackinnon, pp. 199-205

3. A 36-year-old female typist complains of numbness in the little and ring finger in both of her hands. On physical examination, her pinch and grip strength are normal, but she has increased cutaneous pressure threshold for static two-point discrimination at 3 mm. What would the most appropriate treatment be?

A. Ulnar nerve surgical decompression
B. Dynamic splinting at work
C. Night splinting with the elbow between 10 and 30 degrees of flexion
D. Three months of short-term disability

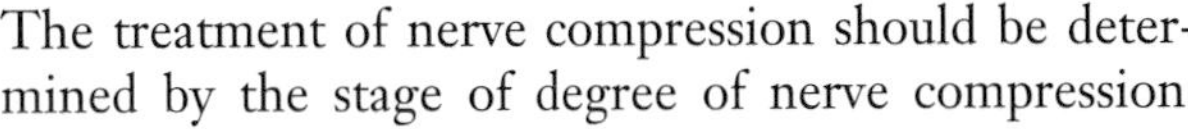

The treatment of nerve compression should be determined by the stage of degree of nerve compression.

Neurosensory and motor testing permit staging. If two-point discrimination is still normal and there is little weakness, the staging is "mild" in degree of compression, and nonoperative regimens should be used. Night splinting is a conservative treatment technique.

Answer: **C**
Dellon, 2000, pp. 127-136

4. A 36-year-old female typist complains of numbness in the little and ring finger in both of her hands. On physical examination, her pinch and grip strength are abnormal, but she has increased cutaneous pressure threshold for static two-point discrimination at <u>8 mm</u>. What would be the most appropriate treatment?

A. Submuscular ulnar nerve transposition
B. Dynamic splinting while at work
C. Night splinting with the elbow between 10 and 30 degrees of flexion
D. Three months of short-term disability

The treatment of nerve compression should be determined by the stage of degree of nerve compression. Neurosensory and motor testing permit staging. If two-point discrimination is abnormal, **axonal loss** has occurred, and according to Dellon, the degree of compression is too advanced for conservative treatment, thus indicating surgical intervention. The surgical intervention in this case is a submuscular ulnar nerve transposition.

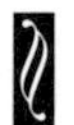

Answer: **A**
Dellon, 2000, pp. 127-136

5. Which sensory receptor is responsible for detecting a sensation of a gentle breeze blowing against the skin?

A. Ruffini end organs
B. Pacinian corpuscle
C. Merkel cell
D. None of the above

The Pacinian corpuscle is a sensory receptor that is innervated by a single, quickly adapting nerve fiber. The Pacinian corpuscle is large and located in subcutaneous tissue. It is extremely sensitive to mechanical stimuli and therefore is responsible for detecting a very gentle breeze blowing across the skin.

Answer: **B**
Dellon, 1997, p. 20
Refer to Fig. 4-1

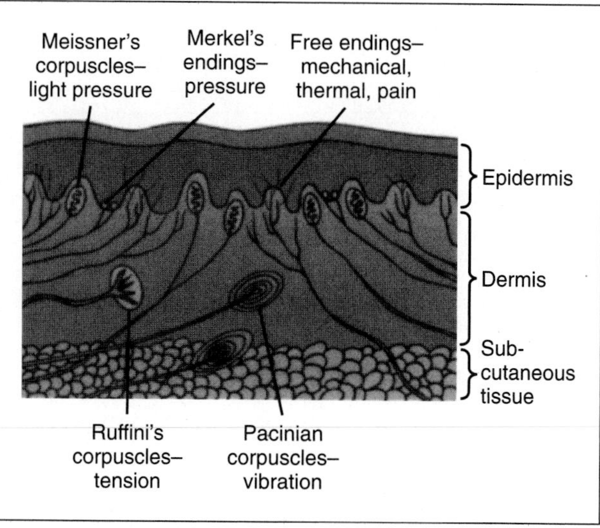

Fig. 4-1 ■ From Lindsay DT: *Functional human anatomy,* St Louis, 1996, Mosby.

6. 30-Hertz vibration is perceived by which of the following?

A. Slowly adapting Ruffini end organs
B. Quickly adapting Meissner corpuscles
C. Quickly adapting Pacinian corpuscles
D. Slowly adapting Merkel cells

30 Hertz (Hz) vibration and movement are perceived by quickly adapting A-ß fibers known as *Meissner corpuscles.* 256-Hz vibration and movement are perceived by the quickly adapting A-ß fibers known as *Pacinian corpuscles.* Both receptors are found in glabrous (non-hairy) skin and are encapsulated (see Fig. 4-1).

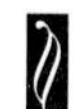

Answer: **B**
Dellon, 1997, pp. 10, 11

7. Constant-touch pressure is perceived by which of the following?

A. Large myelinated A-β fibers slowly adapting
B. Large myelinated A-β fibers quickly adapting
C. Large myelinated A-d fibers quickly adapting
D. Large myelinated A-a fibers slowly adapting

A-ß fibers are called *neuroreceptive afferents,* which may be either slowly or quickly adapting nerve fibers. Constant-touch pressure is perceived by slowly adapting, large, myelinated A-ß fibers. Constant touch is perceived by the Merkel cells found in the glabrous skin and the Ruffini end organs in hairy skin.

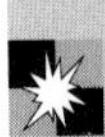
Answer: **A**
Dellon, p. 10

CLINICAL GEM:
The following is a quick reference chart to correlate receptors, functions, and applicable tests:

Specialized receptors	Functions	Applicable tests
Merkel cell	Constant-touch pressure	Semmes-Weinstein monofilament Static two-point discrimination Tuning fork
Pacinian corpuscle	256-Hertz Movement and vibration	Tuning fork
Meissner corpuscle	30-Hertz Movement and vibration	Tuning fork Moving two-point discrimination

8. Which of the following types of sequential neurosensory testing determines the earliest sign of nerve compression?

A. Cutaneous thermal threshold
B. Cutaneous pressure threshold for one-point static touch with nylon monofilaments with Seems Weinstein monofilament (SWM)
C. Cutaneous vibratory threshold
D. Cutaneous pressure threshold for static two-point discrimination with pressure-specified sensory device (PSSD)

Thermal thresholds are the last to change with nerve compression, whereas those for pressure and touch are the earliest to change. In a regression analysis with a neurosensory device that measures the pressure required to discriminate one from two static touch stimuli, the earliest sign of nerve compression was determined to be the change in the threshold for static two-point discrimination.

Answer: **D**
Dellon, 1999, pp. 697-715

9. You are treating a 41-year-old woman who sustained a median nerve injury at the wrist level. A nerve repair was performed. The patient's repair was protected for 3 weeks; next, range of motion and early sensory reeducation were initiated. You would like to progress to object recognition or late-phase sensory reeducation. Which would be the best screening test for determining whether your patient is ready to start late-phase reeducation?

A. Perception of pinprick
B. 256-Hertz vibration
C. Detection of hot or cold
D. 30-Hertz vibration

The recovery sequence begins with pain and temperature because these sensations are perceived through unmyelinated and thinly myelinated fibers. Next, the large myelinated fibers begin to receive 30 Hz by the Meissner corpuscles, which are easy to reinnervate because any of the nine different nerves may innervate this receptor from any direction. After this, moving touch is perceived, followed by constant touch. Next, a 256-Hz stimulus is perceived by means of a single, quickly adapting nerve fiber, which can enter through either end of the large, football-shaped Pacinian corpuscle. When your patient can detect 256 Hz, she is ready for object recognition or late-phase reeducation. If you begin object recognition before the detection of 256 Hz, it will most likely be uneventful, and you and the patient will become frustrated.

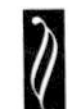
Answer: **B**
Dellon, 1997, pp. 20, 249-250, 262

CLINICAL GEM:
The following is a quick reference list of the order of sensory return.

- Pain and temperature
- 30-Hz vibration
- Moving touch
- Constant touch
- 256-Hz vibration
- Touch localization
- Two-point discrimination
- Stereognosis

10. After an anterolateral surgical approach to the forearm, a patient experiences numbness on the lateral (radial) aspect of his forearm. Which structure is most likely affected?

A. Anterior interosseous nerve
B. Axillary nerve
C. Posterior interosseous nerve
D. Lateral antebrachial cutaneous nerve

The lateral antebrachial cutaneous nerve crosses the elbow and enters the forearm between the biceps and the brachialis. This nerve is at risk in the anterolateral and anterior surgical approaches to the forearm.

Answer: **D**
Hoppenfeld, de Boer, pp. 93, 96
Refer to Fig. 4-2

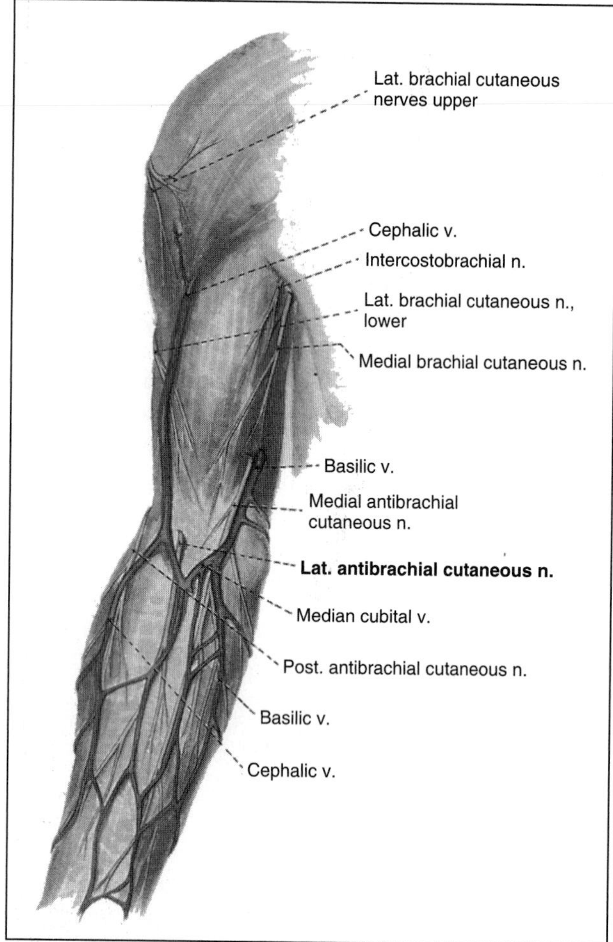

Fig. 4-2 ■ From Mackin EJ, Callahan AD, Skirven TM, et al: *Rehabilitation of the hand and upper extremity*, ed 5, vol 1, St Louis, 2002, Mosby.

11. A 42-year-old man complains that his hands have become weak, and as an auto mechanic he has burned and sometimes cut his fingertips without knowing it until he looked at his fingers. On physical examination, he has intrinsic muscle weakness, and some wasting of the first dorsal interosseous, with normal two-point discrimination in his index and little fingers. What is his most likely diagnosis?

A. Cervical stenosis
B. Peripheral neuropathy, small fiber type
C. Bilateral carpal and cubital tunnel syndrome
D. Syrinx

A syrinx is a cyst in the spinal canal. It usually grows anteriorly. The posterior long tracts, which transmit perception of touch and pressure, are preserved. The ventral motor neurons are damaged early, resulting in intrinsic muscle wasting when the syrinx is located in the cervical spine region. The anterolateral spinal thalamic tracts are usually damaged early in the course of this process, giving deficits in the perception of pain and temperature.

Answer: **D**
Dellon, 1997, pp. 10-15

12. A 30-year-old man presents with inability to flex the tip of the thumb and index finger. Physical examination also identifies weakness in the deltoid. He has no history of injury; rather, the onset was sudden and associated with pain in the shoulder. He can recall working out in the gym the week before symptoms occurred. What is his likely diagnosis?

A. Anterior interosseous nerve (AIN) syndrome
B. Quadrangular space syndrome
C. Schwanoma, upper trunk of brachial plexus
D. Parsonage-Turner syndrome

Anterior interosseous nerve palsy occurs most often in the setting of trauma, or comes on slowly with no history of pain. Additionally, AIN syndrome has no correlation with shoulder pain. When the onset of palsy is rapid and is associated with pain but no trauma, an inflammatory plexopathy such as Parsonage-Turner syndrome must be considered. Electrodiagnostic testing is crucial to document a "spotty" pattern of plexus muscle involvement. The natural history is most often spontaneous resolution.

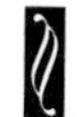
Answer: **D**
Wong, Dellon, pp. 536-539

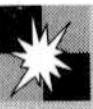

Clinical Gem:
A group of lesions, categorized as idiopathic or cryptogenic brachial plexus neuritis, actually presents a spontaneous entrapment in the brachial plexus. Many of these lesions fall into the category of what Spinner called the *Parsonage-Turner syndrome* (Rockwood, Matsen, p. 143).

13. A 21-year-old wrestler has pain in his anterior shoulder after having a shoulder arthroscopy approach to repair his rotator cuff. His range of shoulder motion is limited by anterior shoulder pain. He can localize the pain to the site of the arthroscopy portal anteriorly. What is his most likely diagnosis?

A. Axillary nerve injury, cutaneous branch
B. Neuroma supraclavicular nerve
C. Bursitis
D. Acromioclavicular impingement

The supraclavicular nerve, from C3-C5, innervates the region of the anterior shoulder skin that is often the site for orthopedic surgery intervention. A painful scar can be caused by a neuroma of these little nerve branches. The sensory portion of the axillary nerve innervates the lateral deltoid region.

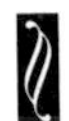

Answer: **B**
Mackinnon, Dellon, p. 68

14. True or False: Pain receptors are in encapsulated cells.

Pain and temperature are perceived by free nerve endings. Receptors for pain and temperature are located on our body surface area through the skin. Pain and temperature receptors are thinly myelinated A-d fibers and unmyelinated C fibers, which conduct at a slow rate compared with the encapsulated cells such as A-β sensory and A-a motor fibers, which are thickly myelinated.

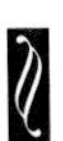

Answer: **False**
Dellon, 1997, pp. 6, 9-13

15. In what is the cell body of the sensory neuron located?

A. Spinal cord
B. Dorsal root ganglion
C. Brain
D. A and B are correct
E. All are correct

The most basic unit of the nervous system is the neuron. The neuron is the functional and structural unit that initiates and conducts impulses. In the peripheral nervous system, there are motor and sensory neurons. The cell body of the motor neuron is located in the ventral horn of the spinal cord. The cell body of the sensory neuron is located in the dorsal root ganglion, outside the central nervous system. The sensory neuron's axon extends to skin.

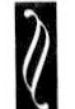

Answer: **B**
Dellon, 1997, p. 2
Refer to Fig. 4-3

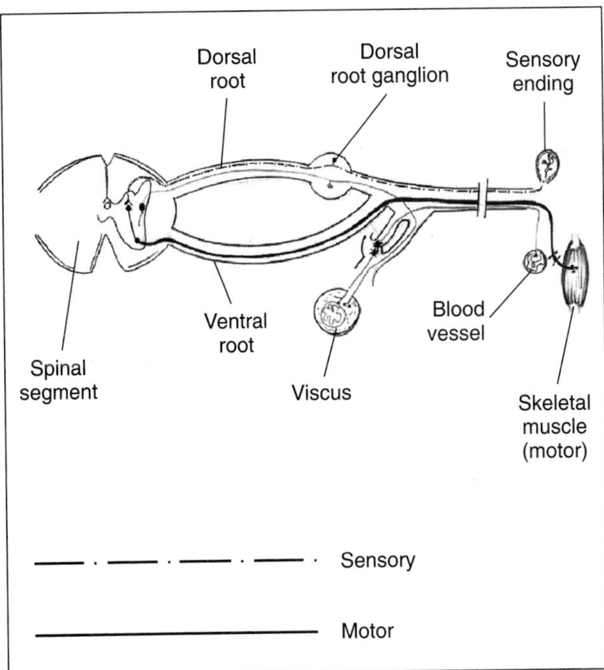

Fig. 4-3

16. True or False: Schwann cells are located in the central nervous system.

Schwann cells are located in the peripheral nervous system and create the myelin sheath around the axon. For axons to conduct fast impulses, an insulation or myelin is required. Myelin is a lipoprotein. The slower conducting axons within the peripheral nervous system are not myelinated. Schwann cells serve an extremely important functional role for the peripheral nervous system. They make nerve growth factor, which enables the peripheral nerve to regenerate. The central nervous system does not have Schwann cells; the analogous cells in this system are oligodendrocytes and astroglia.

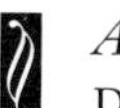

Answer: **False**
Dellon, 1997, p. 4

17. Match Sunderland's five numerical classifications of peripheral nerve injury with their definitions.

Degree

1. First
2. Second
3. Third
4. Fourth
5. Fifth

Definition

A. Transection of the entire trunk
B. Local conduction block with minimal structural disruption
C. Disruption of the axon, endoneurium, and perineurium. The epineural tissue is spared.
D. Disruption of axon only, leaving the endoneurium intact; a neuroma-in-continuity
E. An intact perineurium surrounding a disruption of the axon and endoneurium

Answers: **1, B; 2, D; 3, E; 4, C; 5, A**
Skirven, Callahan in Mackin, Callahan, Skirven, et al, p. 601
Butler, p. 176

18. True or False: The epineurium surrounds the entire nerve.

A nerve is composed of nerve fibers bound together in bundles or fascicles. The perineurium is the connective tissue layer surrounding the fascicle. The endoneurium is the space within the fascicle. The internal (interfascicular) epineurium is the connective tissue lying between the fascicles facilitating gliding. The structure that surrounds the entire nerve is called the *external epineurium.*

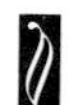

Answer: **True**
Dellon, 1997, p. 6
Brushart in Green, Hotchkiss, Pederson, p. 1382
Butler, p. 8
Refer to Fig. 4-4

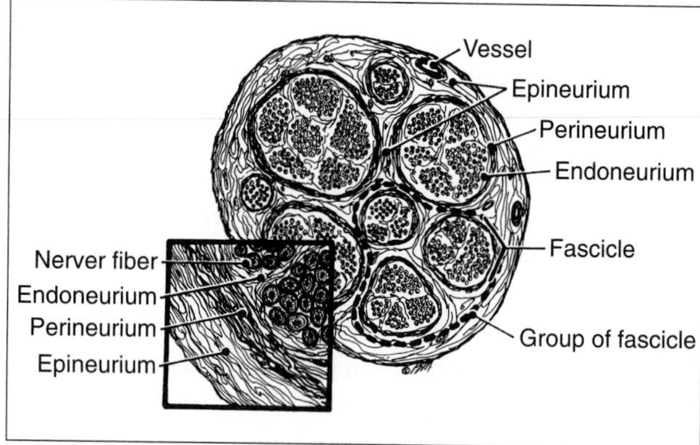

Fig. 4-4 ■ Cross-section of normal peripheral nerve. Peripheral nerve fibrosis of the epineurium constricts the nerve anatomy and metabolism of the axon flow, thus resulting in altered functional and sensory patterns. ■ (Copyright, Elizabeth Roselius, 1993. From Wilgis EFS, Brushart TM: Nerve repair and grafting. In Green DP, Hotchkiss RN, eds: *Operative hand surgery,* vol 2, ed 3, New York, 1993, Churchill Livingstone. Used with permission.)

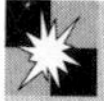

CLINICAL GEM:
The fascicle is the smallest unit of nerve structure that can be manipulated surgically.

19. The perineurium has the following function:

A. Protects the contents of the endoneural tubes
B. Surrounds each fascicle
C. Acts as a diffusion barrier
D. All of the above

The perineurium is a strong, elastic tissue that surrounds each fascicle and protects the contents of the endoneural tubes. It has an important role as a diffusion barrier. The perineurium aids in keeping certain substances out of the intrafascicular environment (see Fig. 4-4).

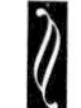

Answer: **D**
Butler, pp. 8, 23-24

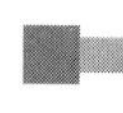

20. Match the medical terminology with the sympathetic function for that term.

Terminology

1. Vasomotor
2. Sudomotor
3. Pilomotor
4. Trophic

Sympathetic Function

A. Gooseflesh response
B. Hair growth and nail changes
C. Skin color and skin temperature changes
D. Sweat

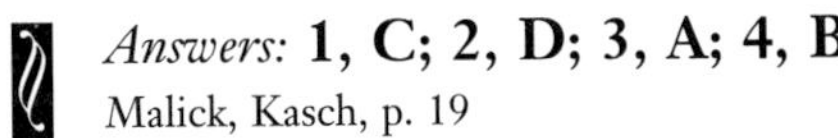

Answers: **1, C; 2, D; 3, A; 4, B**
Malick, Kasch, p. 19

21. How does the median nerve usually enter the forearm?

A. Superficial to the lacertus fibrosis
B. Between the two heads of the supinator
C. Between the two heads of the pronator teres
D. Posterior to the brachial artery

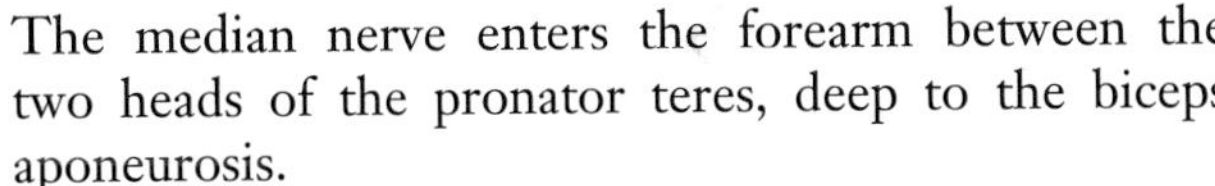

The median nerve enters the forearm between the two heads of the pronator teres, deep to the biceps aponeurosis.

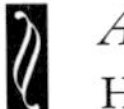

Answer: **C**
Hoppenfeld, de Boer, p. 121

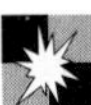

CLINICAL GEM:
Each major peripheral nerve enters the forearm through a two-headed muscle: the median nerve enters through the pronator teres, the radial nerve through the supinator, and the ulnar nerve through the flexor carpi ulnaris.

22. One year after a carpal tunnel decompression, a 50-year-old woman is still complaining of numbness in the thumb and index finger. Her scar is not tender. She has an increased cutaneous pressure threshold in the volar base of the thumb and thenar eminence. She also has abnormal sensibility in her index finger and thumb. What is her most likely diagnosis?

A. Recurrent carpal tunnel syndrome
B. Radial sensory nerve compression
C. Pronator syndrome
D. C7 Radiciculopathy

With the pronator syndrome, there is compression of the median nerve proximal to the wrist. The palmar cutaneous branch of the median nerve arises proximal to the wrist, and it innervates the base of the volar thumb and the thenar eminence. Abnormal sensibility will occur at the base of the thumb and thenar eminence **only** when the compression site is proximal to the wrist due to pathology of the palmar cutaneous branch. Palmar cutaneous branch injury can occur when this branch has been cut by the surgeon's carpal tunnel incision.

Answer: **C**
Rosenberg, Conolley, Dellon, 2001, pp. 258-265

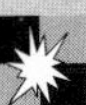

CLINICAL GEM:
A quick way to rule out carpal tunnel syndrome is to assess the thenar eminence. If the sensation is impaired in this area, carpal tunnel is ruled out. The palmar cutaneous branch branches off the main nerve (median nerve) before it passes below the retinaculum, resulting in impaired sensation in the thenar eminence with proximal compression such as in pronator syndrome.

23. After ulnar nerve transposition, the patient complains of pain in the medial aspect of the elbow. On examination, the little and ring finger have normal sensibility, but the skin around the incision is dysesthetic and has a painful trigger point. The most likely cause for these observations is which of the following?

A. Recurrent ulnar nerve compression
B. Injury to the ulnar nerve
C. Neuroma of the palmar cutaneous branch of the median nerve
D. Neuroma of the medial antebrachial cutaneous nerve

The medial antebrachial cutaneous nerve has a posterior branch, which crosses the site for the incisions used for most ulnar nerve transpositions. A painful scar after this surgery must be considered as having a neuroma of this nerve. If the little and ring finger are also numb, recurrent ulnar nerve compression may also be present, as the medial antebrachial cutaneous nerve does not go to the little and ring finger.

Answer: **D**
Dellon, 2002, pp. 158-160
Refer to Fig. 4-2

24. A woman sustains an electrical injury while cleaning her living room rug with a rented rug washing machine. The electric shock knocks her to the floor and leaves her right arm tingling. This tingling persists for 3 months and disturbs her sleep, and her hand becomes clumsy. She most likely has which of the following?

A. Reflex sympathetic dystrophy
B. Cervical disc injury at C6, C7, and C8
C. Compression of the median and ulnar nerve
D. Thoracic outlet syndrome

Electrical energy travels through the body by the line of least resistance, usually muscle and blood vessels. At the wrist and elbow, there is little muscle mass, and the resistance increases, which means there is increased heat energy at these locations. This places the medial and ulnar nerves at risk for compression.

Answer: **C**
Smith, Muehlberger, Dellon, pp. 137-144

25. When you put on a pair of gloves, which receptor perceives stimuli until the glove is removed?

A. Merkel cells
B. Meissner corpuscles
C. Free nerve endings
D. Pacinian corpuscles

The large, myelinated, A-β slowly adapting fibers perceive the constant touch of your gloves. The Merkel cells begin to transmit impulses immediately and continue to transmit them until you remove the gloves.

Answer: **A**
Dellon, 1997, p. 10

26. A 29-year-old woman who is a professional flute player is referred to you for evaluation and treatment. Her complaints range from aching shoulders to coldness and numbness in the whole hand and occasional tingling in the little and ring fingers. The evaluation reveals no intrinsic wasting. The referring physician has ruled out carpal tunnel syndrome, cubital tunnel syndrome, tumors, temporomandibular joint pathology, and cervical disc disease. Which exercise program would you choose?

A. Stretching the wrist and elbow muscles and strengthening the pectoralis minor and scalene muscles
B. Stretching the middle and lower trapezius and strengthening the pectoralis major and minor muscles
C. Stretching the pectoralis minor, upper trapezius, and scalene muscles and strengthening the middle and lower trapezius, serratus anterior, and levator scapulae muscles
D. A and B
E. B and C

After careful examination and discussion with the referring physician, you would conclude that this patient has thoracic outlet syndrome. If the term "thoracic outlet" is taken literally, confusion may occur. Some authors and clinicians refer to thoracic outlet syndrome as brachial plexus compression in the thoracic inlet; thoracic outlet syndrome, by name, implies that the diaphragm is restricted because the thoracic outlet is the region between the thorax and the abdomen.

Thoracic outlet syndrome is accepted among surgeons and neurologists in the following two situations: 1) when the patient presents with a cervical rib, which can cause either subclavian artery or vein occlusion; or 2) when the patient presents with intrinsic muscle wasting and numbness of the little finger. The latter is confirmed with electromyography. These two conditions are uncommon and require surgical intervention. Fortunately, the majority of cases do not fall into these categories and can be managed conservatively.

In this case study, the therapist should observe the patient playing her flute, adjust her practice schedule, change her positioning, and teach exercises to strengthen the patient's shoulder girdle muscles and to relax or stretch the other musculature. The therapist should design a program to strengthen the middle and lower trapezius, serratus anterior, and levator muscles while stretching or relaxing the pectoralis minor, upper trapezius, and scalene muscles. One way to stretch the pectoralis minor and strengthen the serratus is to perform wall push-ups while facing a corner, using both walls.

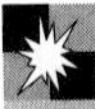

Answer: **C**
Dellon, 1997, pp. 506-539

CLINICAL GEM:
A helpful reference book to recommend to musicians with musculoskeletal pathologies is Richard Norris: *The Musician's Survival Manual: A Guide to Preventing and Treating Injuries in Instrumentalists,* St Louis, 1993, International Conference of Symphony and Opera Musicians.

27. True or False: The concentration of potassium is higher on the inside of a cell in normal muscle and nerve tissue.

To understand the physiology of normal cell excitability, it is important to understand active and passive diffusion through the cell membrane. Muscle and nerve cells are encased in a membrane that separates a charge from the inside and the outside of a cell. This charge has a resting membrane state of approximately −60 millivolts (MV). The inside of the cell is negative in comparison to the outside of the cell. In normal muscle and nerve tissue, potassium (K^+) ions are higher on the inside of the cell, and sodium (Na^+) is higher on the outside of the cell.

The concentration differences are maintained by an active pump across the membrane. This pump helps the cell eliminate sodium ions while receiving potassium ions. In addition, a passive diffusion of ions across the membrane attempts to equalize the ion concentration.

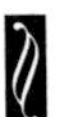

Answer: **True**
Hunter, Mackin, Callahan, pp. 1508-1509
Refer to Fig. 4-5

28. A 32-year-old male sustained a median nerve laceration at the level of the elbow 6 months ago. The nerve was repaired. Manual muscle testing revealed a 4+/5 for the pronator teres and a 3/5 for the flexor digitorum superficialis. Which muscle would you expect to return next?

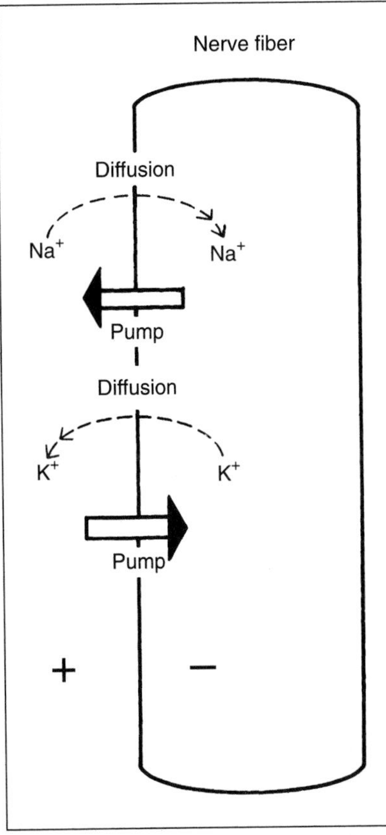

Fig. 4-5 ■ From Hunter JM, Mackin EJ, Callahan AD: *Rehabilitation of the hand: surgery and therapy,* ed 4, St Louis, 1995, Mosby.

A. Flexor digitorum profundus to the first and second digits
B. Flexor digitorum profundus to the second and third digits
C. Pronator quadratus
D. Palmaris longus
E. Palmaris brevis

The median nerve (Fig. 4-6, *B*) arises from the lateral cord (C6, C7) and the medial cord (C8, T1) of the brachial plexus. The median nerve enters the forearm between the two heads of the pronator teres, innervating them, and then innervates the flexor carpi radialis. The next muscle innervated along the course of the median nerve is the palmaris longus, followed by the flexor digitorum superficialis, the flexor digitorum profundus to the index and middle finger (second and third digits), the flexor pollicis longus, and the pronator quadratus. The first muscle that the nerve innervates after crossing the wrist is the abductor pollicis brevis, followed by the opponens pollicis and the flexor pollicis brevis; the nerve terminates in the first and second

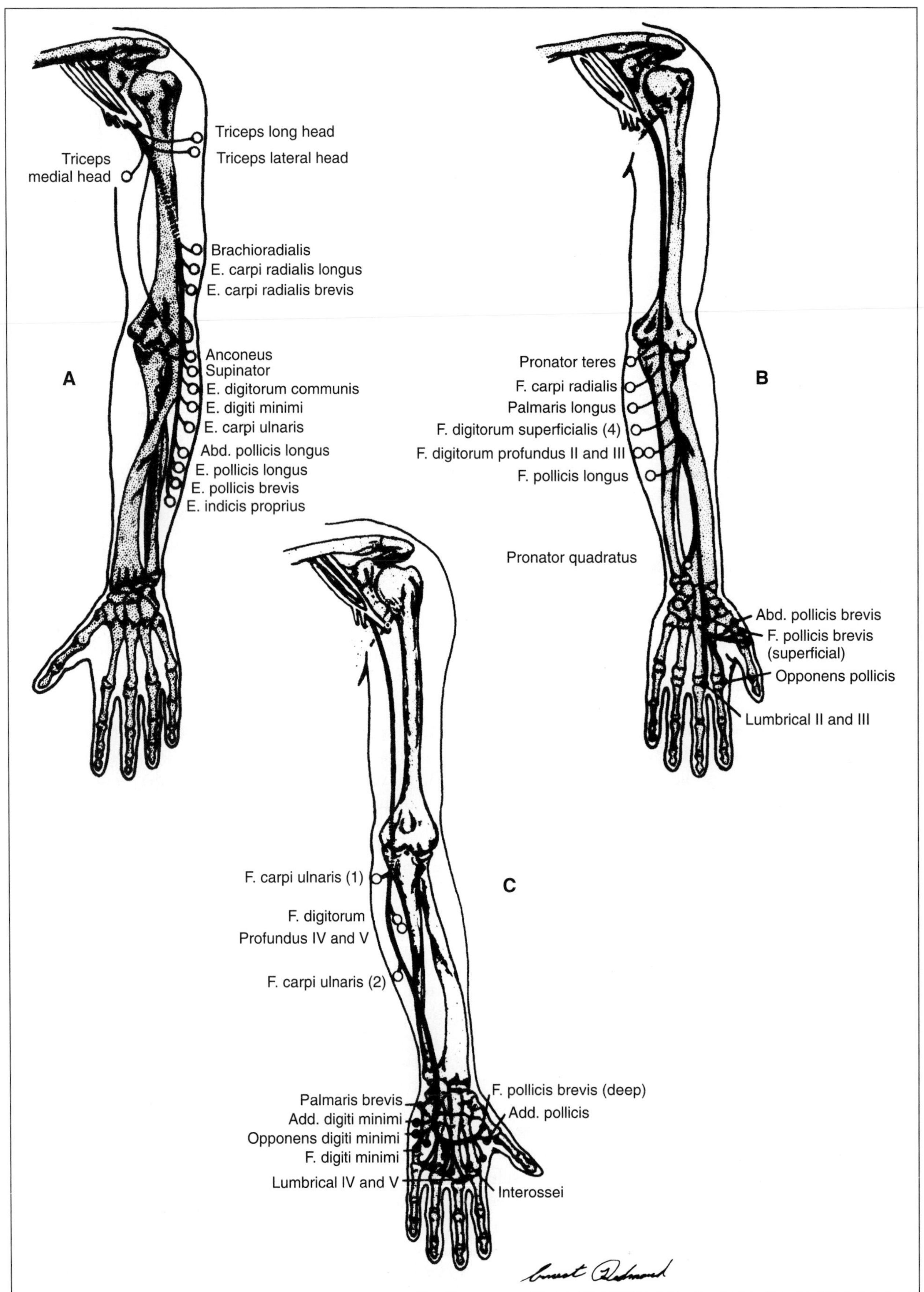

Fig. 4-6 ■ Terminal branches of the **(A)** radial, **(B)** median, and **(C)** ulnar nerves. (Redrawn from the American Society for Surgery of the Hand: *The hand, examination and diagnosis*, Aurora, CO, 1978, The Society.)

lumbricals. Answer A, the first and second digits, refers to the thumb and index fingers.

Answer: **B**

Hunter, Mackin, Callahan, pp. 70, 765
Aulicino in Mackin, Callahan, Skirven, et al, p. 137
Skirven, Callahan in Mackin, Callahan, Skirven, et al, p. 605
Colditz in Mackin, Callahan, Skirven, et al, p. 630

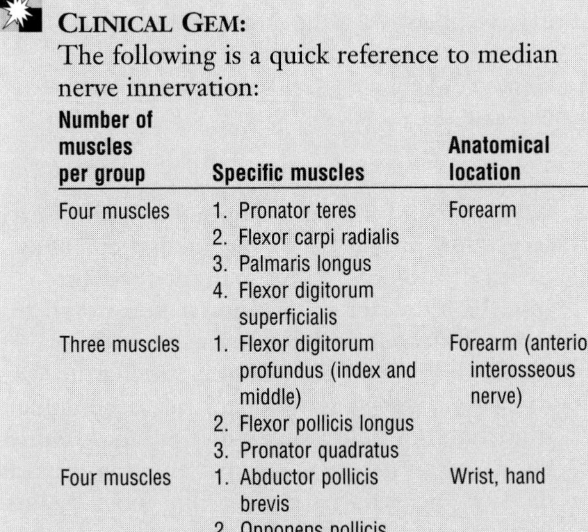

Clinical Gem:

The following is a quick reference to median nerve innervation:

Number of muscles per group	Specific muscles	Anatomical location
Four muscles	1. Pronator teres 2. Flexor carpi radialis 3. Palmaris longus 4. Flexor digitorum superficialis	Forearm
Three muscles	1. Flexor digitorum profundus (index and middle) 2. Flexor pollicis longus 3. Pronator quadratus	Forearm (anterior interosseous nerve)
Four muscles	1. Abductor pollicis brevis 2. Opponens pollicis 3. Flexor pollicis brevis 4. Lumbricals (one and two)	Wrist, hand

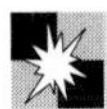

Clinical Gem:

At the mid-forearm, the median nerve branches into the AIN. The AIN innervates the flexor digitorum profundus to the index and middle fingers, the flexor pollicis longus, and the pronator quadratus, and then innervates the volar wrist capsule. When the AIN is damaged, a patient cannot form an O with the thumb and index fingers (see Fig. 18-23).

29. An 18-year-old male sustained an injury to the posterior cord of the brachial plexus. Initially, return of the triceps was observed. Eight months later the patient is able to radially deviate his wrist and slight forearm supination is observed. Which muscle would you expect to return next?

A. Brachioradialis
B. Extensor carpi ulnaris
C. Extensor digitorum communis
D. Extensor indicis

The radial nerve is a continuation of the posterior cord of the brachial plexus. Its roots emerge from C6, C7, C8, and T1 levels. The radial nerve innervates the triceps, anconeus, and brachioradialis as it winds posteriorly on the humerus. Next, the motor branch innervates the extensor carpi radialis longus and extensor carpi radialis brevis and enters the forearm between the two heads of the supinator. At this point, the motor and sensory nerves divide into the superficial sensory branch and the deep branch. There is controversy as to when the radial nerve becomes termed the posterior interosseous nerve (PIN). In about 55% of extremities, the radial nerve supplies the extensor carpi radialis brevis; in the other 45%, the extensor carpi radialis brevis is supplied by the PIN. The PIN supplies the supinator, extensor digitorum communis, extensor digiti minimi, extensor carpi ulnaris, abductor pollicis longus, extensor pollicis longus, extensor pollicis brevis, and extensor indicis proprius (see Fig. 4-6, *A*).

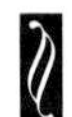

Answer: **C**

Tubiana, Thomine, Mackin, p. 266
Aulicino in Mackin, Callahan, Skirven, et al, p. 137
Colditz in Mackin, Callahan, Skirven, et al, p. 630

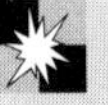

Clinical Gem:

The following is a quick reference to radial nerve innervation:

Muscle	Nerve
Triceps	Radial nerve
Anconeus	
Brachioradialis	
Extensor carpi radialis longus	
Extensor carpi radialis brevis	Radial nerve or posterior interosseous nerve
Supinator	Posterior interosseous nerve
Extensor digitorum communis	
Extensor digiti minimi	
Extensor carpi ulnaris	
Abductor pollicis longus	
Extensor pollicis longus	
Extensor pollicis brevis	
Extensor indicis proprius	

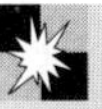

Clinical Gem:

With respect to nerve innervation order, some authors place the anconeus muscle after the triceps and others place it after the extensor carpi radialis brevis.

30. A patient with Type II diabetes complains of numbness in the right thumb, index, and middle finger, and has night-time awakening. Early thenar wasting is present, and static two-point discrimination is 8 mm in the thumb. The most likely diagnosis is which of the following?

A. Diabetic neuropathy only
B. Diabetic neuropathy with carpal tunnel syndrome
C. Diabetic neuropathy with ulnar nerve compression
D. Carpal tunnel

Carpal tunnel syndrome is present in more than 20% of diabetics with neuropathy. When neuropathy is present, there is a symmetrical sensory change in all fingers of both hands. When there is asymmetry in either ulnar versus median or left versus right, and a positive Tinel sign is present, it is likely that a superimposed nerve compression exists in the patient with diabetes.

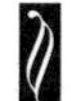
Answer: **B**
Aszmann, Kress, Dellon, pp. 816-822

31. After a nerve repair at the wrist, the best way to evaluate early success of the surgery and whether reoperation and nerve grafting are indicated is to do which of the following?

A. Electromyography (EMG)
B. Nerve conduction velocity studies
C. Neurosensory testing
D. Distal latency with inching technique

Traditional electrodiagnostic studies are painful to most patients, while neurosensory testing is not. For this reason alone, neurosensory testing should be the method of choice. Remyelination is never complete after a nerve repair and is not a good indication. Sensory recovery occurs before motor recovery, and so tests of motor latency and EMG will lag behind those of cutaneous pressure measurements.

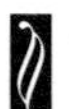
Answer: **C**
Cohen, Dellon, pp. 501-505

32. During sensory nerve regeneration, the first large fiber (group A-β) sensation to recover is that of movement. Which of the following tests of sensibility *cannot* measure this perception threshold?

A. Nylon monofilament (SWM)
B. Pressure-Specified Sensory Device (PSSD)
C. Tuning fork at 30 Hz
D. Stroking the fingertip pulp with examiner's finger

The nylon monofilament is designed to flex at a certain force and is held still while that force is applied and does not assess perception of movement. Vibration and stroking the fingertip pulp stimulates the quickly adapting fibers that transmit perception of movement. The PSSD can measure both one point moving threshold, which is the first perception to occur after a nerve repair, and moving two-point discrimination, which recovers later in the course of nerve regeneration, as more nerve fibers reach the target skin territory.

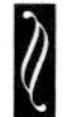
Answer: **A**
Cohen, Dellon, pp. 501-505
Refer to Fig. 4-7

33. A 56-year-old woman sustained an ulnar nerve laceration just distal to the medial epicondyle of the humerus. The patient presented 2 months after her initial injury. You noted full wrist flexion and ulnar deviation with gravity eliminated. The patient was unable to flex the wrist against gravity, and no other ulnar-innervated muscles were functioning. A month later you note that the patient can ulnarly deviate the wrist and flex the wrist against gravity and can tolerate minimal resistance. Knowing the course of the ulnar nerve, which function/motion would indicate that the ulnar nerve is regenerating?

A. Having the patient spread the fingers apart
B. Having the patient bring fingers back together
C. Having the patient perform a hook fist
D. Having the patient pinch a piece of paper

The ulnar nerve arises from the medial cord of the brachial plexus. Its roots emerge from C7, C8, and T1. The ulnar nerve does not innervate any part of the upper extremity until it crosses the elbow and enters the forearm between the two heads of the flexor carpi ulnaris, followed by the flexor digitorum profundus to the fourth and fifth digits. If your patient is able to perform a hook fist (flexing the tips of the fingers), this would indicate regeneration of the ulnar nerve to the flexor digitorum profundus.

The ulnar nerve then crosses the wrist and innervates the following: the abductor digiti minimi, the opponens digiti minimi, the flexor digiti minimi, the third and fourth lumbricals, the palmar interossei, the dorsal interossei, the deep head of the flexor pollicis brevis, and the adductor pollicis. The order of innervation after the ulnar nerve crosses the wrist varies according to different authors (see Fig. 4-6, *C*).

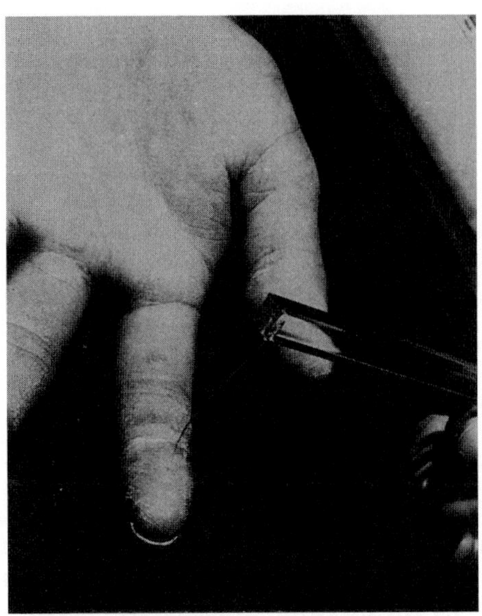

Fig. 4-7 ■ From Hunter JM, Schneider LH, Mackin EJ, et al: *Rehabilitation of the hand,* St Louis, 1978, Mosby.

Answer: **C**
Tubiana, Thomine, Mackin, p. 275
Hunter, Mackin, Callahan, p. 70
Aulicino in Mackin, Callahan, Skirven, et al, p. 137
Colditz in Mackin, Callahan, Skirven, et al, pp. 624-626

CLINICAL GEM:
The following is a quick reference to ulnar nerve innervation:

Flexor carpi ulnaris Flexor digitorum profundus (fourth and fifth digits)	Forearm
Abductor digiti minimi	Wrist and hand muscle (order varies)
Opponens digiti minimi	NOTE: Hunter, Mackin, and Callahan
Flexor digiti minimi	indicate that the first dorsal interosseus
Lumbricals (three and four)	is the last muscle to be innervated.
Interossei (palmar and dorsal) Flexor pollicis brevis (deep) Adductor pollicis	

34. Which of the following potential testing modalities is the first to recover after a nerve repair?

A. One-point static touch
B. One-point moving touch
C. Two-point static touch
D. Two-point moving touch

After recovery of pain and temperature perception, which is caused by the small unmyelinated and small myelinated fibers, large fiber regeneration occurs. The first perception to recover is that of one-point moving touch, then one-point static touch, then two-point moving touch, and finally two-point static touch.

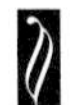

Answer: **B**
Cohen, Dellon, pp. 501-505

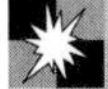

CLINICAL GEM:
According to Dellon's studies, the first parameter to become abnormal with chronic nerve compression is the pressure threshold for static two-point discrimination.

35. At about 6 months after median nerve reconstruction with a neural conduit at the level of the wrist, the patient complains of aching and pain in the palm and hand. The scar, however, is not tender. Which of the following nerve conduits would require removal because it is the likely cause of nerve compression?

A. Vein
B. Silicone tube
C. Neurotube (polyglycolic acid, bioabsorbable)
D. Muscle

Silicone tubes used as conduits are not absorbed; they are permanent. Silicone tubes can become a source of nerve compression and indeed in experimental models are used to create nerve compression. Bioabsorbable nerve conduits such as the polyglycolic acid neurotube are absorbed and cannot cause nerve compression. Compression of nerve by vein and muscle has not been reported to date.

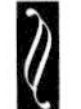

Answer: **B**
Dellon, 1994, pp. 271-272

36. The presence of an ipsilateral Horner's syndrome in a patient with a traction lesion of the brachial plexus indicates which of the following?

A. Infraganglionic lesion involving C8
B. Supraganglionic lesion involving T1
C. Dorsal root injury at C8
D. Cervical stenosis at C8-T1

Horner's syndrome is contraction of the pupil, partial ptosis (drooping), enophthalmos (recession of eyeball into orbit), and sometimes loss of sweating over the affected side of the face. An ipsilateral Horner's syndrome in a patient with a brachial plexus traction injury indicates a supraganglionic lesion involving the T1 nerve root, through which sympathetic fibers enter the plexus. A poor prognosis is associated with root damage at this level.

Answer: **B**

Whitenack, Hunter, Read in Mackin, Callahan, Skirven, et al, p. 727
Koman, Smith, Smith in Mackin, Callahan, Skirven, et al, p. 1700

37. You are treating a patient after ulnar nerve repair at the wrist; no tendons were involved. How long should the nerve be protected by immobilization?

A. 1 day
B. 7 to 10 days
C. 4 weeks
D. 6 to 8 weeks

After nerve repair, immobilization should be required for approximately 7 to 10 days. However, some authors promote 3 weeks of protection after nerve repair before mobilization is initiated. During the period of nerve regeneration, therapy should focus on keeping the affected area supple, mobile, and ready to accept the growing axons. Sensory reeducation programs should be initiated when appropriate reennervation occurs. It is the therapist's responsibility to ensure end organ protection through splinting, gentle range of motion, massage modalities, and protective techniques to maximize functional outcome.

Answer: **B**

Hunter, Mackin, Callahan, p. 622
Hayes, Carney, Wolf, et al, in Mackin, Callahan, Skirven, et al, p. 655

38. True or False: The suprascapular nerve arises from the middle trunk of the brachial plexus.

The suprascapular nerve arises from the upper trunk, from C5 and C6 nerve roots. The suprascapular nerve innervates the supraspinatus and infraspinatus muscles, and sensation to the shoulder capsule (Fig. 4-8).

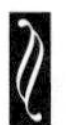

Answer: **False**

Bednar, Wurapa in Mackin, Callahan, Skirven, pp. 1307-1308

39. True or False: Hansen's disease belongs in the family of peripheral nerve diseases and disorders.

Hansen's disease, also known as *leprosy*, is an infectious bacterial disease. This disease damages the nerves (especially in the limbs and facial areas) and can cause skin damage. If the disease is caught early, severe deformity can be prevented. Damage occurs to the peripheral nerves and this causes most of the deformities seen in patients with Hansen's disease.

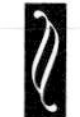

Answer: **True**

Bell-Krotoski, p. 133

40. The lower two thirds of the dermatome that covers the deltoid muscle are derived from which nerve root?

A. C4
B. C5
C. C6
D. C7
E. C8

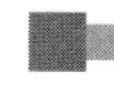

The deltoid is motored by the axillary nerve, which is derived from the brachial plexus roots C5 and C6. The cutaneous nerve supplying sensory innervation to the skin over the lower two thirds of the deltoid is derived from the superior lateral brachial cutaneous nerve (C5 nerve root), branching from the axillary nerve.

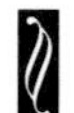

Answer: **B**

Bednar, Wurapa in Mackin, Callahan, Skirven, et al, p. 1308
Butler, p. 111
Refer to Fig. 4-9

41. Which of the following functions is not mediated from the sympathetic nervous system (SNS)?

A. Sudomotor
B. Vasomotor
C. Trophic
D. Pilomotor
E. All of the above are mediated from the SNS.

The SNS mediates vasomotor (skin color and skin temperature), sudomotor (sweat), pilomotor (gooseflesh), and trophic (skin texture, soft-tissue atrophy, nail

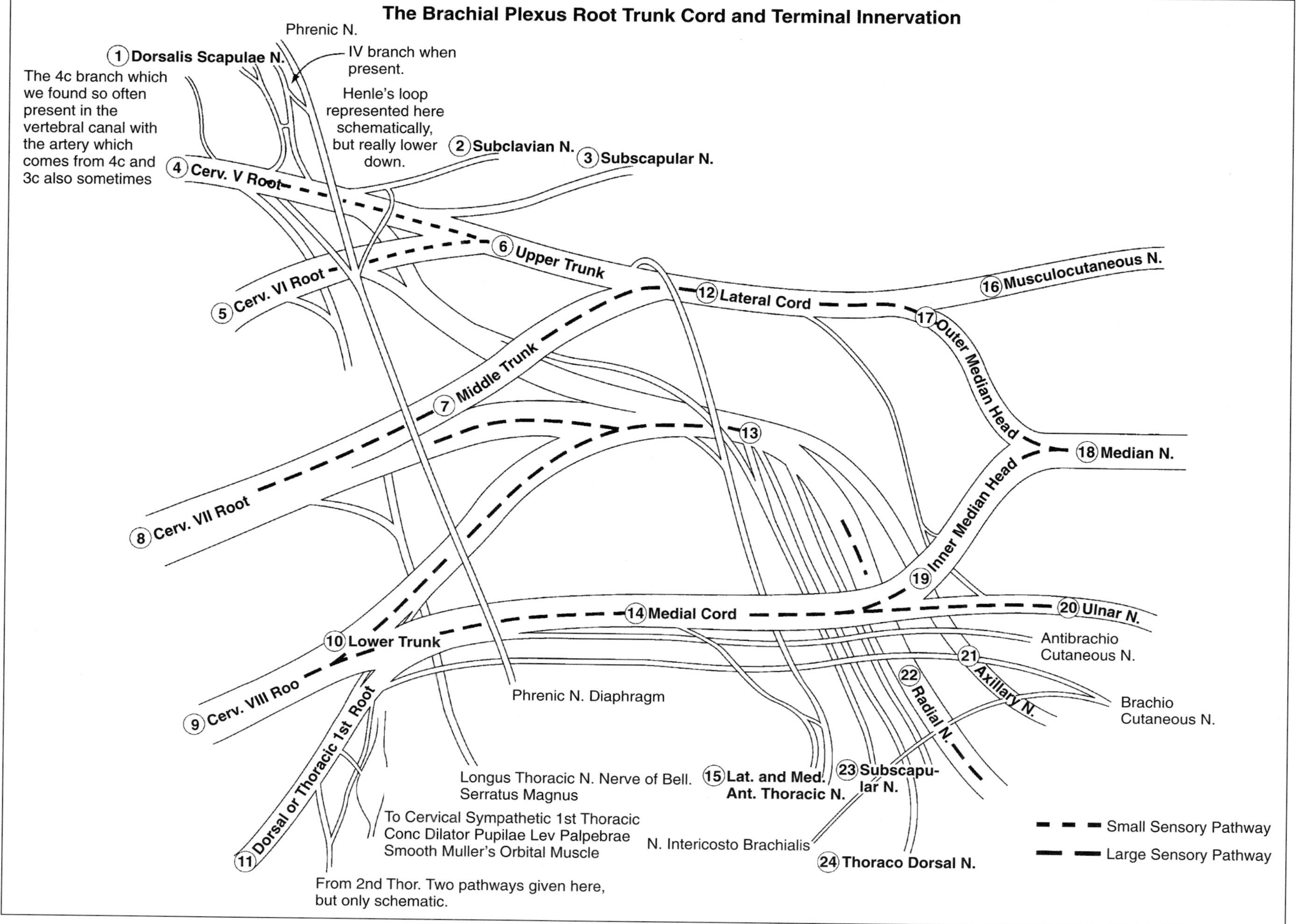

Fig. 4-8 ■ The Stevens diagram of the brachial plexus (Modified from Stevens JH with assistance from Kerr AT: Brachial plexus paralysis. In Codman EA, ed: *The shoulder*, Malabar, FL, 1934, Robert E. Krieger. Used with permission.)

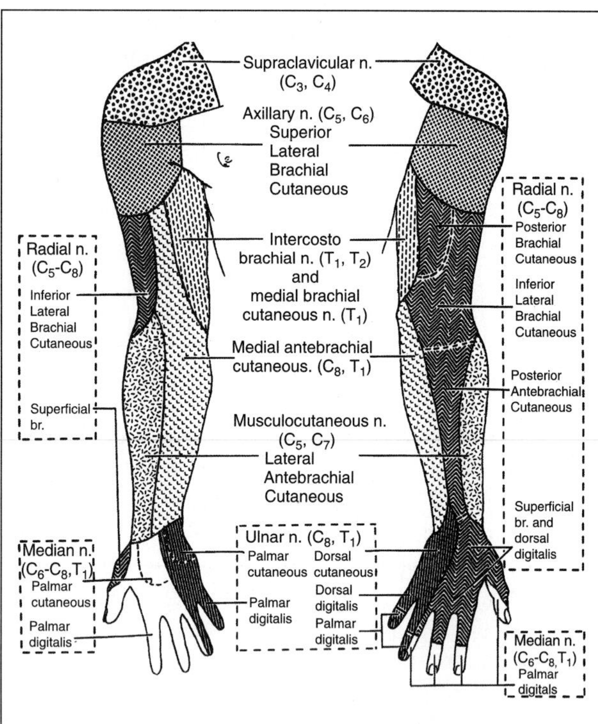

Fig. 4-9 ■ Adapted with permission from Netter FH: *The atlas of human anatomy,* ed 2, Summit, NJ, 1997, CIBA-GEIGY Corp.

changes, hair growth, and rate of healing) functions. After nerve injury, early sympathetic changes include rosy, warm, and dry skin without gooseflesh. Trophic changes include soft, smooth skin texture with hair falling out or becoming longer and finer. Late changes after sympathetic nerve injury include mottling or cyanosis and cool skin with no pilomotor function. The skin is nonelastic; the patient develops curved (talon-like) nails; and hair continues to fall out and become longer and finer.

To treat sympathetic dysfunction, the therapist must return moisture to the skin with daily soaking and oil massage, inspect the patient daily for pressure areas, and use tools or splints that assist in injury prevention.

Answer: **E**
Malick, Kasch, pp. 19, 26

42. Your patient injured her hand on the volar aspect of the palm at the metacarpal head on the radial side of the index finger, 6 inches from her fingertip. She is experiencing sensory loss. How long would you anticipate the nerve to take for her feeling to return after digital nerve repair?

A. 3 weeks
B. 3 months
C. 6 months
D. 12 months
E. One cannot know unless the hand surgeon performs diagnostic testing.

The rate of nerve regeneration is inversely proportional to the distance from the cell body. A Tinel's sign is one way to measure a regenerating axon. When Wallerian degeneration occurs, rates of regeneration vary according to body part (e.g., in the upper arm, regeneration occurs at 8.5 mm/day, whereas 1 to 1.5 mm/day [1 inch/month] has been reported and accepted in the forearm and hand). In this case study, your patient injured herself roughly 6 inches from her fingertip. Nerve regeneration would be expected in approximately 6 months because the distance to the fingertip is roughly 6 inches.

Interestingly, the traditional concept that regenerating axons take 3 weeks to cross the suture line and another 3 weeks to establish function once the distal end of the axon reaches its target end organ is now viewed as incorrect by some authors.

Answer: **C**
Hunter, p. 618
Dellon, pp. 38-43

43. The controversy over how hard to press the prongs when doing two-point discrimination testing has been resolved by an instrument that records the pressure at which the patient can distinguish one from two points. What is the instrument?

A. WEST device
B. Current perception threshold device (neurometer)
C. EAST device
D. PSSD

The WEST device is a form of the nylon monofilaments and cannot measure two-point discrimination. There is no EAST device. The neurometer introduces electrical wave forms as a stimulus and cannot measure pressure thresholds. The unique property of the PSSD is that it measures the pressure required to distinguish one from two points pressing against the skin. These points can be moving or static.

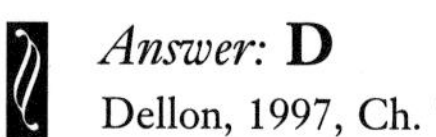

Answer: **D**
Dellon, 1997, Ch. 7

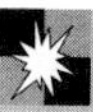

CLINICAL GEM:

The PSSD became available in 1989. It detects a different sequence of sensory loss in chronic nerve compression. It is an instrument designed to measure touch threshold (one-point static, one-point moving, two-point static, and two-point moving).

44. A 52-year-old man is referred to you for sensory reeducation. Your examination reveals that he cannot perceive 256 Hertz (Hz), but is able to perceive 30 Hz. He exhibits difficulty with localization and touch recognition. Which treatment modality would help with early sensory reeducation?

A. Stroke an eraser end across the targeted area.
B. Have your patient identify a variety of objects placed in a bag.
C. Occlude your patient's vision and have him identify various coins.
D. All of the above are excellent tools for early sensory reeducation.

Early sensory reeducation may begin when 30 Hertz and moving touch are perceived. Your goal in early reeducation is to correct false localization and have the patient learn to distinguish constant from moving touch. Early reeducation can be accomplished by stroking or pressing an object (e.g., an eraser end of a pencil or a cotton-ball) to the targeted area. This is completed first with the patient's eyes opened, thus allowing the patient to observe the process. Next, the patient's eyes are closed, and the patient is told to concentrate on the stimulus. Afterward, the patient should open his eyes to observe the stimulus. Having the patient verbalize the location of perceived movement or pressure when his eyes are opened and closed is helpful. A patient will perceive stroking first, followed by constant touch and pressure.

Dellon invented the terms *early* and *late sensory reeducation* in 1970. Answers B and C are performed in late-phase reeducation, which is reeducation of object identification. Attempting object recognition before all sensory submodalities have regenerated to the fingertip is pointless. Keep in mind that some authors divide sensory reeducation into protective and discriminative rather than early and late phases.

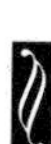

Answer: **A**

Skirven, Callahan in Mackin, Callahan, Skirven, et al, p. 615
Fess in Mackin, Callahan, Skirven, et al, pp. 635-639
Dellon, 1997, pp. 20, 246-295

45. A patient who is being followed in therapy for recovery after a nerve injury has a change in his or her cutaneous pressure threshold with the Semmes-Weinstein nylon monfilaments that goes from a 3.17 to a 5.07. This change demonstrates that the patient has become which of the following?

A. About 2 mg worse
B. About 2 mg worse
C. About 2 mg/mm^2 worse
D. About 100 times worse

The numerical marking on the nylon monofilament introduced by Sidney Weinstein and Josephine Semmes is the logarithm to the base 10 of the force in tenths of milligrams. Thus the difference between markings of 3 and of 5 is one hundred fold—or ten to the second power.

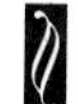

Answer: **D**

Dellon, Mackinnon, Brandt, pp. 756-757

46. A patient has neurosensory testing that stages his degree of cubital tunnel syndrome as mild. The therapist begins nonoperative treatment with splinting and activity of daily living (ADL) modifications. The patient is followed for 3 months. What percentage chance does the patient have for improving?

A. 80%
B. 50%
C. 25%
D. 10%

It has been demonstrated that 80% of patients who change their ADLs for 3 months can resolve their cubital tunnel syndrome complaints without surgical decompression. The success of nonoperative treatment decreases with increasing degrees of nerve compression.

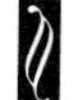

Answer: **A**

Dellon, Hament, Gittelsohn, pp. 1673-1677

47. If the posterior cord of the brachial plexus were injured, paralysis would be expected in which of the following muscles?

A. Latissimus dorsi
B. Deltoid

C. Extensor carpi radialis longus/extensor carpi radialis brevis
D. Coracobrachialis
E. A and D
F. A, B, and C

The posterior cord receives contribution from all three trunks in the brachial plexus. The posterior cord gives rise to the following five nerves: 1) the upper subscapular nerve, which supplies the subscapular muscle; 2) the lower subscapular nerve, which supplies the teres major and a branch of the subscapularis; 3) the thoracodorsal nerve, which supplies the latissimus dorsi; 4) the axillary nerve, which supplies the deltoid muscle and teres minor; and 5) the radial nerve, which supplies the extensors of the elbow, wrist, and digits. The coracobrachialis muscle is innervated by the musculocutaneous nerve, which is part of the lateral cord (see Fig. 4-8).

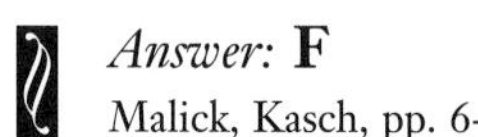
Answer: **F**
Malick, Kasch, pp. 6-9
Hunter, Mackin, Callahan, pp. 888-891, 1875

48. A 32-year-old man sustained a brachial plexus injury. He cannot control shoulder abduction or forward elevation. He can extend his elbow but cannot actively flex his elbow. He is experiencing sensory loss in the thumb and index fingers. The middle finger sensation is intact. Which nerve roots are damaged?

A. C5 and C6
B. C5, C6, and C7
C. C6, C7, and C8
D. C7 and C8

The brachial plexus anatomy is formed by the anterior primary rami of C5, C6, C7, C8, and T1 and their terminal outflow of the peripheral nerves. Injury to the brachial plexus involves commonly observed patterns. In this case study, the lesion involves the C5 and C6 roots. The paralysis of the deltoid and lateral rotators of the humerus and elbow flexors indicates this particular level of injury. In addition, the sensory loss of the thumb and index fingers is the result of C5 and C6 root damage; the middle finger (C7) is spared (see Fig. 4-8).

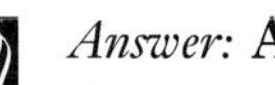
Answer: **A**
Hunter, Mackin, Callahan, p. 636
Whitenack, Hunter, Read in Mackin, Callahan, Skirven, et al, pp. 703-719
Hunter, Whitenack in Mackin, Callahan, Skirven, et al, pp. 733-734

49. After carpal tunnel decompression using an open technique, the patient complains of pain sensation in the scar near the wrist. The pain does not radiate to any of the fingers and finger sensibility is normal. No significant improvement has occurred after 6 months of desensitization techniques, including massage, steroid iontophoresis, and fluidotherapy. What would be the appropriate treatment at this point?

A. Neurolysis of median nerve
B. Nerve graft of median nerve
C. Further therapy
D. Resection of the palmar cutaneous branch of the median nerve

If there is normal sensibility in the thumb and index finger, no treatment is required for the median nerve. In this case the symptoms are from a neuroma of the palmar cutaneous branch of the median nerve. This nerve must be resected and the proximal end placed in a quiet location away from the skin and wrist joint movements.

Answer: **D**
Evans, Dellon, pp. 203-206

50. After a nerve repair at the wrist, when can "final" evaluation of nerve recovery be assessed?

A. 6 months
B. 2 years
C. 4 to 5 years
D. The nerve is in perpetual recovery.

After a nerve suture or nerve graft at the wrist, nerve regeneration to the fingertips occurs by 1 year. After another year of sensory reeducation, final assessment can be performed at 2 years after surgical nerve repair.

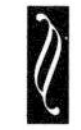
Answer: **B**
Dellon, pp. 38-43

51. After resection of the radial sensory and lateral antebrachial cutaneous nerves and implantation of these nerves into the brachioradialis muscle, a patient complains of paresthesia in the dorsoradial aspect of the wrist. What is the best explanation for a patient's complaints?

A. Recurrent neuroma pain
B. Regeneration of the resected nerves
C. Collateral sprouting from adjacent normal nerves
D. Reflex sympathetic dystrophy/complex regional pain syndrome (RSD/CRPS)

The nerve growth factor released from the distal portion of the resected nerve can stimulate neural regeneration into this region from uninjured adjacent nerves. This is termed *collateral sprouting*. It is a short-lived protective mechanism that will benefit from further desensitization and sensory reeducation. Therefore, collateral sprouting is the best answer.

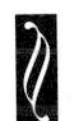

Answer: **C**
Dellon, Aszmann, Muse, pp. 520-525

52. When one is evaluating the upper limb in a patient with a brachial plexus injury, care should be taken during examination of the shoulder joint. To prevent stress on the roots of the brachial plexus, which maximal shoulder abduction should be allowed?

A. 25 degrees
B. 45 degrees
C. 60 degrees
D. 90 degrees

In brachial plexus injuries, the therapist should be careful not to increase tension on the brachial plexus roots. Coronal abduction—especially coronal abduction combined with lateral rotation—may cause tension on the brachial plexus roots if the arm is abducted above 90 degrees. Because the rotator cuff often is paralyzed, which may result in humeral subluxation and abduction, shoulder motion beyond 90 degrees puts additional stress on the capsule and should be avoided.

Answer: **D**
Hunter, Mackin, Callahan, p. 648
Walsh in Mackin, Callahan, Skirven, et al, pp. 742-750

53. The goals of therapy during treatment of a patient experiencing brachial plexus injuries include which of the following?

A. Protecting the limb from additional trauma
B. Preventing contractures
C. Monitoring sensory recovery
D. Addressing psychological issues
E. All of the above

A brachial plexus injury is a devastating, complex event that requires a team approach to treatment. Both psychological distress and physical involvement affect the functional outcome. The healthcare team should help with psychological issues related to functional loss, depression, or difficulty dealing with the loss. In addition, the goals of therapy are to protect the limb from additional trauma, prevent contractures, and monitor sensory and motor recovery.

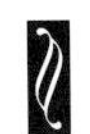

Answer: **E**
Hunter, Mackin, Callahan, pp. 647-655
Walsh in Mackin, Callahan, Skirven, et al, pp. 742-760

54. The term *Klumpke palsy* refers to which brachial plexus level of injury?

A. (C5), C6, C7
B. C6, C7
C. C7, C8
D. (C7), C8, T1

Klumpke palsy is an uncommon lesion in the adult population. It involves the (C7), C8, and T1 nerve-roots. The shoulder, elbow, and wrist extension are intact. Loss of finger flexion, extension, and intrinsic function of the hand is observed. The sensory loss may be severe and usually involves the little finger, ring finger, and medial aspect of the forearm (see Fig. 4-8).

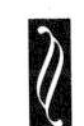

Answer: **D**
Kozin, Ciocca, Speakman in Mackin, Callahan, Skirven, et al, p. 836

55. You are treating a patient 4 weeks after distal fingertip amputation. Primary healing has occurred. He describes extreme hypersensitivity and also reports that the fingertip feels as if it is going to burst. Which contact particle or texture would be best for this patient during initial treatment?

A. Velcro hook
B. Burlap texture
C. Cotton balls
D. High-cycle continuous vibration

Desensitization programs should be initiated at the level of vibration texture and contact medium that the patient can tolerate. A patient with extreme hypersensitivity, as described in this situation, would not be able to tolerate Velcro hook, burlap texture, or high-cycle continuous vibration. Initiating treatment with moleskin texture, felt, or cotton would be more appropriate for this patient. This patient probably would benefit from retrograde massage during the early stage of hypersensitivity. The patient also should work on a home program that uses contact particles and dowel textures to assist with desensitization. Vibration often is more uncomfortable initially, but according to Janet Waylett-Rendall, vibration eventually is preferred over any other desensitization media. Hand-held, battery-operated vibrators can be issued for home use.

Answer: **C**
Hunter, Mackin, Callahan, pp. 698-699
Mackin, Callahan, Skirven, et al
Refer to Fig. 4-10

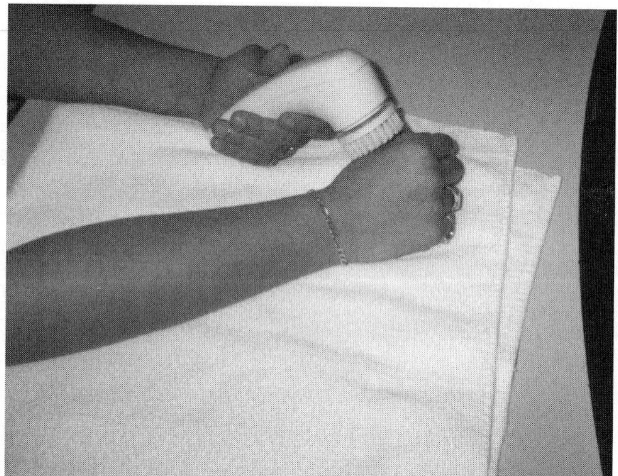

Fig. 4-10

56. A patient who complains of complete loss of sensation in the ring and little finger and along the medial forearm has loss of sensation caused by:

A. C8 nerve-root damage
B. Cubital tunnel compression
C. Guyon canal compression
D. C7 nerve-root damage

Each dorsal root innervates a particular area of skin called a *dermatome*. This patient has *loss* of sensation from C8 dorsal nerve-root damage. The dermatome for C8 is the ring finger, little finger, and the medial forearm. A relationship exists between dermatomes and areas innervated by peripheral nerves. The ulnar nerve and the antebrachial cutaneous nerve are the peripheral nerves that correspond to the C8 dermatome. Sensory changes associated with cubital tunnel compression usually are confined to the ulnar aspect of the hand and the ulnar one and a half digits. In nerve compression syndromes, patients rarely have a complete loss of sensation. Alterations of sensitivity result in nerve compression syndromes rather than complete loss (see Fig. 4-9).

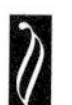

Answer: **A**
Tubiana, Thomine, Mackin, p. 318
Kandel, Schwartz, p. 304

57. Winging of the scapula can result from injury to several different shoulder girdle muscles but is classically attributed to which of the following muscle/nerve combinations?

A. Serratus anterior/suprascapular nerve
B. Serratus anterior/axillary nerve
C. Supraspinatus/long thoracic nerve
D. Serratus anterior/long thoracic nerve

The serratus muscle is innervated by the long thoracic nerve and is the classical cause of winging of the scapula. The suprascapular nerve innervates the supraspinatus muscle which does influence shoulder function. The axillary nerve innervates the deltoid, which also influences shoulder function (see Fig. 10-3).

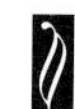

Answer: **D**
Disa, Wang, Dellon, pp. 79-84

58. True or False: Neural gliding to the affected arm is an appropriate treatment for a patient in the irritable phase of thoracic outlet syndrome.

When a patient is in an irritable state (constant pain that is easily provoked and may take a long time to settle), treatment should revolve around rest, with activities limited to those functions that produce minimal or no discomfort. Between rest periods, the patient must avoid activities and postures that strain or aggravate the tissue. Patients initially may need the support of a sling, pillow, or abduction wedge for the shoulder to reduce pain. When irritability is reduced to a moderate or minimal level, neural gliding exercises may be initiated to the unaffected extremity; examples would include neural gliding on the uninvolved arm or a straight leg raise.

Nonirritable neural restrictions can be treated with nerve gliding techniques. The upper limb tensioning techniques, as proposed by Butler, restore neural motion in patients who are in a nonirritable state. Nerve gliding must begin without development of tension in the involved extremity, especially in patients who previously were highly irritable. Patients can be progressed to increased neural tension and postural ergonomic instructions in preparation to return to activities. Next, strengthening conditioning should ensue for return to full activity.

Answer: **False**
Whitenack, Hunter, Read in Mackin, Callahan, Skirven, et al, pp. 723-724
Butler, pp. 104-105

59. When a patient is evaluated for complaints of numbness in the thumb and index finger *after* a carpal tunnel decompression, it is important to consider a more proximal site of compression for the median nerve, instead of recurrent carpal tunnel syndrome. What proximal compression site would you suspect?

A. Deep head of the pronator teres or the lacertus fibrosis
B. The arcade of Froshe
C. The medial head of the triceps
D. Fascia between the brachioradialis and extensor carpi radialis longus

The Arcade of Froshe is a fascial covering of the supinator muscle that compresses the posterior interosseous nerve. The medial head of the triceps can compress the ulnar nerve proximal to the elbow. The radial sensory nerve can be compressed as it exits fascia adjacent to the brachioradialis tendon. The median nerve can be compressed in the forearm beneath the deep head of the pronator teres, the lacertus fibrosis, or the ligament of Struthers (not "arcade").

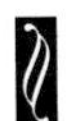
Answer: **A**
Rosenberg, Conolley, Dellon, pp. 258-265
Refer to Fig. 4-11

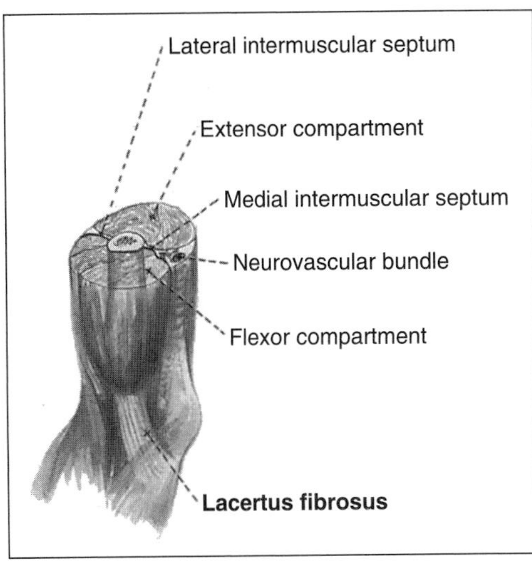

Fig. 4-11 ■ From Mackin EJ, Callahan AD, Skirven TM, et al: *Rehabilitation of the hand and upper extremity,* ed 5, vol 1, St Louis, 2002, Mosby.

60. Which sympathetic function is called *gooseflesh* (Fig. 4-12)?

A. Vasomotor
B. Pilomotor
C. Sudomotor
D. Trophic

Pilomotor function or the "gooseflesh" response is of the skin in the upper extremity. Fig. 4-12 depicts an exaggerated response of one's hair "standing on end."

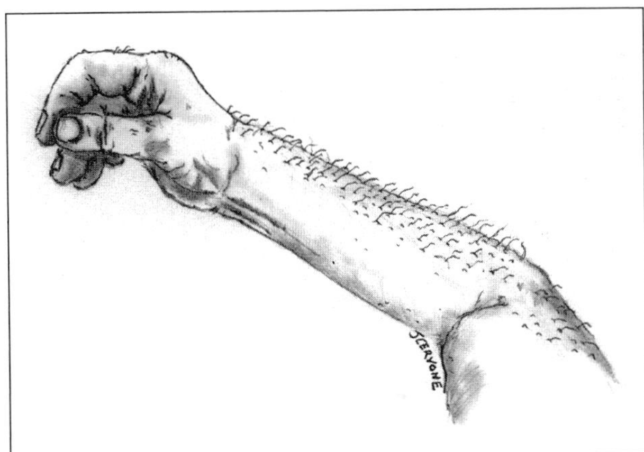

Fig. 4-12

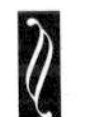
Answer: **B**
Malick, Kasch, p. 19

CLINICAL GEM:
Absence of the "gooseflesh" response occurs when there is complete interruption of sympathetic supply to an area (Mackin, Callahan, Skirven et al, p. 226).

61. Which obstetric palsy most often affects the C5 and C6 nerve roots?

A. Erb's palsy
B. Duval's palsy
C. Seddon's palsy
D. Klumpke's palsy

Obstetric palsy traction injuries are caused by fetal malposition, cephalopelvic disproportion, or the use of forceps.

Erb's palsy is an upper brachial plexus palsy that most often affects the C5 and C6 nerve roots. It includes paralysis of the supraspinatus, infraspinatus, deltoid, biceps, brachialis, and brachioradialis muscles.

Lower brachial plexus injury, known as *Klumpke's* or *Dejerine Klumpke type*, involves the C8 and T1 nerve roots. This injury results in paralysis of the flexors and extensors of the forearm, with sparing of the brachioradialis, supinator, pronator teres, extensor carpi radialis longus, and extensor carpi radialis brevis muscles. The hand intrinsic muscles and part of the triceps are paralyzed. Sensory loss with this injury is severe.

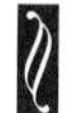

Answer: **A**

Green, p. 1510

Kozin, Ciocca, Speakman in Mackin, Callahan, Skirven, et al, p. 836

62. True or False: In 1943, Seddon introduced a three-part classification of the injured peripheral nerve. The mildest form of nerve injury in Seddon's categorization is referred to as a *neurotmesis.*

The first part of Seddon's three-part classification is the neuropraxic injury, which is the mildest form of nerve injury. The neuropraxic injury is a local conduction block; with this injury the prognosis is excellent because the axonal continuity and nerve conduction is preserved proximal and distal to the injury. The second part, which is called *axonotmesis*, is more severe because axonal disruption leads to Wallerian degeneration of the distal axon. Wallerian degeneration is a degeneration of the distal axon; it takes place over a period of 1 to 2 months. Recovery time varies with axonotmesis and prognosis is good. The most severe type of injury is the third part, called *neurotmesis*, which involves complete transsection of the entire nerve trunk. Prognosis is poor unless surgical repair is performed.

Answer: **False**

Skirven, Callahan in Mackin, Callahan, Skirven, et al, p. 602

Butler, p. 176

63. True or False: Scar tissue may be the culprit in neuroma development.

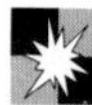

CLINICAL GEM:

The following are nerve injury correlations between Seddon's classification (as described in question 62) and Sunderland's classification (a frequently referenced peripheral nerve injury classification):

Sunderland's classification	Seddon's classification	Injury	Recovery potential
I	Neuropraxia	Axon maintained; stimulation can occur distal to lesion; possible segmental demyelinization	Full
II	Axonotmesis	Loss of axonal integrity with distal axonal degeneration (Wallerian degeneration); endoneurial tube intact	Full
III	Axonotmesis	Endoneurial tube torn; perineurium intact	Slow; incomplete
IV	Axonotmesis	Only epineurium intact	Neuroma-in-continuity is common
V	Neurotmesis	Complete transection of the nerve	None

A neuroma results from a blocked regenerating nerve. This block may have various causes, one of which may be scar tissue. The block causes the regenerating sprouts to become trapped and surrounded by connective tissue. By definition, a neuroma is not painful. When a neuroma is in a vulnerable environment related to tendon or joint movement, the entrapped ends of the failed regenerating axons send painful messages when stimulation occurs from the motion of surrounding tissues. The diagnosis of a neuroma is easy to make because direct tapping over the nerve elicits a painful paresthesia. Conservative treatment consists of iontophoresis, desensitization, protective splinting, ultrasound, transcutaneous electrical nerve stimulation, or steroid injection.

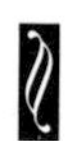

Answer: **True**

Dellon, pp. 44, 45

Herndon in Green, Hotchkiss, Pederson, pp. 1469-1479

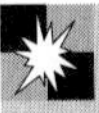

CLINICAL GEM:
The term *neuroma-in-continuity* refers to a neuroma in a nerve that has not been completely severed.

64. Match the following signs with their corresponding descriptions. Note that all relate to ulnar nerve paralysis.

Signs

1. Froment
2. Jeanne
3. Wartenberg
4. Duchenne
5. Egawa
6. Andre-Thomas
7. Masse

Descriptions

A. Clawing of the ring and little finger
B. Hyperextension of the metacarpophalangeal joint of the thumb in pinch grip
C. Pronounced flexion of the thumb interphalangeal joint during adduction toward the index finger (key pinch)
D. Flattening of the metacarpal arch
E. Wrist falls into volar flexion during action of the extensors to the middle finger
F. Inability to adduct the extended little finger to the extended ring finger
G. Inability of the flexed middle finger to abduct radially and ulnarly and to rotate at the metacarpophalangeal joint

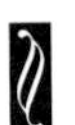

Answers: **1, C; 2, B; 3, F; 4, A; 5, G; 6, E; 7, D**

Tubiana, Thomine, Mackin, p. 280

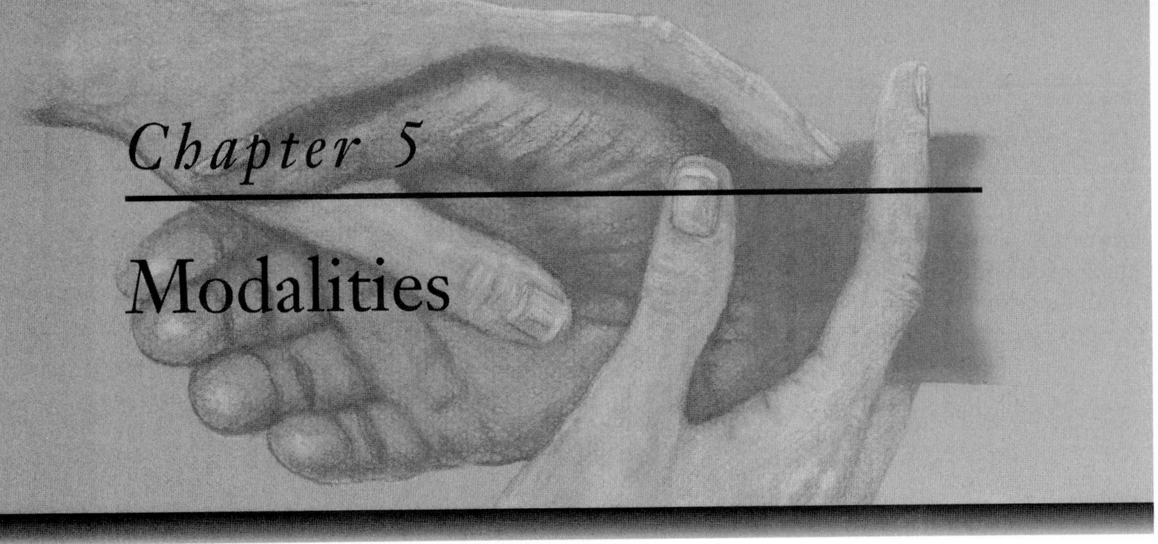

Chapter 5

Modalities

1. Match each of the following modalities to the correct temperature application.

Modality

1. Paraffin
2. Hot pack in hydrocollator
3. Fluidotherapy
4. Whirlpool

Temperature Application (F)

A. 102° to 118°
B. 113° to 129°
C. 158° to 167°
D. 96° to 104°

The temperature of the material that provides the heat is not necessarily the crucial factor in the amount of heat transmitted to the body and the resultant safety of the modality. An increase of 1° or 2° F has dramatic, localized physiologic effects. An increase in temperature of more than 5° F usually results in a burn.

The superficial heating modalities are essentially equivalent in their ability to deliver heat to the body. Water with the greatest specific heat (the amount of heat energy stored at a particular temperature) is delivered at the coolest temperature. Paraffin has a lower specific heat than water and is delivered at a higher temperature, and so on with fluidotherapy.

Moist heat packs are separated from the patient by several layers of toweling because they are kept at the highest temperature in the hydrocollator.

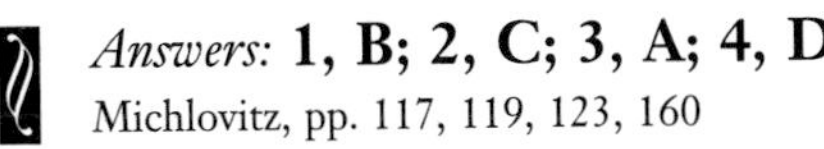

Answers: **1, B; 2, C; 3, A; 4, D**
Michlovitz, pp. 117, 119, 123, 160

2. Ultrasound (US) has been shown to do which of the following?

A. Accelerate healing of soft tissue
B. Decrease muscle tone
C. Decrease calcium deposits in bursae
D. Decrease spasticity

US has been shown to accelerate the healing of soft tissues. Answers B, C, and D are all based on anecdotal evidence only.

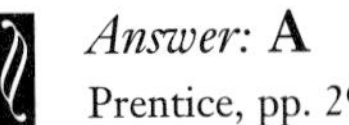

Answer: **A**
Prentice, pp. 293-294

3. Uncomfortable, achy sensations associated with US may be avoided in which of the following ways?

A. Increasing frequency
B. Decreasing intensity
C. Increasing the size of the treatment area
D. All of the above

All of the above can assist with decreasing uncomfortable, achy sensations associated with US. Achy sensations emanate from overheating of the periosteum. Increasing the frequency of US decreases the depth of penetration. Decreasing the intensity decreases the amount of heat generated by US. Increasing the size of the treatment area lowers the spatial averaged intensity of the US and limits the amount of energy received by any given area of underlying periosteum.

Answer: **D**
Prentice, pp. 279-282

4. Which of the following benefits occurs when applying US with the soundhead while the patient's hand is immersed in water, versus direct placement of the body part with the use of gel?

A. Prevention of damage to the soundhead because of poor contact with gel and/or body surfaces
B. Less nonuniformity of intensity to the treatment area
C. Improved transmission of US to deeper tissues
D. More even dosage of US intensity throughout the treatment area
E. Increased nonthermal effects of the US treatment

Prevention of damage to the soundhead caused by poor contact with gel and/or body surfaces can be avoided by performing US in water. The soundhead may be damaged if it is not in contact with transmission gel and the underlying body part. US cannot be transmitted through solids or gases and may reverberate within the soundhead. Water and gel are both excellent transmission media for US, and the physical and physiologic effects of both treatment techniques are virtually equal.

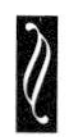
Answer: **A**
Prentice, pp. 289-293

5. The parameters for electrical currents applied to elicit muscle contractions include which of the following?

A. Voltages that never exceed 120 volts
B. Frequencies (pulses per second) of at least 50
C. Frequencies, voltages, and intensities sufficient to elicit action potentials in motor nerves
D. Intensities of at least 50 milliamps

Electric stimulation to elicit muscle contractions could be performed with a virtually infinite number of combinations of frequency, voltage, and intensity. The crucial feature of any given set of parameters is its ability to generate an action potential in a motor nerve, characterized by "strength-duration" curves. Strength-duration curves illustrate the minimal combinations of voltage, intensity, and duration required to generate action potentials, and detailed information on these may be found in any introductory textbook on electrical stimulation.

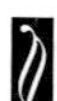
Answer: **C**
Baker, Wederich, McNeal, p. 11

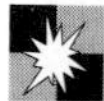
CLINICAL GEM:
Terminology Clarification: *Neuromuscular electrical stimulation (NMES)* is a general term that describes a group of stimulators that use pulsating current to stimulate innervated musculature. This type of stimulation is used for maintaining or gaining range of motion, facilitating a muscle contraction, and substituting for orthoses. The application of electrical stimulation for orthotic substitution is also termed *functional electrical stimulation (FES).*

6. US can facilitate the movement of medications through the skin because of which of the following?

A. Acoustical streaming
B. Minimal impedance
C. Microvibration of pores
D. Hyperfractionation of medication

Acoustical streaming is the term for the overall movement of molecules away from the source of sound; medications placed on the skin are literally pushed into deeper structures, although research has failed to provide strong evidence for this application.

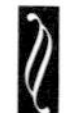
Answer: **A**
Belanger, p. 240

7. Intermittent compression pumping should do which of the following?

A. Be set no higher than 50 mm Hg for the upper extremity
B. Have a ratio of 3 : 1 of inflation to deflation
C. Not exceed the patient's diastolic blood pressure
D. All of the above

Adhering to all of the above guidelines is important when using the intermittent compression pump.

Answer: **D**
Hayes, p. 71
Refer to Fig. 5-1

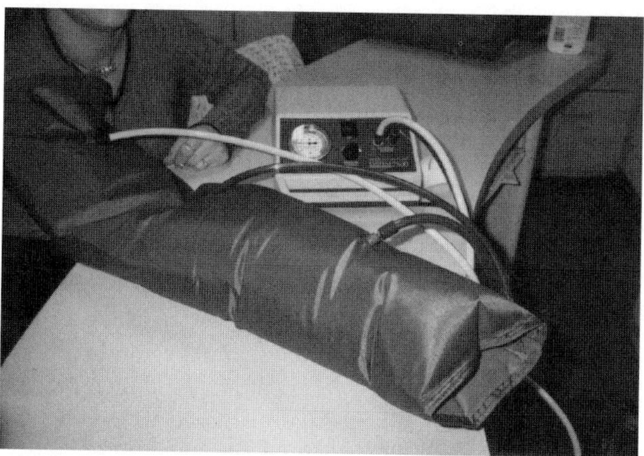

Fig. 5-1

CLINICAL GEM:
Not all schools of thought use intermittent pumps to treat lymphedema. However, if utilized, sequential pumps with gradient pressure are much more effective for treating lymphedema than are one-chamber intermittent pumps.

8. Which of the following is false about cold therapy?

A. It is the thermal agent of choice for the first 24 to 48 hours after injury.
B. It decreases inflammation.
C. It decreases pain.
D. All of the above are true.

All of the above are considered accurate. There is controversy in the literature regarding the effects of cold therapy; therefore further research is warranted.

Answer: **D**
Michlovitz, pp. 84-86

9. At the end of superficial cold applications, the skin is often red. This is evidence of reactive hyperemia, the body's attempt to restore blood flow to an area recently deprived of blood and the oxygen it carries. Therefore when cold is applied to minimize posttraumatic edema, what is the maximum treatment time?

A. 5 minutes
B. 10 minutes
C. 15 minutes
D. 20 minutes

Cold packs to manage posttraumatic edema should be applied for 20 minutes on and 20 minutes off during the first 24 hours after trauma, if possible. Treatment time should *not* exceed 20-minute intervals.

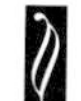

Answer: **D**
Prentice, pp. 211-213

10. True or False: Fluidotherapy is safer than other superficial heating modalities because it can be applied at a much higher temperature.

Fluidotherapy uses particles of cellulose (e.g., sawdust) that are suspended in air as the conductive medium. The specific heat of this combination is *very low*; in other words, the amount of heat energy it contains at any given temperature is much less than that of water and it can therefore be much hotter. So, fluidotherapy is neither safer nor more dangerous than any other type of superficial heating modality. It simply can be hotter because of its low specific heat capacity.

Answer: **False**
Prentice, pp. 233-234
Refer to Fig. 5-2

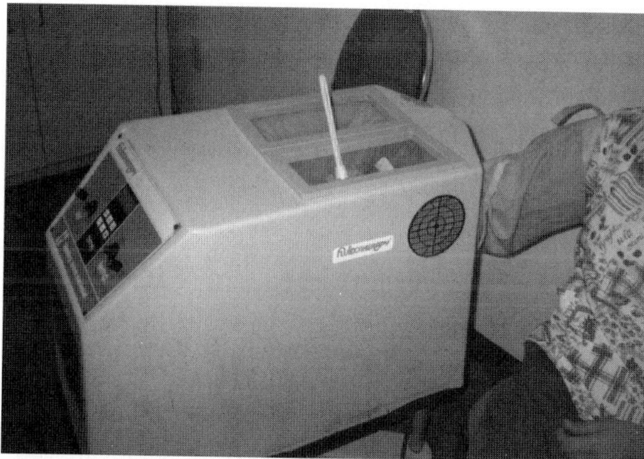

Fig. 5-2

11. Increased tissue temperature is a thermal effect of US. How does this increased temperature affect the blood flow to the treated area?

A. The tissue has a decrease in blood flow.
B. The tissue has an increase in blood flow.
C. The tissue has no change in blood flow.
D. The tissue initially has a decrease in blood flow, followed by an increase in blood flow.

The principal reason for using US for thermal effects is elevated tissue temperature. With increased tissue temperature, a normal response is an increase in blood flow.

Answer: **B**
Michlovitz, pp. 177-179

12. US should be avoided with which of the following types of patient?

A. Under 16
B. Over 55
C. Has a history of hypertension
D. Has a history of cancer in an unrelated location

US has been shown to disrupt epiphyseal plates (growth plates) in long bones; therefore it should be avoided in those who are still growing. There is a potential for US to facilitate metastasis of cancerous lesions, but it is not carcinogenic and may be used on patients with a history of cancer.

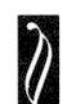
Answer: **A**
Michlovitz, pp. 177-179

13. True or False: It is important to heat US gel for patient comfort and to increase transmission.

Heating US gel is inadvisable because it makes the gel runny and decreases viscosity, which leads to runoff. Gel is an excellent coupling agent for transmission. Using gel helps to decrease air bubbles and friction. Heating increases the oxygen in gel, thus decreasing the coupling medium's effectiveness. Water is an adequate coupling medium; however, increased air bubbles in water reduce transmission.

Answer: **False**
Michlovitz, p. 199

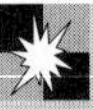
CLINICAL GEM:
A quick reference to gel temperature follows:
Less than 66° F = 90% effective
Greater than 66° F = 73% effective

14. When treating supraspinatus tendonitis with US, which shoulder position is most beneficial?

A. Arm abducted and internally rotated
B. Arm externally rotated and abducted
C. Position of comfort
D. Position that most aggravates pain

When one is using US as a treatment modality for supraspinatus tendonitis, the position of choice is with the arm abducted and internally rotated to expose the supraspinatus tendon from under the acromion process.

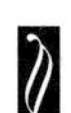
Answer: **A**
Michlovitz, p. 203
Refer to Fig. 5-3

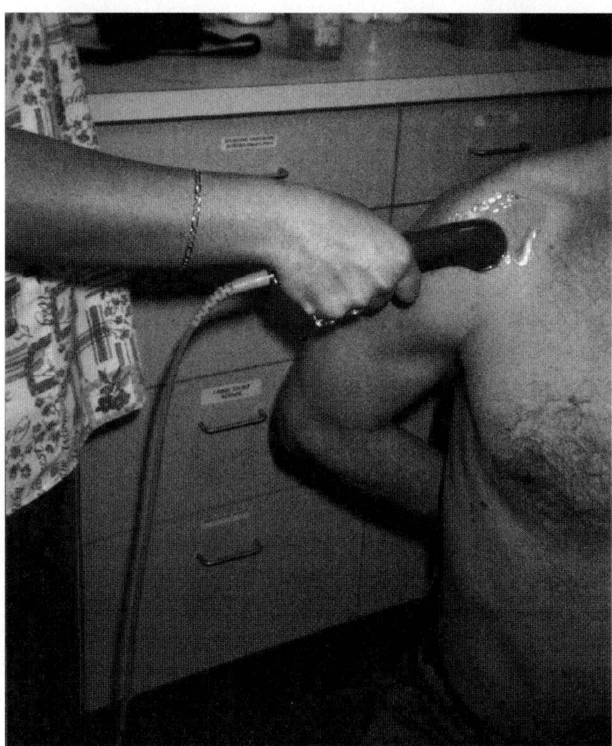

Fig. 5-3

15. You are treating a stiff digit with abundant scar tissue. Which US frequency would be best for elongating the scar?

A. 1 MHz
B. 3 MHz
C. 1.5 w/cm^2
D. 1.0 w/cm^2

When a depth of penetration of up to 2 cm is desired, the therapist should use 3-MHz US, which is ideal for treating hand and wrist pathologies. US has been shown by some authors to be helpful in elongating scar tissue.

A 1-MHz US treatment is best used to treat deeper tissue when desired penetration is up to 5 cm in depth. 1 MHz is ideal for treating the back and lower extremities. Answers C and D are incorrect because they relate to intensity.

Answer: **B**
Hunter, Mackin, Callahan, p. 23
Michlovitz in Mackin, Callahan, Skirven, et al, pp. 1746-1748

16. Intermittent compression pumps may be used with all but which of the following?

A. Postmastectomy lymphedema
B. Venous insufficiency
C. Arterial insufficiency
D. Amputations
E. Traumatic edema

Patients with arterial insufficiency have increased peripheral resistance and compression worsens this condition. Other contraindications include infections, thromboses, cardiac dysfunction, kidney dysfunction, obstructed lymphatic channels, and cancer (see Fig. 5-1).

Answer: **C**
Hayes, p. 71

17. An 80-year-old woman slipped and fell on wet pavement. She landed on an outstretched arm, which resulted in a Colles' fracture of her right wrist. After 6 weeks in a cast, the patient continues to suffer from severe, chronic edema of the wrist and hand. Her treatment included intermittent pneumatic compression (IPC). Necessary chart information for determining progress when treating this condition with IPC would include which of the following?

A. Right wrist muscle strength
B. Pretreatment and posttreatment measurements of girth of the right forearm and wrist
C. Grip strength
D. Active range of motion of right wrist flexion and extension
E. Right forearm and wrist sensation

The comparison of girth measurements before and after treatment and from treatment to treatment is an important clinical indication of the effectiveness of IPC.

Answer: **B**
Hecox, Mehreteab, Weisberg, pp. 424, 427

18. Which of the following explains the usefulness of "spray and stretch" techniques?

A. Spray and stretch is useful because rapid, brief cooling of the skin over a muscle reduces muscle tone.
B. Spray and stretch is useful for facilitating relaxation of muscles in spasm secondary to trauma.
C. Spray and stretch is only useful if performed with proper technique, which includes spraying parallel to muscle fibers, proximal to distal, at a speed of about 10 cm/second.
D. All of the above

D is correct. Spray and stretch, developed by Travell in the 1960s, is a variation of cryotherapy (cold therapy) and has been reported to be useful when specific indications and techniques are employed.

Answer: **D**
Travell, Simons, pp. 65-74, 503-504
Prentice, pp. 219-220
Refer to Fig. 5-4

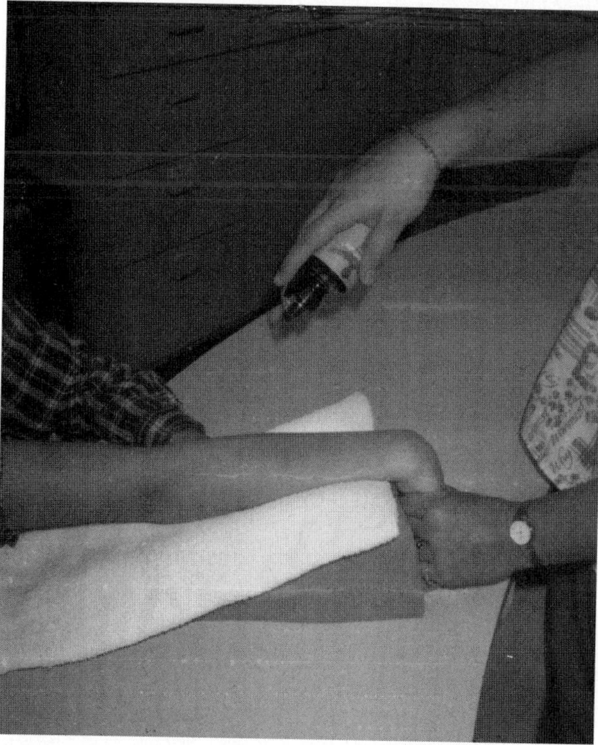

Fig. 5-4

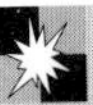

CLINICAL GEM:
Ethyl chloride and fluorimethane are common sprays; however, ethyl chloride is not recommended. Fluorimethane is safer to use but can freeze the skin when a stream is directed on one area for 6 seconds or longer; therefore fluorimethane should be used with caution.

19. The use of the Jobst compression pump is not contraindicated in the presence of which of the following?

A. Infection
B. Vascular damage
C. Pain
D. Fractures
E. It is contraindicated for all of the above.

Compression units should *not* be used when a patient has an active infection, vascular damage, and/or unhealed fractures. If using a compression pump increases the patient's pain level, it should be modified or discontinued; however, *pretreatment pain* is not a contraindication to the use of a compression unit.

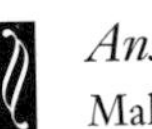

Answer: **C**
Malick, Kasch, p. 98

20. True or False: Melzack and Wall theorized that small-diameter fibers of light touch and proprioception can close the gate to pain fibers.

According to the theory of Melzack and Wall, the "gate" opens to stimuli that approach the central nervous system (CNS) with high speed. Therefore sensations that travel along large-diameter nerve fibers (non-nociceptive) inhibit pain or tend to "close the gate" to pain, especially the throbbing, dull pain typically reported by patients suffering from musculoskeletal trauma. Small-diameter (nociceptive) fibers elicit pain or "open the gate."

Thermal sensations and sensation of electrical stimulation are carried by large-diameter fibers and are the most commonly used physical agents to close the gate in clinical practice.

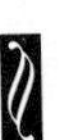

Answer: **False**
Hunter, Mackin, Callahan, p. 1536
Fedorczyk, Barbe in Mackin, Callahan, Skirven, et al, pp. 1729-1730
Mense, Simons, p. 348

21. True or False: You have a patient with hypergranulation tissue on his hand wound. You choose to treat this patient with a lukewarm whirlpool for 15 minutes. This is the best method of treatment.

Hypergranulation tissue, also called *proud flesh*, occurs when granulation tissue continues to form over the original wound. The proper way to treat such a wound is with the application of silver nitrate or corticosteroid cream. A therapist should cease using whirlpool and consider using semipermeable dressings on the wound and decrease the frequency of wound cleansing and dressing changes.

Answer: **False**
McCulloch, Kloth, Feedar, p. 143

22. The use of whirlpool treatments has decreased in past years. This is most likely the result of which of the following?

A. Advances in wound care, including occlusive and semipermeable dressings
B. Increased consciousness of the dangers of transmitting infection from patient to patient
C. Efficacy of medications to enhance peripheral circulation
D. All of the above

The popularity of whirlpool treatments began in an era when they represented the state of the art in cleaning wounds, facilitating healing, and improving peripheral circulation. However, the use of whirlpools has declined for all of the above stated reasons. Refer to Chapter 6, Wounds/Infection, for additional information concerning moist wound healing.

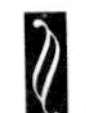

Answer: **D**
Belanger, pp. 347-350

23. Which of the following patients might benefit from contrast baths as a treatment modality?

A. A patient with small-vessel disease secondary to diabetes
B. A patient with arthrosclerotic endarteritis
C. A patient with Buerger's disease
D. A patient who has arthritis of the peripheral joints
E. All of the above patients are poor candidates for contrast baths.

A patient with flexible implant arthroplasties of the metacarpophalangeal joints might benefit from the use of contrast baths. All of the answers except D describe patients who *cannot* use contrast baths as a treatment modality. Caution also should be exercised when using contrast baths for a patient with peripheral vascular disease if the water temperature is set higher than 40° C (104° F).

Contrast baths are used for patients with arthritis of the peripheral joints, joint sprains, and muscle strains and to toughen amputation stumps. Unfortunately, no well-controlled study of the efficacy of contrast baths is available. If a contrast bath is used, the temperature should be between 38° C (104° F) and 44° C (111.2° F) in one basin and 10° C (50° F) to 18° C (64° F) in the other basin. The extremity to be treated should be placed in the warm basin for 10 minutes, then immersed in the cold basin for 1 minute, and then returned to the warm basin for 4 minutes. This cycle should be continued for 30 minutes, with the last immersion being in the warm basin.

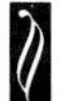

Answer: **D**

Hunter, Mackin, Callahan, p. 1371
Michlovitz in Mackin, Callahan, Skirven, et al, p. 1748
Michlovitz, pp. 161-162

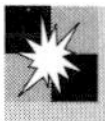

CLINICAL GEM:
For severe edema, some authors advocate ending contrast bath treatment in cold water for 1 minute.

24. True or False: Continuous passive motion (CPM) enhances the healing and regeneration of musculoskeletal tissues.

CPM enhances the healing and regeneration of musculoskeletal tissues, including articular cartilage, synovial membranes, joint capsules, ligaments, and tendons. CPM also is used to overcome joint stiffness and pain, and it minimizes the effects associated with immobilization.

Answer: **True**

Hunter, Mackin, Callahan, p. 1545
LaStayo, Cass in Mackin, Callahan, Skirven, et al, p. 1764
Refer to Fig. 5-5

25. True or False: CPM can provide low-load prolonged stress.

CPM is probably effective in preventing or overcoming joint stiffness because of the machine's ability to provide low-load prolonged stress (LLPS) to tissues. The phenomenon of LLPS is best explained by Atkinson and others, who state that "the fibroblasts of the fibrous connective tissue matrix apparently respond to physical forces by a homeostatic biofeedback loop to maintain the proper balance of tissue constituents." LLPS addresses structural changes in the tissues after trauma and stiffness after immobilization. Understanding of the mechanics of LLPS and its effects on connective tissue is still somewhat speculative.

Answer: **True**

Hunter, Mackin, Callahan, p. 1546
LaStayo, Cass in Mackin, Callahan, Skirven, et al, pp. 1766-1767

26. For which of the following is CPM contraindicated?

A. Burn patients
B. Capsulotomies
C. Fractures with open reduction internal fixation
D. Unstable fractures

CPM is indicated for fractures that are stable after open reduction internal fixation. CPM is not indicated for an unstable fracture. It is, however, indicated in surgical release of joints, capsules, tendons, and extraarticular scar adhesions. CPM has indications for use with surgical repair of tendons or repair of ligaments. Other indications include overcoming joint stiffness, inflammatory conditions, pain, burns, and total joint replacements.

Answer: **D**

Hunter, Mackin, Callahan, pp. 1548-1551
LaStayo, Cass in Mackin, Callahan, Skirven, et al, p. 1768

27. For lateral epicondylitis, the best form of cold therapy for local anesthesia to facilitate the performance of active and/or passive range of motion (ROM) treatment is which of the following?

A. Cold pack
B. Ice massage
C. Cold bath
D. Controlled cold-compression units

A

B

C

Fig. 5-5 ■ Examples of CPM devices used in treating the upper extremity patient. **A,** JACE S600 shoulder chair-mount CPM; **B,** JACE H440 hand rehabilitation system; **C,** JACE W550 portable wrist CPM. (Courtesy JACE Systems, Cherry Hill, NJ.)

An ice massage is the best technique for treating a small area such as in lateral epicondylitis. Ice massage also is helpful when treating a muscle belly, bursa, or trigger point. An area 10 × 15 cm can be covered in 5 to 10 minutes. When ice massage is performed, it is not uncommon for a patient to experience cold followed by burning, then aching, and finally numbness or analgesia.

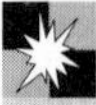

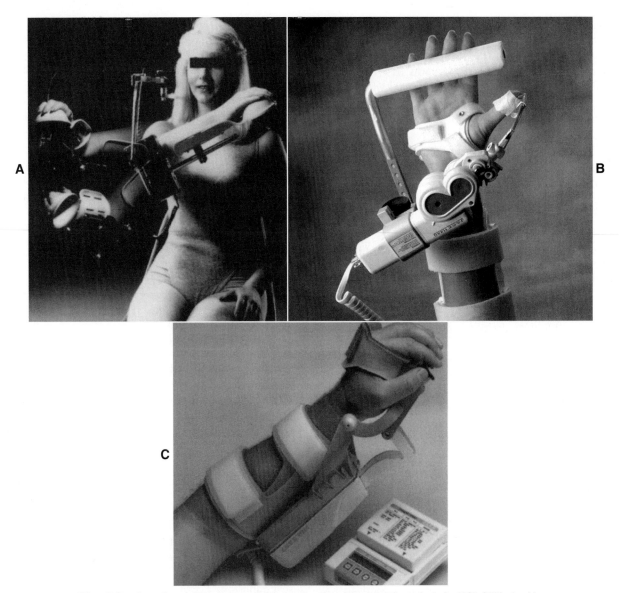

CLINICAL GEM:
A quick way to remember the order of physiological events during ice massage is to think of CBAN: *C*old; *B*urning, *A*ching; *N*umbness.

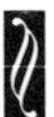

Answer: **B**
Michlovitz, pp. 99-100
Refer to Fig. 5-6

28. Match each electrical stimulation parameter to the corresponding word(s):

Parameter

1. Amplitude
2. Pulse duration

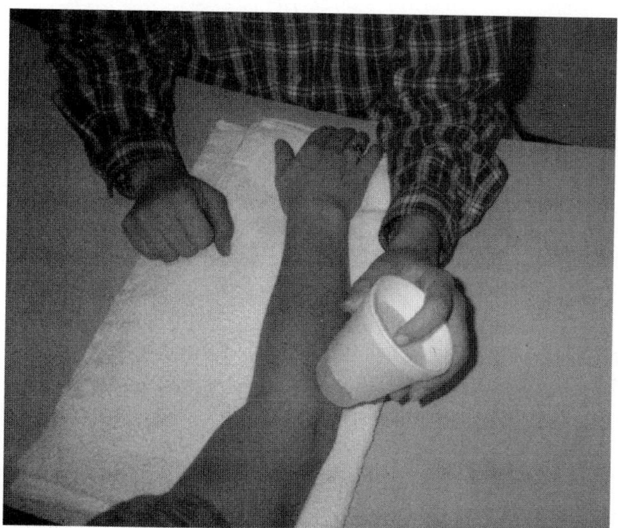

Fig. 5-6

3. Frequency
4. Rise time
5. On time/off time

Word(s)

A. Rate, pulse/second, Hz
B. Width
C. Duty cycle
D. Intensity
E. Ramp/surge

Answers: **1, D; 2, B; 3, A; 4, E; 5, C**
Hunter, Mackin, Callahan, p. 1512
Michlovitz in Mackin, Callahan, Skirven, et al, p. 1753

29. During use of electric stimulation to elicit muscle contractions, increasing the ________ will increase the strength of the contraction.

A. Intensity (amperage)
B. Pulse rate
C. Rise, or surge, time
D. Duty cycle

Many parameters relate to electrical stimulation for muscle contraction. Although nonlinear, they may be summarized as follows: with all other factors held equal, increasing the intensity of current results in increased strength of contraction. Increasing the pulse rate above 20 pulses per second results in a smoother contraction. Increasing the pulse rate from 20 to 80 yields a slight increase in strength but also induces more rapid onset of fatigue. Rates higher than 80 produce no known benefit.

The duty cycle—or on/off time adjustment—has profound effects on fatigue. Duty cycles of 10 seconds on to 10 off (a 1:1 ratio) tend to fatigue muscles within several minutes. In contrast, duty cycles that use a 1:5 ratio (e.g., 15 seconds on and 75 seconds off) allow the muscles to be active for 30 minutes longer.

The rise time, or surge time, is the length of time from the onset of the current until its highest intensity. A gradual rise in intensity (long rise time) yields a gradual increase in muscle strength.

Answer: **A**
Baker, Wederich, McNeal, pp. 91-105

30. Match each wave form to the corresponding current:

Wave Form

1.

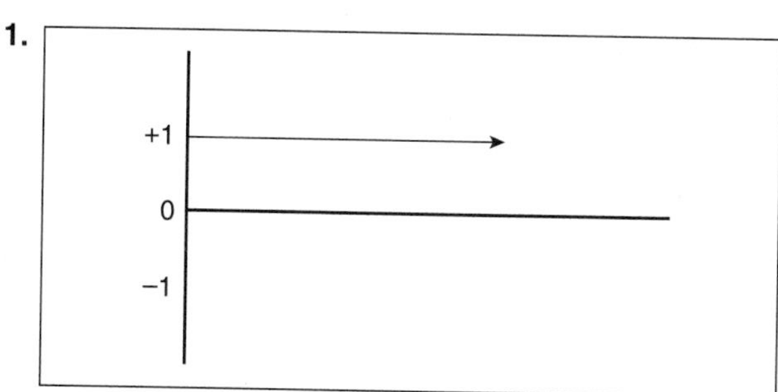

2.

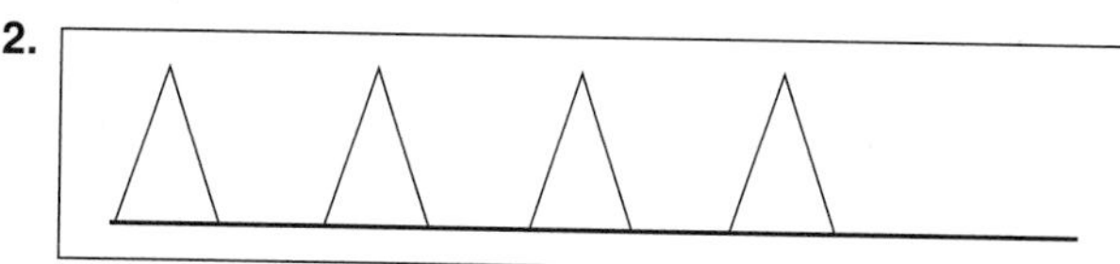

3.

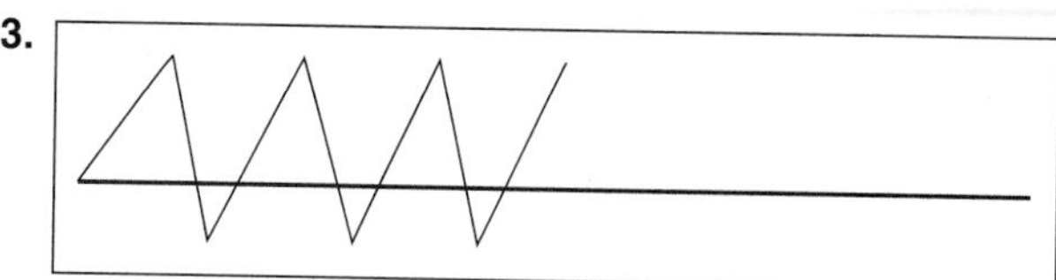

4.

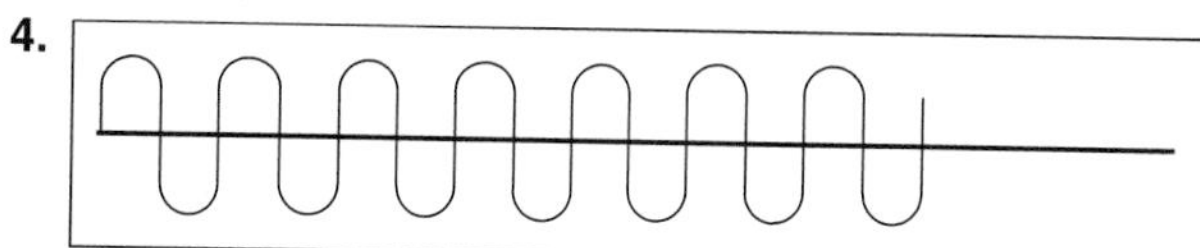

Current

A. Biphasic short duration current
B. Direct current
C. Polyphasic sinusoidal alternating current
D. Monophasic short duration current

Answers: **1, B; 2, D; 3, A; 4, C**

Hunter, Mackin, Callahan, p. 1511
Michlovitz in Mackin, Callahan, Skirven, et al, pp. 1752-1753

31. True or False: You are treating a patient after flexor tendon repair with electrical stimulation to increase the pull-through of his flexor digitorum profundus (FDP) to the middle finger. You notice with your current electrode placement that you are only getting the flexor digitorum superficialis to fire. One option would be to move the electrodes further apart to result in deeper penetration of current.

Although correct in theory, an increase in the distance between electrodes in practice often does little to increase depth of penetration. A more effective strategy for eliciting contractions of deeper muscles is the placement of one electrode over a superficial aspect of a motor nerve, and the other electrode over the muscle belly. In this example, an electrode placed in the cubital fossa will elicit contractions of the portion of the FDP that activate the second and third digits, and an electrode placed over the ulnar nerve will elicit contractions of the portion of the FDP that activate the fourth and fifth digits.

Answer: **True**

Baker, Wederich, McNeal, pp. 144-146

32. Strength-duration tests help determine the excitability of nerve and muscle tissues. Test results are plotted on log paper with the stimulus intensity on the Y axis and duration on the X axis. The relative position of the curve and the rheobase and chronaxie are identified on the graph. Answer true or false to the following statements:

A. Rheobase is the minimum intensity required to elicit a minimally visible contraction when the duration is infinite.

B. Chronaxie is the duration required for a stimulus with twice the rheobase intensity to elicit a visible contraction.

C. The strength-duration curve of a denervated muscle requires a lower intensity for a given duration than does an innervated muscle.

D. Sensory nerve tissue has a higher threshold than muscle tissue.

Rheobase is the minimum intensity required to elicit a minimally visible contraction when the duration is infinite and the chronaxie is twice the rheobase. Although it is excitable tissue, denervated muscle requires a stimulus of higher amplitude and longer duration than does a normally innervated muscle. Sensory nerve tissue responds more quickly than a motor (muscle) nerve and requires a lower intensity and shorter duration than muscle tissue.

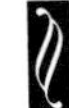

Answers: **A, True; B, True; C, False; D, False**

Hecox, Mehreteab, Weisberg, pp. 277-278
Meyer, pp. 124, 225
Refer to Fig. 5-7

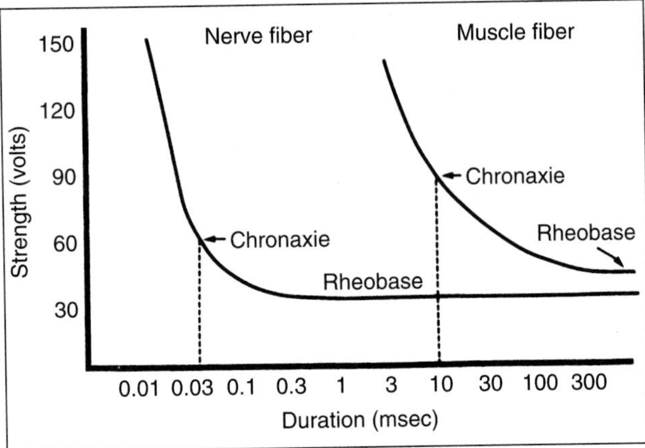

Fig. 5-7 ■ Strength duration curve of nerve and muscle fiber. (From Hunter JM, Mackin EJ, Callahan AD: *Rehabilitation of the hand: surgery and therapy*, ed 4, St Louis, 1995, Mosby.)

33. True or False: Most commercially available muscle stimulators require that the cathode (negative pole) be placed on the motor point, and the anode (positive pole) be placed distally.

Most commercially available stimulators are biphasic, or alternating, current stimulators. This means that each electrode alternates between positive and negative polarity throughout the treatment.

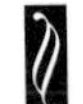

Answer: **False**

Belanger, Wederich, McNeal, pp. 347-350

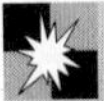

CLINICAL GEM:

One way to remember polarity is to recall that A+ (anode+) is a better grade than C– (cathode–).

34. Which type of current should be used with denervated muscle tissue (pick the best answer)?

A. Direct current
B. Any current with a long-pulse duration (>1000 microseconds)
C. Alternating current
D. All of the above

Long-pulse durations are required to overcome the capacitance of muscle fibers—that is, their ability to resist depolarization by artificial means. Electrical stimulation (ES) to elicit muscle contractions actually works by depolarizing motor nerve fibers. In the 1950s, long-duration currents were only available in combination with direct currents; therefore many therapists relying on textbooks of that era assume that A is the correct answer.

Unfortunately, long-pulse durations evoke significantly more skin impedance than short ones, thus heating of the skin. Increases in skin temperature easily lead to burns if the skin is denervated, which often accompanies denervation of muscles.

Because of the high risk of burns, very few manufacturers produce ES devices with durations long enough to elicit contractions of denervated muscle.

Answer: **B**
Baker, Wederich, McNeal, pp. 85-86

35. A 33-year-old active tennis player developed a gradual onset of extensor tendonitis in the right forearm and is unable to play tennis secondary to severe, sharp pain at the common extensor tendon origin when extending his wrist. Iontophoresis has been indicated as a treatment option. Which solution is the most appropriate choice for this diagnosis?

A. Copper sulfate
B. Saline
C. Lidocaine
D. Dexamethasone

This patient has developed lateral epicondylitis. Dexamethasone is the most appropriate solution to use with iontophoresis. Dexamethasone is an antiinflammatory and is effective for treating arthritis, bursitis, and tendonitis with iontophoresis.

Answer: **D**
Hecox, Mehreteab, Weisberg, p. 297
Hunter, Mackin, Callahan, p. 1517
Michlovitz in Mackin, Callahan, Skirven, et al, pp.1755-1758

36. Iontophoresis is chosen to treat edema and pain on the dorsum of a wrist. Which of the following is incorrect with regard to setting up iontophoresis treatment?

A. Clean skin and perform a sensation assessment.
B. Use an interrupted direct current generator.
C. Use an active electrode with the opposite polarity of the ion to be delivered.
D. Place a second, larger dispersive electrode on a distant area.
E. Electrodes should be buffered by the manufacturer.

An active electrode with the *same* polarity as the ion to be delivered is necessary. The ions are delivered to the tissues while they are repelled by an electrode with the same polarity. All of the other answers are correct statements regarding iontophoresis.

Answer: **C**
Hecox, Mehreteab, Weisberg, pp. 296-297
Michlovitz in Mackin, Callahan, Skirven, et al, pp. 1757-1758
Refer to Fig. 5-8

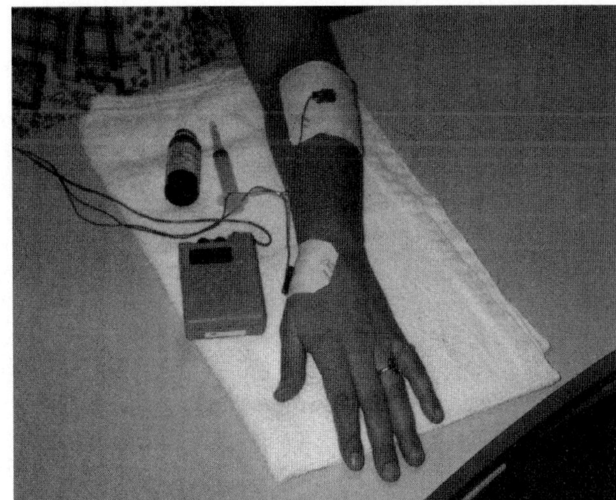

Fig. 5-8

CLINICAL GEM:
Medications used for iontophoresis

Drug	Preparation strengths	Polarity	Clinical identification
Dexamethasone	4 mg/ml	Negative	Inflammatory conditions (tendonitis, bursitis, arthritis)
Lidocaine	4%-5% solution	Positive	Analgesia
Salicylate	10% trolamine salicylate ointment or 2%-3% sodium salicylate solution	Negative	Arthritis

Adapted from Ciccone CD: *Pharmacology in rehabilitation*, ed 2, Philadelphia, 1996, FA Davis. In Mackin EJ, Callahan AD, Skirven TM, et al: *Rehabilitation of the hand and upper extremity*, ed 5, St Louis, 2002, Mosby.

37. A 25-year-old man presents with pain of the left wrist 2 days after playing in a racquetball contest. Which of the following treatment parameters is most appropriate for decreasing pain during treatment that uses ES?

A. Continuous, high voltage at 50 to 120 Hz for 10 to 30 minutes
B. Surged, Russian stimulation at 2500 Hz for 30 to 60 minutes
C. Interrupted, low voltage at 5 Hz for 20 minutes
D. None of the above is appropriate.

To help reduce acute pain, high-voltage ES is often used, with a rate of 50 to 120 Hz for 10 to 30 minutes. A continuous mode is most effective because the patient can comfortably tolerate an ongoing, unmodified series of pulses. This mode allows muscle relaxation and a reduction in pain.

Answer: **A**
Meyer, p. 215
Hecox, Mehreteab, Weisberg, pp. 266-267

38. Which of the following transcutaneous electrical nerve stimulation modes is appropriate when painful procedures (e.g., debridement) are performed on a patient?

A. Conventional
B. Low-rate
C. Brief, intense
D. All of the above

The brief intense technique involves a brief and intense high-rate (above 100 pulses/second) and high-width (above 200 microseconds) current at an intensity as high as the patient can tolerate. Brief intense transcutaneous electrical nerve stimulation produces a tetanic contraction and results in surface analgesia for 10 to 15 minutes. This is a noxious stimulus and is best used with and before painful procedures such as burn debridement, passive stretching, or minor surgery.

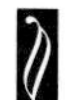

Answer: **C**
Hecox, Mehreteab, Weisberg, p. 302
Refer to Fig. 5-9

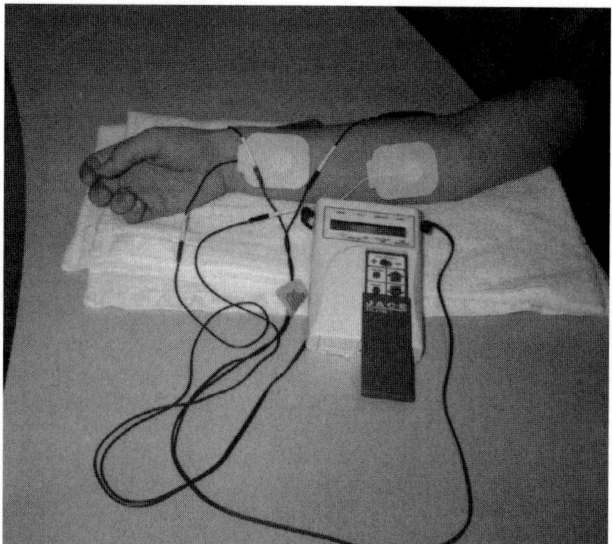

Fig. 5-9

39. Which of the following is true about using ES for the acceleration of wound healing?

A. It is still considered experimental.
B. It is no longer considered useful.
C. It is considered an adjunctive therapy by the Centers for Medicare and Medicaid Services (CMS).
D. It is useful only if the patient has poor sensation.

According to the CMS, very good evidence suggests that ES can accelerate the healing of most types of wounds, although the use of ES—or lack thereof—is far from the most crucial factor in wound healing. It is far less important than the presence or absence of infection, intact circulation, and good overall nutritional status.

Answer: **C**
Medicare coverage issues manual, Transmittal 166

40. The ideal parameters for treating wounds with ES include which of the following?

A. Direct currents of 75 to 100 volts
B. Pulse rate of ~100
C. Positive electrode over the wound to stimulate epithelialization
D. Negative electrode over the wound to stimulate formation of granulation tissue
E. All of the above

All of the above are correct. Although there is much room for variation depending on available technology and/or patient comfort, these guidelines are based on large-scale, multicenter studies of the past decade.

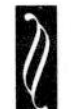

Answer: **E**
Kloth, McCulloch, p. 305

41. Electromyographic (EMG) biofeedback is most useful for which of the following?

A. Training patients to better control the neural activation of skeletal muscle
B. Strength-training
C. Desensitizing patients who have extreme fear of moving after painful injury
D. Increasing the speed of reinnervation after traumatic injury to motor nerves

EMG biofeedback is a technique to collect and display the neural signals that activate skeletal muscle. Although teaching patients to increase the level of activation may result in strength gains, the primary usefulness is to teach control of neural activation of skeletal muscle. Hence EMG biofeedback might be useful after cerebrovascular accident and in cases of autogenic inhibition secondary to pain, or to teach patients how to keep their activation consistent to minimize tremor.

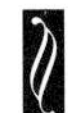

Answer: **A**
Prentice, p. 151

CLINICAL GEM:
Terms to remember
EMG stands for *electromyography.*
Electro- means *electrical activity.*
Myo- means *muscle.*
-Graphy means *graphical representation.*

42. Mr. X has carpal tunnel syndrome and is referred for "cold" laser treatment. What is your therapeutic intervention?

A. US with cold pack
B. ES with ice pack
C. Low-level laser therapy (LLLT)
D. All of the above

LLLT has been successfully used around the world for more than 25 years. The Food and Drug Administration (FDA) recently cleared LLLT for carpal tunnel syndrome. LLLT reduces inflammation, stimulates nerve function, develops collagen and muscle tissue, helps generate new and healthy cells and tissues, increases blood supply, and reduces acute and chronic pain. LLLT is a painless, sterile, noninvasive, drug-free treatment that is used to treat a variety of pain syndromes, neurologic conditions, and pathologies.

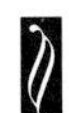

Answer: **C**
Batter, et al, pp. 171-178

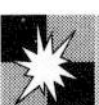

CLINICAL GEM:
The Microlight 830 is a state-of-the-art LLLT device that was designed by a team of doctors and leading medial engineers to harness the therapeutic application of advanced low energy laser technology. Visit www.laserhealthproducts.com for more information.

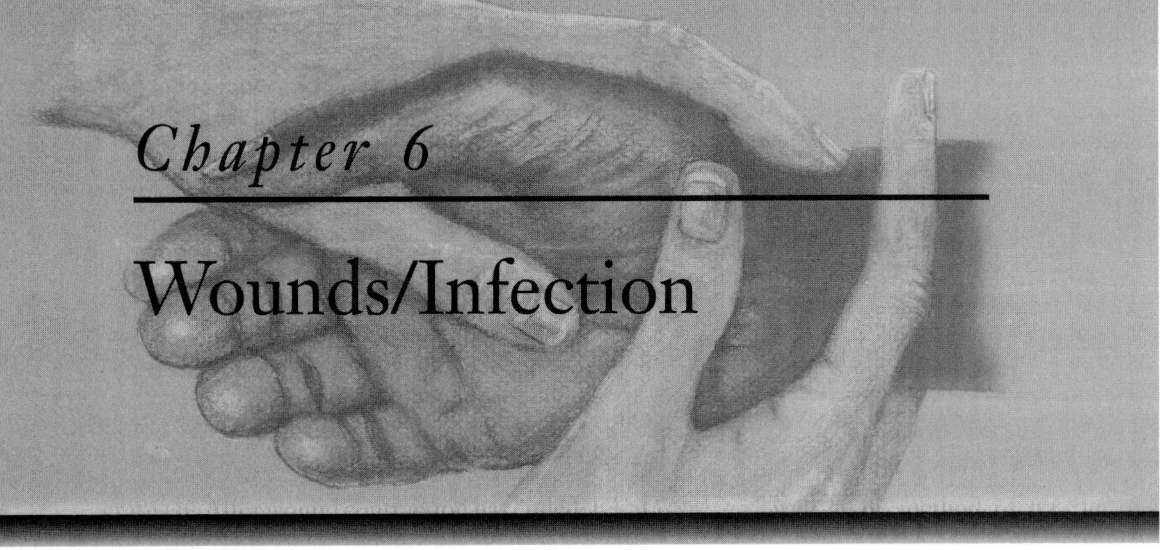

Chapter 6

Wounds/Infection

1. Match the following term with the appropriate definition.

Term

1. Autolytic
2. Debridement
3. Denuded
4. Eschar

Definition

A. Leathery thick necrotic tissue, often dry and black
B. Loss of epidermis
C. Removal of necrotic tissue
D. Disintegration or liquefaction of tissue or cells by the body's own mechanisms

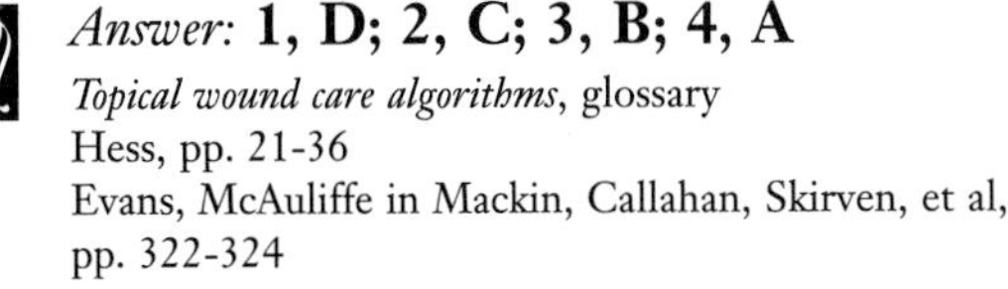

Answer: **1, D; 2, C; 3, B; 4, A**

Topical wound care algorithms, glossary
Hess, pp. 21-36
Evans, McAuliffe in Mackin, Callahan, Skirven, et al, pp. 322-324

2. All but which of the following are terms used for the inflammatory stage of wound healing?

A. Exudative
B. Proliferative
C. Lag
D. Substrate

Exudative, *lag*, *substrate*, and *inflammatory* are all terms for the first stage of wound healing; proliferative, fibroblastic, and reparative are all names for the second stage of wound healing. The first stage of wound healing is a complex arena of cellular activity; this stage begins with injury and usually lasts 3 to 5 days. Stage two lasts until day 21 and is termed *proliferative* with respect to collagen deposition and connective tissue. An infected wound cannot progress to stage two of wound healing. Stage three (the remodeling stage) generally begins around day 21 and may last for 24 months. This stage focuses on contraction and collagen degradation. It is important to understand that the three stages of wound healing overlap and are influenced by many variables. These variables include—but are not limited to—diet, age, infection, and other medical conditions. All of these factors can alter wound-healing time frames.

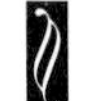

Answer: **B**

Hunter, Mackin, Callahan, p. 228
Evans, McAuliffe in Mackin, Callahan, Skirven, et al, p. 323
Smith, Price in Mackin, Callahan, Skirven, et al, p. 331
McCulloch, Kloth, Feedar, p. 3
Refer to Fig. 6-1

3. Autolysis is the method of debridement that occurs naturally and can be facilitated by moist wound dressings. Which of the following wounds would be suitable for this method of debridement?

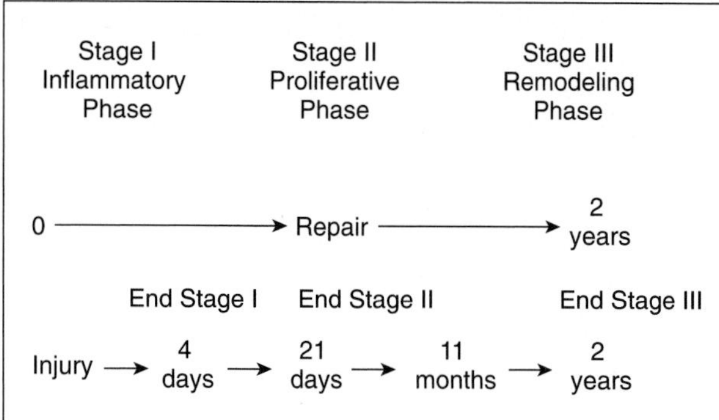

Fig. 6-1 ■ Time frame of wound healing stages.

A. A dry eschar-covered wound
B. A patient who cannot tolerate surgical debridement
C. A patient who has a coagulation disorder
D. All the above

All of the above are appropriate candidates for autolytic debridement. Autolytic debridement allows the body to break down necrotic tissue by using the body's enzymes and defense mechanisms. Autolytic debridement is accomplished by using a variety of moist wound healing dressings, which can help maintain a moist wound environment and thereby promote reepithelialization. They also have been shown to reduce pain and provide a barrier to infection. Many moist wound-healing dressings that will promote autolysis are available.

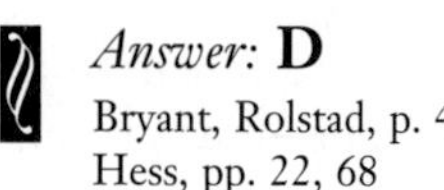
Answer: **D**
Bryant, Rolstad, p. 4
Hess, pp. 22, 68

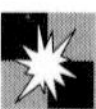
Clinical Gem:
Hydrocolloid, alginate, or hydrogel dressings can be used to achieve natural autolytic cleansing.

4. The inflammatory stage in an untidy wound is completed in how many days?

A. 2 days
B. 5 days
C. 10 days
D. The length of this stage is indefinite.

In a clean (tidy) wound, the inflammatory stage often lasts 5 days. In an untidy wound, the inflammatory stage lasts indefinitely until debris is cleaned from the wound. Severe trauma to the tissues, infection, excessive manipulation of the tissue in surgery, aggressive therapy, and inappropriate wound management are among the causes of a prolonged inflammatory stage.

Answer: **D**
Hunter, Mackin, Callahan, pp. 237-238
Smith, Price in Mackin, Callahan, Skirven, et al, pp. 331-332

5. Match each of the following terms with the correct definition.

Term

1. Collagen
2. Chemotaxis
3. Dehiscence
4. Exudate
5. Ground substance

Definition

A. Accumulation of a fluid in a cavity, matter that penetrates through vessel walls into adjoining tissue, or the production of pus or serum
B. A fibrous, insoluble protein found in connective tissues that represents about 30% of total body protein
C. The bursting open of a wound
D. The fluid, semifluid, or solid material that occupies the intercellular space in fibrous connective tissue, cartilage, or bone
E. The movement of additional white blood cells to an area of inflammation in response to the release of chemical mediators by neutrophils, monocytes, and injured tissue

Answers: **1, B; 2, E; 3, C; 4, A; 5, D**
Taber's cyclopedic medical dictionary
Evans, McAuliffe in Mackin, Callahan, Skirven, et al, pp. 311-328

6. A diagnosis of malnutrition can be made if which of the following is true?

A. Patient receives tube feedings
B. Serum albumin levels are below 3.5 mg/dl
C. Total lymphocyte count is above 1800 mm^3
D. Weight is appropriate for patient's height

Table 6-1

Markers of Malnutrition

Marker	Normal value	Mild depletion	Moderate depletion	Severe depletion
Percent of usual body weight	100%	85% to 95%	75% to 84%	<75%
Albumin, g/dl	≥3.5	2.8 to 3.4	2.1 to 2.7	<2.1
Prealbumin, mg/dl	16 to 30	10 to 15	5 to 9	<5
Transferrin, mg/dl	>200	150 to 200	100 to 149	<100
Total lymphocyte count, mm^3	2500	<1500	<1200	<800

From Hess CT: *Clinical guide to wound care*, ed 4, Philadelphia, 2002, Lippincott, Williams & Wilkins.

Nutrition is an important element in maintaining healthy skin and tissues and affecting repair when damage has been done. Malnutrition impairs the immune system. Total lymphocyte counts are a reflection of immune competence and as a guideline should be >1800 mm^3. A consultation with a dietitian should be made when the patient has inadequate dietary intake, has a drop in weight of 5%, or has serum albumin below 3.5 mg/dl. Vitamin C and zinc in a multivitamin may also assist wound healing where deficiencies exist (Table 6-1).

Answer: **B**

Sussman, Bates-Jensen, p. 261
Hess, pp. 38-39

7. Which of the following choices is true with regard to wound healing and nicotine consumption?

A. Collagen production is increased in smokers.
B. Cigarette smoking increases the risk for needing microvascular surgery.
C. Nicotine decreases platelet adhesion.
D. Nicotine has significant vasoconstrictive effects; however, these effects resolve immediately on completion of smoking.

Cigarette smoking dramatically increases the risk of needing microvascular surgery. Most studies are derived from animal studies to show the effects of smoke and tobacco on wound healing. Collagen production is decreased in smokers, and nicotine increases platelet adhesion, thus increasing the risk of thrombus formation in the microvasculature. Nicotine inhibits red blood cell proliferation, macrophages, and fibroblast activity. Significant vasoconstrictive effects from smoking can be present up to 50 minutes after completion of smoking.

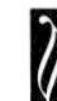

Answer: **B**

Jorgensen, Kallehave, Christensen, pp. 450-455
Chang, Buncke, Slezak, pp. 467-474
Kwiatkowski, Hanley, Ramp, pp. 590-597
Jensen, Goodson, Hopf, pp. 1131-1134

8. Wound healing occurs by primary, secondary, or tertiary intention. Patient Mr. Z has had a wound abscess drained; packing is instituted after review of culture; and surgery is planned for a surgical closure. This type of wound healing is classified as which of the following?

A. Primary
B. Secondary
C. Tertiary

Primary closure refers to surgical closure after planned surgery or insertion of sutures after trauma. Secondary closure involves leaving the wound "open" until it heals, as in the case of a venous or pressure ulcer. Tertiary closure is appropriate for the example given in the question—left open for a while then surgically closed.

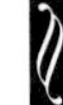

Answer: **C**

Hess, pp. 4-15
Jarvis, p. 39
Levin, Moorman, Heller in Mackin, Callahan, Skirven, et al, pp. 345-347

9. True or False: Most open wounds of the hand require antibiotics.

Most open wounds do not require antibiotics. Antibiotics should be reserved for wounds in which there is a high risk for infection, such as bite wounds, penetrating wounds, crush injury wounds, highly contaminated wounds, and wounds that have a delay of a few hours before debridement occurs. Because of the widespread use of antibiotics in the past, many bacteria populations currently are now able to resist the medicine; therefore, it is recommended that antimicrobial therapy be delayed until laboratory results are known. One alternative treatment for infection is the use of a hyperbaric chamber.

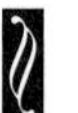

Answer: **False**

Green, p. 1545
McCulloch, Kloth, Feedar, p. 81

10. True or False: Research has shown that moist wound dressings impede healing and increase the risk of infection.

A moist wound healing environment actually promotes reepithelialization and healing. Drying wounds by exposure to air impedes healing by making migration of new cells difficult. Much research has been done that demonstrates that moisture in the wound does not increase the risk of infection.

Answer: **False**

Jarvis, p. 46
Evans, McAuliffe in Mackin, Callahan, Skirven, et al, p. 320

11. An open crush injury is classified as which type of wound?

A. Tidy wound
B. Untidy wound
C. High-level wound
D. Low-level wound

A tidy wound is defined as a clean laceration with minimal tissue injury and contamination; examples include surgical incisions, flaps, and grafts. An untidy wound has a significant amount of soft-tissue injury with a high degree of contamination and an unknown amount of deeper structure viability. Delayed primary closure or secondary wound healing is used for untidy wounds because of the higher degree of contamination associated with them. Answers C and D are incorrect because these categories do not exist.

Answer: **B**

Clark, Wilgis, Aiello, pp. 1-3
Evans, McAuliffe in Mackin, Callahan, Skirven, et al, pp. 313-314

12. True or False: Collagen synthesis usually begins between 3 and 5 days after an injury.

Collagen synthesis begins during the second stage of wound healing. This stage typically begins 3 to 5 days after an injury and ends between the 14th and 28th day. Fibroblasts produce collagen molecules that are complex helical structures. It is the collagen molecule that provides the strength and rigidity of scar tissue.

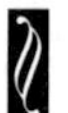

Answer: **True**

Ablove, Howell, p. 166
Smith, Price in Mackin, Callahan, Skirven, et al, p. 331

13. True or False: Platelets and macrophages release growth factors essential for tissue repair.

Both platelets and macrophages release growth factors essential for tissue repair. Platelets most likely are the first cells at an injury site. They attempt to form a balance or a hemostatic environment. Platelets release growth factors that contribute to fibrin deposition, fibroplasia, and angiogenesis. Platelets assist in clot formation, which stops bleeding.

Macrophages are essential regulatory cells in the repair process and they release growth factors essential for tissue repair. The macrophage performs phagocytosis of bacteria, dead cells, foreign bodies, and damaged tissue.

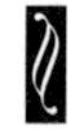

Answer: **True**

McCulloch, Kloth, Feedar, pp. 10, 17-18
Smith, Price in Mackin, Callahan, Skirven, et al, pp. 314-318

14. Match each wound definition with the correct classification. Each classification is used twice.

Definition/Term

1. Serosanguinous drainage
2. Necrotic tissue
3. Surgical debridement
4. Thick, creamy exudate
5. Macrophages attempting to clean exudate
6. Wound may appear clean or pink to bright red or may be composed of dark red granulation tissue

Classification

A. Red wound
B. Yellow wound
C. Black wound

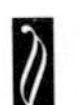

Answers: **1, A; 2, C; 3, C; 4, B; 5, B; 6, A**

Hunter, Mackin, Callahan, pp. 222-225

Evans, McAuliffe in Mackin, Callahan, Skirven, et al, pp. 317-319

Refer to Table 6-2

15. Why is ice contraindicated on an open wound?

A. Vasodilation
B. Vasoconstriction
C. Hypersensitivity
D. Hyposensitivity

Cold therapy causes vasoconstriction and reduces metabolism. Lundgren concluded that a 20% decrease in wound tensile strength occurs in wounds (rabbits) with cold therapy. It is recommended that cold therapy be avoided for the first 3 weeks after wounding because of the physiologic effects of cold therapy. Also, keep in mind that a major precaution with cold therapy is cold hypersensitivity or urticaria. Cold hypersensitivity may create areas of wheals, with reddened borders and blanched centers, accompanied by histamine release, which may cause an increase in heart rate, decreased blood pressure, and syncope. So with all modalities or treatments, monitor your patients for adverse reactions.

Answer: **B**

Michlovitz in Mackin, Callahan, Skirven, et al, pp. 1748-1749

16. The maximal strength of healed skin is which percentage of the strength of normal tissue?

A. 30%
B. 50%
C. 75%
D. 100%

At week 3, a normal sutured wound has less than 15% to 25% of its normal strength. Reorganized collagen reaches a maximal strength of 70% to 80% of original tissue.

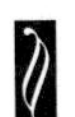

Answer: **C**

Ablove, Howell, p. 166

17. True or False: One of the leading causes of impaired wound healing is diabetes mellitus.

Patients with diabetes are predisposed to diseases such as atherosclerosis and renal failure. Atherosclerosis leads to major vessel (macrovascular) and small vessel (microvascular) disease. Hyperglycemia contributes to the altered healing in diabetic wounds at a cellular level; increased availability of nutrients for bacteria and impaired leukocyte function participate in making diabetic wounds a challenge.

Answer: **True**

Hess, pp. 10-14

18. True or False: A keloid is classically considered a raised scar within the boundaries of the original wound.

A keloid scar results from excessive collagen deposition during the healing process. This imbalance occurs when collagen synthesis (production) exceeds collagen lysis (breakdown). Keloids are more common in areas of increased skin tension (e.g., trunk, shoulders, earlobes). Keloids migrate beyond the boundaries of the wound, whereas hypertrophic scars stay within those boundaries. However, not all authors accept this definition, which distinguishes the keloid from the hypertrophic scar. Some authors suggest that the only difference between the two is that the keloid is an extreme variant of a hypertrophic scar.

Answer: **False**

McCulloch, Kloth, Feedar, p. 27

Richards, Staley, pp. 381-382

Herndon, pp. 388-389

19. Which level of organism is indicative of sepsis?

A. 10 organisms per gram of tissue
B. 10^2 organisms per gram of tissue
C. 10^3 organisms per gram of tissue
D. 10^7 organisms per gram of tissue

Wound sepsis (infection) is determined by bacterial contamination *exceeding* 10^5 organisms per gram of tissue. This level can be determined only by tissue biopsy. Estimates suggest that 10^3 organisms per gram of tissue normally are present in skin. The US Institute of Surgical Research recommends that wounds with more than 10^5 organisms per gram of tissue heal by secondary intention to reduce bacterial count.

Table 6-2

Simplifying Clinical Decision Making for Open Wounds

	Black wound	Yellow wound	Red wound
Description	Covered with thick necrotic tissue or eschar	Generating exudates; looks creamy; contains pus, debris, and viscous surface exudate	Uninfected, properly healing with definite borders, may be pink or beefy red, granulated tissue and neovascularization
Cellular activity	1. Autolysis, collagenase activity 2. Defense, phagocytosis 3. Macrophage cell	1. Immune response, defense 2. Phagocytosis 3. Macrophage cell	1. Endothelial cells—angiogenesis 2. Fibroblast cells—collagen and ground substance 3. Myofibroblast—wound contraction
Debridement	1. Surgical, preferred 2. Mechanical, whirlpool, dressings 3. Chemical, enzymatic digestion	Separate wound debris with aggressive scrubs, irrigation, or whirlpool	N/A—Avoid any tissue trauma or stripping of new cells
Cleansing	1. Irrigation 2. Soap and water scrubs 3. Whirlpool	1. Use no antiseptics 2. Soap and water 3. Surfactant-soaked sponge 4. Polaxmer 188, Pluronic F-68	1. No antiseptics 2. Ringer's lactate 3. Sterile saline, sterile water
Topical treatment	Topical antimicrobials with low WBC or cellulitis	1. Topical antimicrobials to control bacterial contamination 2. Silver sulfadiazine, bactroban, neomycin, polymixin B, Neosporin	1. N/A For simple wounds 2. Vitamin A for patients on steroids 3. Antimicrobials for immunosuppressed patients
Dressing	1. Proteolytic enzyme to debride 2. Synthetic dressing, autolysis 3. Dress to soften eschar 4. Wet-to-dry for necrotic tissue	1. Wet-to-dry—wide mesh to absorb drainage 2. Wet-to-wet—saturated with medicants 3. Hydrocolloid or semipermeable foam dressings, hydrogels	1. Occlusive or semiocclusive dressings; semipermeable films 2. Protect wound fluids and prevent desiccation
Desired goal	1. Remove debris and mechanical obstruction to allow epithelialization, collagen deposition to proceed 2. Evolve to clean, red wound	1. Light debridement without disrupting new cells 2. Exudate absorption 3. Bacterial control 4. Evolve to red wound	1. Protect new cells 2. Keep wound moist and clean to speed healing 3. Promote epithelialization, granulation tissue formation, angiogenesis, wound contraction

From Evans RB: An update on wound management, *Hand Clin* 7(3):418, 1991.
N/A, Not applicable; *WBC*, white blood cell.

Answer: **D**

Green, pp. 1545, 1713
McCulloch, Kloth, Feedar, pp. 114, 126
Nathan, Taras in Mackin, Callahan, Skirven, et al, p. 360

20. True or False: Hyperbaric oxygen therapy (HBO) may be used to treat limb crush injuries and/or compartment syndrome.

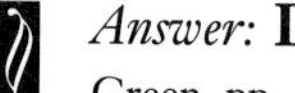

Crush injury can produce severe traumatic ischemia, thus compromising the limb's soft tissue and circulation and resulting in necrosis. After severe crush injury and/or compartment syndrome, ischemia may be caused by either large or small vessel disruption. HBO is theorized to maintain tissue oxygen tensions at a viable level despite low tissue perfusion. Edema reduction is another major benefit of HBO. HBO increases tissue oxygenation to foster wound healing by supporting white blood cell bacterial destruction, thus allowing fibroblasts to proliferate and build collagen and to develop new epithelial tissue.

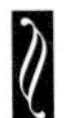
Answer: **True**
Kindwall, Gottlieb, Larson, pp. 898-908
Hess, pp. 16, 77

21. True or False: HBO is the same as topical oxygen therapy.

HBO refers to the form of treatment in which the entire patient is placed in a chamber and breathes oxygen at increased atmospheric pressure. Topical oxygen therapy is used when a limb is encased in a container with oxygen applied topically. Topical oxygen therapy therefore has little physiologic relation to HBO.

Answer: **False**
Kindwall, Gottlieb, Larson, pp. 898-908

22. Cellulitis involving the fold of soft tissue around the fingernail is which type of infection?

A. Felon
B. Collar button infection
C. Lymphangitis
D. Paronychia

A paronychia (Fig. 6-2) occurs after the introduction of staph *(Staphylococcus)* into a hangnail. This may occur to one side of the nail or it may surround the nail plate. It is the most common infection that occurs in the hand. In the early phase, it can be treated successfully with warm saline soaks, oral antibiotics, and rest. Surgical drainage is indicated for a more extensive lesion. After surgery, the packing is removed at 48 to 72 hours and warm saline soaks are initiated. These are discontinued when the inflammatory reaction ceases.

A felon is a suppurative abscess on the fat pad of the finger that often decompresses spontaneously. Surgical drainage is indicated if a felon is present for more than 48 hours. A collar button infection occurs in the web space through a fissure (break) in the skin and is treated with surgical drainage. Lymphangitis is a serious and rapidly progressing infection that is characterized by fine, red streaks extending from the infection site to the groin or axilla along the pathways of the lymphatics. Fever, chills, myalgia (pain in muscles), and headaches often are reported and prompt medical attention is necessary.

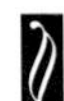
Answer: **D**
Green, pp. 1022-1023
Mosby's medical, nursing & allied health dictionary
Kasdan, p. 463
Nathan, Taras in Mackin, Callahan, Skirven, et al, pp. 361-362

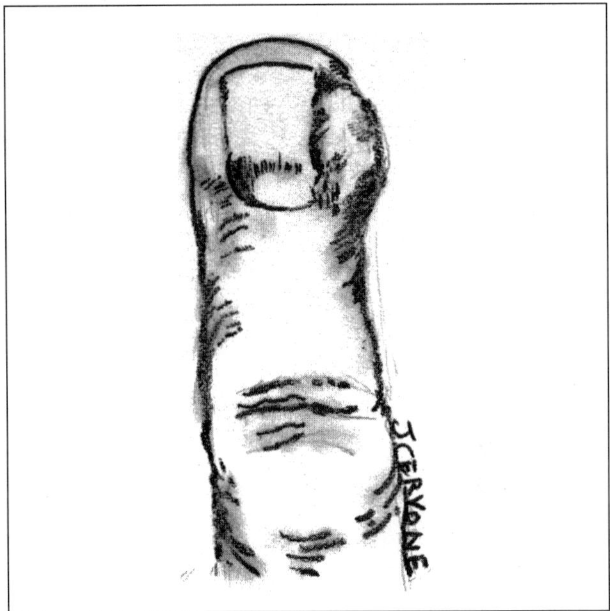

Fig. 6-2

23. True or False: Pus always is a sign of infection.

Pus (purulence) is not necessarily an indication of active infection. During stage one of wound healing a complex orchestra of vascular and cellular activities occurs. A neutrophil is a leukocyte that is classified as a polymorphonuclear granulocyte. Neutrophils migrate into a wound through chemotactic attraction immediately after an injury. The survival of neutrophils is short-lived (from 6 hours to several days). Neutrophils are present when a wound is contaminated. Simply put, pus is a large amount of dead, engorged neutrophils at the wound site. If laboratory results are negative for sepsis, the pus is called *sterile pus*; therefore pus is not a cardinal sign of infection.

Answer: **False**
McCulloch, Kloth, Feedar, pp. 6-9
Evans, McAuliffe in Mackin, Callahan, Skirven, et al, p. 316

24. True or False: High-pressure injection injuries may result in amputation.

High-pressure injection injuries usually are innocuous in appearance; however, these can be devastating injuries that may result in amputation and disfigurement. These injuries occur when paint, grease, or diesel fuel is accidentally injected into a worker during use of airless spray or grease guns. These injuries may be invasive and require prompt medical attention for optimal results. A visual assessment cannot determine the level of injury; surgical exploration and debridement are necessary.

Answer: **True**
Kasdan, p. 465

25. Which of the following is contraindicated with infection?

A. Antimicrobial therapy
B. Retrograde massage
C. Immobilization
D. Heat

Retrograde massage should not be used when a patient has an active infection because it might cause the infection to spread proximally. Immobilization is used during active infection to prevent spreading. It is important to immobilize only the affected areas. Heat can increase blood flow, as well as assist in the delivery of antibiotics and therefore is helpful with the treatment of superficial infections.

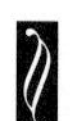

Answer: **B**
Hunter, Mackin, Callahan, p. 252
Nathan, Taras in Mackin, Callahan, Skirven, et al, p. 360

26. Which animal bite is most common?

A. Dog
B. Cat
C. Bird
D. Human

Most animal bites are inflicted by dogs. However, bites from cats are associated with more complications. Interestingly, human bites may contain as many as 42 species of bacteria. A bite from a human may have a bacteria count of 10^8.

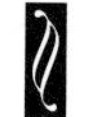

Answer: **A**
Hunter, Mackin, Callahan, et al, p. 256
Nathan, Taras in Mackin, Callahan, Skirven, p. 364

27. Your patient, who is a fisherman, presents with an obvious hand infection. Which organism might be present?

A. *Pasteurella multocida*
B. *Escherichia coli*
C. *Neisseria gonorrhoeae*
D. *Mycobacterium marinum*

M. marinum is a species of mycobacterium that is found in warm-water environments. A person with an open wound may be exposed while working in water or while swimming at the beach or in a lake, river, or pool. Most often the skin, flexor tendon sheaths, carpal canal or extensor tendons is affected. The infection may present as chronic skin ulceration or a localized tenosynovitis.

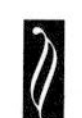

Answer: **D**
Green, p. 1036
Nathan, Taras in Mackin, Callahan, Skirven, et al, p. 365

28. What is one of the four cardinal signs of Kanavel?

A. Extreme tenderness over the proximal interphalangeal joint
B. Severe pain on attempted passive extension of a digit
C. Isolated swelling at the proximal interphalangeal joint
D. Involved digit postures in full extension

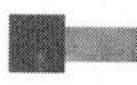

Tenosynovitis of the tendon sheath can be identified by the four cardinal signs of Kanavel, which are as follows: 1) uniform swelling of the digit; 2) digit held in a flexed posture; 3) tenderness over the affected tendon sheath; and 4) severe pain with passive extension/hyperextension of the digit. Flexor tenosynovitis is a serious infection that requires immediate medical attention. The treatment most commonly includes surgical decompression and drainage along with intravenous antibiotics.

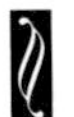

Answer: **B**

Kasdan, p. 467
Nathan, Taras in Mackin, Callahan, Skirven, et al, p. 363
Refer to Fig. 6-3

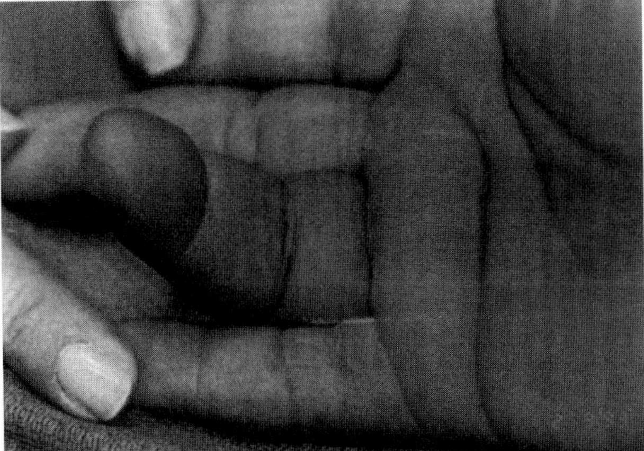

Fig. 6-3 ■ From Mackin EJ, Callahan AD, Skirven TM, et al: *Rehabilitation of the hand and upper extremity,* ed 5, vol 1, St Louis, 2002, Mosby.

29. Which of the following is most compatible with wound healing?

A. Saline
B. Hydrogen peroxide (H_2O_2)
C. Povidone-iodine
D. Chlorhexidine gluconate (Hibiclens)

Of the above answers, saline is the most compatible with wound healing. Wound specialists say the only solution that should be placed in a wound is one that can safely be poured into the eye. Many wound specialists condemn the use of antiseptics. Studies have shown that all antiseptic agents are cytotoxic. Hydrogen peroxide has minimal bacterial effect and is often misused along with povidone-iodine and Hibiclens. Some wound therapists believe that the pH of saline is too acidic for wounds and recommend lactated Ringer's solution because it is more compatible with the wound environment.

Answer: **A**

Hunter, Mackin, Callahan, pp. 226-228
Evans, McAuliffe in Mackin, Callahan, Skirven, et al, pp. 320-322
McCulloch, Kloth, Feedar, p. 145

CLINICAL GEM:
When recommending home wound cleansing with saline, you can substitute with contact lens solution. It is cheap, sterile, and effective. In fact, the spray can solution is particularly effective in home wound care.

32. Which of the wound dressings does the following: 1) effectively kills *Staphylococcus, Pseudomonas,* and *Proteus;* 2) can be used prophylactically to protect grafts from infection; 3) modulates the metalloproteinase activity and returns it to normal levels from the abnormally high levels found in chronic wounds; and 4) should be kept moist with sterile water rather than saline?

A. Silver sulfadiazine
B. Topical triple antibiotic wet to dry
C. Acticoat 7
D. Xeroform gauze

Acticoat 7 is a Smith and Nephew, Inc., product that consists of two layers of absorbent, rayon/polyester inner core sandwiched between layers of silver-coated polyethylene netting. This sustained release of broad-spectrum ionic silver actively protects the dressing from bacterial contamination, and the inner core maintains the moist environment needed for wound healing. Acticoat 7 delivers 7 days of uninterrupted antimicrobial activity. Acticoat 7 is indicated to prevent infection in partial- and full-thickness wounds, including first- and second-degree burns, grafts, and donor sites. It may also be used over debrided and grafted wounds.

Answer: **C**

Wounds: a compendium of clinical research and practice, 13(2), supplement b
Hess, pp. 415-417

31. What is the most common source of replant failure?

A. Arterial insufficiency
B. Venous insufficiency
C. Vasospasm
D. None of the above

Three types of vascular compromise may cause replant failure: vasospasm, arterial insufficiency, and venous insufficiency. Vasospasm can occur from manipulation of the replant, often during dressing changes. Conservative measures are employed to relieve vasospasm; these measures include gentle massage, vasodilators, analgesics, warm compresses, and regional anesthetic blocks to assist in restoring circulation to the part. Arterial insufficiency is noted when the digit remains pale. Reexploration must be immediate to salvage the failing replant. Venous insufficiency is probably the most common cause of replant failure. Congestion is identified by the dusky hue present in the replant. If no adequate veins are available during surgery, the surgeon may try to achieve venous drainage through other means. The nail bed can be removed and heparin soaks can be applied to maintain a constant ooze from the part while venous channels are reestablished. Leeches also have been used under such conditions and have proved helpful in sustaining "the artery-only replant."

Answer: **B**

Hunter, Mackin, Callahan, p. 1084
Jones, Chang, Kashani in Mackin, Callahan, Skirven, et al, pp. 1440-1443

32. True or False: Vitamin A gel can be used in the treatment of wound patients who take steroids.

The inflammatory phase of wound healing is related to the body's immune system response to an injury. This inflammatory phase usually lasts 3 to 7 days. Steroids counteract inflammation and topical application of vitamin A will counteract the steroid and restart the inflammatory process in the chronic wound.

Answer: **True**

Sussman, Bates-Jensen, p. 44
Evans, McAuliffe in Mackin, Callahan, Skirven, et al, p. 317
Refer to Table 6-2

33. Negative pressure therapy with vacuum-assisted closure (VAC) is contraindicated in which of the following?

A. Stage 3 to 4 pressure ulcers
B. Dehisced surgical incisions
C. Mesh grafts and tissue flaps
D. Wounds with necrotic tissue

A VAC device assists in wound closure by applying localized negative pressure to the wound. VAC negative pressure is applied to a special porous dressing positioned in the wound cavity or over a flap or graft. This porous dressing distributes negative pressure throughout the wound and helps remove interstitial fluids from the wound. The mini-VAC provides adjustable negative pressure therapy in a battery-powered ambulatory device, which you may see more often in hand and upper extremity wounds.

The four major contraindications for VAC are cancer in surrounding wound or tissues, fistulas to major organs or body cavities, untreated osteomyelitis, and wounds with necrotic tissue.

A VAC stretches the wound bed cells and in so doing causes epithelial cells to multiply rapidly; therefore it is contraindicated if cancer is present. Negative pressure on vital organs or fistulas could lead to trauma. Osteomyelitis must first be treated with appropriate antibiotic protocol; then VAC may be used. Necrotic tissue in the wound bed impedes the inflammatory and proliferative phases of wound healing progression and increases the bioburden risk. Necrotic tissue is removed prior to application of VAC therapy.

Answer: **D**

Mendez-Eastman, pp. 20-24
Hess, pp. 429-431
Evans, McAuliffe in Mackin, Callahan, Skirven, et al, pp. 324-325

34. You have a patient with a mild crush injury from a printing press. A minimal amount of serous drainage is observed from the healthy, granulating tissue. Which dressing would you use?

A. Dry, sterile dressing (DSD)
B. Wet-to-dry dressing
C. Adaptic dressing
D. Coban dressing

Your goal is to promote the healing process. Adaptic dressing, classified as an impregnate, allows reepithelialization and prevents adherence of the secondary dressing. You would not choose a DSD alone because it would interrupt the healing process by disturbing the wound bed when removed. In current practice, wet-to-dry dressing has limited use because of the aggressive nature of debridement, which affects both healthy and unhealthy tissue. A wet-to-dry technique is not recommended for wounds with less than 70% necrotic tissue, for wounds with tendon exposures, when it causes bleeding or pain, or when infection is present.

Answer: **C**

McCulloch, Kloth, Feedar, p. 152

35. Patient Mr. B has a dehisced surgical incision on the dorsal aspect of his left hand with exposed tendon and tunneling of 1 cm at 12 o'clock. The orthopedic surgeon has prescribed VAC therapy to promote granulation tissue. True or False: VAC therapy with black foam at 125 mm Hg continuous suction would be appropriate.

White foam is used for a tunneling wound. Black foam has larger pores and is considered to be most effective at stimulating granulation tissue and wound contraction. White or soft foam is indicated for tunnels because it is denser with less likelihood of shredding during removal from a tunnel. White foam is indicated to cover the tendon during VAC therapy because it affords more protection to the delicate tendon structures and growth of granulation tissue into the foam will be restricted.

Answer: **False**
VAC reference manual, pp. 5-12
Hess, pp. 429-431

36. A 25-year-old male patient is sent to hand therapy for evaluation and treatment after flexor digitorum superficialis/flexor digitorum profundus repair of the ring finger. The patient has minimal drainage from the wound with 2 mm of exposed tendon. Which dressing would you choose?

A. Coban (elastic wrap)
B. Tegaderm (semipermeable film [SPF])
C. Kaltostat (calcium alginate dressing)
D. Kerlix (DSD)

Exposed tendons *must* be protected to prevent desiccation. The best choice is an SPF such as Tegaderm, Op-Site, or Bioclusive. These SPFs help regulate the wound environment by preventing dehydration without maceration. SPFs are contraindicated for infected or moderately heavy exuding wounds. Coban and Kerlix are not appropriate because they would not protect the tendons or keep a moist environment. Kaltostat is used for debridement and for moderate-to-heavy exuding wounds.

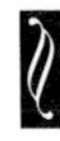
Answer: **B**
McCulloch, Kloth, Feedar, p. 163

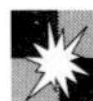
CLINICAL GEM:
If leakage, nonadherence, or maceration occurs with the use of an SPF, a possible solution is to use a pouch dressing. This is a type of SPF that can collect exudate. A therapist also may choose to use a more absorbent dressing or change the wearing schedule to allow for more frequent dressing changes.

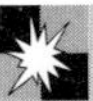
CLINICAL GEM:
Biolex wound gel (Bard Patient Care) with mesh dressings is a newer product that provides a moist, acidic environment to maintain humidity for an exposed tendon.

37. A 24-year-old, right-hand-dominant mill worker arrives in the emergency room 3 hours after sustaining blunt trauma to his left forearm. The patient's radiographs are normal. The patient complains of severe, progressive pain in the forearm. Physical examination reveals swelling of the proximal one third of the forearm with pain on deep palpation and pain with passive muscle stretches. The hand is warm and pink. Radial and ulnar pulses are normal. Two-point discrimination is normal over all five digits. Which of the following is the most appropriate next step in management?

A. Immobilization and inpatient observation
B. Gallium scan
C. Immediate fasciotomy
D. Immobilization and outpatient observation
E. Technetium scan

Compartment syndrome is a surgical emergency. Muscle that is ischemic for 4 hours is irreparably damaged. The diagnosis of compartment syndrome is made during clinical examination. Compartment pressures of more than 45 mm Hg also are diagnostic, but this test is not necessary when the history, signs, and symptoms are consistent. The hallmark of muscle and nerve ischemia is pain. The pain is persistent, progressive, and unrelieved by immobilization. In this patient, the muscle compartments are swollen; distal pulses and distal perfusion are not affected because the radial and ulnar arteries pass adjacent to and between muscle compartments, not through them. In this case, the appropriate next step in management is emergency decompression through fasciotomy.

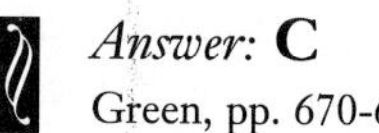

Answer: **C**
Green, pp. 670-673

38. Mr. X returns to the clinic with 50% red granulation and 50% slough ratio in his wound. The physician prepares the wound bed with a topical anesthetic prior to debridement with a curette. Which form of debridement is this?

A. Chemical
B. Sharp
C. Autolytic
D. Mechanical

Chemical or enzymatic debridement uses enzymes to debride slough or necrotic tissue from the wound bed. Sharp debridement is with a sterile instrument such as a curette or forceps and scissors. This can be done in the clinical setting or the operating room.

Autolytic debridement allows the body's own enzymes to break down devitalized tissue. A moist wound dressing facilitates liquefaction of necrotic tissue. The drawback is that this is a slow process in comparison with other more aggressive debridement methods.

Mechanical debridement in the form of a wet to dry dressing is not used as much because it causes trauma to new cell growth as well as the targeted devitalized tissue.

Answer: **B**
Jarvis, p. 45
Hess, pp. 18-22
Evans, McAuliffe in Mackin, Callahan, Skirven, et al, p. 317
Refer to Table 6-2

39. You are treating a 75-year-old woman who had an olecranon fracture treated with open reduction internal fixation. The hardware was removed at 2 weeks after surgery because of ulnar nerve complications and the patient was immobilized for an additional 4 weeks. When the cast is removed, a yellow wound measuring 2.5 cm wide, 2.0 cm long, and 1.5 cm deep is noted on the elbow. The wound is infected and has moderate amounts of thick, creamy exudate. Which dressing would you choose?

A. Hydrogel dressing (HGD)
B. Calcium alginate dressing (CAD)
C. Hydrocolloid dressing (HCD)
D. SPF dressing

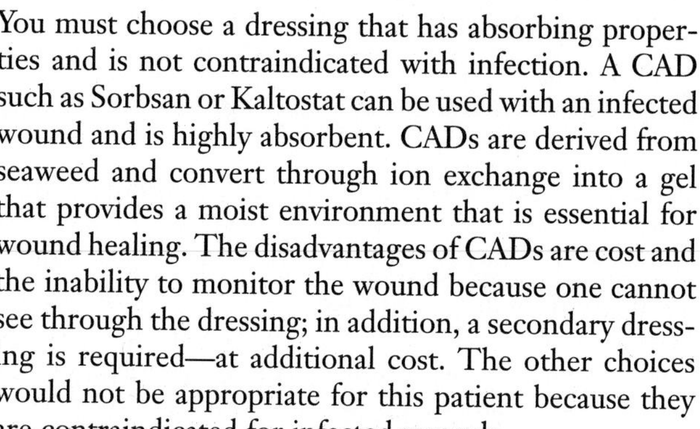

You must choose a dressing that has absorbing properties and is not contraindicated with infection. A CAD such as Sorbsan or Kaltostat can be used with an infected wound and is highly absorbent. CADs are derived from seaweed and convert through ion exchange into a gel that provides a moist environment that is essential for wound healing. The disadvantages of CADs are cost and the inability to monitor the wound because one cannot see through the dressing; in addition, a secondary dressing is required—at additional cost. The other choices would not be appropriate for this patient because they are contraindicated for infected wounds.

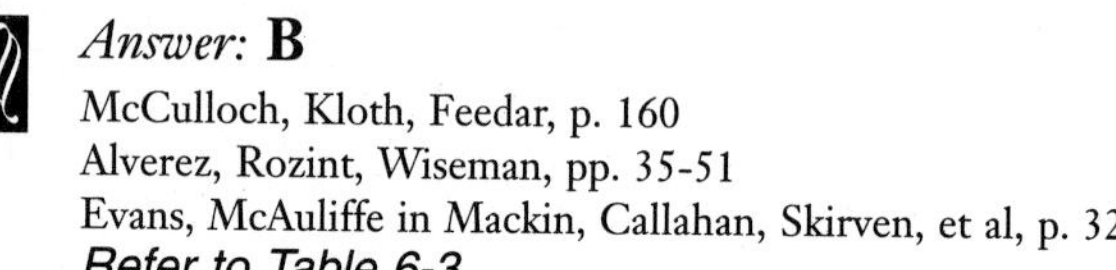

Answer: **B**
McCulloch, Kloth, Feedar, p. 160
Alverez, Rozint, Wiseman, pp. 35-51
Evans, McAuliffe in Mackin, Callahan, Skirven, et al, p. 321
Refer to Table 6-3

40. A patient presents with a bright red to dark red wound. You notice granulating tissue. Which would be the best treatment for this patient?

A. Whirlpool
B. Wet-to-dry dressing
C. Protect the wound; keep it moist
D. Clean the wound of eschar

A red wound is a healthy, healing wound. Your goal is to protect the fragile, budding, granulating tissue by keeping it moist and protected. A whirlpool is contraindicated because it can disturb granulating tissue; the same is true of a wet-to-dry approach (dead matter or necrosed tissue). Eschar is not present in a healthy, red wound.

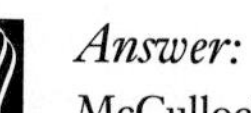

Answer: **C**
McCulloch, Kloth, Feedar, pp. 138-143
Evans, McAuliffe in Mackin, Callahan, Skirven, et al, p. 317
Refer to Table 6-2

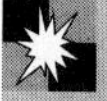

CLINICAL GEM:
Remind your patients not to over-apply ointments for moist wound healing. Over-applying will cause the surrounding healthy tissue to become macerated.

Table 6-3

Properties, Indications, and Precautions for Microenvironmental Dressings*

	Semipermeable film	Semipermeable foam	Semipermeable hydrogel	Hydrocolloid
Commercial name	Bioclusive Blisterfilm Ensure-It Omniderm Oproflex Opsite Polyskin Tegaderm Uniflex	Coraderm Lyofoam Lyofoam C Primaderm Synthaderm	Geliperm Intrasite Scherisorb Spenco Secondskin Vigilon	Biofilm Comfeel ulcus Demiflex Duoderm Granuflex Intact J & J Ulcer Dressing Restore
Indications	Clean, minimally exudative wound; red wound, sutured wounds, donor graft sites (split-thickness grafts), superficial burns, IV site dressing, superficial ulcers	Yellow wound, moderate to high exudates, skin ulcers, odiferous cancers, venous ulcers when combined with stockings or pressure dressings	Donor sites, superficial operation sites, chronic damage to epithelium, yellow exudating wounds; may apply over topical antimicrobials	Yellow wounds, friction blisters, postoperative dermabrasions, decubitus ulcers, venous stasis ulcers, cutaneous ulcers
Characteristics	Semiocclusive, occlusive, nonabsorbent, transparent, thin, adhesive, resistant to shear, low friction, does not control temperature, permeable to O_2 gas and water, impermeable to water and bacteria	Hydrophilic properties on wound side, hydrophobic on other side; limited absorbent capacity; permeable to water vapor and gas; polyurethane foams with a heat- and pressure-modified wound contact surface	Three-dimensional hydrophilic polymers that interact with aqueous solutions, swell and maintain water in their structure; insoluble in water; conform to wound surface; permeable to water vapor and gas, impermeable to water; tape required for fixation	Combines benefits of occlusion and absorbency; absorbs moderate to high exudate: expands into wound as exudate is absorbed to provide wound support; vision occluded; atraumatic removal; outer layer impermeable to gas, water, bacteria
Function	Mimics skin performance, protects from pathogens, decreases pain, maintains wound humidity, enhances healing by protecting wound fluids, protects from pressure, shear, and friction	Maintains wound humidity, absorbs excess exudates, maintains warmth, decreases pain, cushions wound while averting "strikethrough"	Maintains wound humidity; facilitates autolytic debridement; absorbs excess exudates; allows evaporation without compromising humidity; removes toxic components from wound; maintains warmth; decreases pain	Absorbs exudates to form a gel that swells; applies firm pressure to the floor of a deep ulcer; autolytic debridement maintains wound humidity; maintains warmth; removes toxic compounds; decreases wound site
Precautions	Only for uninfected, red wounds; apply to dry periwound area; frame wound by 2 in; break in seal allows microbes to enter wound from dressing margins	Visual monitoring occluded, low adherence, must tape	Permeable to bacteria, for moderate exudates, dehydrates easily, nonadhesive	Vision occluded; do not use on hairy surfaces

From Mackin EJ, Callahan AD, Skirven TM, et al: *Rehabilitation of the hand and upper extremity*, ed 5, vol 1, St Louis, 2002, Mosby.

*Disclaimer/contraindications: All environmental dressings must be used in accordance with product information, which provides guidelines for indications, application, and contraindications. Some contraindications are wounds ulcerated into the muscle, tendon, or bone; third-degree burns; edge-to-edge eschar; wounds associated with osteomyelitis and active vasculitis; ischemic ulcers; and infected wounds. These products are all-inclusive and are not necessarily endorsed by the author or publisher but are provided as a source for further study.

41. You are treating a patient with an external fixation device. You notice a heavy crusted exudate around the pins. How do you provide pin care?

A. Soap and water
B. Hydrogen peroxide
C. Neosporin
D. Hibiclens

Pin care is a very important aspect of hand therapy that is necessary to prevent infection. Hydrogen peroxide would be the best choice in this example to remove the crust; however, after the wound exhibits new granulation tissue, its use is discontinued or it is diluted because of its cytotoxic effects. Hibiclens, another wound cleaner, also is known to have cytotoxic effects. Neosporin is advocated by some; however, it may seal the area, thus preventing drainage. Soap and water is not as effective as hydrogen peroxide on a crusted wound.

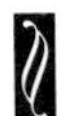
Answer: **B**
Hunter, Mackin, Callahan, p. 226
Evans, McAuliffe in Mackin, Callahan, Skirven, et al, p. 320

42. Mr. B is status post a traumatic hand injury and is awaiting wound closure with a skin graft. The ulcer presents with beefy red granulation tissue and minimal exudate; recent tissue culture demonstrates a microbial count of 10^6 colony forming units (CFUs). True or False: This ulcer is ready for grafting.

Granulating wound studies show that wounds are ready for grafting when tissue biopsies are $\leq 10^5$ CFU. $\leq 10^5$ Has a 94% take; those that had less than 20% take had CFU counts of higher than 10^5 CFU. Therefore Mr. B is not ready for grafting of his ulcer at this time.

Answer: **False**
Heggers, p. 26

43. An emergency room doctor calls a hand surgeon to consult about a patient regarding possible replantation. Which of the following individuals is the least likely candidate for replantation?

A. A 68-year-old retiree with an amputated thumb
B. A 9-year-old child with an amputated index finger through the proximal interphalangeal joint
C. A 22-year-old musician with an amputation of the small finger through the metacarpophalangeal joint
D. A 39-year-old laborer with an amputated index finger through the proximal interphalangeal joint

Replantation requires the ability to reliably repair small vessels using microvascular techniques. The best candidates for replants are patients who have sustained sharp lacerations. The time that has elapsed since injury is crucial, especially for more proximal injuries in which the ischemic part contains muscle. Contraindications include multiple levels of injury, avulsions, and a prolonged warm ischemic interval. Acceptance criteria for replantation vary from center to center and among surgeons. Most microsurgeons would question the advisability of a single finger replant except under certain circumstances (e.g., thumbs or in children or patients with special requirements, such as musicians). In the above example, the 39-year-old laborer would be best served by amputation; time off from work is minimized, and the index finger is the most expendable because of the seamless integration of the long finger for tasks involving fine grip. Replanted digits often are stiff and in the way, and can be cold-intolerant and painful for prolonged periods.

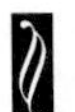
Answer: **D**
Green, pp. 1085-1102

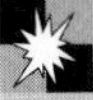
CLINICAL GEM:
The maximal warm ischemic time (when the amputated part is not cooled) is 12 hours for digit replantation and 6 hours for proximal replantation (proximal to the carpus).
The maximal cold ischemic time is 24 hours for digit replantation and 12 hours for proximal amputation.

44. Mrs. X has an open wound with 90% red granulating tissue, 5% yellow, and 5% black. What would be your treatment intervention strategy?

A. Enzyme ointment to debride black wound
B. Hydrogen peroxide
C. Saline
D. Tegaderm

The three-color concept classifies wounds as red, yellow, or black. As stated earlier, red is a healthy granulating wound. Yellow indicates the presence of exudates or slough and the need for wound cleaning, and the black wound indicates the presence of eschar. If a wound displays two or even all three colors at once it is often referred to as a *mixed wound.* According to the *Clinical Guides of Wound Management*, when a wound is mixed you should base your intervention on the least desirable color present. For example, in our question you have a red, yellow, and black wound. Therefore you should base your strategy on the black wound. An enzyme ointment can be used to treat the black portion of the wound. You can choose an antimicrobial ointment for the yellow portion and a simple wound gel for the red portion. Some facilities classify mixed wound colors by percentages, as we did in our question. The mixed wound may be treated with different wound products for each wound color area.

Answer: **A**

Hess, pp. 94, 275
Evans, McAuliffe in Mackin, Callahan, Skirven, et al, p. 317
Smith, Price in Mackin, Callahan, Skirven, et al, p. 338

Clinical Gem:
Make sure your enzyme ointment does not touch the healthy red granulation tissue.

Disclaimer/contraindications: All environmental dressings must be used in accordance with product information, which provides guidelines for indications, application, and contraindications. Some contraindications are wounds ulcerated into the muscle, tendon, bone, third-degree burns, edge-to-edge eschar, wounds associated with osteomyelitis and active vasculitis, ischemic ulcers, and infected wounds. The products presented in this chapter are all-inclusive and are not necessarily endorsed by the author or publisher but are provided as a source for continued study.

Chapter 7

Flaps/Grafts/Thermal Conditions

1. True or False: Most burns that occur from an electrical short are not actual conductive electrical burns but are more commonly flash burns.

Contrary to popular belief, many electrical injuries occur from an electrical short that results in flash thermal burns of the hands. This causes a variety of depth burns to the palmar or dorsal skin, which may be spotty or patchlike. They are usually superficial and are treated similarly to thermal burns.

True electrical burns, however, are completely different. The burns consistent with a true electrical current injury, or electrocution, would be characterized more by a discrete entrance and exit wound on usually widely separated parts of the body. They are characterized by damage to multiple tissue layers—including muscles, nerves, and vessels—as well as edema and necrosis of subfascial tissues. They are ominous in that there is damage to functional tissues throughout the extremity. They may also require fasciotomy and debridement and may develop compartment syndrome.

Answer: **True**
Achauer in Green, Hotchkiss, Pederson, p. 2051

2. A wound of the dorsal hand with exposed tendon and/or bone is best treated with which of the following procedures?

A. Open wound care and dressing changes
B. A skin graft
C. A local flap of skin
D. All of the above procedures are equally good.

The coverage of a wound with exposed tendon or bone requires tissue that brings its own blood supply with it. A skin graft by definition requires the blood supply of the wound site in order to survive. It carries with it no intact vascularity. Because of this, a skin graft will not work well on tendon or bone because of inadequate blood supply in those tissues.

It is best to provide vascularized coverage for exposed tendon or bone using a flap. Either a local flap from the dorsal hand in the form of a transposition or rotation flap may be used, or a pedicled flap, such as a radial forearm flap, may be employed. The radial forearm flap provides more versatile coverage to wounds that do not have readily available adjacent skin. The dorsal hand has enough skin laxity that many smaller dorsal wounds may be closed with rotation or transposition flaps of dorsal skin.

The use of simple wound care in such a wound would not be expected to readily heal the wound and could result in desiccation and necrosis of exposed tendon or bone and/or infection of those areas.

Answer: **C**
Lister, Pederson in Green, Hotchkiss, Pederson, p. 1783

3. Which of the following is not a commonly used local flap for wound closure?

A. Z-plasty
B. V-to-Y advancement
C. Moberg advancement flap
D. Lateral arm free flap

The Z-plasty (Fig. 7-1), V-to-Y advancement (Fig. 7-2), and Moberg flap (Fig. 7-3) all rely on tissues that are immediately adjacent to the wound. These techniques depend on the availability of sufficient local tissue for coverage of the adjacent wound.

The two other large categories of flaps include pedicled flaps, such as the radial forearm flap or the Littler neurovascular island flap, and the free tissue transfer, which can occur from a great variety of different donor sites. When local tissue is insufficient, the pedicled or free flaps allow tailored placement of specialized tissues where necessary by the means of vascular dissection or microvascular anastomosis.

Answer: **D**

Lister, Pederson in Green, Hotchkiss, Pederson, pp. 1783-1840

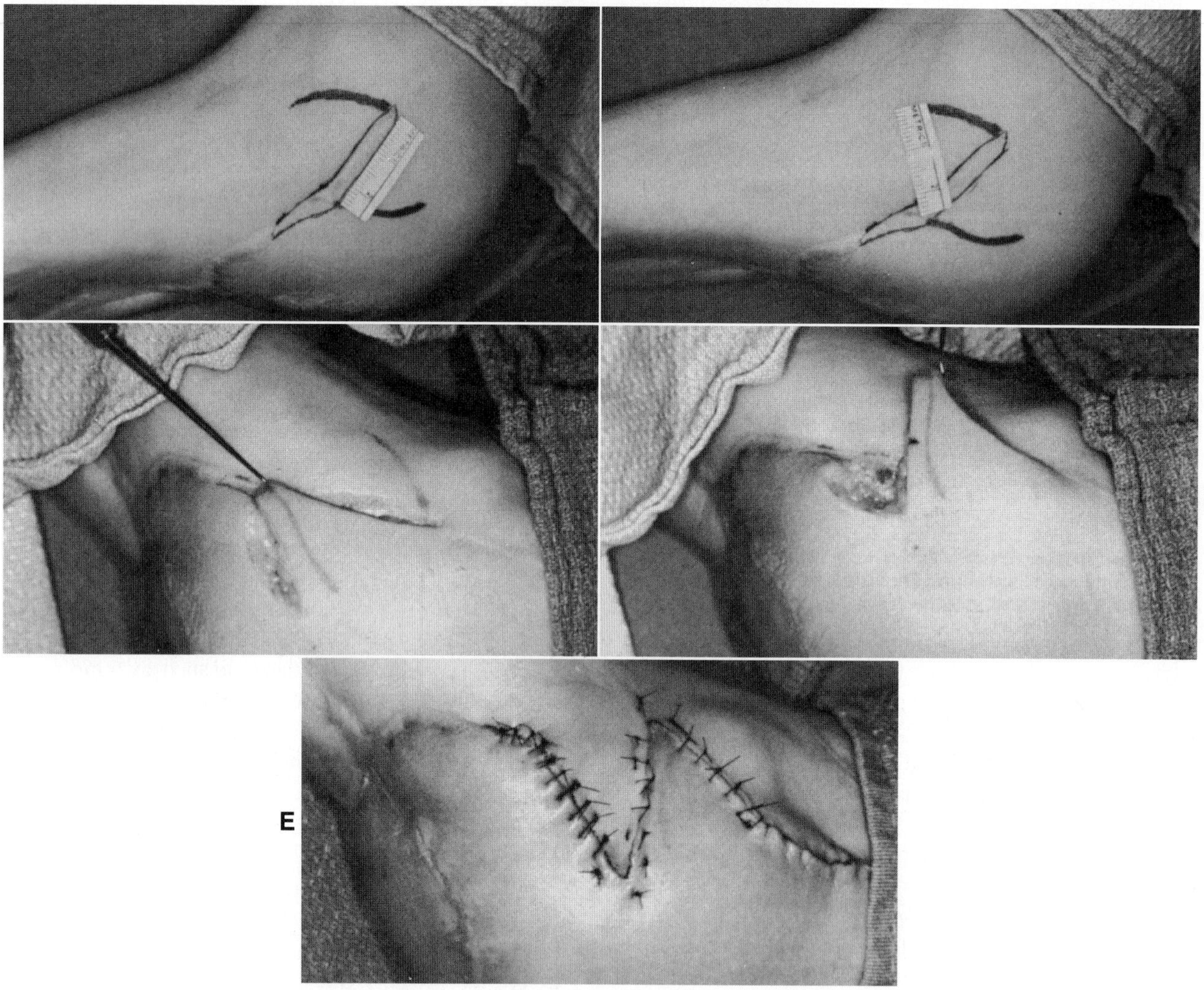

A

B

C

D

E

Fig. 7-1 ■ **A** through **E,** Z-plasty. (From Green DP, Hotchkiss RN, Pederson WC: *Green's Operative hand surgery,* ed 4, New York, 1999, Churchill Livingstone.)

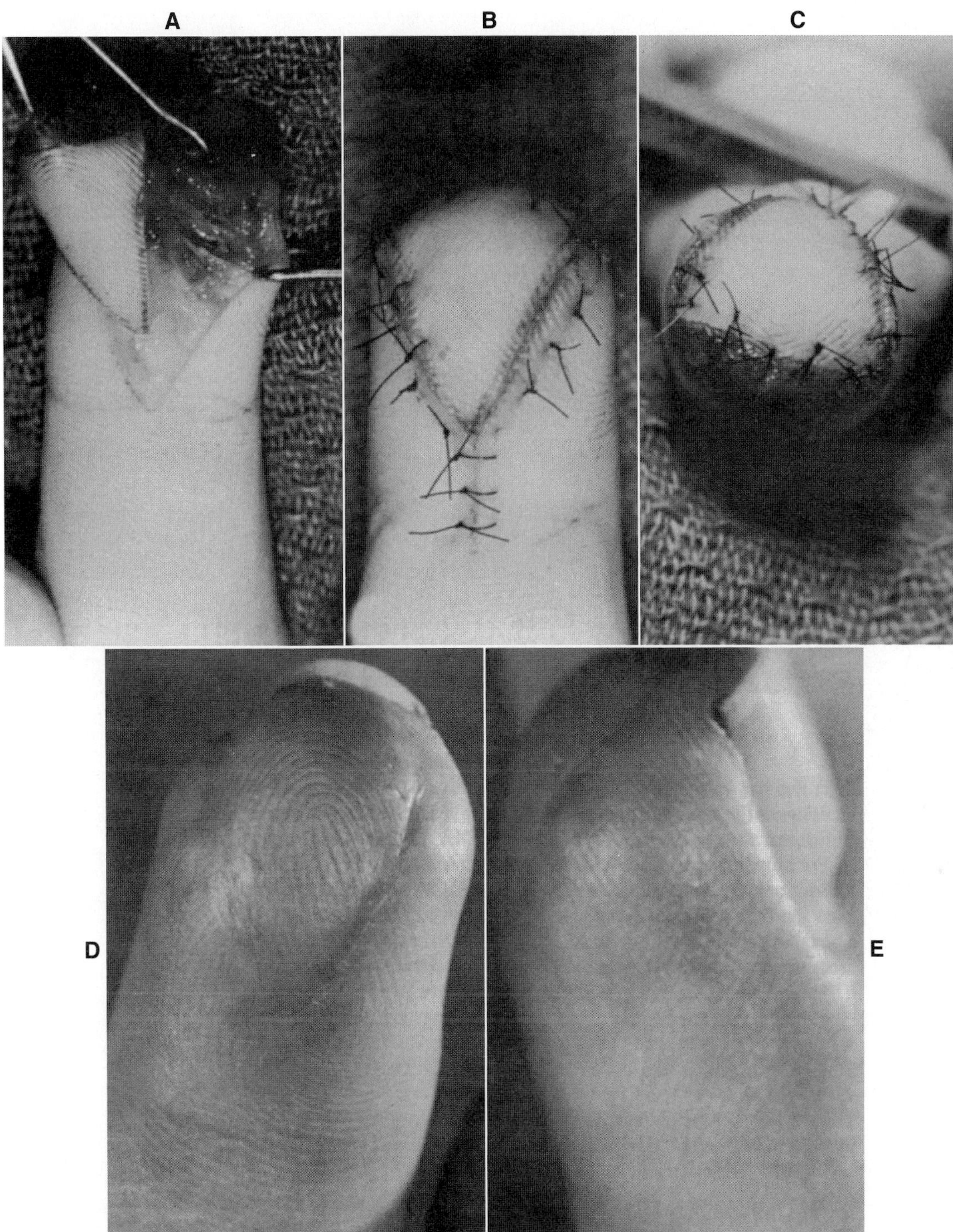

Fig. 7-2 ■ **A** through **E**, V-Y advancement. (From Green DP, Hotchkiss RN, Pederson WC: *Green's Operative hand surgery*, ed 4, New York, 1999, Churchill Livingstone.)

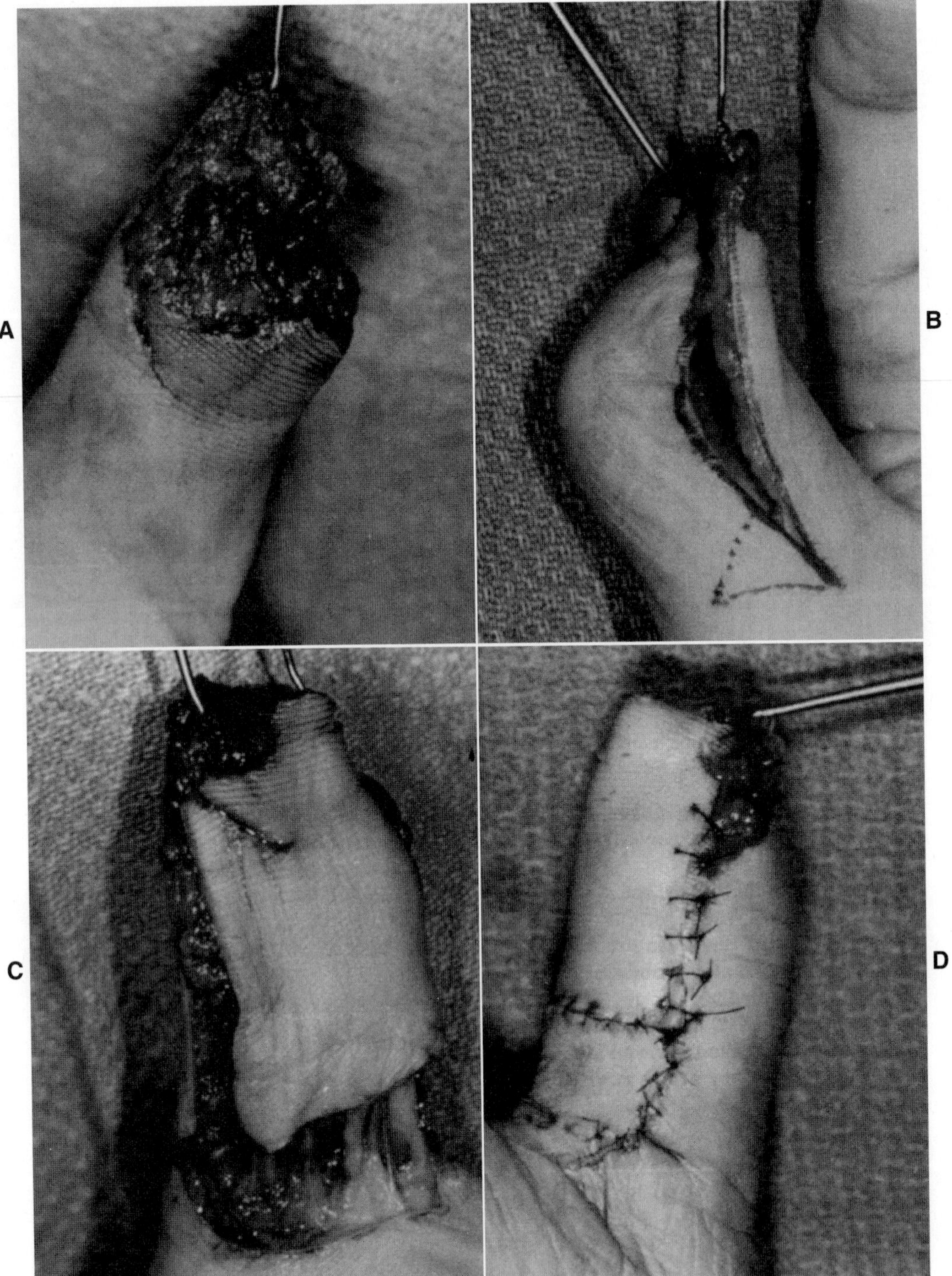

Fig. 7-3 ■ **A** through **D**, Moberg advancement. (From Green DP, Hotchkiss RN, Pederson WC: *Green's Operative hand surgery*, ed 4, New York, 1999, Churchill Livingstone.)

4. Which of the following should be avoided when treating a patient status post grafting, with edema?

A. Home exercise program
B. Active range of motion (AROM)
C. Whirlpool
D. All of the above should be avoided.

The use of a whirlpool should be avoided because it requires the arm to be placed in a dependent position, which leads to increased edema.

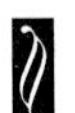
Answer: **C**
Vasudevan, Melvin, pp. 520-523

5. Which of the following is the most effective and accessible method for preventing and reducing edema?

A. Jobst pressure garments
B. Retrograde massage
C. Elevation
D. Coban wrap

All of the above can be used to manage edema. Elevation is the most effective and accessible method for preventing and reducing edema because it requires no assistance.

Answer: **C**
Vasudevan, Melvin, pp. 520-523

6. True or False: Edema is synonymous with oedema.

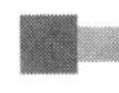

Oedema is the spelling used in Great Britain. The terms are synonymous.

Answer: **True**
Taber's cyclopedic medical dictionary

7. True or False: Raynaud's disease occurs with a causative disease.

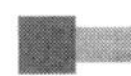

Raynaud's disease (idiopathic Raynaud's phenomenon) occurs without a specific causative disease. It occurs most often in young women and presents bilaterally, with an absence of primary disease. Raynaud's syndrome or Raynaud's phenomenon, in contrast, is associated with a disease process. Some of the causes of Raynaud's phenomenon may include connective tissue disorders (rheumatoid arthritis or scleroderma), arterioocclusive disorders, and late sequelae to cold injury. Vibratory trauma to the digits from power tools is also associated with Raynaud's phenomenon.

Answer: **False**
Hunter, Mackin, Callahan, pp. 972-973
Taras, Lemel, Nathan in Mackin, Callahan, Skirven, et al, p. 892

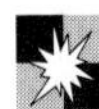
CLINICAL GEM:
85% of patients with scleroderma will manifest symptoms of Raynaud's phenomenon.

8. The first color response in patients with Raynaud's phenomenon is which of the following?

A. Cyanosis
B. Erythema
C. Pallor
D. No color changes occur with Raynaud's phenomenon.

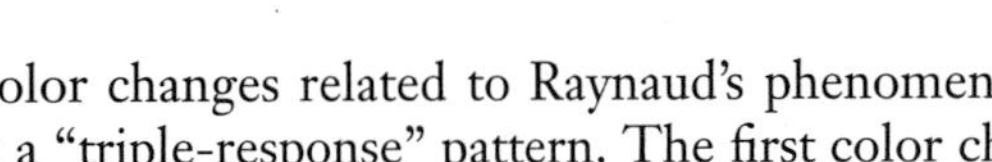

Color changes related to Raynaud's phenomena occur in a "triple-response" pattern. The first color change is ischemic pallor, which is followed by cyanotic coloring; as blood flow returns, a reactive erythema is noted.

Answer: **C**
Hunter, Mackin, Callahan, p. 962
Taras, Lemel, Nathan in Mackin, Callahan, Skirven, et al, p. 882

9. True or False: A good choice for treatment of Raynaud's phenomena is thermal biofeedback.

Thermal biofeedback is an excellent modality for pain relief and for learning rewarming techniques for patients experiencing Raynaud's phenomenon. It is especially helpful in reducing attacks in Raynaud's disease.

Answer: **True**
Hunter, Mackin, Callahan, p. 1567
Taras, Lemel, Nathan in Mackin, Callahan, Skirven, et al, p. 893

10. Which of the following is not a commonly used choice for first webspace contracture release?

A. Skin graft
B. First dorsal metacarpal artery transposition flap
C. Five-flap Z-plasty
D. Neurovascular island flap

The five-flap Z-plasty is actually a combination of two symmetrically opposing Z-plasties and a Y-to-V advancement flap designed to increase the length of the skin in the first webspace. It is a common technique for first webspace contracture.

The skin graft is functional in the first webspace in that it allows for a direct increase in the amount of skin available for first webspace expansion.

The first dorsal metacarpal artery transposition flap is dissected from the dorsal radial aspect of the proximal index finger and is based on the artery near the metacarpal head. This is ideally positioned for placement into the first webspace. However, the donor site requires skin grafting.

Although the neurovascular island flap is a possible donor for the first webspace, it is not commonly used because it is a much more specialized flap that attempts to carry with it not only skin but also sensate tissue usually used for resurfacing of a fingertip or the thumb tip.

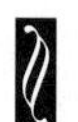

Answer: **D**

Lister, Pederson in Green, Hotchkiss, Pederson, pp. 1791-1796

11. Which of the following is not an acceptable donor site for a full-thickness skin graft?

A. The volar wrist crease
B. The ulnar hypothenar eminence
C. The groin or lower abdomen
D. The posterior ear skin
E. The medial ankle

Donor sites for full-thickness skin grafts are multiple, and they vary between sources in the palm of the hand or wrist and more remote sources. Palmar skin from the hand or the foot is often best for replacing palmar skin on the hand. It is more similar in nature, including color, skin appendages, and skin thickness.

Skin from the groin or the ear is often used for reconstructive purposes. There may be problems with hair growth from groin skin on the palm, and there is a difference in quality of the skin from those areas. The key element in all donor sites for full-thickness grafts is the availability of enough surrounding skin to close the donor site wound.

The leg and ankle would be unusual donor sites because of the relative paucity of extra skin in those areas. Nonetheless, plantar skin from the instep is a reasonable choice for the hand.

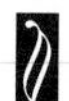

Answer: **E**

Browne in Green, Hotchkiss, Pederson, p. 1773

12. Which of the following is an advantage of a meshed split-thickness skin graft?

A. Mesh openings in the graft allow drainage of blood or exudates.
B. Meshed skin grafts contract minimally in comparison to sheet grafts or full-thickness grafts.
C. A meshed skin graft tends to have a more naturally skinlike appearance when it is healed.
D. The donor site from a split graft heals more quickly than the donor site from a full-thickness graft.

The primary advantages of a meshed split-thickness skin graft are that the meshing allows openings, which will drain fluid or exudate. If exudate or blood is not allowed to drain, it can tent up the graft and keep it from adhering to the vascular bed. The other advantage of a split graft is that the meshing allows for expansion of the graft itself. The pattern of meshing consists of multiple small slits cut into the graft. This allows it to expand into a netlike pattern, which allows for greater area of coverage. In the hand, there is usually plenty of donor site skin available, and expansion is not usually necessary. The advantages to a nonmeshed skin graft include less contraction and a more normal healed appearance.

Answer: **A**

Browne in Green, Hotchkiss, Pederson, pp. 1771-1772
Simpson, Gartner in Mackin, Callahan, Skirven, et al, p. 1479
Refer to Fig. 7-4

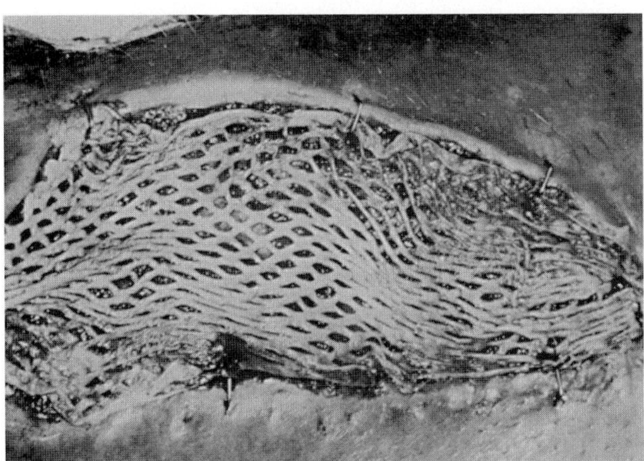

Fig. 7-4 ■ From Green DP, Hotchkiss RN, Pederson WC: *Green's Operative hand surgery*, ed 4, New York, 1999, Churchill Livingstone.

13. What is the mildest type of cold injury?

A. Chilblains
B. Frostbite
C. Immersion injuries
D. All of the above are mild types of injuries.

Chilblains are the mildest form of cold injury. They occur when individuals are exposed repeatedly to the cold with limited protection. Acute forms often are resolved within a week, but the condition can become chronic.

Immersion injuries occur from exposing an extremity to wet cold at a temperature above freezing. Common sequelae from immersion injuries are Raynaud's phenomenon, hyperhidrosis, muscle wasting, and cold sensitivity. Frostbite results from a crystallization of tissue water and occurs with exposure to temperatures below freezing. (Tissue freezes at approximately −2° C; the body's normal core temperature is 37° C or 98.6° F.)

Answer: **A**
Hunter, Mackin, Callahan, pp. 1295-1296
Byl, Merzenich in Mackin, Callahan, Skirven, et al, p. 1527
House, Fidler in Green, Hotchkiss, Pederson, p. 2061

14. True or False: The Hunting reaction is a protective reaction to cold exposure.

The Hunting reaction is a cyclic vasodilation and constriction that occurs with exposure to water or air at about 0° C (32° F). However, if an individual experiences prolonged cold exposure, the protective Hunting reaction will be overcome and the tissues will freeze.

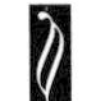

Answer: **True**
Hunter, Mackin, Callahan, p. 1296

15. True or False: Rewarming treatment after frostbite should be performed slowly.

Years ago physicians advocated rewarming the extremity slowly, first with cold water baths, or by allowing the extremity to thaw at room temperature. Evidence has shown that rapid rewarming at 40° to 44° C (104° to 112° F) is the most important step in salvaging the tissue and function of a frostbitten limb. Rewarming usually occurs within 30 minutes. The treatment may be very painful and require the use of intravenous (IV) analgesics. Blisters appear within hours after warming, and their treatment is controversial.

Answer: **False**
Green, p. 2034
House, Fidler in Green, Hotchkiss, Pederson, p. 2062
Brown, Hamlet, Feehan in Mackin, Callahan, Skirven, et al, p. 1531
Refer to Fig. 7-5

16. All but which of the following should be used in the management of a patient with acute frostbite?

A. Daily whirlpool treatment
B. Range of motion exercises
C. Resting splints if needed
D. Always remove blisters.

All of these options should be used in the management of frostbitten patients, except for the removal of *all* blisters. The removal of blisters is a controversial topic; it is not *always* necessarily the best choice for treatment. Some physicians believe that early removal reduces tissue damage. Others propose that the intact blister provides protection and therefore should be left alone.

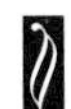

Answer: **D**
Hunter, Mackin, Callahan, p. 1299
Brown, Hamlet, Feehan in Mackin, Callahan, Skirven, et al, pp. 1531-1533

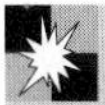

CLINICAL GEM:
The most common long-term symptoms after cold injury are excessive sweating, pain, cold extremities, numbness, abnormal skin color, and stiff joints.

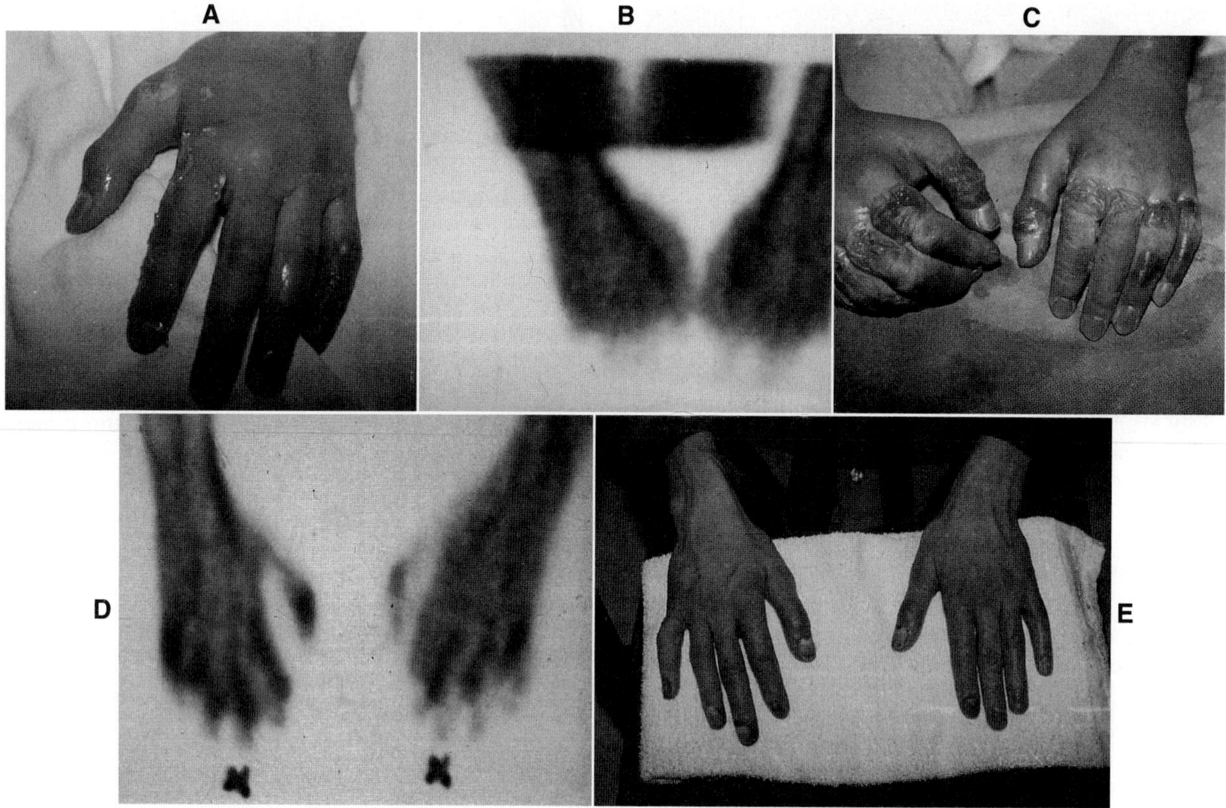

Fig. 7-5 ■ **A,** A 25-year-old patient with schizophrenia with both hands frozen. After rapid rewarming, there was no digital blood flow on Doppler examination. **B,** No digital perfusion—second phase of Tc99 scan. **C,** Two days after administration of 60 mg intravenous tissue plasminogen activator (TPA), digital flow was restored. Blisters are apparent on thumb and fingers. **D,** Repeat triple-phase Tc99 scan 7 days after TPA—digits are perfused. **E,** All digits survived, with good functional recovery of the hand. (Case courtesy John Twomey, MD, Hennepin County Medical Center, Minneapolis, MN; From Green DP, Hotchkiss RN, Pederson WC: *Green's Operative hand surgery*, ed 4, New York, 1999, Churchill Livingstone.)

17. True or False: The American Burn Association classifies a hand burn as a major injury.

The American Burn Association has established criteria for defining major burns that require hospitalization or care in a burn center. A burn to the hand is included among the definitions of a major burn. After a burn injury, mobility of the hand must be preserved; function must be restored; and soft-tissue coverage must be stable and soft. A failure to achieve these objectives can result in the individual not returning to work or functional independence. Burn center personnel have experience in treating critical hand burns and can assist patients in achieving good, functional outcomes.

Answer: **True**

Herndon, p. 506
Richards, Staley, pp. 114-115

18. According to the "rule of nines," the hand constitutes which percentage of total body surface area?

A. 1%
B. 3%
C. 5%
D. 7%

During evaluation of a burn wound, an estimate of the size of the wound is made. This helps assess the severity of the injury and determine the patient's prognosis. Knowing the size of the wound also helps establish treatment protocols for fluid resuscitation, nutritional support, and surgery. Burn size is estimated by calculating the total body surface area (TBSA) covered by the wound. Only partial- and full-thickness wounds are used in estimation. The percentage of TBSA covered by a burn is most often determined with a diagram that divides the body into 11 segments, with each one representing 9% TBSA. With this method, called the "rule of nines," a hand is calculated to be approximately 3% of an individual's TBSA. Therefore a circumferential burn to the hand would be classified as a 3% burn.

Answer: **B**

Richards, Staley, pp. 109-110
Herndon, p. 35
Pillet, Mackin in Mackin, Callahan, Skirven, et al, p. 1475
Refer to Fig. 7-6

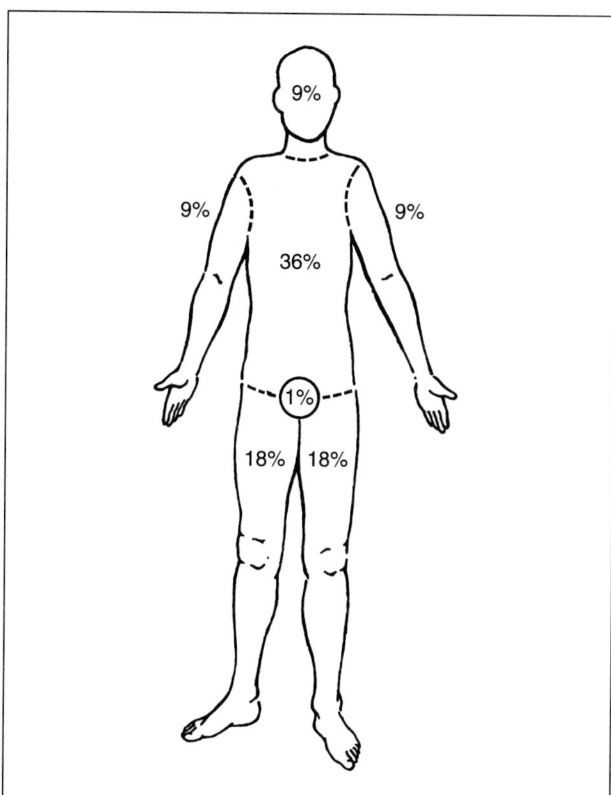

Fig. 7-6 ■ Rule of nines. (From Pedretti LW, Early MB: *Occupational therapy: practice skills for physical dysfunction*, ed 5, St Louis, 2001, Mosby.)

19. True or False: Full-thickness (third-degree) burns are quite painful.

Full-thickness (third-degree) burns destroy the full thickness of the skin, which may include the muscle, tendon, and bone. Initially, these burns often are pain-free and insensitive to pinprick because of the loss of nerve endings in the skin. However, most third-degree burns are surrounded by second-degree burns, which are very painful.

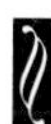

Answer: **False**

Hopkins, Smith, pp. 571-572
Simpson, Gartner in Mackin, Callahan, Skirven, et al, p. 1477

CLINICAL GEM:
The severity of a burn is determined by the temperature of the source, time of contact, thickness of the skin, and depth of the burn at the injury level. These factors will help determine whether excision and grafting are needed.

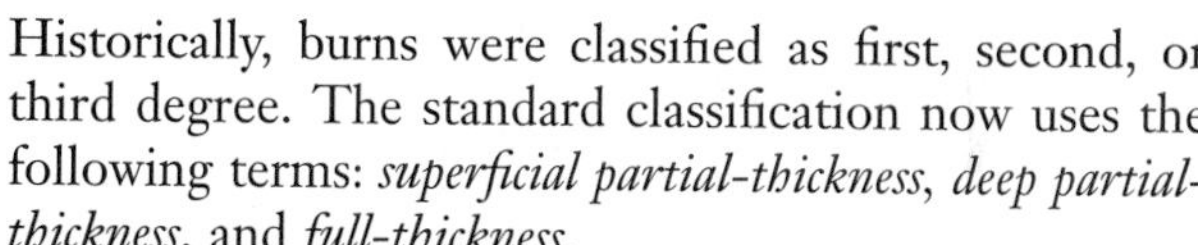

20. A patient in the clinic presents with an erythematous and blistering burn on his right thumb. How would you classify this burn?

A. First-degree
B. Superficial partial-thickness
C. Deep partial-thickness
D. Full-thickness

Historically, burns were classified as first, second, or third degree. The standard classification now uses the following terms: *superficial partial-thickness, deep partial-thickness,* and *full-thickness.*

Superficial partial-thickness burns involve the epidermis and also may involve the upper dermis. They are characterized by erythema, blister formation, and pain. The skin heals spontaneously by reepithelializaiton in 2 weeks or less, with normal functional ability and appearance. These burns are more painful and present with blisters and subcutaneous edema. The patient in this question falls into this classification.

Deep partial-thickness burns involve the epidermis, the papillary and reticular layers of the dermis, and sometimes the fat domes of the subcutaneous layers. These burns can be waxy-white looking, mottled, or erythematous, but they are pliable and will blanch if pressed lightly. Healing time is 21 to 35 days for these burns as long as the wound is free from infection. These burns may develop hypertrophic scars. These cases are treated with grafting procedures to prevent poor functional outcome and cosmesis.

Full-thickness burns destroy the full thickness of the skin. The skin varies from a dry, leathery appearance to charred skin, depending on burn severity. Full-thickness burns can be subcategorized as minor, moderate, or severe. The patient may experience minimal to no pain because nerve endings have been burned. Most large areas require grafting. If these areas are left to heal on their own, they may take many months. Hypertrophic scarring can be severe.

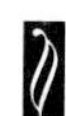

Answer: **B**

Hopkins, Smith, pp. 571-572
Richards, Staley, pp. 110-112
deLinde, Knothe in Mackin, Callahan, Skirven, et al, p. 1492

21. True or False: A keloid scar has distinct characteristics that distinguish it from a hypertrophic scar.

Controversy regarding the difference between a keloid scar and a hypertrophic scar has continued for almost 200 years. The keloid was first described in 1802. Hypertrophic scars were defined in 1847. Since then, their differences have been questioned. A keloid historically has been characterized as a scar that extends beyond the boundaries of the original wound. This definition continues to be used by some authors. However, some studies suggest little difference between these two types of scars and argue that a keloid may be an extreme variant of a hypertrophic scar. Further research is needed to solve this complex issue.

Answer: **False**

Richards, Staley, pp. 381-382
Herndon, pp. 388-389
Hunter, Mackin, Callahan, p. 1269

22. How long does a hypertrophic scar take to fully mature?

A. 1 month
B. 3 months
C. 5 months
D. 6 months or longer

During the first 6 to 12 weeks of wound healing, biomechanical and cellular changes accelerate and hypertrophic scars begin to appear. Collagen synthesis is active during this healing phase. Attempts to alter the scar are most effective between the sixth and twelfth weeks. A hypertrophic scar takes approximately 6 months to 2 years to reach maturity. A mature scar is less dense to the touch and more pliable. To determine whether a scar is mature, remove the pressure garment for a day or two and examine whether any changes in the scar's appearance occur. Return to normal skin color is *not* expected.

Answer: **D**

Richards, Staley, pp. 383-385
Hunter, Mackin, Callahan, p. 1273

CLINICAL GEM:
Silicone gel sheets have been shown to be effective in both the prevention and treatment of hypertrophic scars and keloids. The mechanism of action of silicone gel sheets has been investigated but remains unknown. It is effective with and without the use of pressure dressings.

23. True or False: The application of superficial heat can be beneficial in the treatment of a burned hand after wound closure.

Therapeutic heat can increase blood flow, reduce pain caused by passive stretching, and decrease muscle spasms. When connective tissue is heated and stretched simultaneously, its ability to lengthen increases. Heating the burn wound after wound closure can help temporarily elongate scar tissue. Moist hot packs, fluidotherapy, or paraffin can be used to decrease hand stiffness and increase the extensibility of tissues. It is important to remember that applying heat before wound closure is contraindicated because it may increase edema or cause hemorrhaging.

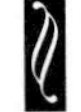

Answer: **True**

Richards, Staley, pp. 420-421, 568

24. When can exercises be safely initiated after a burn injury?

A. First 48 hours
B. 4 to 5 days
C. 7 to 10 days
D. 2 to 3 days

Edema formation, which is the body's initial response to a burn injury, occurs within the first 8 to 12 hours and peaks at 36 hours. Exercise programs for burn injury must be initiated as soon as possible (in the first 48 hours) after injury. Exercises are designed to help reduce edema, increase circulation, and assist with wound healing. Exercises are progressed to address passive range of motion (PROM), strength deficits, and functional loss and to provide resistance against the contracting scar in later stages. Forceful or aggressive exercises are not needed and can do more harm than good by constantly reinjuring fragile tissue and resulting in more collagen deposition with increased scar formation.

Answer: **A**

Hunter, Mackin, Callahan, p. 1271
deLinde, Knothe in Mackin, Callahan, Skirven, et al, pp. 1499-1500
Herndon, p. 453
Richards, Staley, pp. 324-329

25. All of the following are factors that influence the development of scar tissue. Which one is most important in predicting hypertrophic scar development?

A. Race
B. Burn depth
C. Age
D. Length of time for wound closure

All of the above factors affect hypertrophic scar development.

AGE: Most hypertrophic scars develop in individuals 30 years of age and younger, perhaps because this age group has a higher incidence of trauma and a higher rate of collagen synthesis when compared with older individuals.

RACE: Races with darker pigmentation (Black and Asian) have a higher incidence of hypertrophic scar development in comparison with Caucasians. One study found that Black populations have twice the incidence of hypertrophic scar development that Caucasians have.

BURN DEPTH: Hypertrophic scars develop from deep wounds that involve the reticular dermis. The reticular dermis is a deep plane in which collagen fibers are thicker and numerous elastic fibers form undulating (up-and-down) patterns. These wounds take longer than 3 weeks to heal, thus contributing to scar hypertrophy.

LENGTH OF TIME FOR WOUND CLOSURE: Hypertrophic scars develop from wounds that take longer than 3 weeks to close. If a wound is open for an excessive amount of time, greater amounts of collagen are deposited, making the length of time for wound closure *the most important factor* in predicting hypertrophic scarring. Collagen deposition results in the formation of thick, rigid scar tissue. Seventy-eight percent of wounds that take longer than 21 days to close develop hypertrophic scars.

Answer: **D**

Richards, Staley, pp. 385-387
Hunter, Mackin, Callahan, pp. 1268-1271

26. A patient in the clinic presents with a dorsal hand burn. In which position should she be splinted?

A. Wrist neutral, metacarpophalangeal joints at 20 degrees flexion, and interphalangeal joints flexed
B. Wrist neutral, metacarpophalangeal joints at 40 degrees flexion, and interphalangeal joints at 30 degrees flexion
C. Wrist at 15 degrees extension, metacarpophalangeal joints at 60 degrees flexion, and interphalangeal joints extended
D. Wrist at 30 degrees extension, metacarpophalangeal joints extended, and interphalangeal joints extended

Because of edema and wound tightness, the unsupported hand will position itself in a claw deformity of wrist flexion, metacarpophalangeal joint hyperextension, and interphalangeal flexion. To prevent this deformity, the wrist should be placed in slight extension, with the metacarpophalangeal joints at 60 to 70 degrees of flexion and the interphalangeal joints in full extension. If the thumb is involved, it should be splinted in abduction, with the interphalangeal joint slightly flexed. Splinting the hand in this position helps preserve the extensor mechanism and assists in preventing collateral ligament tightness.

Answer: **C**

Hunter, Mackin, Callahan, p. 1273
Richards, Staley, p. 283
Herndon, p. 446
deLinde, Knothe in Mackin, Callahan, Skirven, et al, pp. 1498-1499
Refer to Fig. 7-7

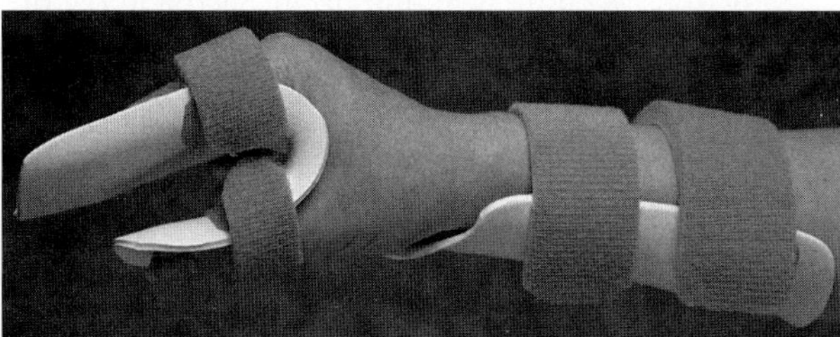

Fig. 7-7 ■ A resting hand splint. The hand is in an antideformity (intrinsic plus) position. (From Coppard BM, Lohman H: *Introduction to splinting: a critical-thinking and problem-solving approach,* St Louis, 1996, Mosby.)

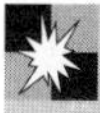

CLINICAL GEM:
In a literature review, more than 40 descriptions that stated how to splint dorsal hand burns were found.

27. Which of the following flaps does not require a second stage for division of the flap?

A. Thenar flap
B. Cross-finger flap
C. Groin flap
D. Latissimus dorsi free flap

The first three options all are characterized by the creation of a pedicle flap, which is attached to the recipient site and is left attached to the donor site for a variable period of time. All three of these flaps require dividing at a second stage. A free flap does not require a second stage for division.

Answer: **D**
Lister, Pederson in Green, Hotchkiss, Pederson, pp. 1802, 1810, 1825, 1833

28. Which of the following postoperative factors is most likely to cause failure of a flap?

A. Poor diet
B. Infection
C. Anticoagulant therapy
D. An overly compressive dressing or splint

Flap blood supply is known to be fragile. A cast or dressing that is applied too tightly can cut off blood supply or venous outflow and cause flap failure.

Anticoagulants, diet, and infection are not usually the cause of a flap failure, although an untreated infection could damage the flap significantly.

Nutrition certainly is an important factor in overall healing but is not usually the cause of the loss of a flap.

Answer: **D**
Lister, Pederson in Green, Hotchkiss, Pederson, pp. 1842-1843

29. True or False: Any muscle can be transferred via a free-flap technique for virtually any wound.

Muscle flaps are categorized generally by the vascular anatomy of the muscle. Categories that are amenable to free tissue transfer are those in which a single pedicle may support the entire muscle. Examples include the latissimus dorsi with one dominant pedicle and smaller peripheral pedicles, the tensor fasciae latae with one vascular pedicle for the entire muscle, and the dorsalis muscle with one dominant pedicle plus one other minor pedicle. Other muscles cannot be transferred successfully because they have a segmental blood supply in which one pedicle alone will not supply the entire muscle.

The anatomy of the vascular supply as well as the size and thickness of the muscle determine its ability for use as a muscle flap. Every muscle cannot be transferred via a free-flap technique.

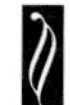

Answer: **False**
Lister, Pederson in Green, Hotchkiss, Pederson, p. 1822

30. A 21-year-old woman is referred to therapy with a hand burn. She has limited motion; you choose joint mobilization to increase finger flexion. When can you begin joint mobilization techniques after a burn injury?

A. During the acute phase
B. After reduction of edema
C. During the scar maturation phase
D. After wound closure

A burn scar must have good tensile strength to tolerate the friction that occurs during joint mobilization. Therefore joint mobilization should not be performed until the scar maturation phase; complications may occur if this technique is used earlier.

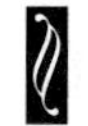

Answer: **C**
Richards, Staley, p. 336

31. A 7-year-old boy sustained an amputation of the tip of his nondominant ring finger. The resulting healthy, red wound measures 1 cm in diameter. No bone is exposed at the base of the wound. Which of the following would be the most appropriate form of management with the least chance of complications and minimal costs?

A. Healing by secondary intention
B. Full-thickness skin graft from the groin
C. Cross-finger flap
D. Thenar flap
E. Atasoy V-Y advancement flap

Healing by secondary intention is the most appropriate management of this injury. It provides good, functional results with few complications at a low cost. The primary disadvantage is an extended period of healing. Although skin grafting would require a shorter period of healing, additional procedures would be necessary, and the overall cost would be higher. In addition, no evidence suggests that skin grafting results in improved function. Grafting is more appropriate for volar oblique amputations.

A flap should be considered if pulp loss is greater than 1.5 cm in diameter and bone remains intact. Local flaps, such as the V-Y advancement flap, usually provide good sensibility but are difficult to mobilize when more than 1 cm of tissue is required. Cross-finger flaps and thenar flaps are excellent for reconstruction of the volar fingertip but are not necessary for small, uncomplicated injuries. Although the cross-finger flap causes less flexion contracture of the proximal interphalangeal joint, the thenar flap provides more tissue bulk and is consistently more successful in reconstructing large injuries.

Answer: **A**

Yaremchuk, p. 125
Levin, Moorman, Heller in Mackin, Callahan, Skirven, et al, p. 345

32. When nerves, blood vessels, and tendons are not injured and a healthy recipient bed is present, which of the following is the most appropriate form of reconstruction of the dorsal hand?

A. Skin graft
B. Cross-finger flap
C. V-Y advancement flap
D. Free flap

Treatment alternatives for soft-tissue coverage of the hand should be considered logically. Options range from simple (primary closure or skin grafts) to complex (flap or free-tissue transfer). The simplest method that will preserve form and function should be used. In this example, a skin graft would be the best choice because of its simplicity in the presence of a healthy recipient bed.

Answer: **A**

American Society for Surgery of the Hand, pp. 281, 287

33. True or False: The part of a flap that provides the blood supply is termed the *pedicle.*

A flap is skin with varying amounts of underlying tissue that is used to cover a defect. A flap receives its blood supply from a source other than the tissue in which it is placed. The part of the flap that provides the blood supply is termed the *pedicle.* All flaps have pedicles of varying types.

Answer: **True**

Green, p. 1741

34. The most common cause of skin graft failure is which of the following?

A. Excessive pressure on a fresh graft
B. Infection
C. Hematoma
D. Movement of the grafted area

A hematoma is a mass of clotted blood caused by a break in a blood vessel. The clot resides in the undersurface of the graft, isolated from the endothelial buds of the recipient bed, thus preventing revascularization and causing skin graft failure. Infection is the second most common cause of graft loss and is minimized by proper preparation of the wound bed. The other causes listed also can lead to graft failure and must be prevented.

Answer: **C**

Orenstein, pp. 1-30

35. The most appropriate coverage for a burn wound involving the entire dorsum of the hand is which of the following?

A. Full-thickness skin graft
B. Split-thickness skin graft
C. Primary closure
D. Latissimus dorsi myocutaneous free flap

In this example, a split-thickness skin graft (Fig. 7-8) is the best and simplest solution. The graft can be harvested with minimal donor site morbidity and yields an excellent functional result. A full-thickness skin graft would not be large enough to reconstruct this defect without grafting the donor area. Primary closure is not possible in this large defect. A latissimus dorsi myocutaneous free flap carries a significant donor site morbidity, and its thickness would not be needed in this case.

Answer: **B**
Orenstein, pp. 1-30

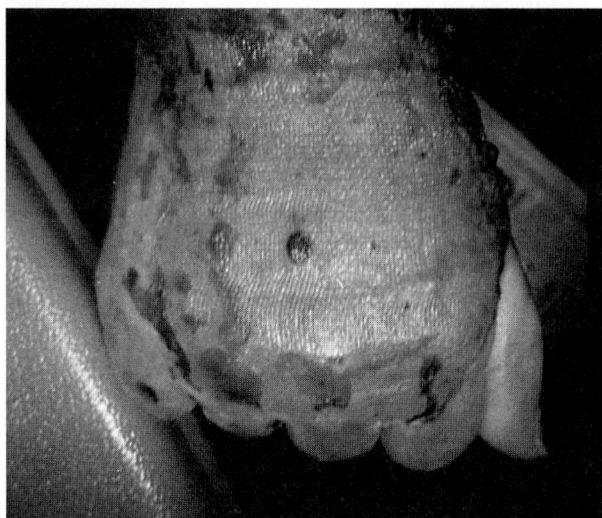

Fig. 7-8 ■ From Mackin EJ, Callahan AD, Skirven TM, et al: *Rehabilitation of the hand and upper extremity,* ed 5, St Louis, 2002, Mosby.

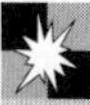

Clinical Gem:
In general, in reference to grafting, immediate debridement and grafting are often possible, and no more than 2 or 3 days should be allowed to pass for the purpose of establishment of a good bed. The principle of allowing a healthy bed of granulation to develop over time is no longer considered correct and should be replaced with the concept of early grafting.

36. True or False: Splinting helps to minimize contractures after skin grafting.

Splinting is essential to minimize the risk of joint contractures after skin grafts. Most surgeons use splinting in the immediate postoperative period. Early mobilization and joint range of motion are also used once the graft has demonstrated good adherence.

Answer: **True**
American Society for Surgery of the Hand, pp. 281-287

37. Which of the following is *not* an appropriate treatment for an open wound of the hand without dead tissue or osteomyelitis?

A. Kaltostat
B. Hydrogel moist wound dressing changes
C. Wound VAC negative pressure wound therapy
D. Leaving the wound open to air so that it can dry out

An open wound without dead tissue is best treated with a moist wound environment, which will help to promote reepithelization. A Hydrogel dressing or Kaltostat may provide a consistent moist environment and have some enzymatic activity. The negative pressure dressing also maintains a moist environment. In addition, it increases blood flow to the area, provides mechanical contraction of the wound, and may decrease bacterial counts as well.

Letting the open wound dry out open to air is probably the least advantageous approach with less inducement to reepithelization.

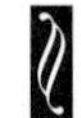

Answer: **D**
Hess, pp. 9-10

38. Primary treatment objectives in fingertip amputations include all but which of the following?

A. Closing the wound
B. Maximizing sensory return
C. Preserving length
D. Maintaining joint function
E. Maintaining cosmetic appearance

Ten percent of all accidents seen in emergency facilities in the United States involve hand and fingertip amputations. The first four choices are primary treatment objectives; cosmetic appearance is of secondary concern.

Answer: **E**
Orenstein, pp. 1-30

39. Match each graft with the appropriate definition.

Graft

1. Autograft
2. Isograft
3. Allograft
4. Xenograft (heterograft)

Definition

A. Graft tissue is transferred from a member of one species to a member of another species.
B. Transplant tissue is transferred between two genetically dissimilar members of the same species.
C. A graft is transferred between people who are identical in histocompatibility antigens (e.g., identical twins).
D. A graft is taken from a donor site and placed in a different site in the same person.

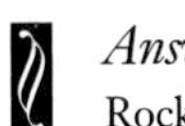

Answers: **1, D; 2, C; 3, B; 4, A**

Rockwood, Green, p. 159
Taber's cyclopedic medical dictionary

40. True or False: After receiving skin grafting to a burn wound on the dorsum of the hand, a patient is likely to have some degree of sensory loss.

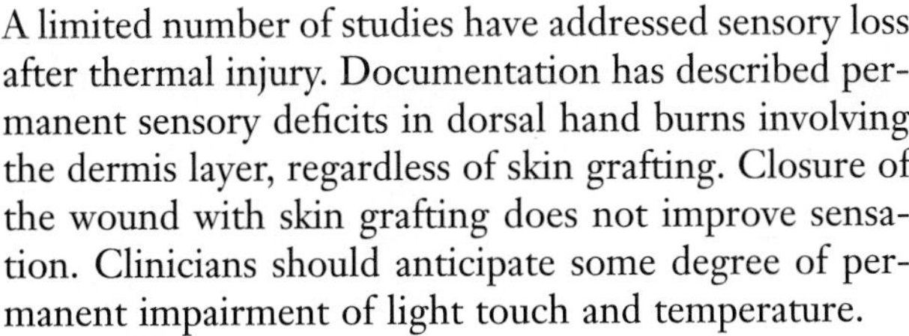

A limited number of studies have addressed sensory loss after thermal injury. Documentation has described permanent sensory deficits in dorsal hand burns involving the dermis layer, regardless of skin grafting. Closure of the wound with skin grafting does not improve sensation. Clinicians should anticipate some degree of permanent impairment of light touch and temperature.

Answer: **True**

Richards, Staley, pp. 540-541
deLinde, Knothe in Mackin, Callahan, Skirven, et al, p. 1521

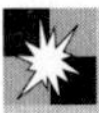

CLINICAL GEM:
An explanation for diminished sensation is that increased scar formation impedes axon regeneration in skin grafts. It may take a year or two to achieve final sensory recovery.

41. Which of the following is *not* an example of an interim pressure technique?

A. Co-wrap
B. Isotoner glove
C. Pressure bandages
D. Custom fit garment

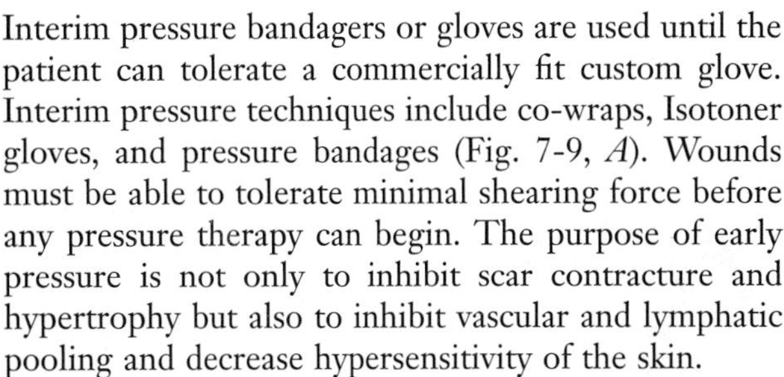

Interim pressure bandagers or gloves are used until the patient can tolerate a commercially fit custom glove. Interim pressure techniques include co-wraps, Isotoner gloves, and pressure bandages (Fig. 7-9, *A*). Wounds must be able to tolerate minimal shearing force before any pressure therapy can begin. The purpose of early pressure is not only to inhibit scar contracture and hypertrophy but also to inhibit vascular and lymphatic pooling and decrease hypersensitivity of the skin.

When commercially fit gloves (Fig. 7-9, *B*) (not an interim pressure technique) are applied, the wounds should be no larger than the size of a quarter, with minimal edema and adherent grafts. If gloves are forced on a patient too early, the friction caused by the material can result in blister formation and skin breakdown.

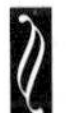

Answer: **D**

Richards, Staley, p. 393
Herndon, p. 449
Hunter, Mackin, Callahan, pp. 282, 1281-1282
deLinde, Knothe in Mackin, Callahan, Skirven, et al, pp. 1496, 1510

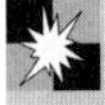

CLINICAL GEM:
Open-fingertip gloves are recommended for day wear and closed-tip gloves are recommended initially for night use.

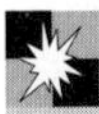

CLINICAL GEM:
Custom gloves are worn continuously and a new fit is needed around every 2 months to ensure adequate pressure is provided.

42. Which of the following is the optimum capillary pressure for the reduction of hypertrophic scar?

A. 5 mm Hg
B. 10 mm Hg
C. 25 mm Hg
D. 45 mm Hg

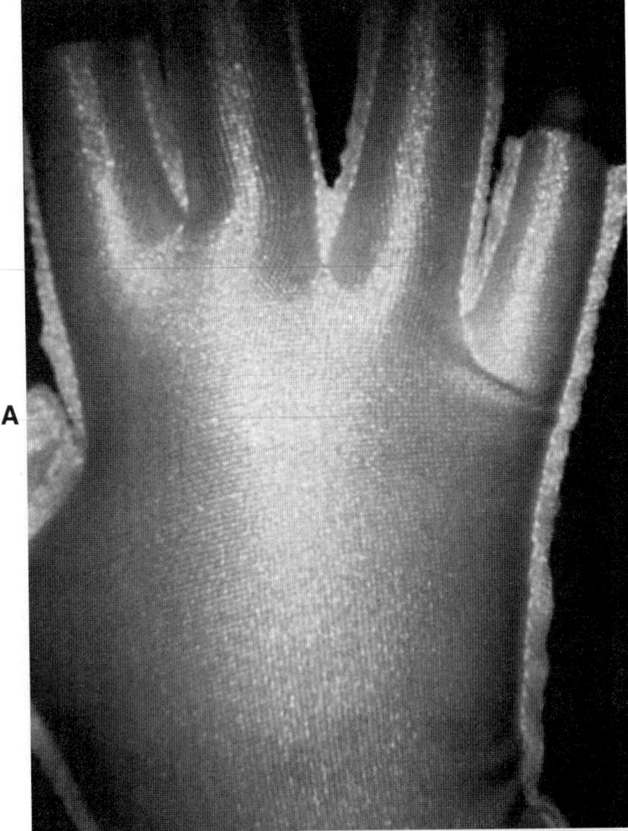

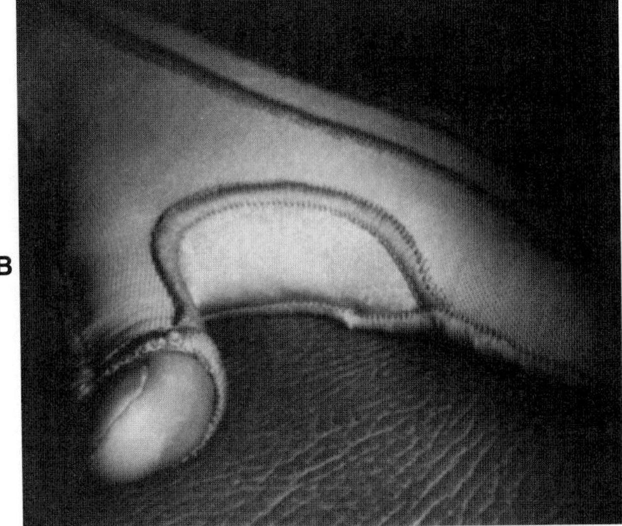

Fig. 7-9 ■ **A,** Interim pressure glove constructed of 3:1 stretch swimsuit Lycra (non-custom fit). **B,** Bio-Concepts glove. (From Mackin EJ, Callahan AD, Skirven TM, et al: *Rehabilitation of the hand and upper extremity,* ed 5, St Louis, 2002, Mosby.)

Many studies are examining the amount of pressure needed to alter scar maturation. Studies have shown that the application of compression with pressures greater than 15 mm Hg has a positive influence on scars; however, pressures greater than 40 mm Hg can macerate a scar. Twenty-five mm Hg is thought to be necessary to reduce blood flow to collagenous tissue; this amount of pressure results in a smoother, flatter, and more pliable scar. Another viewpoint is that pressure only causes dehydration of the scar and that the temporary diminished size of the scar after pressure application is caused by the close approximation of collagen cross-linking. In summary, despite the lack of objective data, the therapist can take advantage of the positive effects seen with pressure on scar tissue.

Answer: **C**

Richards, Staley, pp. 393-394
Hunter, Mackin, Callahan, p. 1282
deLinde, Knothe in Mackin, Callahan, Skirven, et al, p. 1510

43. What is the optimal wound technique closure for a deep palmar wound?

A. Full-thickness skin graft (FTSG)
B. Meshed split-thickness skin graft
C. Split-thickness skin graft (STSG)
D. Primary closure

FTSGs (Fig. 7-10) placed on palmar burns are reported to be more durable, with less contraction in comparison with STSGs. FTSGs require less therapy and a shorter wearing time of pressure garments.

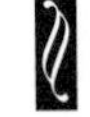

Answer: **A**

Hunter, Mackin, Callahan, p. 1278
Richards, Staley, p. 195

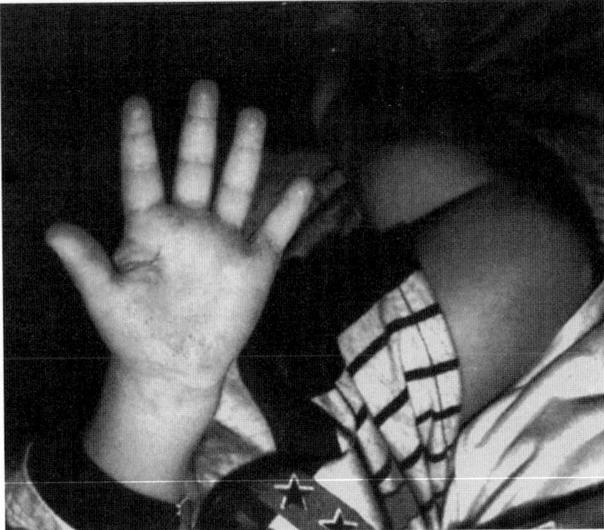

Fig. 7-10 ■ Full-thickness skin graft on the palm of a pediatric patient who was treated for a contact burn. The patient required minimal therapy. (From Mackin EJ, Callahan AD, Skirven TM, et al: *Rehabilitation of the hand and upper extremity,* ed 5, St Louis, 2002, Mosby.)

44. True or False: FTSGs contract more postoperatively than STSGs.

Approximately 95% of skin is composed of dermis; the other 5% is epidermis. An FTSG includes the epidermis and dermis. An STSG contains epidermis and partial dermis. The greater the proportion of dermis included in the graft, the greater the power of the graft to *inhibit* contraction; consequently, FTSGs contract less postoperatively. After wound contraction has ended, FTSGs are able to grow, whereas STSGs tend to remain in a fixed, contracted state and grow minimally, if at all.

Answer: **False**

Orenstein, pp. 1-30

45. True or False: The cross-finger flap is used primarily to cover digital defects.

Crouier first described the cross-finger flap for fingertip reconstruction in 1951. It brings durable cover to exposed bone, joint, and/or flexor tendons when local advancement flaps do not suffice. Blood supply of the cross-finger flap is random and based on the subdermal plexus of an adjacent digit. The dorsum of the proximal or middle phalanx of the long finger is the most common source of flap tissue.

Answer: **True**

Smith, Aston, p. 868
Orenstein, pp. 1-30
Levin, Moorman, Heller in Mackin, Callahan, Skirven, et al, p. 349
Refer to Fig. 7-11

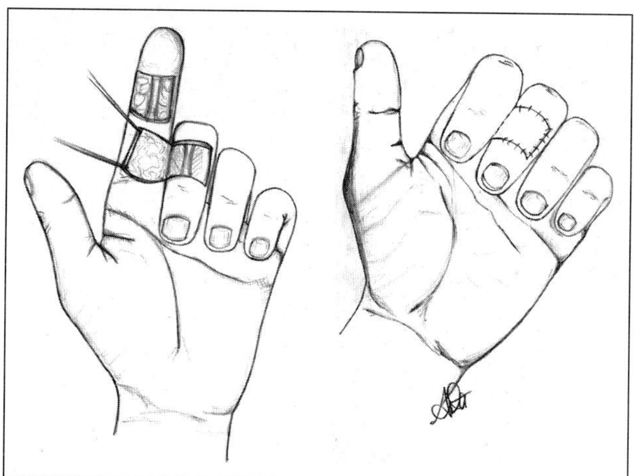

Fig. 7-11

46. Which of the following is an example of a random pattern flap?

A. Groin flap
B. Thoracoabdominal flap
C. Scapular flap
D. Temporoparietal flap

Flaps can be classified into axial and random types as well as by method of transfer, destination, geometry, and tissue composition. The thoracoabdominal flap is an example of a random pattern flap. Choices A, C, and D are axial-pattern flaps. Axial-pattern flaps are single-pedicle flaps that receive their blood flow from a single, constant vessel, whereas random pattern flaps receive their blood supply from many vessels of the subdermal or subcutaneous plexus.

Answer: **B**

Hodges, pp. 1-30
Green, pp. 1741-1742

47. A 45-year-old woman has loss of skin and subcutaneous tissue of the volar aspect of the distal third of the dominant thumb; the distal phalanx is exposed. Which of the following procedures would be best for soft-tissue coverage of this crush injury?

A. Dressing changes and healing by secondary intention
B. Full-thickness groin skin graft
C. Split-thickness hypothenar skin graft
D. Index cross-finger flap
E. Volar advancement flap

The most appropriate management for this thumb defect is coverage with a double neurovascular thumb volar advancement flap, which was first proposed by Moberg to treat amputations of the thumb that occurred distal to the interphalangeal joint. This volar advancement flap provides stable sensate coverage of the wound, using adjacent tissue that is similar in color and texture. Coverage can be augmented by temporarily flexing the interphalangeal joint, by creating an island flap using V-Y advancement, or by skin grafting of the proximal defect.

Dressing changes and healing by secondary intention are appropriate only for injuries of 1 cm or less. Full-thickness groin skin grafts result in diminished sensory recovery and poor match of color and texture. STSGs applied directly to exposed bone provide inadequate coverage and little padding. The index cross-finger flap is inappropriate and would unnecessarily traumatize an adjacent digit, further impairing hand function.

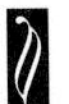

Answer: **E**

Levin, Moorman, Heller in Mackin, Callahan, Skirven, et al, p. 348
Yaremchuk, p. 143
Refer to Fig. 7-12

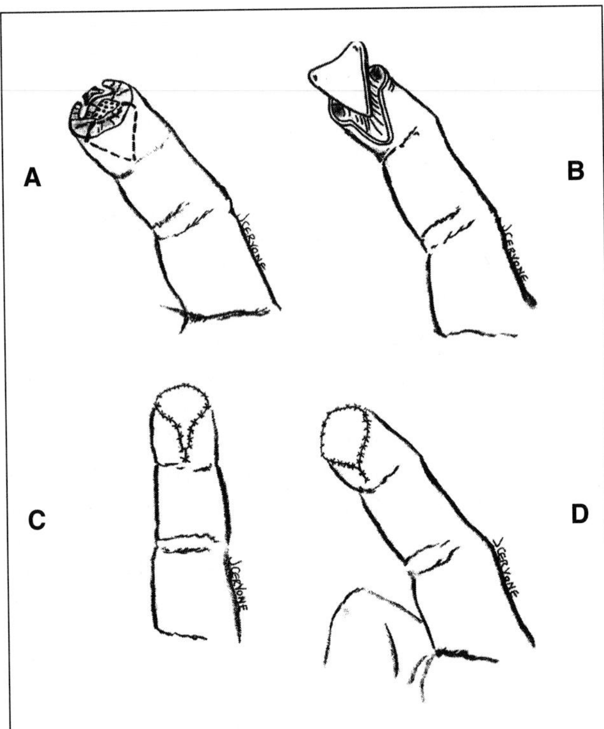

Fig. 7-12 ■ **A**, Plan. **B**, Advancement. **C**, Front view **D**, Oblique view.

48. True or False: Full-thickness or deep partial-thickness burns of the hand can benefit from early excision and grafting.

Most authors advocate early excision and grafting after the extent of a burn is known. This reduces edema formation and permits early joint motion. The hand should be splinted with the metacarpophalangeal joints flexed and the interphalangeal joints extended. The use of STSGs or FTSGs helps to minimize joint contracture. Early aggressive occupational therapy can help obtain optimal function.

Answer: **True**

Smith, Aston, pp. 857-887
Orenstein, pp. 1-30

49. All but which of the following are true statements about thenar flaps?

A. They are most commonly used for coverage of the distal phalanx of the index or long finger.
B. A proximal interphalangeal joint flexion contracture can occur as a result of flap design and positioning.
C. A thick flap is raised in the subcutaneous tissue plane near the volar metacarpophalangeal crease.
D. This flap can be surgically performed in a single stage.

Choices A, B, and C are correct. This flap can be proximally, distally, or laterally based, overlying the metacarpophalangeal joint crease. The flap is inset and the finger is protected with a splint. The pedicle is transected during the second surgical stage, usually 14 days after insetting. A proximal interphalangeal joint contracture can occur, especially in older individuals. Some surgeons use this flap only in younger patients due to risk of proximal interphalangeal joint flexion contractures.

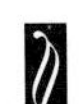

Answer: **D**

Smith, Aston, pp. 870-873

50. True or False: The radial forearm flap can be used for coverage of major dorsal tissue losses of the hand.

The radial forearm flap is a fasciocutaneous flap based on the radial artery and its nerve and located in the lateral intermuscular septum. The radial artery supplies blood to most of the skin of the forearm. The radial forearm flap may be raised as a distally based island axial flap (Fig. 7-13, *A*) or as a free neurovascular transfer. This flap may be used for complex tissue losses where there is exposed tendon, bone, or joints. The flap is inset (Fig. 7-13, *B*) and the donor site is closed with a skin graft in a one-stage procedure. A bone segment from the radius also can be incorporated when bone is needed for reconstruction.

Answer: **True**

Smith, Aston, pp. 870-880
Levin, Moorman, Heller in Mackin, Callahan, Skirven, et al, p. 350

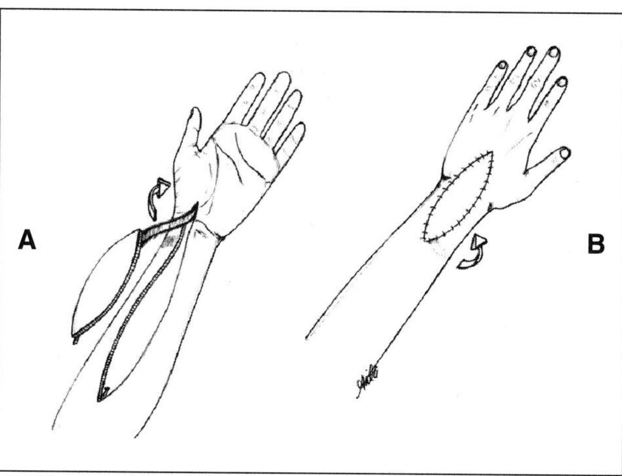

Fig. 7-13

51. True or False: The temporoparietal fascia free flap is ideally suited for coverage of hand defects requiring soft-tissue bulk.

This flap is obtained from the temporoparietal area of the skull, which is located between the subcutaneous tissues and the temporalis muscle fascia. The superficial temporal artery and vein provide the blood supply. The flap is thin and vascular and is an excellent means of palmar reconstruction. The donor scar usually is well hidden. Maximum dimensions of the flap usually do not exceed 13 cm by 9 cm. This flap is used as a free flap transfer and usually is skin-grafted after insetting; it is not appropriate for defects that require significant tissue bulk.

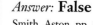

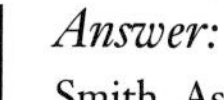

Answer: **False**

Smith, Aston, pp. 875-883
Levin, Moorman, Heller in Mackin, Callahan, Skirven, et al, pp. 354-355

52. All but which of the following are true about the groin flap?

A. It is an axial-pattern flap based on the superficial circumflex iliac artery.
B. It may be used as a pedicle flap or a free neurovascular transfer.
C. The most common associated complication is infection.
D. It may be used for coverage of complex open wounds of the hand and wrist.

Infection is not the most common complication associated with the groin flap. A primary concern is if the groin flap will "take." Answers A, B, and D are true statements about the groin flap.

The groin flap may be used as a free neurovascular transfer; however, the variable arterial and venous anatomy may limit its use. Other more commonly used free flaps for hand coverage are the radial forearm flap, the lateral arm flap, and the temporoparietal fascia flap. Each of these can provide thin, supple, well vascularized coverage of difficult wounds.

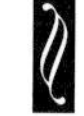

Answer: **C**

Smith, Aston, pp. 875-878

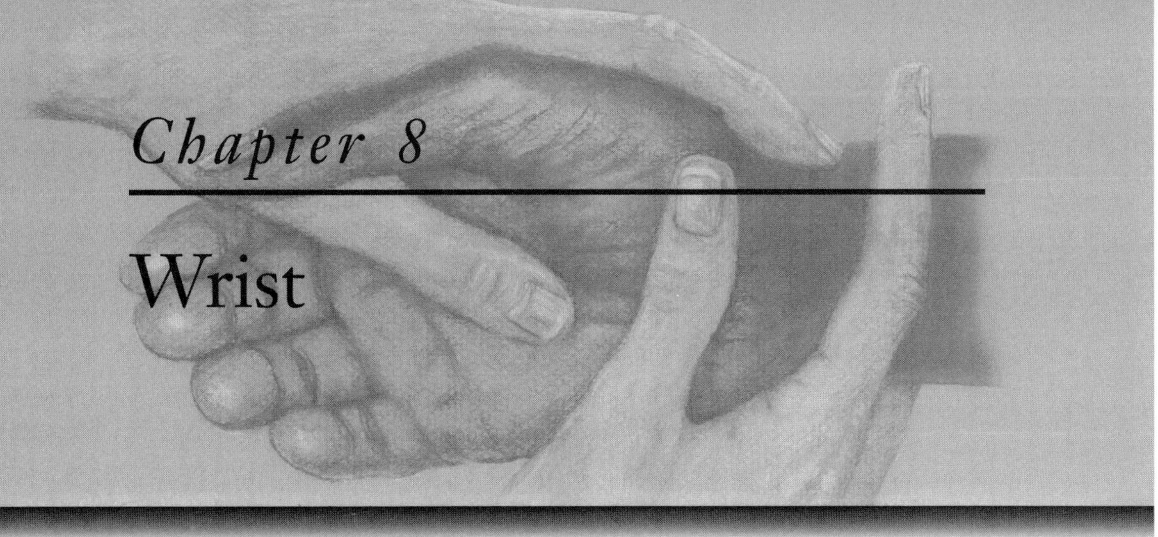

Chapter 8

Wrist

1. What is the structure indicated in Fig. 8-1?

A. Ulnotriquetral ligament
B. Ulnolunate ligament
C. Ulnar collateral carpal ligament
D. Articular disc of wrist
E. None of the above

The arrow in Fig. 8-1 depicts the articular disc of the wrist. This articular disc is a fibrocartilaginous structure about the distal radioulnar (DRU) joint. The articular disc of the wrist is known as the *triangular fibrocartilage* (TFC), which is part of the triangular fibrocartilage complex (TFCC). The TFC provides a smooth mobile gliding surface for the ulna side of the wrist and stability of the DRU joint. Portions of the articular disc (central) endure compressive forces between the ulnar head and triquetrum during grip and do not contribute to the stability of the DRU joint. *Isolated* degenerative and traumatic tears to the TFC can occur but will not affect the stability of the DRU joint. However, if the pathology includes the TFCC, instability is noted.

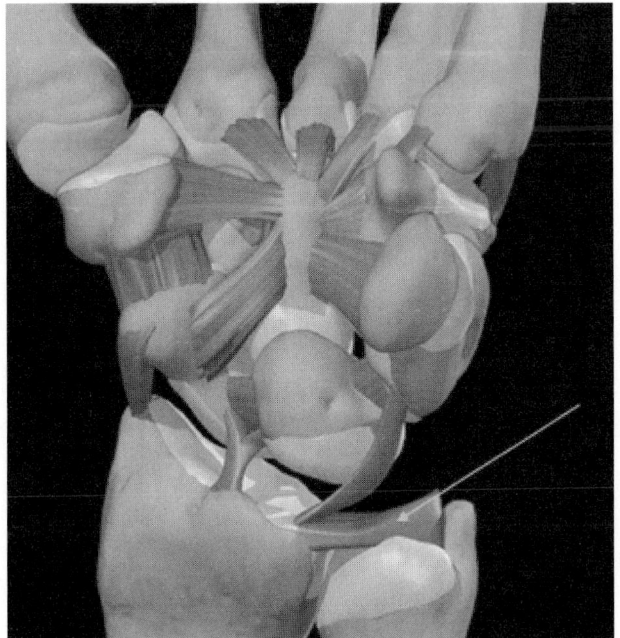

Fig. 8-1 ■ Courtesy Judy C. Colditz, OTR/L, CHT, FAOTA, HandLab, a Division of RHRC, Inc.

The ulnotriquetral and ulnolunate are part of the extrinsic volar ligaments about the wrist. The ulnolunate ligament connects the TFC to the lunate. The ulnar collateral carpal ligament is part of the ulnocarpal ligament structure. This is a strong ligament that extends from the ulna and is often considered part of the joint capsule.

Answer: **D**

Taleisnik, 17-21
Frykman, Watkins in Mackin, Callahan, Skirven, et al, p. 1125
LaStayo in Mackin, Callahan, Skirven, et al, pp. 1156-1170
Dell, Dell in Mackin, Callahan, Skirven, et al, pp. 1171-1184
LaStayo, pp. 1156-1184

2. The major stabilizer of the DRU joint is which of the following?

A. Pronator quadratus muscle
B. Extensor retinaculum
C. Concave shape of the sigmoid notch
D. Volar radioulnar ligament
E. TFCC

Although all the structures listed contribute to DRU stability, the TFCC with its thickened periphery (DRU ligaments) has the greatest effect on its stability, particularly in pronation. This supports the notion that pronation is an important component in TFC disruptions.

Answer: **E**

Gupta, Allaire, Fornalski, et al, pp. 854-862
Jaffe, Chidgey, LaStayo, pp. 129-138
Refer to Fig. 8-2

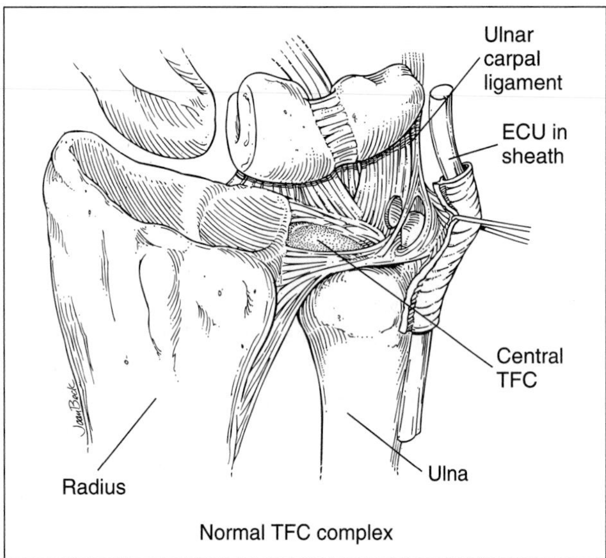

Fig. 8-2 ■ From Cooney WP, Linscheid RL, Dobyns JH: *The wrist: diagnosis and operative treatment*, St Louis, 1998, Mosby.

3. Which of the following is true about negative ulnar variance?

A. It excessively loads the ulnocarpal articulation.
B. It is positively correlated with Kienbock's disease.
C. It decreases the force transmission through the radiocarpal joint.
D. A and C
E. All of the above

Ulnar variance is a measure (obtained radiographically) of the distance that the ulnar head extends below (negative) or above (positive) the articular surface of the radius, with the latter increasing forces through the ulnocarpal articulation and the former increasing forces through the radiocarpal articulation; hence its association with Kienbock's disease (see Fig. 8-12).

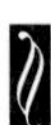

Answer: **B**

Chung, Spilson, Kim, pp. 494-499
LaStayo in Mackin, Callahan, Skirven, et al, pp. 1156-1170

4. A hand surgeon shows you a posteroanterior (PA) radiograph in which there is no visible joint between the lunate and the triquetrum. The patient has no surgical scar and no history of trauma. Which of the following statements is true with regard to this condition?

A. It is less common than a similar condition that involves the capitate and hamate.
B. It is associated with restricted wrist motion.
C. It is caused by an incomplete separation of the embryological carpal cartilage.
D. It is rarely seen in people of African descent.
E. It is usually associated with more serious congenital anomalies.

This patient has a lunotriquetral (LT) coalition (Fig. 8-3). A *coalition* refers to an incomplete separation of the embryological cartilage. One large bone appears without an articulation between two bones. When only two bones are involved, the condition usually is not associated with other congenital anomalies. An LT coalition usually is an incidental finding; it does not affect range of motion (ROM) and typically has no symptoms. However, the referenced article cites one symptomatic case.

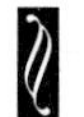

Answer: **C**

Simmons, McKenzie, pp. 190-193

5. Your patient with symptomatic carpal instability resulting from a fall on an outstretched hand (FOOSH) 2 weeks ago is referred to you with evaluation and treatment orders. Which of the following would be considered appropriate treatment?

A. Splinting
B. High-grade joint mobilization
C. Putty-gripping exercises
D. A and C
E. All of the above

Vigorous ROM or resistance activities are contraindicated during the early protective phase of healing (~6 weeks). High-grade joint mobilization is also not advised when dealing with an instability. Stability can sometimes be restored with wrist splinting and avoidance of axial loading (resistive fisting), but surgical stabilization is often required.

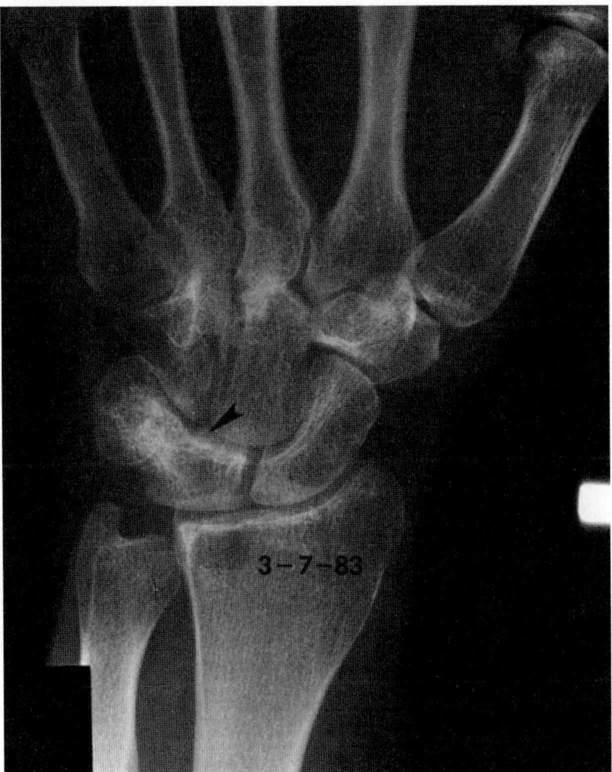

Fig. 8-3 ■ From Cooney WP, Linscheid RL, Dobyns JH: *The wrist: diagnosis and operative treatment*, St Louis, 1998, Mosby.

Answer: **A**

LaStayo, Michlovitz, pp. 321-348
Wright, Michlovitz, pp. 148-156

6. What is the most commonly fractured carpal bone?

A. Trapezium
B. Capitate
C. Hamate
D. Scaphoid
E. Lunate

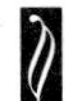

The most commonly fractured carpal bone is the scaphoid. This fracture is common in young adult males. Reports have indicated that these fractures account for 60% to 70% of all carpal injuries. Unfortunately, scaphoid nonunions are not uncommon because of the scaphoid's dependence on a single interosseous blood supply that often is disrupted after fracture. Other carpal fractures include the trapezium (1% to 5% of all carpal injuries), capitate (1% to 2%), hamate (2% to 4%), pisiform (1% to 3%), triquetrum (3% to 4%), trapezoid (less than 1%), and lunate (2% to 7%).

Answer: **D**

Prosser, Herbert, p. 139
Kozin, 2001, pp. 515-524
Refer to Fig. 8-4

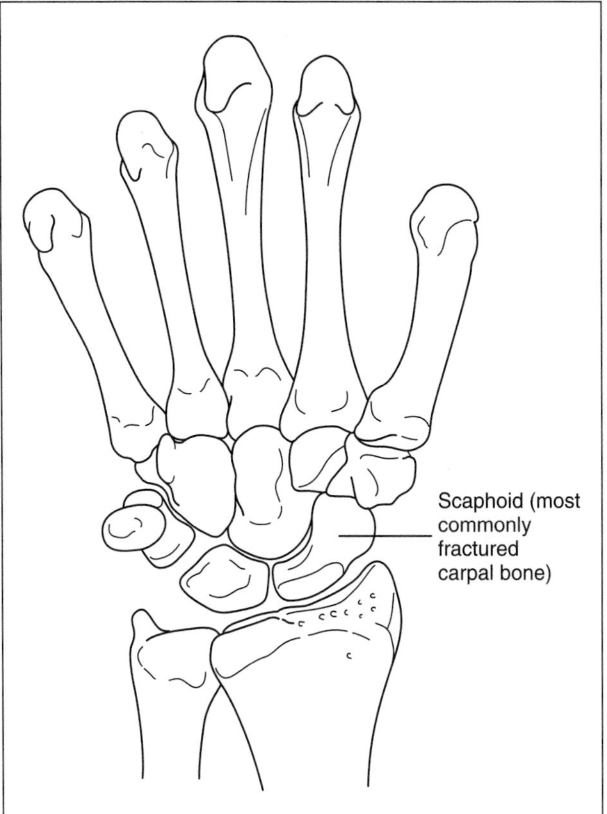

Fig. 8-4 ■ Palmar aspect of distal radius and ulna, carpus, and metacarpals. (From Taleisnik J: *The wrist*, New York, 1985, Churchill Livingstone.)

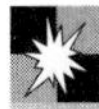

CLINICAL GEM:
The proximal pole of the scaphoid is poorly vascularized; therefore it is notorious for delayed healing. Fortunately, only about 10% of scaphoid fractures are through this proximal pole; 80% are through the waist. The remainder is at the tuberosity or distal pole.

Cooney, Linscheid, Dobyns, p. 395

7. What percentage of force is transmitted across the radiocarpal joint when the wrist is loaded in the neutral position?

A. 80%
B. 60%
C. 40%
D. 20%
E. 10%

Eighty percent of force is transmitted at the radiocarpal joint, and the remaining 20% is transmitted across the ulnocarpal joint. With pronation, the ulnocarpal force transmission increases to 37%; with ulnar deviation, the ulnocarpal force increases to 28%.

Answer: **A**

Berger, p. 92
Palmer, pp. 929-971

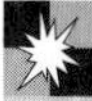

CLINICAL GEM:
With supination, the ulnocarpal force transmission decreases; therefore when structures need to be unloaded on the ulnar side, a supinated position will decrease the ulnocarpal force. Clinicians should also consider a supinated position to start grip-strengthening exercises in those with ulnar impaction syndrome.

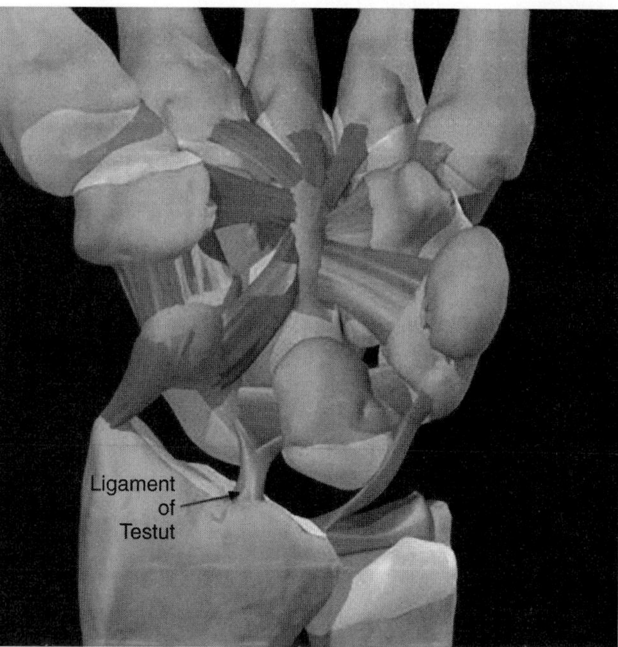

Fig. 8-5 ■ Courtesy Judy C. Colditz, OTR/L, CHT, FAOTA, HandLab, a Division of RHRC, Inc.

8. Which ligament is known as a ligament of Testut?

A. Deltoid ligament
B. Radioscapholunate ligament
C. Radioscaphocapitate ligament
D. Radiotriquetral ligament
E. Ulnar lunate ligament

The radioscapholunate ligament (Fig. 8-5) is also known as the *ligament of Testut*. This ligament has been described as a remnant of vascular ingrowth to the carpus. The ligament of Testut perhaps is more appropriately classified as a mesocapsule rather than a ligament. It is part of the extrinsic ligamentous system. Extrinsic ligaments are extracapsular and pass from the radius or metacarpals to the carpal bones; intrinsic ligaments are intracapsular and originate from and insert on adjacent carpal bones. The intrinsic ligaments are thicker and stronger volarly than they are dorsally.

Answer: **B**

Bednar, Osterman, pp. 10, 11
Cooney, Linscheid, Dobyns, p. 82

9. After a limited carpal fusion of the following bones—capitate, hamate, lunate, and triquetrum—you would expect which of the following?

A. A 50% reduction in wrist ROM
B. A relatively high nonunion rate
C. Recovery of 75% to 80% of normal forearm rotation
D. A and C
E. All of the above

There is some discrepancy regarding the contribution of each wrist joint to specific wrist motions. Functionally, however, it is safe to say that both the radiocarpal and midcarpal joints contribute to flexion, extension, and deviations of the wrist; clinically, both of these joints need to be addressed when attempting to restore wrist motion. Limited carpal fusions that cross one of the wrist joints will result in approximately 50% loss of wrist ROM, with forearm rotation being unaffected. Grip strength should approximate 75% to 80% of the uninvolved side.

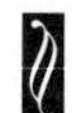

Answer: **A**

Mih, pp. 615-625
Moojen, Snel, Ritt, pp. 81-87
Ruby, Cooney, An, pp. 1-10

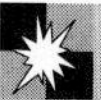

CLINICAL GEM:
Fusions that comprise greater surface area of bone (e.g., four bones as described above) will have relatively low nonunion rates in comparison with two- or three-bone limited carpal fusions.

10. Which of the following carpal bones acts as a sesamoid bone?

A. Trapezium
B. Trapezoid
C. Pisiform
D. Hamate
E. Scaphoid

The pisiform is considered a carpal bone but functions as a sesamoid bone, onto which the flexor carpi ulnaris tendon inserts. The definition of a *sesamoid bone* is an oval nodule of bone or fibrocartilage embedded in a tendon or joint capsule. The patella is the largest sesamoid bone. The pisiform is a rounded carpal bone that lies over the triquetrum. Although anatomically the pisiform is located in the proximal carpal row, it does not participate in either the radiocarpal or midcarpal joints. It is a sesamoid bone whose sole function appears to be to increase the moment arm of the flexor carpi ulnaris muscle as its tendon courses over the pisiform. It also, however, is a site (pisotriquetral joint) for degenerative joint changes. The flexor carpi ulnaris inserts into the pisiform with prolongations to the hamate and the fifth metacarpal.

Answer: **C**

Cooney, Linscheid, Dobyns, p. 66
Taber's cyclopedic medical dictionary
Yamaguchi, Viegas, Patterson, pp. 600-606

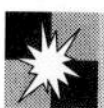

CLINICAL GEM:
The pisiform is the only carpal bone with a tendon insertion from a forearm muscle.

11. What is the normal radial inclination and palmar tilt in the wrist?

A. Radial inclination of 33 degrees and palmar tilt of 20 degrees
B. Radial inclination of 22 degrees and palmar tilt of 12 degrees
C. Radial inclination of 13 degrees and palmar tilt of 21 degrees
D. Radial inclination of 10 degrees and palmar tilt of 10 degrees
E. Radial inclination of 41 degrees and palmar tilt of 25 degrees

Typically the radial inclination is 22 to 23 degrees (Fig. 8-6, *A*) and the palmar tilt is 11 to 12 degrees (Fig. 8-6, *B*). With a loss of normal palmar tilt, dorsal angulation can occur. The wrist may appear deformed, forces are shifted to the ulnar-sided tissues (thus causing ulnar wrist pain), and ROM deficits are noted. Loss of radial inclination has been correlated with decreased grip strength and ROM. If the anatomy is not restored, the functional use of the arm may be limited or painful.

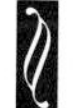

Answer: **B**

Cooney, Linscheid, Dobyns, pp. 328, 570
Laseter, Carter, pp. 117-118
LaStayo in Mackin, Callahan, Skirven, et al, pp. 1156-1170

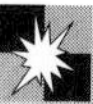

CLINICAL GEM:
Patients who are referred to therapy after a distal radius fracture inevitably have a loss of normal angulation and/or inclination. Patients who are lucky enough to get normal anatomy restored after their fractures typically do not have impairments that require therapy (i.e., they do not get referred to therapy).

12. Which fracture describes a distal radius fracture with dorsal displacement?

A. Colles'
B. Smith's
C. Palmar Barton's
D. All of the above present with a dorsal displacement.
E. Reverse Colles'

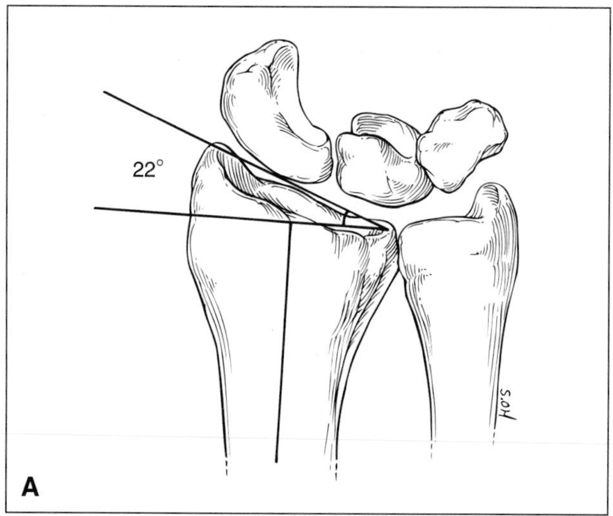

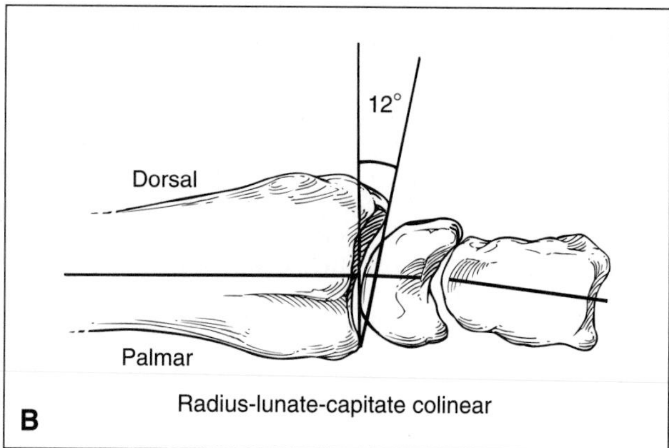

Fig. 8-6 ■ **A** and **B** From Cooney WP, Linscheid RL, Dobyns JH: *The wrist: diagnosis and operative treatment,* St Louis, 1998, Mosby.

A Colles' fracture (Fig. 8-7) is a distal radius fracture with dorsal displacement. A Smith's fracture, also known as a *reverse Colles'*, presents with palmar angulation of the distal radius. A Barton's fracture is a fracture-dislocation in which the rim of the distal radius is displaced dorsally or palmarly along with the hand and carpus. A Barton's fracture is different from both Colles' and Smith's fractures because the *dislocation* is the most obvious radiographic abnormality; a fracture of the radius is noted secondarily.

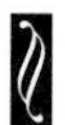

Answer: **A**

Laseter, Carter, p. 114
Cooney, Linscheid, Dobyns, p. 315

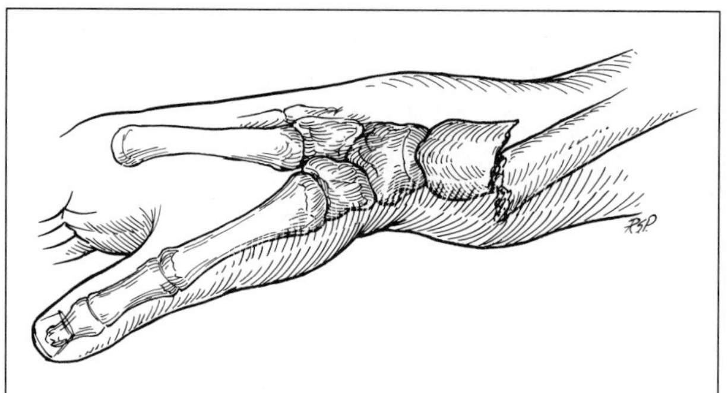

Fig. 8-7 ■ From Malone TR, McPoil TG, Nitz AJ: *Orthopedic and sports physical therapy*, ed 3, St Louis, 1997, Mosby.

13. A distal radius fracture patient shows you his X-ray film, and you see a healed extraarticular fracture of the distal radius which has shortened by 3 mm, is dorsally angulated, and the DRU joint space is narrowed. Which of the following might you expect?

A. A loss of forearm rotation
B. An increase in force transmission across the ulnocarpal articulation
C. Ulnar wrist pain
D. A and C
E. All of the above

After the immobilization and fracture healing of the distal radius, wrist extension and forearm rotation (commonly supination) often are limited, and pain is experienced at the extremes of motion. An increase in force transmission across the ulnocarpal articulation occurs, and grip strength is reduced by more than 50%. Overcoming wrist stiffness and a return of functional wrist motion is a priority. This is complicated, however, by the fact that over 50% of extraarticular (and 35% of intraarticular distal radius fractures) can have TFCC lesions and ulnar wrist pain.

Answer: **E**

Jupiter, Fernandez, pp. 203-219
Laseter, Carter, pp. 117-118
LaStayo in Mackin, Callahan, Skirven, et al, pp. 1156-1170
Richards, Bennett, Roth, pp. 772-776

14. One of the most important objectives of distal radius fracture rehabilitation is the restoration of which of the following?

A. Digit extension
B. Digit flexion
C. Supination
D. Isolated wrist extension
E. Pronation

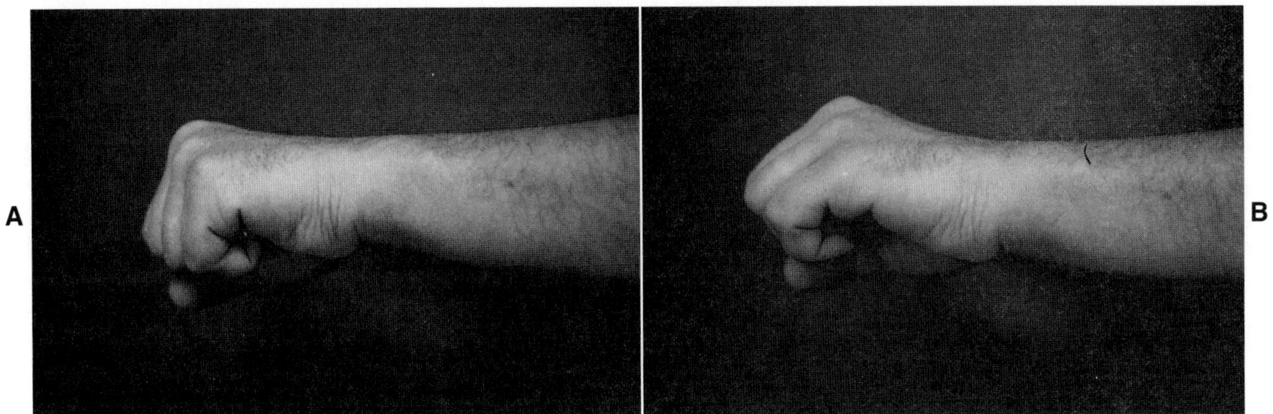

Fig. 8-8 ■ From Mackin EJ, Callahan AD, Skirven TM, et al: *Rehabilitation of the hand and upper extremity*, ed 5, vol 2, St Louis, 2002, Mosby.

The patient who has been immobilized in some degree of wrist flexion for several weeks often develops a substitution pattern of using digital extensors to implement wrist extension. It is extremely important to reestablish independent wrist extension and overcome this pattern to improve function. Obviously it is also important to overcome the other ROM impairments, but one must not underestimate the importance of reconstituting active wrist extension via the extensor carpi radialis longus (ECRL) and extensor carpi radialis brevis (ECRB) (Fig. 8-8). To do this, it often is necessary to have the patient hold something so that he or she can concentrate on the wrist rather than on the digits during extension.

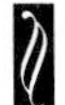

Answer: **D**
Laseter, Carter, pp. 112-124
LaStayo, Michlovitz, pp. 321-348

15. The most common tumor in the wrist is which of the following?

A. Dorsal wrist ganglion
B. Lipoma
C. Giant cell tumor
D. Hemangioma
E. Fibrosarcoma

The word *tumor* can be misleading. It should be recalled that "tumor" is generic and refers to swelling or enlargement; it does not necessarily imply a solid growth. Commonly seen dorsal wrist ganglions arise from the scapholunate (SL) interosseous ligament and are intimately involved in the dorsal capsule (Fig. 8-9). Patients may complain of pain and weakness of the wrist. Some physicians treat ganglions with arthroscopy. Transilluminescence with a penlight over the ganglion can quickly allay the fear of a solid tumor. Malignant tumors (sarcomas) in the wrist and hand are very rare. Giant cell tumors commonly are seen in the fingers. Lipomas occasionally are seen in the wrist.

Answer: **A**
Dorland's illustrated medical dictionary
Nelson, Sawmiller, Phalen, pp. 1459-1464
Smith, pp. 432-433

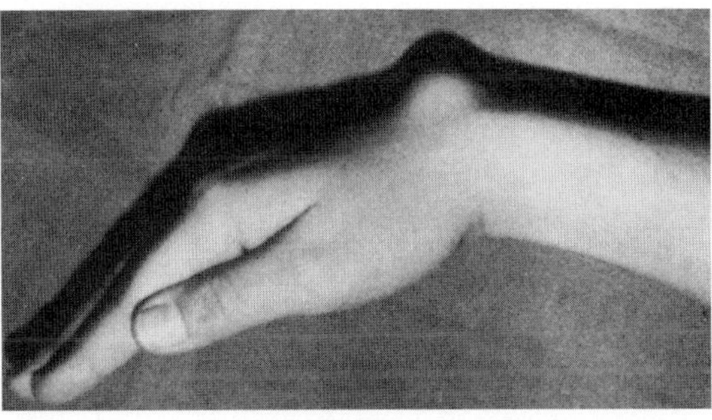

Fig. 8-9 ■ From Smith P: *Lister's The hand: diagnosis and indications*, ed 4, London, 2003, Churchill Livingstone.

16. All but which of the following are true about a scapholunate advanced collapse (SLAC) wrist?

A. It is characterized by degenerative changes at the triquetral-hamate joint.
B. It is characterized by the pronounced impairment of pain, which is exacerbated by axial loading (gripping) and radial deviation.
C. It is based on degenerative changes between the scaphoid, lunate, capitate, and radius.
D. It can result from a scaphoid nonunion.
E. It can result from an SL ligament disruption.

Instability of the scaphoid (via nonunion or a ligamentous disruption) can be associated with the SLAC wrist condition. SLAC wrist pathology is a pattern of degenerative changes that are based on and caused by articular alignment problems between the scaphoid, lunate, capitate, and the radius and that are exacerbated by axial loading (gripping) and radial deviation. The triquetral hamate joint is not involved in SLAC wrist.

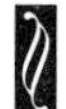

Answer: **A**

Watson, Weinzweig, Zeppieri, pp. 39-49
Wright, Michlovitz, pp. 148-156

17. You are asked to evaluate a 60-year-old patient with a Colles' fracture. In the typical distal radial fracture, treated by traction and percutaneous pinning, you would most likely identify a loss of which motion 6 months after the fracture?

A. Volar flexion
B. Dorsiflexion
C. Flexion lags of the index and long fingers
D. Radial deviation
E. Ulnar deviation

The typical Colles' fracture displaces the articular surface dorsally. Often this can result in as much as 30 to 40 degrees of dorsal articular tilt. Most fractures treated with traction and pinning restore the articular tilt to neutral. It is difficult to restore the 10 to 15 degrees of volar articular tilt seen on the lateral view. Because the articular tilt is neutral, the wrist most likely lacks complete volar flexion, but dorsiflexion actually may increase in comparison with the unaffected extremity. Flexion lags of digits can be seen and commonly are associated with "fracture disease;" they usually are not a result of pinning technique.

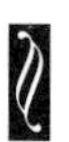

Answer: **A**

Rayhack, pp. 287-300

CLINICAL GEM:
"Fracture disease" is a constellation of symptoms caused by prolonged immobilization. It can lead to a vicious pain cycle, unresolved edema, muscle atrophy, and osteoporosis. It is not a necessary part of fracture management and can be avoided or prevented with early digital motion and edema management.

18. True or False: An SL dissociation produces a volar intercalated segment instability (VISI).

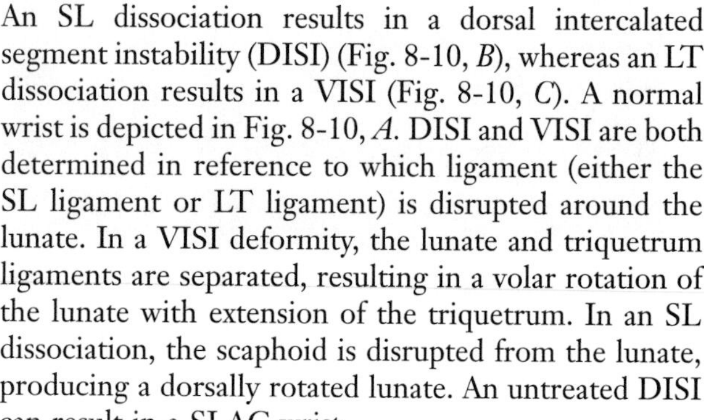

An SL dissociation results in a dorsal intercalated segment instability (DISI) (Fig. 8-10, *B*), whereas an LT dissociation results in a VISI (Fig. 8-10, *C*). A normal wrist is depicted in Fig. 8-10, *A*. DISI and VISI are both determined in reference to which ligament (either the SL ligament or LT ligament) is disrupted around the lunate. In a VISI deformity, the lunate and triquetrum ligaments are separated, resulting in a volar rotation of the lunate with extension of the triquetrum. In an SL dissociation, the scaphoid is disrupted from the lunate, producing a dorsally rotated lunate. An untreated DISI can result in a SLAC wrist.

Answer: **False**

Bednar, Osterman, p. 12
Wright, Michlovitz in Mackin, Callahan, Skirven, et al, pp. 1186-1188
Hunter, Mackin, Callahan, p. 329
Wright, Michlovitz, pp. 148-156

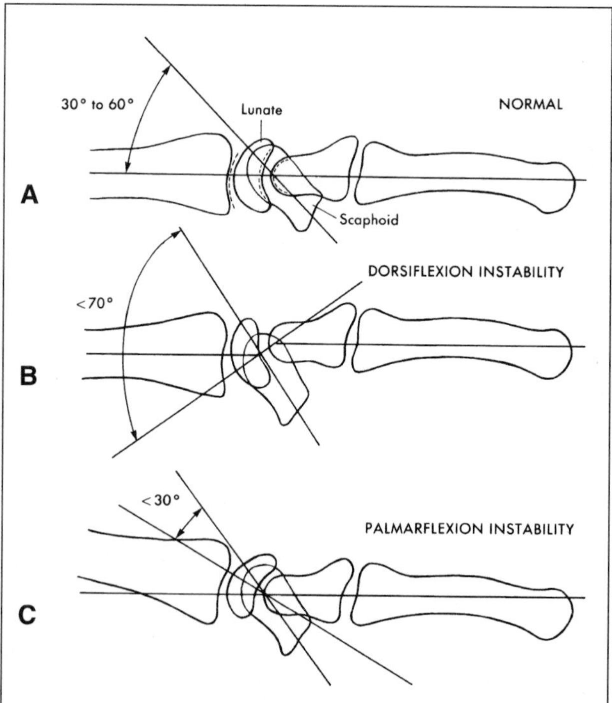

Fig. 8-10 ■ **A,** Normal wrist with the lunate properly aligned. **B,** DISI pattern. The lunate is dorsally rotated (or looking up in extension). **C,** VISI pattern. The lunate is volarly rotated (or looking down in flexion). (From Hunter JM, Mackin EJ, Callahan AD: *Rehabilitation of the hand: surgery and therapy,* ed 4, St Louis, 1995, Mosby.)

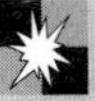

CLINICAL GEM:
An SL gap has been called the *Terry Thomas sign*. This refers to a British actor with a wide gap between his front teeth (Fig. 8-11).

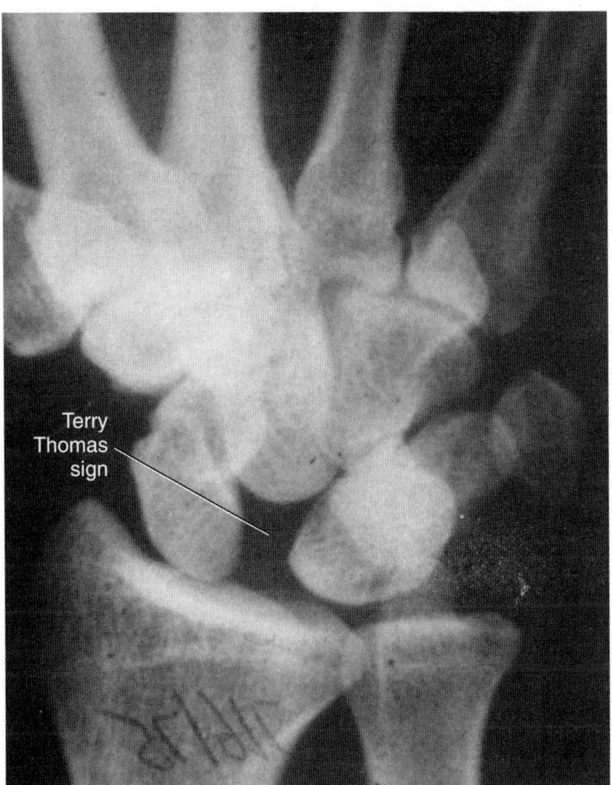

Fig. 8-11 ■ From Hunter JM, Mackin EJ, Callahan AD: *Rehabilitation of the hand: surgery and therapy*, ed 4, St Louis, 1995, Mosby.

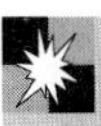

CLINICAL GEM:
Another important term to be familiar with is *carpal instability dissociative*, which is an instability between the carpal bones or through the carpal bones in the same carpal row (proximal or distal). This occurs as a result of intrinsic ligament damage, most commonly of the SL or LT ligaments.

A carpal instability nondissociative (CIND) is a fairly uncommon form of wrist pathology that involves instability *between* the carpal rows rather than within a single carpal row. CIND often is seen in individuals with ligament laxity and often is called a *midcarpal instability*.

19. The most notable clinical characteristic of a midcarpal row instability is which of the following?

A. Radially based wrist pain
B. Tenderness at the ulnar styloid
C. The abrupt carpal shift (which can produce a clunking sound) that occurs with ulnar deviation
D. The abrupt carpal shift (which can produce a clunking sound) that occurs with radial deviation
E. None of the above

Midcarpal row instability is a nondissociative type of carpal instability and is typically difficult to diagnose because static imaging studies are often unremarkable. The typical patient has lax ligaments at the wrist and other joints. If excessive laxity is noted, the tests for dissociative conditions within the proximal row (i.e., the scaphoid shift and ballottement tests) may produce false positives. Perhaps the most notable clinical characteristic of midcarpal instability is the abrupt carpal shift that occurs with ulnar deviation during the catch-up clunk test.

Answer: **C**

LaStayo in Mackin, Callahan, Skirven, et al, pp. 1156-1170
Wright, Michlovitz in Mackin, Callahan, Skirven, et al, p. 1187
Wright, Dobyns, pp. 550-568

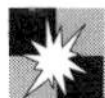

CLINICAL GEM:
Typically, midcarpal instability is noticed first on clinical examination and then confirmed with cineradiography.

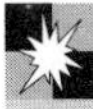

CLINICAL GEM:
The patient performs the catch-up clunk test for midcarpal instability in the following way:

- Active wrist radial to ulnar deviation and back.
- A positive test will result in a clunk or thud and pain at a point just beyond neutral as the wrist moves into ulnar deviation.
- A positive test indicates instability but not specifically whether it is at the midcarpal or radiocarpal joint or at both levels. A similar clunk may be heard in the presence of SL or LT instability.

20. A fracture of the radial head combined with DRU joint dislocation is classified as which of the following?

A. Colles' fracture
B. Essex-Lopresti fracture dislocation
C. Barton's fracture dislocation
D. Piano-key fracture
E. Chauffeur fracture

A radial head fracture combined with a DRU joint dislocation is termed an *Essex-Lopresti fracture dislocation.* The interosseous membrane tears in this injury result in proximal migration of the radius. An ulnar plus variance of 2 to 3 mm often develops in patients after this injury; however, this becomes symptomatic enough to warrant treatment in only a minority of the cases. Radial head replacements with silicone prostheses may be of temporary help in stabilizing the radius, but angulation, fragmentation, capitellar erosion, and particulate synovitis frequently are seen as adverse reactions. An ulna resection is a better choice, but persistent radial migration can occur along with other problems. Ulnar head resection is a last resort.

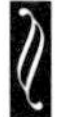

Answer: **B**
Cooney, Linscheid, Dobyns, pp. 851-852
Stabile, Pfaeffle, Tomaino, pp. 195-204

21. Which of the following is true about the gripping rotatory impaction test (GRIT)?

A. It is used to identify patients with ulnar impaction (abutment).
B. It requires the use of a grip dynamometer and a radiograph.
C. It is positive when the supinated : pronated grip strength is significantly greater than 1.0.
D. A and C
E. All of the above

The GRIT assessment is the clinical assessment corollary to the radiographic image of the pronated-gripped forearm/wrist but does *not* require an X-ray. That is, the GRIT can quantitatively identify wrists with symptomatic ulnar impaction in the clinic with the use of a dynamometer by first unloading the symptomatic ulnocarpal structures in supination, thus decreasing the pain response and allowing greater grip force production. Second, the GRIT increases the load to the symptomatic ulnocarpal structures in pronation, increasing the pain response and preventing maximum grip force. Therefore the supinated : pronated grip strength ratio is greater than 1.0.

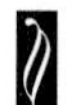

Answer: **D**
LaStayo, Weiss, pp. 173-179

22. You are treating a patient with undiagnosed wrist pain. The patient reports pain in the wrist, weakness, and diminished motion. Radiographs reveal an ulnar minus variance. What might the diagnosis be for this patient?

A. Preiser's disease
B. Kienböck's disease
C. Madelung's deformity
D. None of the above
E. All of the above

In 1910, Kienböck described a condition that was characterized by pain, stiffness, and swelling in the wrist. Kienböck's disease tends to occur in young active adults in the third or fourth decades of life. It usually occurs in the dominant extremity but can occur bilaterally. The ulnar minus variance noted in 1928 by Hulten is observed in only 23% of radiographs of normal wrists but is present in 78% of patients with Kienböck's disease. The etiology of the disease remains controversial. Some authors have proposed that the ulnar minus variance subjects the lunate to a greater compression or shear stress. This compression or shear stress has been coined the "nutcracker effect."

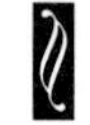

Answer: **B**
Almquist, p. 141
Refer to Fig. 8-12

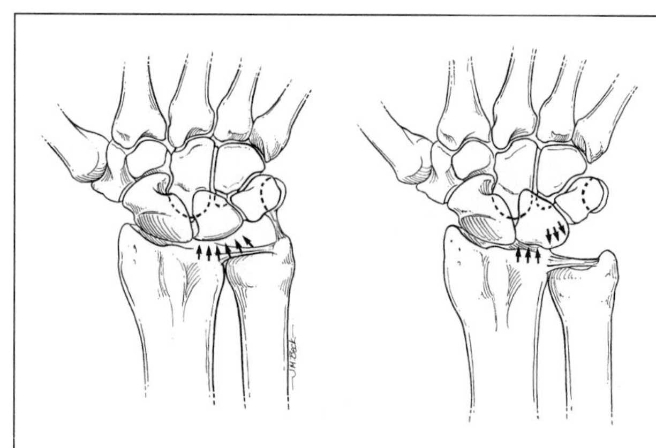

Fig. 8-12 ■ The lunate in a normal wrist is almost completely supported by the distal radius (*left*). In Kienböck's disease, the lunate is not as well covered by the radius and thus is more susceptible to uneven compression (*right*). (From Cooney WP, Linscheid RL, Dobyns JH: *The wrist: diagnosis and operative treatment,* St Louis, 1998, Mosby.)

23. True or False: Ligamentotaxis is the goal of external fixation for distal radius fractures.

Ligamentotaxis is the principle of molding fracture fragments into alignment as a result of tension, via an external fixator, applied across a fracture by the surrounding intact soft tissues. Using an external fixator to establish ligamentotaxis restores anatomic alignment and maintains fracture reduction during healing.

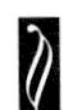

Answer: **True**

Kaempffe, pp. 205-209

24. All but which of the following are possible treatment options for patients with Kienböck's disease who have a 3-mm negative ulnar variance?

A. Scaphoid, trapezium, trapezoid arthrodesis
B. Radial shortening
C. Ulnar lengthening
D. LT fusion
E. Capitate shortening

The goal of leveling procedures used to treat Kienböck's disease is to decrease the biomechanical pressure on the lunate. LT fusion would not be effective in decreasing the lunate load. Capitate shortening has been advocated as a treatment option, but some physicians doubt its ability to decrease biomechanical load. The other three procedures do appear to decrease lunate biomechanical load.

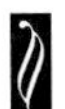

Answer: **D**

Allan, Joshi, Lichtman, pp. 1281-1336
Coe, Trumble, pp. 417-429

25. Weightlifters and gymnasts tend to repetitively hyperextend and forcefully load their wrists. A specific nerve injury in these individuals can cause development of perineural fibrosis and pain, without sensory changes. Which nerve is associated with this phenomenon?

A. Palmar cutaneous nerve
B. Radial sensory nerve
C. Posterior interosseous nerve
D. Deep branch of the ulnar nerve
E. Superficial dorsal branch of the ulnar nerve

The posterior (dorsal) interosseous nerve is the terminal branch of the radial nerve. It has no cutaneous sensory innervation. This nerve is located on the floor in the fourth compartment and is accompanied by the posterior branch of the anterior interosseous artery. Irritation of the posterior interosseous nerve often is associated with dorsal wrist ganglia. Less well known is its irritation by repetitive, forceful hyperextension, which causes perineural fibrosis (abnormal scarring around a nerve).

Answer: **C**

Aulicino, pp. 455-466
Refer to Fig. 18-8

CLINICAL GEM:
The posterior interosseous nerve does not have sensory innervation but does provide proprioceptive innervation to the wrist joint. Therefore this nerve can cause a painful wrist.

26. Your patient complains of pain in the LT area. The patient reports a painful clicking and point tenderness. Which of the following tests is helpful to assess the LT ligament?

A. Watson's shift test
B. Ballottement test
C. Piano-key test
D. All of the above are appropriate tests.
E. None of the above is an appropriate test.

When a patient complains of pain in the LT area, a helpful test is the ballottement test, as described by Reagan (Fig. 8-13, *A* and *C*). The lunate is stabilized firmly with the thumb and index finger of one hand while the pisotriquetral unit is rocked with the other hand. A positive test results in pain, crepitus, and laxity. A modification of this test is the "shear" test, as described by Kleinman (Fig. 8-13, *B*). To perform this test, the patient rests the elbow on the table with the forearm in neutral rotation. The examiner's contralateral thumb is placed over the dorsal aspect of the lunate just beyond the medial edge of the distal radius. With the lunate stabilized, the examiner uses his or her opposite thumb to load the pisotriquetral joint from a palmar to dorsal plane, thus creating a shearing force at the LT joint and causing pain. Although these are good tests, they are less specific at determining LT involvement than we would like. These tests can produce a false positive because of other pathologies.

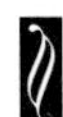

Answer: **B**

Green, pp. 894-896
Cooney, Linscheid, Dobyns, pp. 531-533
LaStayo, Howell, pp. 10-17

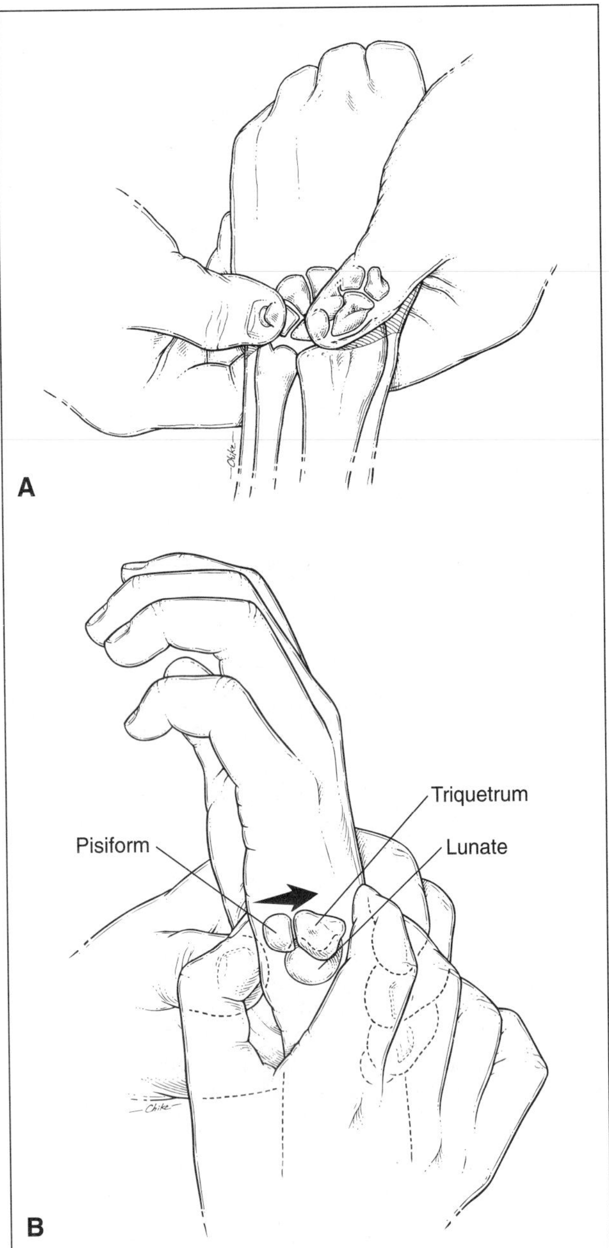

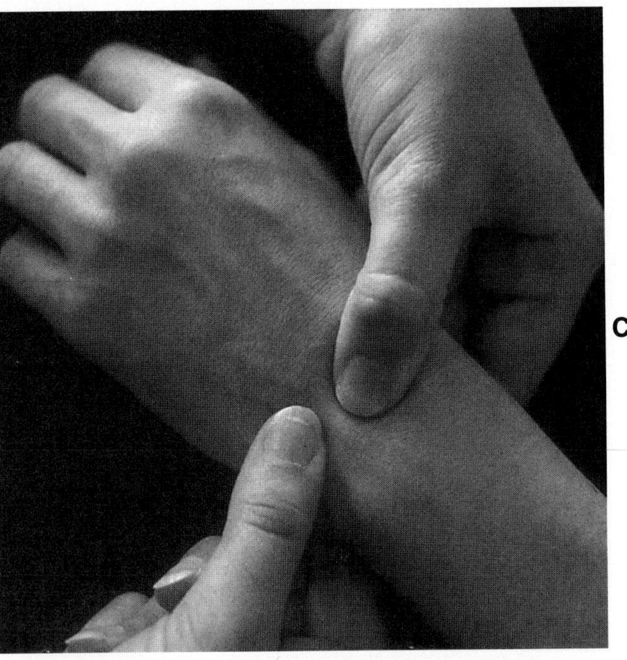

Fig. 8-13 ■ LT stress test. **A,** Ballottement test. The purpose of the test is to rock or "ballotte" the lunate against the triquetrum to demonstrate pain related to instability, cartilage loss, or local synovitis. Both hands are used to grasp the lunate and triquetrum and to stress up and down the LT interval. **B,** LT shear test. The purpose of the test is to place a dorsal shear force by lifting the pisiform and triquetrum dorsally on the fixed lunate. The examiner's hands support the lunate dorsally (examiner's contralateral thumb) while the opposite hand (ipsilateral thumb) directly loads the pisotriquetral joint from a palmar to dorsal direction. **C,** LT ballottement test. (**A** and **B** From Cooney WP, Linscheid RL, Dobyns JH: *The wrist: diagnosis and operative treatment,* St Louis, 1998, Mosby; **C** from Mackin EJ, Callahan AD, Skirven TM, et al: *Rehabilitation of the hand and upper extremity,* ed 5, St Louis, 2002, Mosby.)

27. You are treating a patient who fell on his outstretched hand several months ago. The patient presents with pain and tenderness dorsally over the midwrist region. You perform a scaphoid shift (also known as Watson's) test, and it is positive. Which injury might you suspect?

A. TFCC tear
B. LT tear
C. SL tear
D. Distal radius fracture
E. Radial head fracture

The scaphoid shift test is used to assess SL ligament competence. To perform this test, the wrist is placed in ulnar deviation and the examiner's thumb is placed on the scaphoid tuberosity. As the wrist is brought into radial deviation, the normal flexion of the scaphoid is blocked by the examiner's thumb. If there is an instability, a dorsal subluxation of the scaphoid occurs. A click or snap is noted as the scaphoid reduces back to the wrist when the pressure is released from the tuberosity. This diagnosis is further confirmed with a clenched-fist radiograph to assess the size of the gap between the scaphoid and the lunate (see Fig. 8-11).

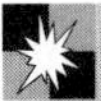

Answer: **C**

Wright, Michlovitz, p. 150
Cooney, Linscheid, Dobyns, pp. 256-258
LaStayo, Howell, pp. 10-17
Refer to Fig. 8-14

CLINICAL GEM:
Up to 30% of healthy wrists will exhibit a false positive response to the scaphoid shift test due to excessive laxity in the wrist. To eliminate the false positives in this situation, the examiner can perform a dynamic scaphoid shift test by asking the patient to make a fist while performing the test.

28. True or False: The SL and LT ligaments are homogenous structures.

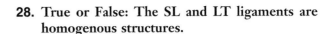

These ligaments are made up of three heterogeneous structures/regions. The three parts (volar, dorsal, and middle membranous) do not have the same tensile strength. The volar and dorsal components are the most resistant to tear forces, whereas the middle membranous portion is made up of fibrocartilage and is approximately five times less resistant to tear. Therefore structurally, the volar and dorsal portions of the complex are the most important for stability.

Answer: **False**

Berger, pp. 32-40

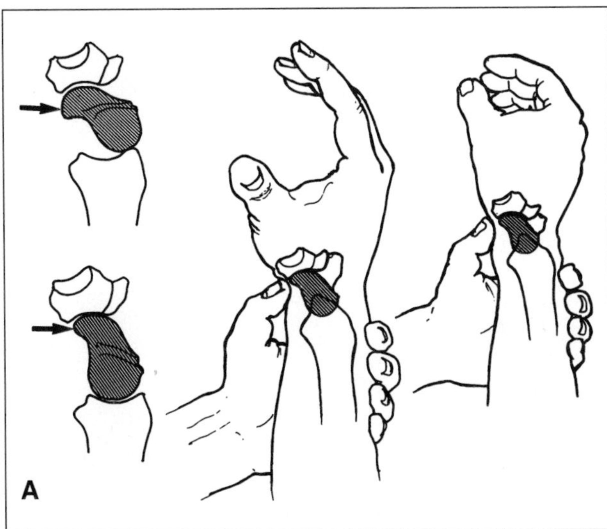

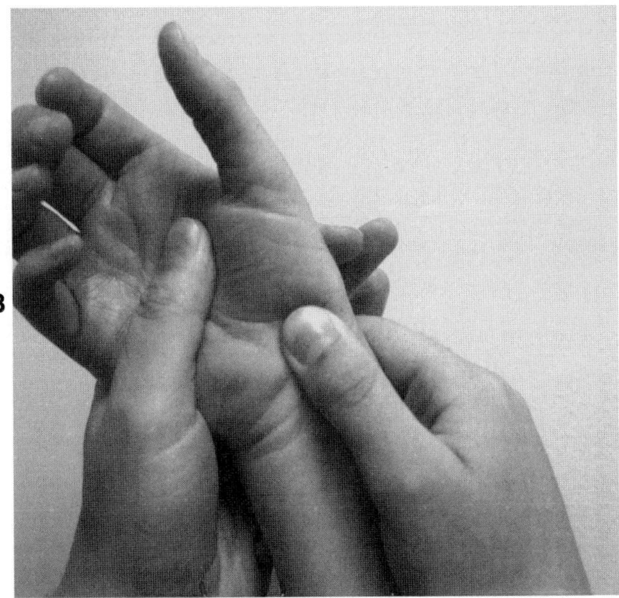

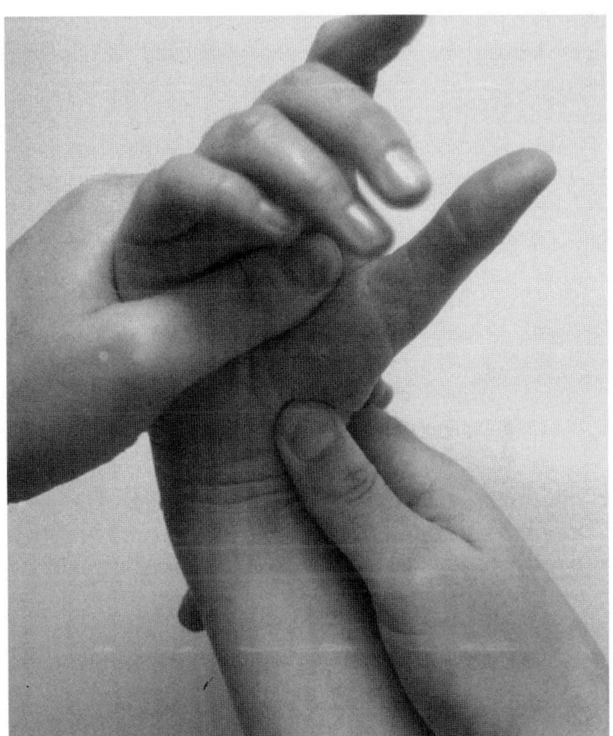

Fig. 8-14 ■ **A,** Scaphoid displacement test is performed by pushing upward on the scaphoid tuberosity while the hand is in ulnar deviation. This tends to cause the scaphoid to ride out of the radial fossa over the dorsal rim, at times producing a painful snap. The test might be positive in loose-jointed individuals and requires clinical and radiologic correlation. **B** and **C,** Watson's test. (**A** From Cooney WP, Linscheid RL, Dobyns JH: *The wrist: diagnosis and operative treatment,* St Louis, 1998, Mosby; **B** and **C** from Mackin EJ, Callahan AD, Skirven TM, et al: *Rehabilitation of the hand and upper extremity,* ed 5, St Louis, 2002, Mosby.)

29. A patient with an acute onset of wrist pain has a soft-tissue opacity on a lateral carpal radiograph. The patient is treated with indomethacin, and the pain quickly resolves. A follow-up radiograph 2 weeks later demonstrates nearly complete disappearance of the amorphous, well-circumscribed opacity. The most likely diagnosis is which of the following?

A. SLAC with osteoarthritis
B. Gout
C. Acute calcium soft-tissue deposition
D. Rheumatoid arthritis
E. Pseudogout

This remarkable acute onset of symptoms and equally remarkable resolution with indomethacin and rest is infrequently seen but can occur with acute calcium soft-tissue deposition. Opacities are visualized as fluffy soft-tissue calcium deposits that can disappear on radiographs in as little as 2 weeks.

Pseudogout would show linear calcification in the TFCC that would not resolve in 2 weeks. Calcifications seen with rheumatoid arthritis or gout also would not disappear on radiographs in 2 weeks. Osteophytes are common in degenerative joint disease, but they would not be seen in the soft tissues as fluffy, opaque deposits.

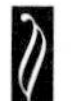
Answer: **C**
Milford, p. 377
Carroll, pp. 422-426

30. The manual maneuver pictured in Fig. 8-15 is a volar and dorsal glide of the ulna on a stabilized radius, first in neutral forearm rotation and then at the extremes of supination and pronation. Which of the following statements are correct?

A. An unstable DRU joint can be identified with this maneuver.
B. In a normal wrist/forearm you would expect greater volar and dorsal translation of the ulna in the extremes of forearm rotation.
C. A too stable (i.e., stiff) DRU joint can be improved with this maneuver.
D. A and C
E. All of the above

To test the stability of the DRU joint and concomitantly the supportive function of the TFCC, one can use this simple provocative maneuver. This technique is a translation maneuver of the ulna on the radius in various positions of forearm rotation. It is performed by stabilizing the radius with one hand and manually translating the ulna volarly and dorsally with the other hand. This should be done initially in neutral forearm rotation, where up to 5 mm of translation may be noted (in both the normal and unstable DRU joint). In the extreme positions of supination and pronation, however, less translation should be noticed as the stabilizing DRU joint bony structures control motion and the TFCC structures tighten. If translation of the ulna at the extremes of rotation equals that of the neutral translation, DRU joint instability is present. If there is hypomobility and limited forearm rotation with this maneuver, it can be used to mobilize the DRU joint.

Answer: **D**
LaStayo in Mackin, Callahan, Skirven, et al, pp. 1156-1170

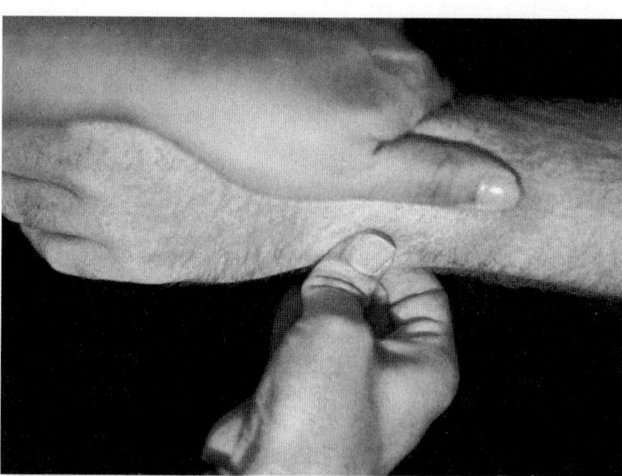

Fig. 8-15 ■ From Mackin EJ, Callahan AD, Skirven TM, et al: *Rehabilitation of the hand and upper extremity*, ed 5, vol 2, St Louis, 2002, Mosby.

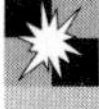
CLINICAL GEM:
This maneuver, because it places tension and stress on stabilizing ligamentous structures, can be used as a joint mobilization technique when those structures have adaptively shortened.

31. You are treating a patient with a 6-week-old distal radius fracture that was fixed with an open reduction internal fixation (ORIF) (dorsal plate). The patient reports that "something snapped in my wrist when I moved it." Finger ROM is normal and the thumb interphalangeal joint can be actively extended to 0 degrees but cannot achieve hyperextension. What is the most likely cause of these symptoms?

A. Breakup of adhesions of the radial carpal joint
B. Incongruity at the radial carpal joint
C. Tenosynovitis of the flexor carpi radialis
D. Extensor pollicis longus rupture
E. Crepitus

The extensor pollicis longus may rupture after a distal radius fracture. A roughened surface and possibly some slight dorsal articular tilting predisposes rupture of the extensor pollicis longus. Vascularity is probably compromised, and the tendon attenuates and ultimately ruptures. The thumb interphalangeal joint often can extend to zero by using the intrinsic muscles of the thumb, but hyperextension will be lacking. Also lacking will be the ulnar border of the snuffbox during the physical examination.

Answer: **D**

Engkvist, Lundburg, pp. 76-86
Tubiana, Thomine, Mackin, p. 312
Hunter, Mackin, Callahan, pp. 60, 551
Skirven, Osterman in Mackin, Callahan, Skirven, et al, pp. 1102, 1103

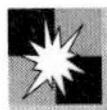

CLINICAL GEM:
With an extensor pollicis longus rupture, the patient is unable to lift his or her thumb off of the table. This motion is termed *retroposition*.

32. A 10-year-old competitive gymnast who landed especially hard on an outstretched hand has complaints of ulnar wrist pain, which was treated conservatively with cast immobilization following negative radiographic findings. Six months later her ulna has apparently stopped growing, and her ulnar negative variance is greater than 4 mm. She had an epiphyseal plate injury of which of the following?

A. Distal radius
B. Radial head
C. Proximal ulna
D. Distal ulna
E. None of the above

Salter and Harris first classified epiphyseal plate injuries according to the pattern on X-ray appearance, which also corresponded to their severity. This is the classification that is most commonly used when describing epiphyseal injuries. Salter and Harris Type V injuries occur when there is a crush injury to the epiphyseal plate. There may be no obvious finding on X-ray, although from the nature of the injury, the clinical signs, and abnormal long bone growth patterns, a serious injury of the growth plate is to be suspected.

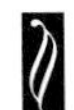

Answer: **D**

Bley, Seitz, pp. 231-237

33. Pain and paresthesias on the ulnar aspect of the hand and at the little finger after a hard swing at a baseball could be caused by which of the following?

A. Scaphoid fracture
B. DeQuervain's tenosynovitis
C. Hook of hamate fracture
D. Keinbock's disease
E. None of the above

Hook of hamate fractures may be hard to document but often occur with racket, club, or batting sports. Missed fractures are common. The patient may have findings of ulnar neuritis or pain. Physical examination may be completely unrevealing; therefore special imaging tests such as computed tomography (CT) can be helpful.

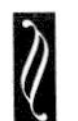

Answer: **C**

Geissler, pp. 167-188

34. A patient with a diagnosis of wrist sprain is referred to you from a general physician for evaluation and treatment. During your evaluation, the patient reveals that he fell from the back of a moving vehicle last week but that the emergency room radiographs were negative. He currently is wearing a prefabricated wrist splint. The patient has exquisite tenderness in the snuffbox during palpation. Which injury might this patient have?

A. TFCC tear
B. Scaphoid fracture
C. LT tear
D. Colles' fracture
E. Pisotriquetral degenerative joint disease

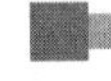

Often early radiographs are reported negative with scaphoid fractures, but this patient's extreme tenderness should alert you to a possible fracture. When the patient is seen immediately after injury, the fracture may not be readily apparent. Negative initial films should be followed up after 2 weeks of cast immobilization with a second radiograph. This allows osteoporosis adjacent to the fracture to develop and provides radiographic evidence of the fracture.

Answer: **B**
Cooney, Linscheid, Dobyns, p. 393

35. An ulnar styloid fracture alone can do which of the following?

A. Compromise the function of the palmar and DRU ligaments of the TFCC
B. Increase the relative force transmission through the radiocarpal joint
C. Cause DRU joint anteroposterior (AP) instability
D. A and C
E. All of the above

A fracture at the ulnar styloid's base and significant displacement of an ulnar styloid fracture can increase the risk of DRU joint instability, likely because of the subsequent impairment of the TFCC.

Answer: **D**
May, Lawton, Blazar, pp. 965-971

36. You are treating a patient who has obvious signs of ulnar abutment after distal radius fracture. The patient has pain with extremes of rotation and ulnar deviation, which are aggravating his discomfort. At times, the patient complains of a clicking sensation, activity-related swelling, and decreased strength and motion. Radiographs reveal an ulnar plus variance of 2.6 mm. Surgery will be performed. What is the surgical treatment of choice, according to Cooney, Linscheid, and Dobyns, when there is minimal DRU joint involvement?

A. Bower's hemiresection
B. Darrach procedure
C. Suave-Kapandji procedure
D. Ulnar resection (shortening)
E. One bone forearm

Each of the procedures mentioned has potential benefit through relieving stress on the ulnar side of the wrist by effectively unloading the ulna. However, each may result in residual symptoms that may bother the patient. According to Cooney, Linscheid, and Dobyns, the ulnar resection (shortening) is the procedure of choice for most cases of ulnar abutment (see Fig. 18-16, *D*). The ulnar shortening has the advantage of maintaining the articular surfaces of the ulnocarpal joint and the DRU joint. Another benefit of ulnar shortening is tightening of the ulnocarpal ligaments and the TFCC, which provides a stabilizing effect for patients with ligament laxity or injury. Postoperatively, the extremity is immobilized in a Muenster-type cast for 6 weeks to control forearm rotation. This is followed by use of a removable, custom-made splint until complete union is obtained.

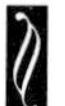
Answer: **D**
Cooney, Linscheid, Dobyns, pp. 776-782
Jaffe, Chidgey, LaStayo, pp. 129-138
Refer to Fig. 8-16

CLINICAL GEM:

- The Suave-Kapandji procedure can lead to instability at the site of pseudoarthrosis (Fig. 8-16, *A*).
- Bower's hemiresection may result in residual impingement at the sigmoid notch (Fig. 8-16, *B*).
- Darrach resection may result in residual weakness and instability (Fig. 8-16, *C*).

37. Fusion of the scaphoid, trapezium, trapezoid (STT) joint, also termed the *triscaphe joint*, is a useful procedure for all but which of the following?

A. Carpal instability
B. Kienböck's disease
C. Triscaphe arthritis
D. Radioscaphoid arthritis
E. TFCC tear

A fusion of the STT joint is best used as a treatment for triscaphe arthritis, carpal instabilities, and Kienböck's disease. An STT fusion would not be used for a patient with radioscaphoid arthritis. In fact, one of the long-term side effects of an STT fusion is radiocarpal arthritis. This often is caused by a failure to achieve scaphoid realignment during fusion. The creation of a four-bone fusion by using the capitate, hamate, lunate, and triquetrum with a scaphoid excision is one possible procedure for radioscaphoid arthritis.

Answer: **D**
Leibovic, pp. 601-613
Watson, Weinzweig, Guidera, pp. 307-315

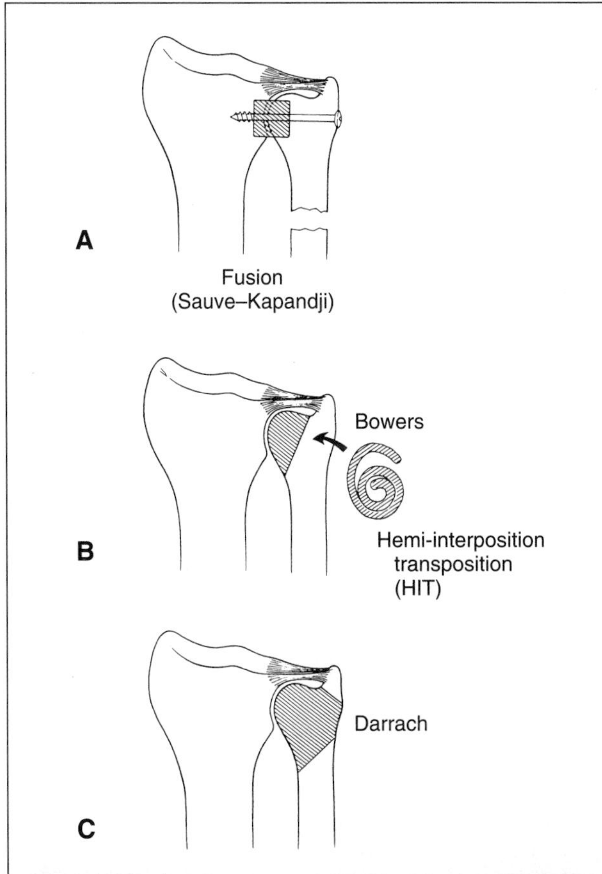

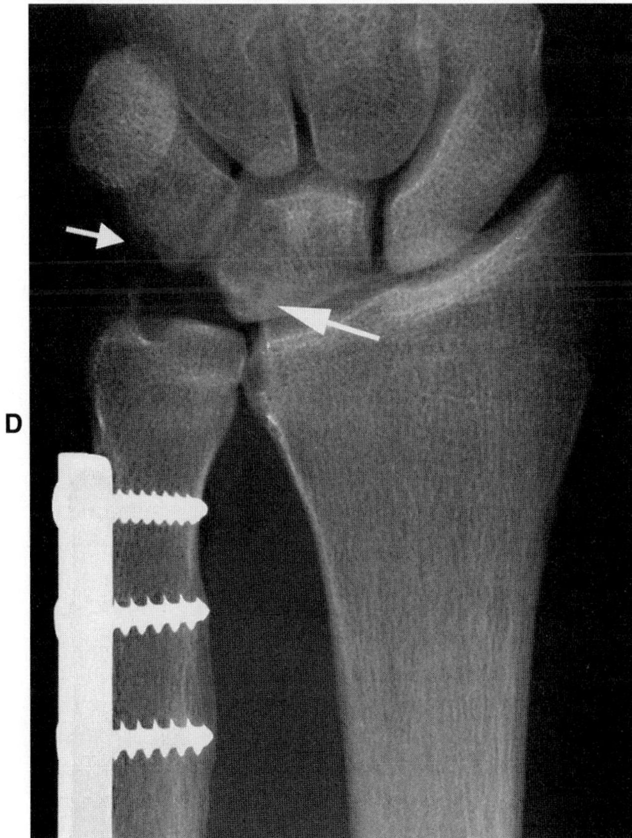

Fig. 8-16 ■ Ulnar shortening. From Cooney WP, Linscheid RL, Dobyns JH: *The wrist: diagnosis and operative treatment*, St Louis, 1998, Mosby.

38. True or False: A peripheral tear of the TFCC almost always occurs secondary to direct force.

A peripheral tear of the TFCC almost always occurs secondary to a direct compressive or shearing force. It often is associated with distal radius fractures. The patient complains of ulnar-sided wrist pain and weakness. Central tears of the TFCC occur traumatically or from deterioration. With a TFCC tear, the patient often complains of pain with resisted forearm rotation and sometimes reports a painful click. The central one third of the TFCC is a cartilaginous weight-bearing area that does not have or require a vascular supply. Central tears are treated with surgical debridement, and peripheral tears most often are treated with surgical repair (see Fig. 8-2).

Answer: **True**

Adams, Samani, Holley, pp. 189-193
Cooney, Linscheid, Dobyns, pp. 720-723

CLINICAL GEM:
Clinical assessment of the central TFCC can be performed with a TFCC load test (Fig. 8-17) in which the examiner ulnarly deviates the patient's wrist and moves the proximal carpal row in a volar/dorsal direction with gentle manual compression over the TFCC. With a TFCC tear, patients typically have pain with forearm pronation, ulnar deviation, and gripping.

39. After a TFCC peripheral tear is treated with surgical repair, when are passive supination and pronation allowed for a patient with limited range?

A. After 2 weeks
B. After 4 weeks
C. After 6 weeks
D. After 10 weeks
E. Never

After a peripheral repair of the TFCC, the patient is immobilized for 1 week in a long-arm cast. This is followed by use of a long-arm Muenster-style splint or sugar tong splint until weeks 2 to 4. Supination and pronation are restricted during this time to limit stress on the repair. During weeks 4 to 6, the patient is in a short-arm splint, and he or she can begin elbow ROM. From week 6 through week 10, active ROM is begun,

8 WRIST

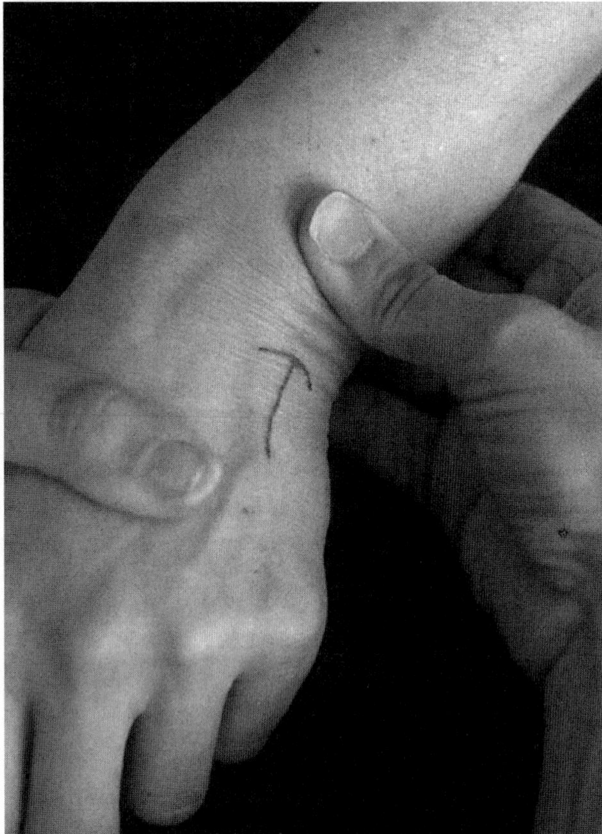

Fig. 8-17 ■ TFCC load test.

but extremes of motion—especially supination and pronation—are avoided so as to prevent stress on the repair. At week 10, no restrictions apply. Gentle passive ROM is initiated if limitations are noted for supination and pronation. Strengthening also is initiated at this time.

Answer: **D**

Jaffe, Chidgey, LaStayo, pp. 129-138
Skirven, pp. 98-105

CLINICAL GEM:

As always, "protocols" are simply guidelines. If the forearm has a pronounced passive limitation of motion (i.e., very stiff), passive ROM may be initiated earlier. Conversely, if forearm rotation exhibits very little limitation of motion, passive ROM may never be required.

40. You are treating a patient with a distal radius fracture. He complains of pain with ulnar deviation of the wrist and with gripping when the forearm is pronated. He is unable to open jars or use a screwdriver without difficulty. Loading the wrist also is painful for him. This patient might be exhibiting symptoms of which of the following?

A. Posterior interosseous neuritis
B. Scaphoid impingement
C. Ulnar impaction syndrome
D. Scaphoid-trapezial arthritis
E. None of the above

Ulnar impaction syndrome commonly occurs after malreduction of distal radius fractures, premature closure of the radial physis, or Madelung's deformity. Ulnar impaction syndrome is a common cause of dorsal ulnar wrist pain; it causes the patient pain with ulnar deviation and loading of the wrist. When the forearm is in pronation, the radius migrates proximally in relation to the ulna, thus increasing the ulnocarpal abutment. Diagnosis is made by testing forearm pronation-supination with the wrist in ulnar deviation as well as by compression of the ulnar side of the wrist against the distal ulna with the forearm pronated. The GRIT is also helpful. Diagnostic procedures to confirm ulnocarpal impingement include a bone scan, an arthrogram, and arthroscopy, after routine and stress radiographs have been taken.

Answer: **C**

Cooney, Linscheid, Dobyns, pp. 244-245
LaStayo in Mackin, Callahan, Skirven, et al, pp. 1156-1170

41. Which of the following tools is used primarily to diagnose ligament injuries of the wrist?

A. Tomography
B. Arthrography
C. Ultrasonography
D. CT scan

Wrist arthrography is used primarily to evaluate the integrity of the wrist ligaments and the TFCC. In a normal wrist, injection of contrast material through arthrography does not produce leakage from one joint to another. If the contrast material crosses from one interval to another, it is consistent with a ligament injury.

Ultrasonography can be helpful in evaluation of the painful wrist, especially if a ganglion cyst is present. Ultrasound also is helpful in evaluating the tendons as well as the tendon sheaths. CT is helpful in evaluating possible DRU joint disruption; it is more accurate than radiographs, especially when the patient is in pain or when cast immobilization makes positioning difficult. CT scans also are helpful in detecting subtle fractures, evaluating the healing fracture, and identifying occult tumors, bone lesions, scaphoid fractures, and Kienböck's disease. Tomography is used for evaluating position alignment and articular involvement of fractures.

One tool not yet mentioned is magnetic resonance imaging (MRI). MRI is useful when assessing a patient with possible osteonecrosis, soft-tissue masses, and neural compression in the carpal tunnel. The primary benefit of MRI for the wrist involves the assessment of avascular changes that may be present in the scaphoid, lunate, or capitate bones.

Answer: **B**
Bond, Berquist, pp. 113-123
Cooney, Linscheid, Dobyns, pp. 272-278

42. A radial styloid fracture is classified as which of the following types of fracture?

A. Smith's fracture
B. Barton's fracture
C. Colles' fracture
D. Chauffeur fracture
E. None of the above

A Chauffeur fracture is one in which the radial styloid is fractured off the radius. This fracture usually can be treated with closed reduction and percutaneous pin fixation. However, if the fracture is displaced more than 3 mm, there may be an associated SL dissociation; in this case, open reduction with repair of the ligament and anatomic reduction of the distal radial styloid is performed.

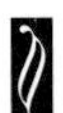

Answer: **D**
Cooney, Linscheid, Dobyns, p. 352
Refer to Fig. 8-18

43. True or False: In ulnar deviation of the wrist, the proximal carpal row extends.

In wrist ulnar deviation, the proximal carpal row extends, glides volarly, and translates radially. The distal carpal row in ulnar deviation flexes, glides dorsally, and translates ulnarly. The reverse occurs in radial deviation.

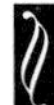

Answer: **True**
Cooney, Linscheid, Dobyns, p. 528
Moojen, Snel, Ritt, pp. 81-87

44. True or False: Complete palmar dislocation of the lunate occurs in the end stages of perilunate dislocation.

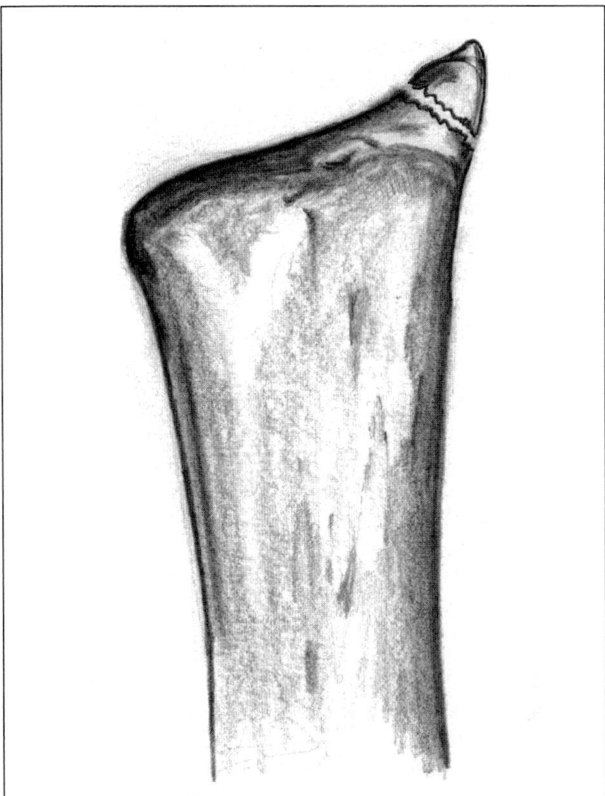

Fig. 8-18

A lunate dislocation is merely the end phase of a perilunate dislocation in which the lunate is spit out volarly, often into the carpal canal. This is considered the most severe form of a perilunate instability—a Grade four carpal injury. Clinically, most lunate dislocations are thought to be caused by wrist dorsiflexion injuries as a result of FOOSH.

Answer: **True**
Cooney, Linscheid, Dobyns, pp. 696-697
Kozin, 1998, pp. 114-120
Refer to Fig. 8-19

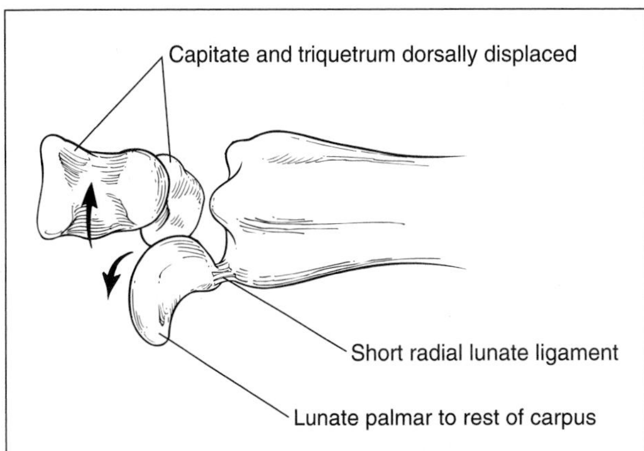

Fig. 8-19 ■ Complete palmar dislocation of the lunate. (From Cooney WP, Linscheid RL, Dobyns JH: *The wrist: diagnosis and operative treatment*, St Louis, 1998, Mosby.)

8 WRIST

45. The most reliable goniometric method for measuring wrist flexion and extension is via which of the following?

A. Radial technique
B. Ulnar technique
C. Volar/dorsal technique
D. Medial technique
E. Lateral technique

The volar/dorsal technique, in which the goniometer is placed volarly for measuring extension and dorsally for measuring flexion, is the most reliable.

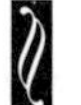

Answer: **C**
LaStayo, Wheeler, pp. 162-174

CLINICAL GEM:
Many factors, however, can effect wrist goniometric measurements (e.g., deformities, swelling, scar). Therefore, although the volar/dorsal technique is the most reliable, the ulnar (i.e., medial) and radial (i.e., lateral) techniques also have clinically acceptable reliability.

46. Ulnar translation of the carpus is *not* associated with which of the following?

A. Severe carpal (wrist) trauma
B. Rheumatoid arthritis
C. Psoriatic arthritis
D. Preiser's disease
E. It is associated with all of the above.

Ulnar translocation commonly occurs after attenuation of ligament support caused by rheumatoid or psoriatic arthritis. On a rare occasion, ulnar translation of the carpus may be seen after severe wrist trauma. The diagnosis is made with radiographs showing abnormal translation of the lunate in an ulnar direction. In a traumatic, rheumatoid, or psoriatic condition, a radiolunate fusion is the best choice for a successful outcome. There is no place for nonsurgical treatment. Preiser's disease is an avascular necrosis of the scaphoid and is not associated with ulnar translation of the carpus.

Answer: **D**
Taleisnik, pp. 305-307

47. You have been asked to fabricate a low-temperature thermoplastic ulnar gutter splint for a patient with a triquetral avulsion fracture. Where would this patient be most tender and swollen?

A. Volarly over the pisiform
B. Over the TFC
C. Laterally over the ulnar collateral ligament attachment
D. On the ulnar side of the dorsum of the carpus over the dorsal triquetral body
E. Over the space of Poirier

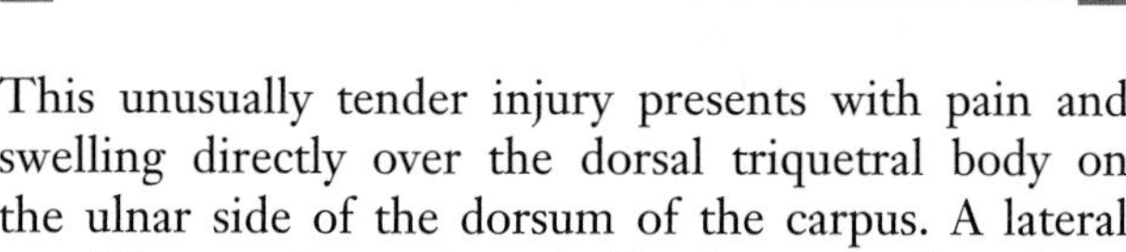

This unusually tender injury presents with pain and swelling directly over the dorsal triquetral body on the ulnar side of the dorsum of the carpus. A lateral or oblique radiograph typically shows small avulsion fracture fragments. Symptoms commonly subside within 3 to 4 weeks of ulnar gutter splinting. Persistence of pain beyond 6 weeks suggests that a more serious intraligamentous injury may be present. The space of Poirier is described in Chapter 1, question 39 (see Fig. 1-23).

Answer: **D**
Taleisnik, pp. 149-151

48. What is considered a functional wrist ROM for performing most activities of daily living?

A. 5 degrees of flexion, 30 degrees of extension, 10 degrees of radial deviation, and 15 degrees of ulnar deviation
B. 40 degrees of flexion and extension and 40 degrees of composite radial and ulnar deviation
C. A and B
D. None of the above is considered functional.

Studies have revealed a range of numbers for functional wrist ROM. Palmer indicates that 5 degrees of flexion, 30 degrees of extension, 10 degrees of radial deviation, and 15 degrees of ulnar deviation are needed for functional use. More recently, Ryu and the Mayo Clinic Group found that 40 degrees of wrist flexion, 40 degrees of wrist extension, and 40 degrees of composite radial and ulnar deviation are needed for functional ROM. Most important to remember is that a person can be functional with less than normal wrist ROM. Our goal is to maximize ROM in a pain-free range.

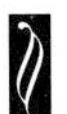
Answer: **C**
Ryu, Cooney, Askew, p. 409
Skirven, pp. 98-105
Watson, Weinzweig in Green, Hotchkiss, Pederson, p. 108
Bednar, Lersner-Benson in Mackin, Callahan, Skirven, et al, p. 1195

49. A patient is referred to you for evaluation and treatment with a diagnosis of wrist sprain. During your evaluation, the patient reveals normal ROM and 50% strength, with tenderness in the TFCC region. Your initial treatment should include which of the following?

A. Splinting the wrist at 0 degrees of extension and activity modification
B. A strengthening program
C. Referral for surgical intervention
D. Ultrasound and hot packs for pain management; no splint
E. Forearm rotation exercises

This patient may have a TFCC tear. Initial treatment for a TFCC injury is conservative. Treatment involves splinting with 0 degrees of wrist extension, antiinflammatory medication, and activity modification. After a trial of 3 to 6 months of conservative measures, surgical intervention may be considered. Before surgical intervention, further diagnostic studies are helpful to confirm the diagnosis of TFCC tear.

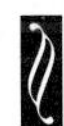
Answer: **A**
Jaffe, Chidgey, LaStayo, pp. 129-135
LaStayo in Mackin, Callahan, Skirven, et al, pp. 1156-1170

50. An LT fusion results in approximately what percentage of flexion loss?

A. 80%
B. 55%
C. 27%
D. 12%
E. 100%

Fusions crossing the radiocarpal joint (e.g., scapho-radiolunate fusion) lose approximately 55% of flexion/extension. Fusions crossing the intercarpal row (e.g., scaphotrapeziotrapezoid fusion) lose approximately 27% of flexion/extension. However, fusions within a single carpal row (e.g., LT fusion) lose approximately 12% of flexion/extension.

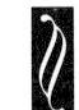
Answer: **D**
Meyerdierks, Werner, p. 528

51. True or False: When pronation and supination are performed, the ulna rotates around the radius.

Pronation-supination is a complex movement. It combines rotation of the radius around the ulna with horizontal and axial translation. The actual movement of the radius on the ulna in pronation-supination is a combination of rolling and sliding. When the arm is pronated, the radius crosses the ulna. In this pronated position, the radius proximally migrates in relation to the ulna, thus leading to a more positive ulnar variance.

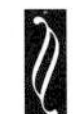
Answer: **False**
Cooney, Linscheid, Dobyns, p. 222

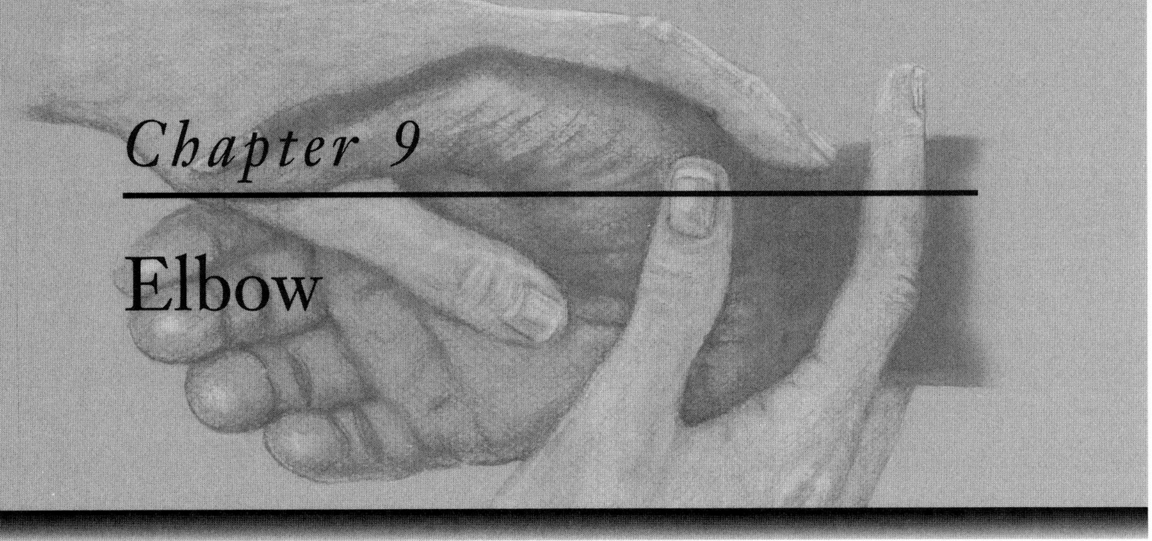

Chapter 9

Elbow

1. A distal biceps rupture typically occurs at which of the following locations?

A. Distal myotendinous junction
B. From the ulna
C. From the coracoid
D. From the radial tuberosity

The distal biceps typically avulses off of the radial tuberosity of the proximal radius as a result of a single traumatic episode. It requires surgical reattachment in most cases.

Answer: **D**
Morrey, 1994, pp. 115-124
Morrey, 2000, pp. 468-469
Refer to Fig. 9-1

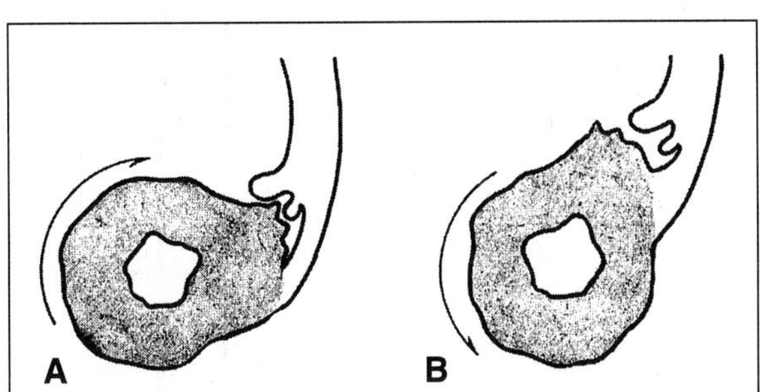

Fig. 9-1 ■ Illustration of the pathophysiology of distal biceps rupture. Hypertrophic changes at the radial tuberosity cause irritation of the tendon, predisposing it to degenerative changes and rupture during pronation and supination. From Davis WM, Yassine Z: An etiologic factor in the tear of the distal tendon of the biceps brachii, *J Bone Joint Surg* [Am] 38:1368, 1956.

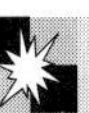

CLINICAL GEM:
Bicep tendon ruptures are a common occurrence in well-conditioned, healthy, competitive weightlifters. Anabolic steroid abuse and the mechanism of injury account for the surprisingly common occurrence.

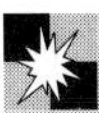

CLINICAL GEM:
Preexisting degenerative changes in the biceps tendon predispose patients to rupture. Hypertrophic changes at the radial tuberosity irritate the tendon, thus predisposing it to degenerative changes and rupture during pronation and supination.

Morrey, 2000, p. 469

2. Lateral epicondylitis of the elbow principally involves degenerative change of what structure?

A. Lateral humeral epicondyle
B. Extensor carpi radialis longus (ECRL)
C. Extensor carpi radialis brevis (ECRB)
D. Supinator

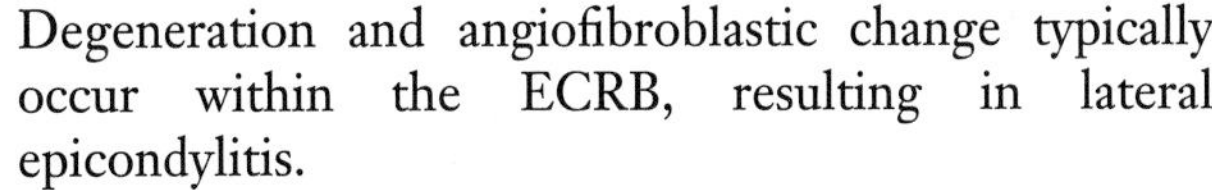

Degeneration and angiofibroblastic change typically occur within the ECRB, resulting in lateral epicondylitis.

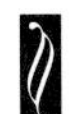

Answer: **C**
Morrey, 1994, pp. 129-138
Lillegard, Butcher, Rucker, p. 150

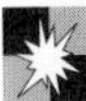

CLINICAL GEM:
Tennis elbow, a common overuse injury of the elbow, can result from repetitive loading of the wrist.

3. Which part of the ulnar collateral ligament (UCL) of the elbow is typically injured in throwers?

A. The posterior bundle
B. The transverse ligament
C. The interosseous ligament
D. The anterior bundle

The anterior bundle of the medial (ulnar) collateral ligament is the crucial component that resists valgus stress during the throwing motion. It is the major stabilizer of the elbow, and throwers often injure it.

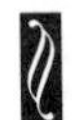

Answer: **D**
DeLee, Drez, Miller, p. 1252
Morrey, 2000, p. 549
Refer to Fig. 9-2

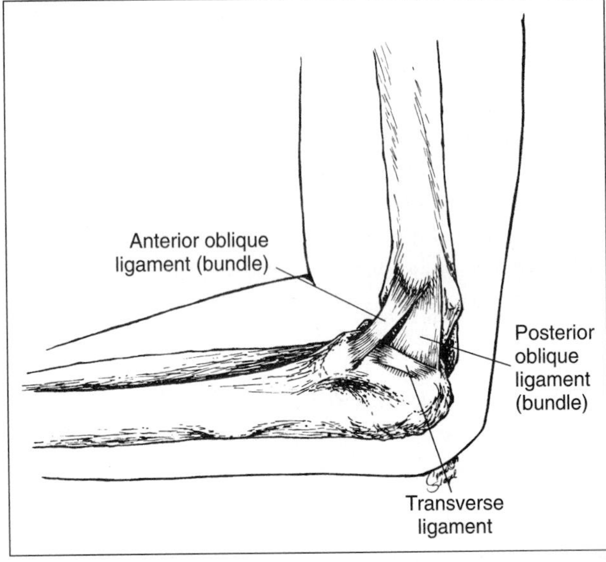

Fig. 9-2 ■ From DeLee JC, Drez D, Miller MD: *DeLee & Drez's Orthopaedic sports medicine: principles and practice,* ed 2, Philadelphia, 2003, WB Saunders.

4. Which clinical sign indicates ulnar neuritis at the elbow?

A. Phalen's test
B. Tinel's test
C. Jobe's test
D. Ulnar relocation test

A Tinel's sign over the cubital tunnel is the hallmark of ulnar neuritis at the elbow.

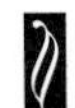

Answer: **B**
Lillegard, Butcher, Rucker, pp. 149-150

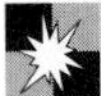

CLINICAL GEM:
Ulnar nerve pathology is often found in throwing athletes but can also be seen with those who play racquet sports, skiers, and weight lifters.

5. Where is radial nerve compression in the forearm typically located?

A. At the radial neck
B. Beneath the extensor digitorum communis
C. Within the supinator at the arcade of Frohse
D. Immediately proximal to the radiocarpal joint

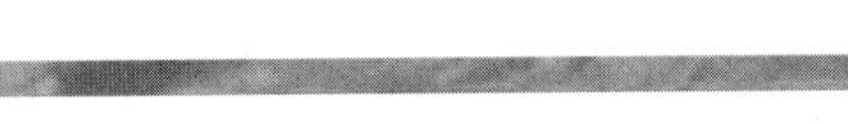

The deep branch of the radial nerve often is compressed at the arcade of Frohse within the supinator muscle.

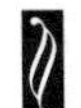

Answer: **C**
Morrey, 1994, p. 201

6. How is the Cozen's test performed?

A. Using electromyographic (EMG)/nerve conduction study
B. Palpation of the lateral humerus
C. Forced supination with resisted elbow extension
D. Resisted wrist extension with proximal ECRB palpation

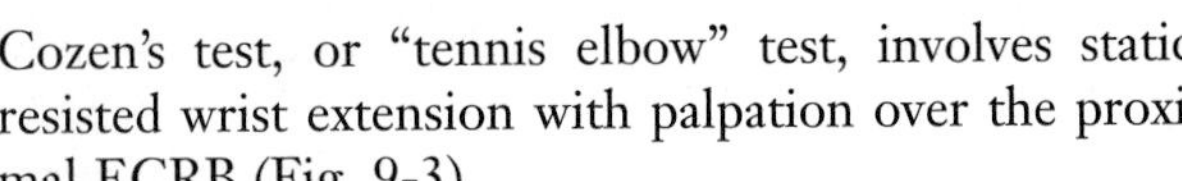

Cozen's test, or "tennis elbow" test, involves static, resisted wrist extension with palpation over the proximal ECRB (Fig. 9-3).

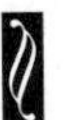

Answer: **D**
Hoppenfeld, p. 57
Fedorczyk in Mackin, Callahan, Skirven, et al, p. 1274

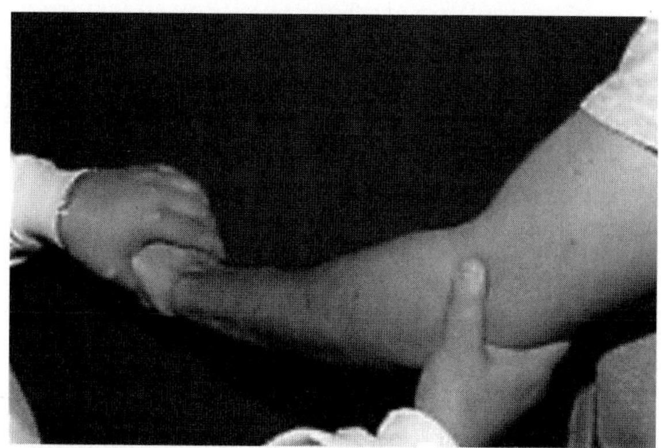

Fig. 9-3 ■ From Mackin EJ, Callahan AD, Skirven TM, et al: *Rehabilitation of the hand and upper extremity*, ed 5, St Louis, 2002, Mosby.

7. What is an Essex-Lopresti lesion?

A. Fracture of the radial head and coronoid
B. Fracture of the capitellum
C. Fracture of the radial head with proximal radial migration
D. Dislocation of the elbow with intraarticular fragments

An Essex-Lopresti lesion involves disruption of the interosseous membrane with proximal radial migration and fracture of the radial head. The Essex-Lopresti injury is a ligamentous injury sustained at the distal radioulnar (DRU) joint at the time of the radial head fracture and is considered an uncommon injury. The radius must be repaired to reestablish congruence of the DRU joint.

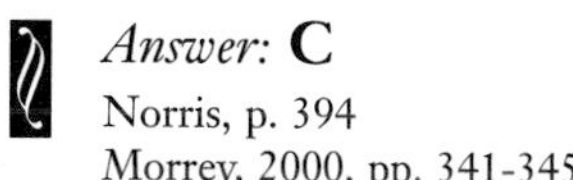

Answer: **C**
Norris, p. 394
Morrey, 2000, pp. 341-345

8. What is Panner's disease?

A. Synovitis of the elbow
B. Osteochondritis of the capitellum
C. Chronic bicipital tendonitis
D. Avulsion of the flexor pronator origin

Panner's disease, or osteochondritis of the capitelum, is a range of disorders from idiopathic osteochondrosis to osteochondritis dissecans with a loose body formation.

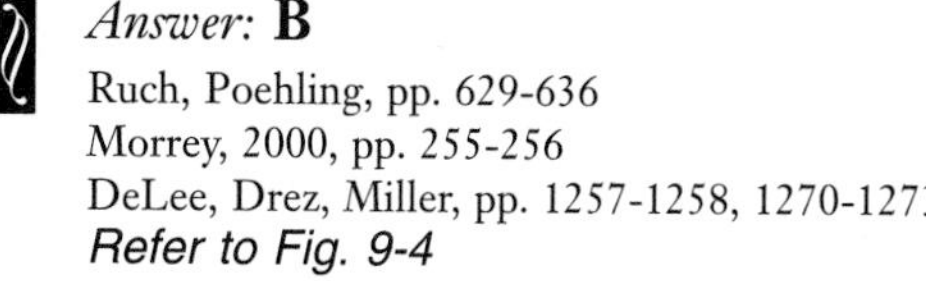

Answer: **B**
Ruch, Poehling, pp. 629-636
Morrey, 2000, pp. 255-256
DeLee, Drez, Miller, pp. 1257-1258, 1270-1273
Refer to Fig. 9-4

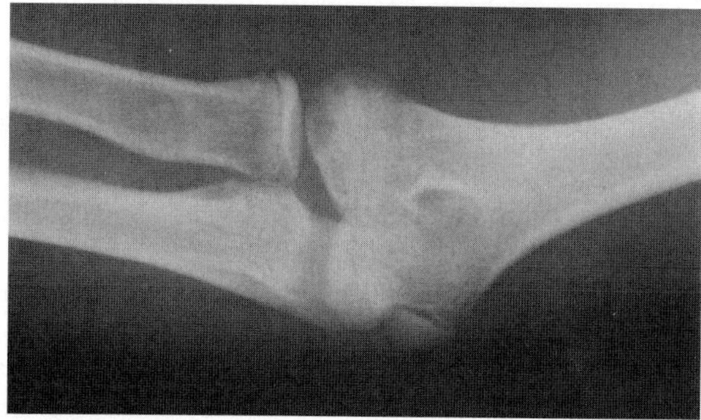

Fig. 9-4 ■ Osteochondrosis of the capitellum in the dominant arm of a young athlete. (From DeLee JC, Drez D, Miller MD: *DeLee & Drez's Orthopaedic sports medicine: principles and practice*, ed 2, Philadelphia, 2003, WB Saunders.)

Clinical Gem:
Osteochondritis is one of the causes of "little league elbow."

9. Which nerve is particularly at risk during elbow arthroscopy?

A. Musculocutaneous
B. Ulnar
C. Median
D. Radial

The radial nerve is only 3 mm away from the anterolateral portal in a cadaver study. Use of blunt cannulae and instruments minimizes risk to the radial nerve during arthoroscopy.

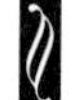

Answer: **D**
Lindenfeld, pp. 413-417

10. Which muscle overlies the anterior bundle of the UCL and therefore may have protective value for this vulnerable structure?

A. Flexor carpi ulnaris (FCU)
B. Flexor digitorum superficialis
C. Pronator teres
D. Flexor carpi radialis

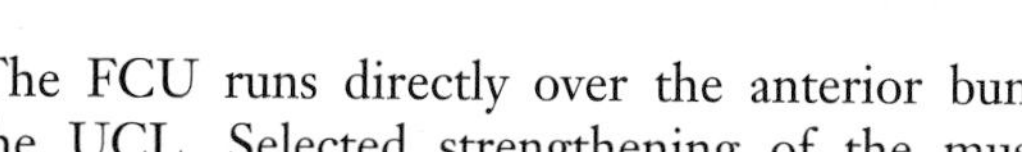

The FCU runs directly over the anterior bundle of the UCL. Selected strengthening of the muscle in throwers may protect against ligament injury.

Answer: **A**
Davidson, Pink, Perry, pp. 245-250

11. Reconstruction of the UCL traverses which structures?

A. Radius—lateral humeral epicondyle
B. Coronoid—medial humeral epicondyle
C. Olecranon—medial humeral epicondyle
D. Radial neck—capitellum

The reconstruction of the UCL entails placing a ligament graft transosseously and spanning the medial humeral epicondyle to the coronoid.

Answer: **B**
Morrey, 1994, pp. 149-169

12. True or False: The elbow joint is a biaxial joint, with 2 degrees of motion, flexion/extension, and supination/pronation.

The elbow joint is made up of two separate joints. The ulnohumeral joint resembles a hinge (ginglymus), which allows elbow flexion and extension. Axial rotation at the radiohumeral and proximal radioulnar joint is a pivoting type of motion (trochoid) rendering joint articulation to be classified as a trochoginglymoid joint (see Fig. 1-27).

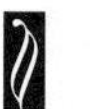

Answer: **False**
Norkin, Levangie, p. 241
Morrey, 2000, pp. 17-21

13. After a thorough examination, you suspect a patient is experiencing cubital tunnel syndrome. You target your treatment to decrease compression of the ulnar nerve as it passes through the tendon of what muscle?

A. FCU
B. Palmaris longus
C. Pronator teres
D. Long head of the triceps

Repetitive forceful contraction of the FCU muscle may compress the ulnar nerve, resulting in cubital tunnel syndrome. This syndrome is characterized by paresthesia in the ulnar nerve distribution of the forearm and hand, usually brought on with sustained elbow flexion. The FCU muscle may be palpated by starting at the medial condyle and moving distally, as it is the most lateral muscle in the wrist flexor and pronator muscle group.

Answer: **A**
Norkin, Levangie, p. 258
Hoppenfeld, p. 44
Magee, p. 144
Morrey, 2000, pp. 848-851

14. True or False: The bicep muscle is the primary elbow flexor with the forearm held in supination as well as pronation.

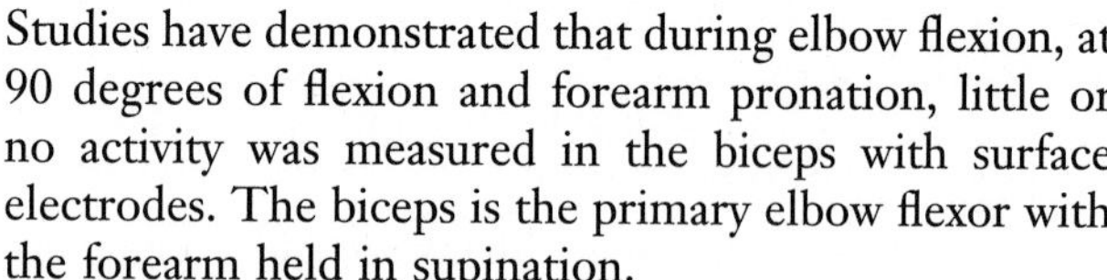

Studies have demonstrated that during elbow flexion, at 90 degrees of flexion and forearm pronation, little or no activity was measured in the biceps with surface electrodes. The biceps is the primary elbow flexor with the forearm held in supination.

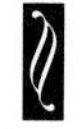

Answer: **False**
Morrey, 2000, p. 56
Refer to Fig. 9-5

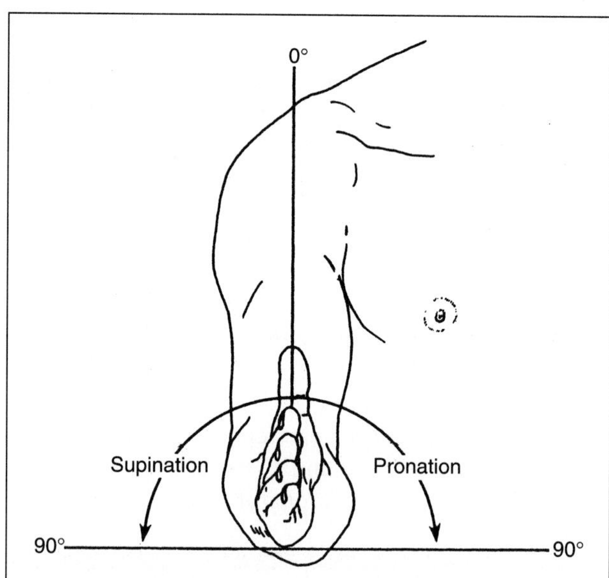

Fig. 9-5 ■ From Magee DJ: *Orthopedic physical assessment*, ed 2, Philadelphia, 1992, WB Saunders.

15. With most elbow patients, an examiner should conduct a clearing of the cervical spine to rule out radicular pain. Match the nerve roots C5, C6, and C7 with their respective muscles to be tested for strength and reflexes.

Nerve Roots

A. C5
B. C6
C. C7

Muscles

1. Triceps, wrist flexion, and finger extension
2. ECRL, ECRB, brachioradialis
3. Biceps

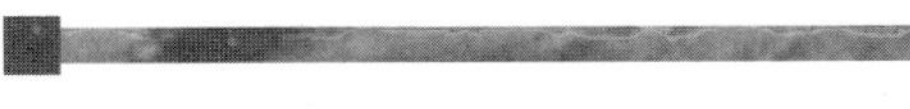

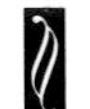

Answer: **A, 3; B, 2; C, 1**
Morrey, 2000, p. 65

16. The shoulder should also be evaluated when examining the elbow. Name the test that is performed by resisted shoulder flexion with the elbow held in supination and extension. A positive test is indicative of bicep tendinitis.

A. Speed's
B. Yeargason's
C. Drop-arm test
D. Supraspinatus test

The above description explains the Speed's test. A positive Speed's test indicates bicep tendinitis with pain elicited over the bicipital groove (Fig. 9-6). NOTE: Yeargason's test also assesses for bicipital tendonitis, but the test is different (Fig. 9-7).

Answer: **A**
Magee, p. 117
Rockwood, Matsen, pp. 1035-1036

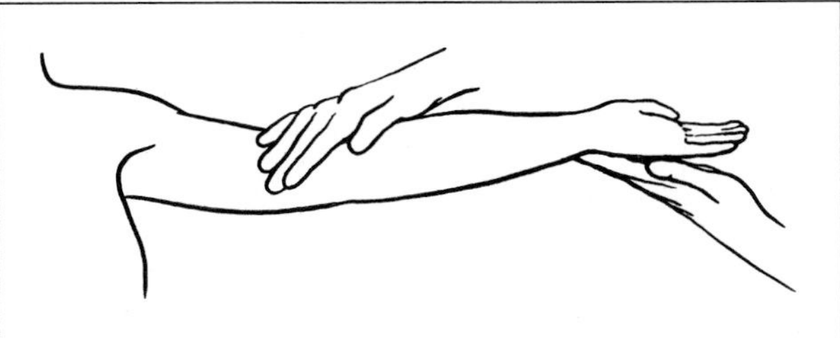

Fig. 9-6 ■ Speed's test. The biceps resistance test is performed with the patient flexing the shoulder against resistance with the elbow extended and the forearm supinated. Pain referred to the biceps tendon area constitutes a positive result. (From Rockwood C, Matsen F: *The shoulder*, Philadelphia, 1998, WB Saunders.)

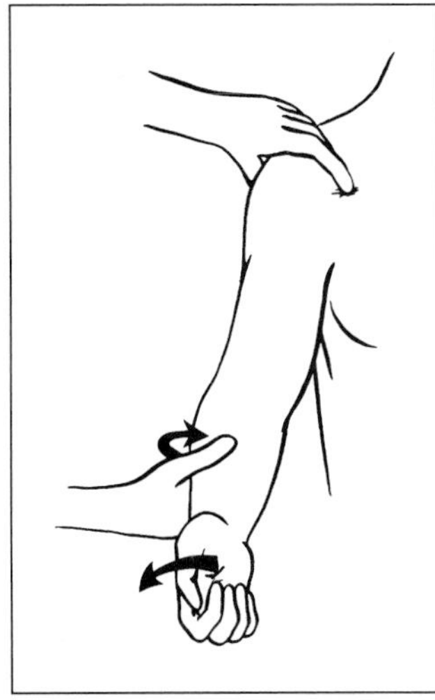

Fig. 9-7 ■ Yergason's sign. With the arm flexed, the patient is asked to forcefully supinate against resistance from the examiner's hand. Pain referred to the anterior aspect of the shoulder in the region of the bicipital groove constitutes a positive result. (From Rockwood C, Matsen F: *The shoulder*, Philadelphia, 1998, WB Saunders.)

17. Mrs. P was referred to you for evaluation and treatment with a diagnosis of lateral epicondylitis of the dominant extremity. She has had two rounds of nonsterioidal anti-inflammatory drugs (NSAIDs) 6 months apart, followed by cessation of sporting activities and causative tasks that elicit pain. The initial goal to reduce pain and inflammation was achieved and patient is now sent to occupational therapy for rehabilitation. Patient reports pain with causative activities at a 3 to a 4 on a scale of 1 to 10. What should your initial plan of care consist of?

A. Begin sports and all activities without restrictions
B. Complete immobilization and rest to continue for 3 more months
C. Continue tissue healing by wearing a counterforce brace, modify activities, begin wrist extensor stretching, and isometric exercises
D. Begin eccentric and concentric exercises with elbow fully extended and a 5-pound weight, wrist extensor stretching, return to sports without modifications

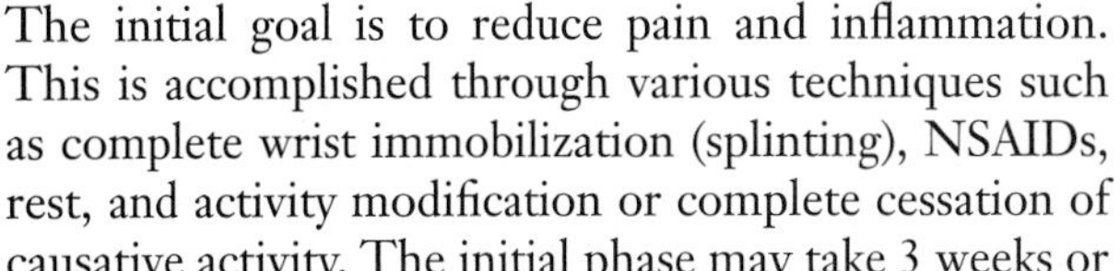

The initial goal is to reduce pain and inflammation. This is accomplished through various techniques such as complete wrist immobilization (splinting), NSAIDs, rest, and activity modification or complete cessation of causative activity. The initial phase may take 3 weeks or longer to accomplish relief of pain and inflammation. Phase two of rehabilitation will continue to focus on tissue healing via avoidance of causative or abusive activities. Counterforce bracing may be used. Rehabilitation is begun with wrist extensor stretches, modification of activities, and isometric exercises with the elbow flexed to decrease the load to the wrist extensors. As pain allows, eccentric and concentric exercises are introduced, beginning with no weight and gradually increasing to add weight. The goal is to increase the demand on the muscles without increasing pain.

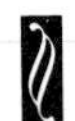

Answer: **C**
Jobe, pp. 431-440

CLINICAL GEM:
Binder studied 125 lateral epicondylitis patients treated nonsurgically who were followed from 1 to 5 years. Ten percent of patients continued to be symptomatic to some degree, 26% had recurrence of symptoms, and more than 40% had minor discomfort that affected some aspect of their activities.

Jobe, p. 436

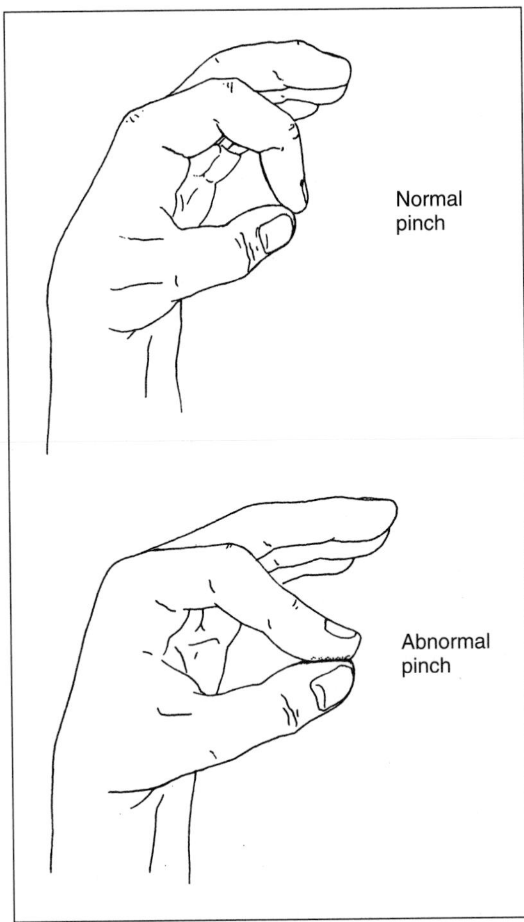

Fig. 9-8 ■ Normal versus abnormal pinch seen in anterior interosseous nerve syndrome. (From Magee DJ: *Orthopedic physical assessment*, ed 2, Philadelphia, 1992, WB Saunders.)

18. You suspect your patient has suffered from an injury to the anterior interosseous nerve. Which of the following tests would you perform?

A. Elbow flexion test
B. Upper limb tension test
C. Pinch grip test
D. Tinel's sign

The pinch grip test is done by having the patient pinch the tips of the index finger and thumb together. If the patient is unable to maintain a tip-to-tip position but rather a finger-to-thumb pad contact, then the test is considered positive.

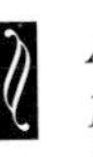

Answer: **C**
Magee, p.154
Refer to Fig. 9-8

19. True or False: Both the long head and the short head of the biceps originate above the glenohumeral joint and insert below the humeroulnar and humeroradial joint.

The long head originates from the tendon that contributes to the supraglenoid tendon, with the short head originating from coracoid process of scapula. They both insert to the radial tuberosity.

Answer: **True**
DeLee, Drez, Miller, p. 1066

20. Nursemaid's elbow or pulled elbow syndrome results from a longitudinal traction of the forearm causing the radial head to separate from which ligament?

A. Lateral collateral
B. Annular
C. Quadrate ligaments
D. Oblique cord

When the radial head separates from the annular ligament, resulting in pain and the inability to rotate the radial head, it is termed *nursemaid's elbow*. In most cases the annular ligament is not ruptured. It is thought that pulled elbow syndrome (nursemaid's elbow) is because of a generalized ligamentous laxity of the elbow.

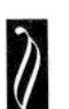
Answer: **B**
Norkin, Levangie, p. 257
Morrey, 2000, pp. 274-275

CLINICAL GEM:
Nursemaid's elbow is most seen in children between 6 months and 3 years. As the radius grows and becomes more ossified, pulled elbow syndrome is less common.

21. A patient fractured his proximal radius and ulna and was casted in 60 degrees of elbow flexion for 8 weeks. His cast was recently removed, and you have received orders for aggressive manual therapy to regain full range. You should contact the physician because you believe this may lead to the formation of ectopic bone and myositis officans if done improperly. True or False?

Additional care needs to be undertaken with aggressive therapy to an elbow after trauma. As optimal restoration of motion is typically a goal of rehabilitation, caution needs to be taken with passive stretching as well as splinting because overly aggressive rehabilitation may result in further complications, one of which may be ectopic ossification about the elbow.

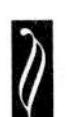
Answer: **True**
Morrey, 2000, p. 437

22. A complete distal bicep tendon avulsion injury is most common in which of the following?

A. Poor-conditioned male
B. Poor-conditioned female
C. Well-conditioned male
D. Well-conditioned female

The literature states that the majority (up to 80%) of avulsion ruptures occur in the right-dominant upper extremity in well-developed males. The mechanism of injury is commonly a sudden extension force to the elbow when the elbow is in 90 degrees of flexion.

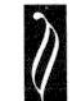
Answer: **C**
Morrey, 2000, p. 468

23. Lateral epicondylitis is accurately described as an acute, inflammatory process of which tendon?

A. ECRB
B. ECRL
C. Extensor carpi ulnaris
D. Extensor digitorum muscle

The pathophysiology dates back to the 1800s, when it was believed that the common extensors were detached because of repeated wrist extension and forearm supination. The current consensus, based on clinical and surgical evidence, suggests a microtear of the ECRB tendon. The ECRB is most often the cause of lateral tendinosis (epicondylitis). This tendon originates along the lateral epicondyle of the humerus as well as the radial collateral ligament and inserts into the third metacarpal.

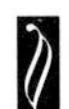
Answer: **A**
Morrey, 2000, p. 523
Jobe, p. 433

CLINICAL GEM:
Tennis elbow has been divided and classified according to anatomic structures. *Lateral tennis elbow* involves the ECRB. *Medial tennis elbow* involves the flexor pronator origin at the medial epicondyle and is often associated with compression neurapraxia of the ulnar nerve; *posterior tennis elbow* involves the triceps at its attachment to the olecranon. Posterior tennis elbow is uncommon but is seen in throwers such as baseball players and javelin athletes. *Combination tennis elbow* has symptoms of both lateral and medial tennis elbow.

Morrey, 2000, p. 523

24. After an open release for medial or lateral tendinosis, with the consideration of no secondary complications, the athlete can expect to return to desired activity competition in what time span?

A. 3 to 5 months
B. 5 to 8 months
C. 8 to 12 months
D. 12 or more months

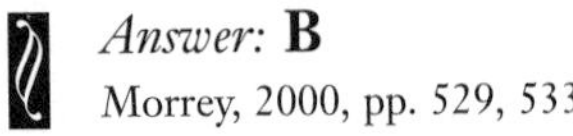

Although time frames for the different surgical options to treat lateral epicondylitis differ, in general, a practical guide for return to sports activities after such a procedure is 5 to 8 months. Rehabilitation should not only focus on the elbow but also include upper arm, shoulder, and back rehabilitation exercises.

Answer: **B**
Morrey, 2000, pp. 529, 533

25. At what time can an athlete return to a throwing program after repair of a torn UCL of the elbow?

A. 4 months
B. 6 months
C. 8 months
D. 10 months

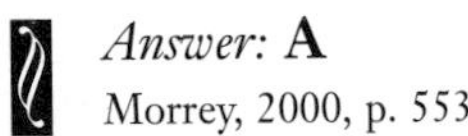

At approximately 4 months postoperative UCL repair a gentle, short throwing program should be implemented into the rehabilitation process.

Answer: **A**
Morrey, 2000, p. 553

26. True or False: The lateral epicondyle, medial epicondyle, and tip of olecranon line up in full elbow extension.

In full extension the above anatomical landmarks are colinear. When the elbow is flexed at 90 degrees, they form an inverted triangle, or an equilateral triangle from a posterior view. These bony landmarks are altered when elbow pathology is present.

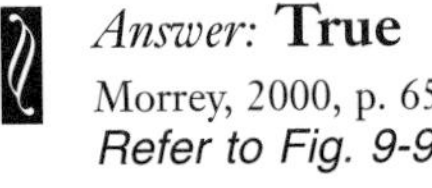

Answer: **True**
Morrey, 2000, p. 65
Refer to Fig. 9-9

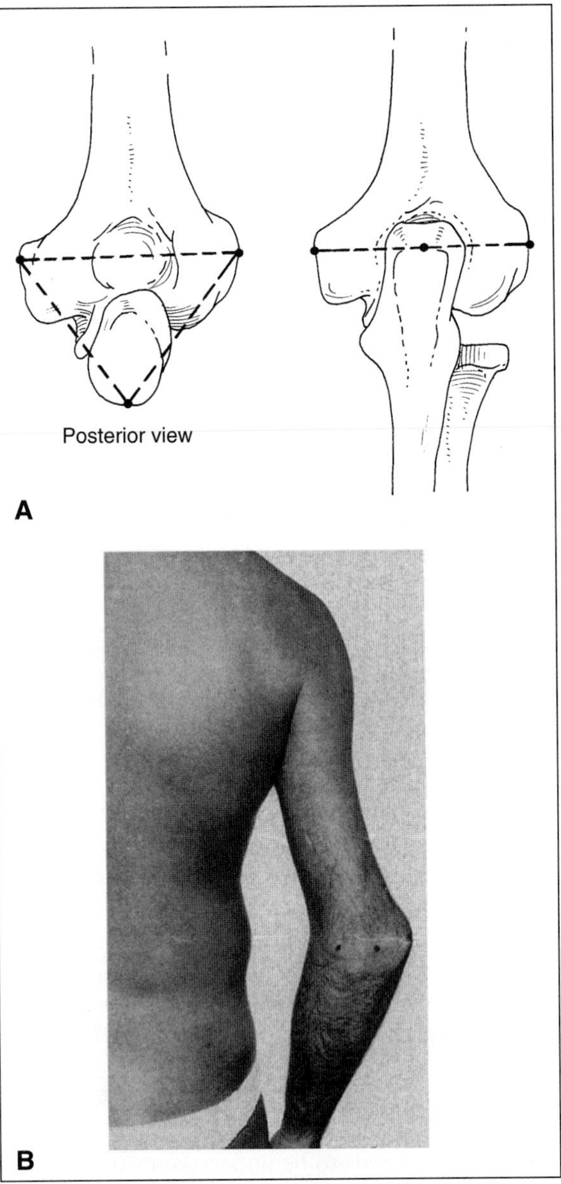

Fig. 9-9 ■ With the elbow flexed to 90 degrees, the medial and lateral epicondyles and tip of the olecranon form an equilateral triangle as viewed from the posterior. When the elbow is extended, this relationship is changed to a straight line that connects these three bony landmarks **(A)**. The relationship with displaced, intraarticular distal humeral fractures is altered **(B)**. (From Morrey BF: *The elbow and its disorders*, ed 3, Philadelphia, 2000, WB Saunders. By permission of the Mayo Foundation for Medical Education and Research. All rights reserved.)

27. True or False: A patient who is experiencing elbow pain may have referred pain from shoulder pathology.

If a patient complains of elbow pain your evaluation must include the shoulder because shoulder pathology may have referred pain to the elbow. Shoulder impingement tendinitis and associated rotator cuff pathology has pain that is manifested in the brachium.

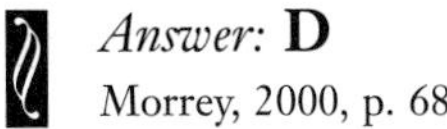

Answer: **True**
Morrey, 2000, p. 65

28. All the following muscles cross the elbow joint except which of the following?

A. Brachioradialis, brachialis, biceps
B. Coracobrachialis, deltoid
C. Pronator teres, extensor carpi ulnaris, FCU
D. Anconeus, triceps

The coracobrachialis and deltoid do not cross the elbow joint.

Answer: **B**
Morrey, 2000, pp. 13-40

29. What is considered normal range of motion for the uninjured elbow?

A. Extension/flexion arc 0 to 145 degrees; pronation/supination 75 degrees/85 degrees
B. Extension/flexion arc 5 to 125 degrees; pronation/supination 60 degrees/75 degrees
C. Extension/flexion arc 5 to 130 degrees; pronation/supination 65 degrees/75 degrees
D. Extension/flexion arc 0 to 120 degrees; pronation/supination 60 degrees/70 degrees

The normal arc of extension/flexion about the elbow is 0 to 145 degrees and 75 degrees for pronation and 85 degrees for supination.

Answer: **A**
Morrey, 2000, p. 67

30. What is considered the functional arc of motion of the elbow (motion necessary to do the majority of activities of daily living)?

A. Extension/flexion arc 0 to 145 degrees; pronation/supination 75 degrees/85 degrees
B. Extension/flexion arc 10 to 125 degrees; pronation/supination 60 degress/60 degrees
C. Extension/flexion arc 10 to 110 degrees; pronation/supination 40 degrees/35 degrees
D. Extension/flexion arc 30 to 130 degrees; pronation/supination 50 degrees/50 degrees

The essential arc of motion of the elbow to carry out most activities is 30 to 130 degrees. Supination requires roughly 50 degrees as well as 50 degrees of pronation for most activities of daily living (ADLs).

Answer: **D**
Morrey, 2000, p. 68

31. Match the elbow ossifications centers in children to the ages of appearance.

Ossification Centers

1. Capitelum
2. Trochlear
3. Radial head
4. Lateral epicondyle
5. Olecranon
6. Medial epicondyle

Age of Appearance

A. 4 years old
B. 5 years old
C. 2 years old
D. 8 years old
E. 9 years old
F. 10 years old

Answers: **1, C; 2, D; 3, B; 4, F; 5, E; 6, A**
Morrey, 2000, pp. 157-161

Clinical Gem:
There are six ossification centers: *c*apitellum, *m*edial epicondyle, *r*adial head, *t*rochlear, *o*lecranon, *l*ateral epicondyle. The order of appearance (CMRTOL) is 2, 4, 5, 8, 9, and 10.

32. When considering pinning on the medial side after closed reduction supracondylar fracture, one must be careful with which neurovascular structure?

A. Median nerve
B. Brachial artery
C. Ulnar nerve
D. Musculocutaneous nerve

Pinning a supracondylar fracture on the lateral side is very safe. If you are considering putting in a pin from the medial side, you should remember that the nerve at highest risk is the ulnar nerve.

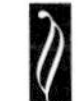

Answer: **C**
Morrey, 2000, pp. 201-206

33. An ulnar shaft fracture that is associated with radial head dislocation is called which of the following?

A. Galeazzi
B. Essex-Lopresti
C. Monteggia
D. Smith's

In 1814 GB Monteggia of Milan first described the injury called the *Monteggia fracture.* The Monteggia fracture is a fracture of the ulna and is associated with anterior dislocation of the radial head.

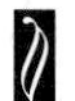

Answer: **C**
Morrey, 2000, p. 403
Refer to Fig. 9-10

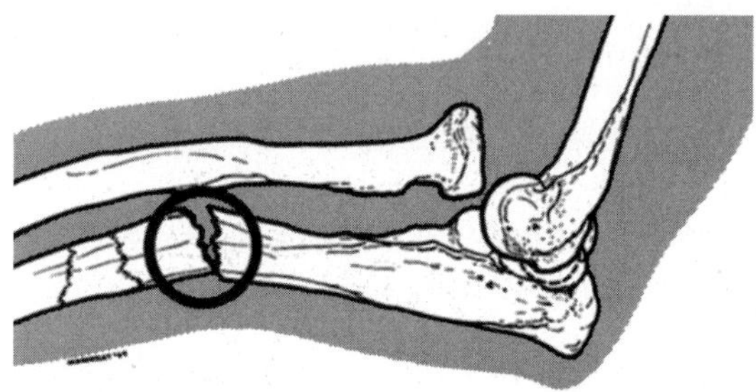

Fig. 9-10 ■ Monteggia lesion type I. (From Reckling FW, Cordell LB: Unstable fracture-dislocations of the forearm: the Monteggia and Galeazzi lesions, *Arch Surg* 96:999, 1968.)

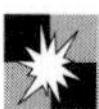

CLINICAL GEM:
The term *Monteggia* was coined in 1814, the same year that Colles coined his fracture.

34. True or False: The forearm consists of two basic compartments.

The volar compartment consists of flexors and pronators, which are further divided into superficial and deep muscle groups. The dorsal compartment consists mainly of the wrist and finger extensors.

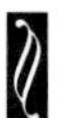

Answer: **True**
Morrey, 2000, pp. 13-15, 35-40, 62

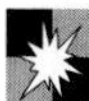

CLINICAL GEM:
The mobile wad of Henry consists of the brachioradialis, ECRL, and ECRB. Some authors refer to the mobile wad of Henry as a separate compartment, and others include it in the dorsal compartment.

35. Compartment syndrome of the forearm is known as which of the following?

A. Perthe's syndrome
B. Dupuytren's disease
C. Volkmann's ischemia
D. Hansen's disease

Another term for compartment syndrome of the forearm is *Volkmann's ischemia.* Therapists should be knowledgeable of the pathology and clinical manifestations of compartment syndrome. A differential diagnosis may be arterial injury.

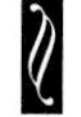

Answer: **C**
Morrey, 2000, pp. 209-211
Refer to Fig. 9-11

36. True or False: Nirschel believes that conservative management of lateral epicondylitis may be successful based on the outcome of a "simple handshake."

Nirschel et al determined which patients may respond to conservative treatment based on the results of the "simple handshake test." This test is performed by having the patient shake the examiner's hand firmly with the elbow extended (Fig. 9-12, *B*) and then supinate the forearm against resistance (Fig. 9-12, *A*). Repeat the handshake with the elbow flexed to 90 degrees. Pain is expected in the region of the lateral epicondyle. The examiner notes how severe the pain is in the elbow with the elbow extended versus when it is flexed at 90 degrees. If reported pain is less when the elbow is flexed at 90 degrees in comparison with when the elbow is extended, conservative management may be more favorable.

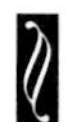

Answer: **True**
Fedorczyk in Mackin, Callahan, Skirven, et al, p. 1275

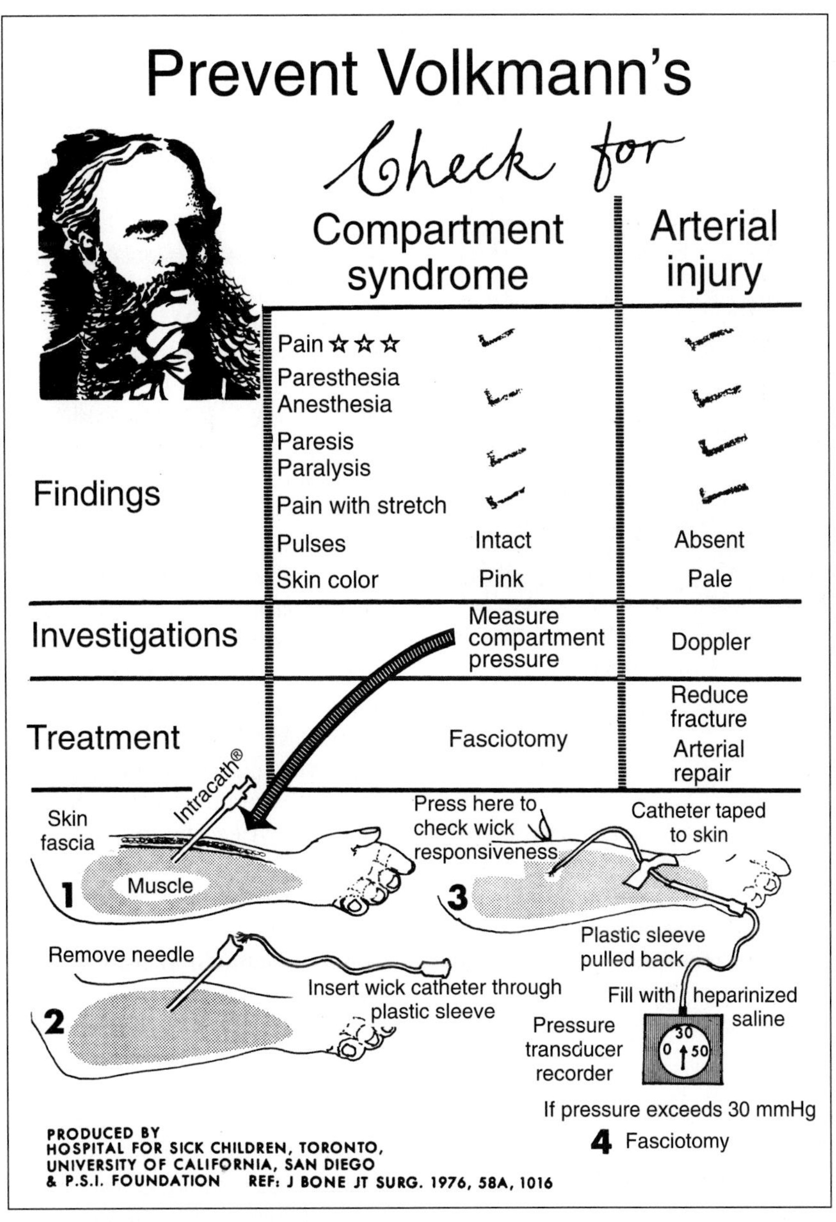

Fig. 9-11 ■ Poster that outlines the clinical findings, investigations, and treatment of compartment syndromes. The poster is used to alert medical and nursing staff to the diagnosis and prevention of Volkmann's ischemic contracture. (From Mubarak SJ, Hargens AR: *Compartment syndromes and Volkmann's contracture*, Philadelphia, 1981, WB Saunders.)

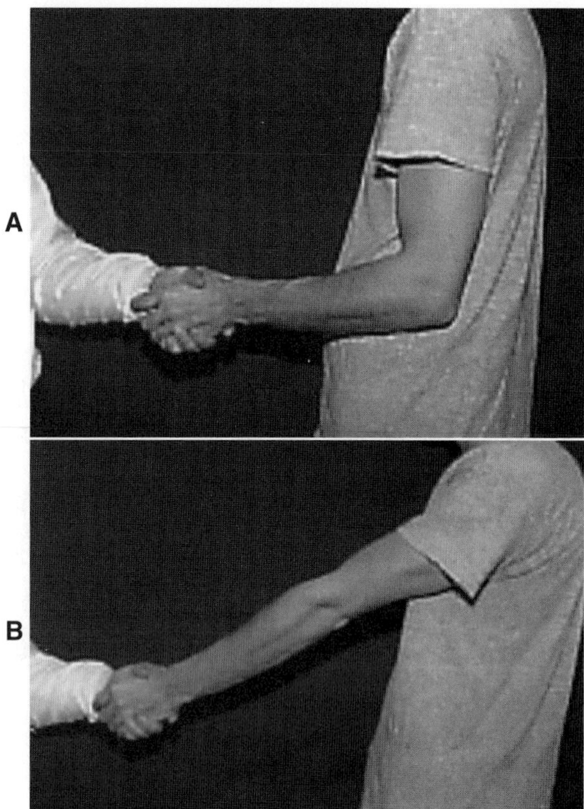

Fig. 9-12 ■ From Mackin EJ, Callahan AD, Skirven TM, et al: *Rehabilitation of the hand and upper extremity*, ed 5, St Louis, 2002, Mosby.

37. Mr. X underwent an anterior transposition of the ulnar nerve to surgically treat cubital tunnel. Mr. X was referred to you at postoperative day 4 with orders to evaluate and treat. However, the patient's treatment was delayed until 3 weeks after surgery due to no insurance authorization until that time. Evaluation reveals the following:

- **Active range of motion (AROM): 50 degrees less full elbow extension**
- **AROM: 130 degrees elbow flexion**
- **Limited finger motion**
- **Hypersensitive scar**
- **Intermittent paresthesias in the little finger**
- **Moderate edema**

What should your treatment plan be comprised of?

A. Compressive wraps around the elbow, aggressive stretching, thermal agents, desensitization techniques

B. Compressive wraps around the elbow, thermal agents, contract-relax exercises of the elbow, aggressive stretching

C. Contract-relax elbow exercises, desensitization, soft tissue massage, manual edema mobilization (MEM), stretching, splinting for protection, return to work education

D. Desensitization techniques, soft tissue massage, MEM, nerve gliding, stretching the elbow, contract-relax exercises of the elbow, edema glove

Initiation of AROM after cubital tunnel release varies greatly within the literature and in therapy clinics. In general, therapy is determined by the surgeon, therapist, and the surgical procedure.

In this example Mr. X underwent an anterior transposition of the ulnar nerve. Beginning AROM within 5 to 10 days postoperatively is not unusual for this procedure. Mr. X is about 3 weeks after surgery with significant elbow AROM limitations; therefore you want to begin stretching—but not aggressively, because of his neurological hypersensitivity. Protective splinting is not indicated at this point and may be discontinued. Compressive wraps around the elbow are *not* indicated because Mr. X's nerve is hypersensitive, and this technique can aggravate the neuritis. However, an edema glove is recommended to help control edema in the hand. MEM can be initiated to control edema; therefore teaching self-MEM is recommended. You may also use thermal agents if edema does not increase. Additionally, contract-relax elbow exercises will be beneficial to help regain elbow flexion and extension. Stretching the elbow is also initiated with good clinical observation to ensure that edema and/or neurological symptoms do not increase. Nerve mobilization can be initiated to glide the ulnar nerve. Desensitization techniques should also be instructed for the patient's home program. In summary, initial goals with Mr. X are the following: regain AROM of the elbow, decrease edema, regain full fist, and control neurological symptoms.

Answer: **D**

Skirven, Callahan in Mackin, Callahan, Skirven, et al, p. 614
Omer in Mackin, Callahan, Skirven, et al, p. 676
Blackmore in Mackin, Callahan, Skirven, et al, pp. 679-689
Walsh in Mackin, Callahan, Skirven, et al, pp. 766-769

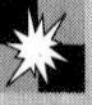

CLINICAL GEM:
Neurologic symptoms (paresthesias) typically diminish over time following surgery. It is not unusual for this process to take up to 12 months or longer. Also note that axonal regeneration will increase discomfort or even pain because pain fibers regenerate fastest. You can give your patient a soft elbow pad to help control the discomfort.

38. Mrs. G, a 42-year-old woman, is referred 6 months status post radial head fracture. She presents with a stiff elbow that is rendering ADLs difficult, if not impossible. Evaluation reveals that the patient can use a keyboard and clean countertops. The patient is slow and awkward with donning and doffing socks, tying shoes, and opening and closing doors. She is unable to wash her face, carry a plate, receive objects in her hand, brush her teeth, or perform pericare. What motion is Mrs. G primarily unable to achieve?

A. Elbow flexion
B. Forearm pronation
C. Forearm supination
D. Elbow extension

Although Mrs. G is having difficulty with all planes of motion, her ADL status is most limited with tasks requiring supination. The following shows the relationship to functional tasks and elbow position:

Forearm supination	Receive objects in palm, carry plates, wash face, high buttoning/fastening, shave, pericare, turning pages
Forearm pronation	Use keyboard/mouse, write, cut food, wipe countertops, pour from a pitcher
Elbow flexion	Fasten top neck button, put objects to mouth, shave, wash face, brush hair, place phone to ear, brush teeth
Elbow extension	Don/doff socks, tie shoes, put arm into coat/blouse sleeve, open/close doors, rise from a chair, reach for a coffee mug or an object on a table

Your plan of care may incorporate static progressive forearm supination splinting such as with the Joint Active Systems (JAS) supination/pronation splint (Fig. 9-13). You want to focus on regaining elbow range of motion—primarily in extension and forearm supination—to restore functional ADLs.

Answer: **C**
Griffith in Mackin, Callahan, Skirven, et al, pp. 1245-1261

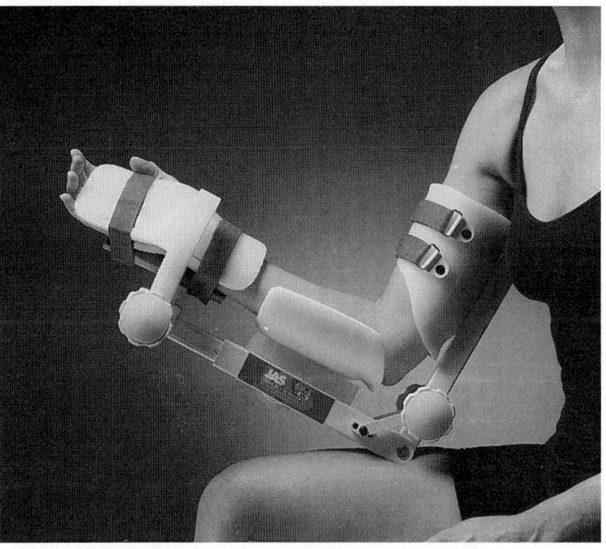

Fig. 9-13 ■ Permission granted from Joint Active Systems (JAS), Effingham, IL.

39. A 38-year-old man sustained extensive third-degree burns over both arms and legs and an open fracture of the tibia. He is unconscious as a result of a fiery motorcycle accident. Three weeks later, he is still comatose but is now physiologically stable. Therapy for his elbows should consist of which of the following?

A. Active assisted motion
B. An aggressive passive range of motion program to minimize contractures
C. Splinting in 30 degrees of flexion to minimize soft-tissue tension on the posterior side
D. Splinting in 90 degrees of flexion to minimize soft-tissue tension on the flexion side
E. Continuous splinting to minimize heterotopic ossification

Burn injuries result in soft-tissue contractures with permanent loss of extension. This is particularly common about the elbow and should be aggressively treated by preventative measures. Although active assisted exercises would be ideal, in a comatose patient this is not a choice, and an aggressive program of passive motion should be undertaken.

Answer: **B**
Cooney, pp. 433-451

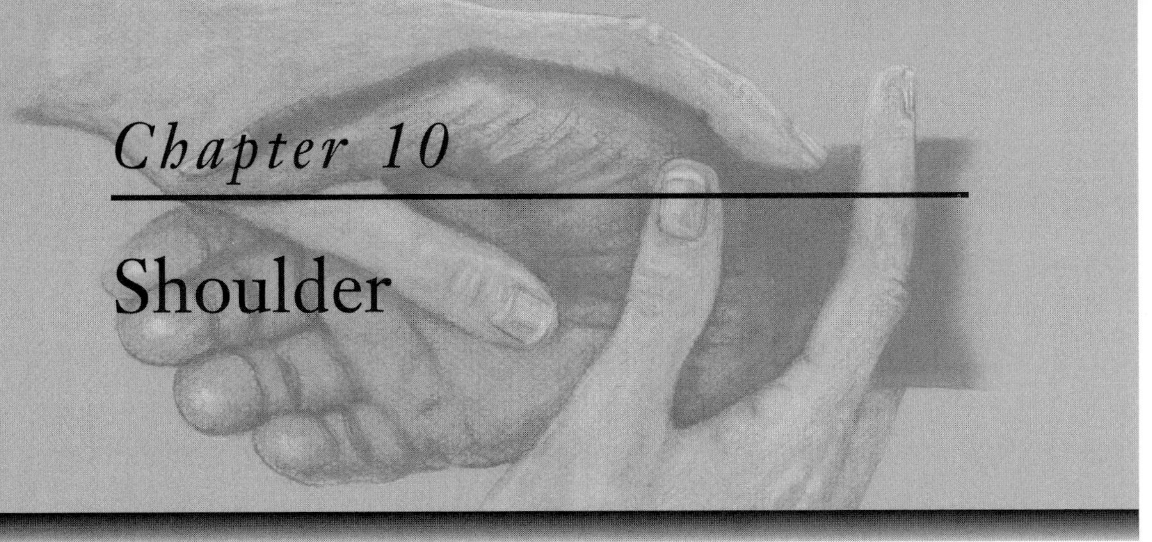

Chapter 10

Shoulder

1. The rotator interval is a potentially pathologic space between which two structures?

A. Teres minor, infraspinatus
B. Supraspinatus, subscapularis
C. Deltoid, pectoralis major
D. Supraspinatus, infraspinatus

The rotator interval is an anatomical space that is variably sized between the supraspinatus and subscapularis. Injury to the rotator interval can result in posteroinferior instability.

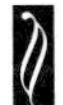

Answer: **B**

Fu, Ticker, Imhoff, p. 12
DeLee, Drez, Miller, pp. 847, 1067
Refer to Fig. 10-1

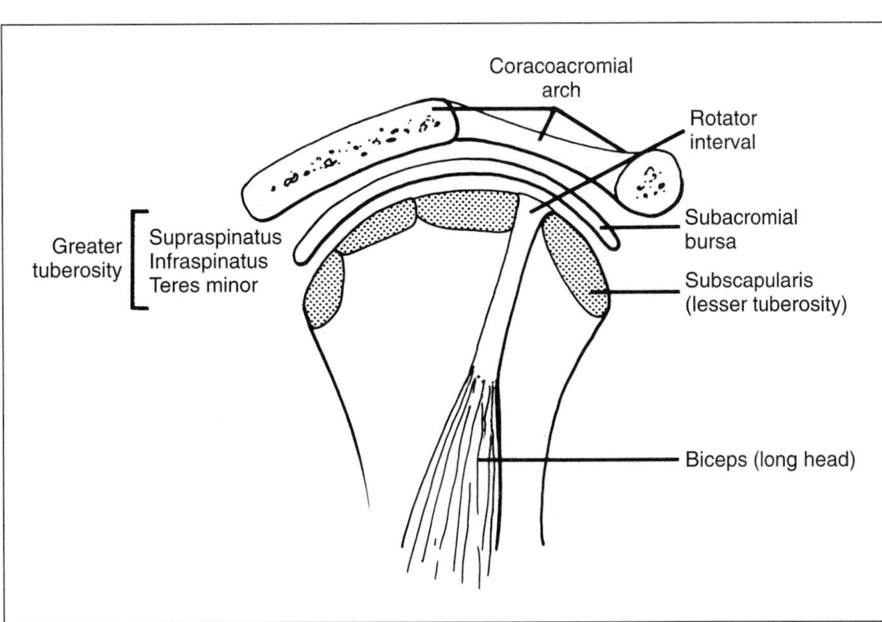

Fig. 10-1 ■ From DeLee JC, Drez D, Miller MD: *DeLee & Drez's Orthopaedic sports medicine*, ed 2, Philadelphia, 2003, Saunders.

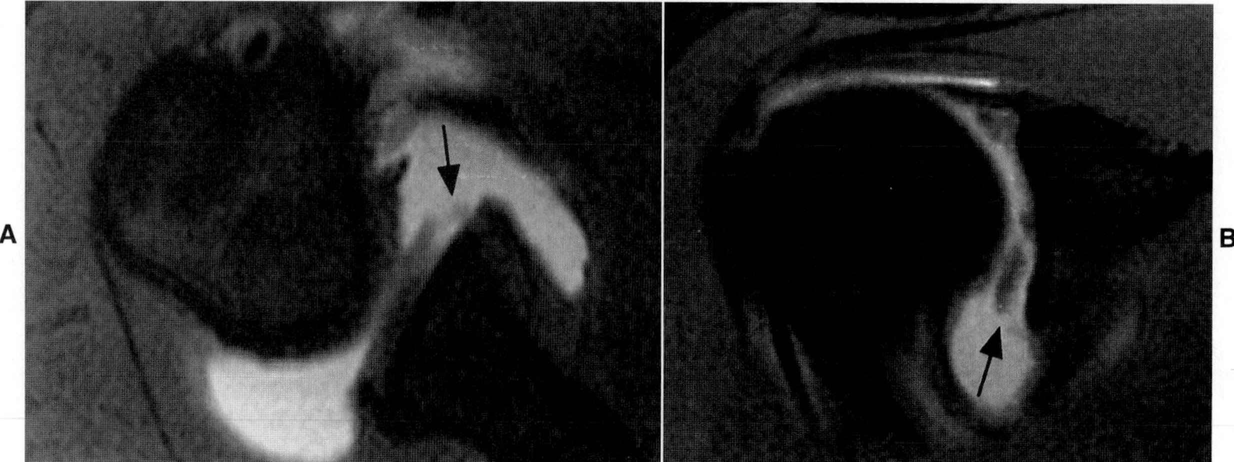

Fig. 10-2 ■ Bankart lesion, magnetic resonance arthrography. Axial **(A)** and oblique coronal **(B)** T_1-weighted images with fat saturation after intra-administration of gadolinium demonstrate disruption of the anteroinferior labrum (*arrows*). The gadolinium distends the joint capsule and the torn and irregular-appearing labrum.

2. Repair of a Bankart lesion involves reattachment of what structures?

A. Deltoid to acromion
B. Anteroinferior labrum to subscapularis
C. Anteroinferior labrum to glenoid
D. Pectoralis to humerus

The anteroinferior labrum is reattached to the glenoid rim in a Bankart repair.

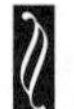

Answer: **C**
Fu, Ticker, Imhoff, p. 71
Refer to Fig. 10-2

3. The scapula "wings" when which muscle is paralyzed or weakened?

A. Subscapularis
B. Serratus anterior
C. Rhomboid major
D. Serratus posterior

During normal scapulohumeral rhythm, the serratus anterior holds the scapula in place as it slides over the rib cage. Winging of the scapula occurs when the serratus anterior muscle becomes weak from an injury to the long thoracic nerve. The muscle originates from ribs 1 through 9 and inserts along the medial border of the scapula.

Answer: **B**
Norris, p. 277
Rockwood, Matsen, pp. 56-57
Greenfield, Syen, pp. 201-207
Refer to Fig. 10-3

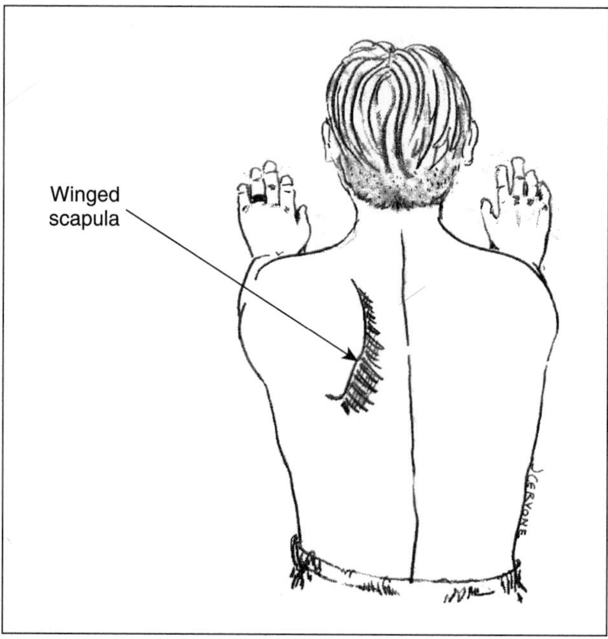

Fig. 10-3 ■ As a pushup is performed, "winging" of the scapula is evident.

4. Two prime retractors of the scapula are the rhomboid major and the rhomboid minor. Name the nerve that innervates these muscles.

A. Thoracodorsal nerve
B. Long thoracic nerve
C. Subscapular nerve
D. Dorsal subscapular nerve

The dorsal scapular nerve is derived from C4 and C5 nerve roots and innervates the rhomboid major, rhomboid minor, and levator scapulae.

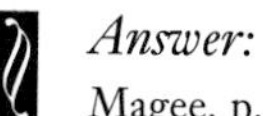

Answer: **D**
Magee, p. 104

5. Match each muscle with the nerve that supplies it.

Muscle

1. Serratus anterior
2. Rhomboid major
3. Latissimus dorsi
4. Trapezius (upper fibers)

Nerve

A. Dorsal scapular
B. Thoracodorsal
C. Accessory
D. Long thoracic

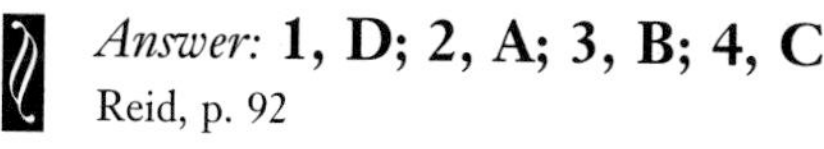

Answer: **1, D; 2, A; 3, B; 4, C**
Reid, p. 92

6. Which test would be appropriate to use when evaluating a patient with suspected anterior shoulder instability?

A. Drop-arm test
B. Apprehension test (crank test)
C. O'Brien's clinical test
D. Empty can test

Anterior and posterior instability are best tested in the supine position with the arm and shoulder on the border of the table. The arm and shoulder are externally rotated. The apprehension test is positive if the patient displays anxiety and muscle defense against the external rotation (Fig. 10-4). This response usually indicates anterior instability.

The other tests listed are used to assess specific shoulder pathologies, such as the rotator cuff (drop-arm and empty can tests) and superior labrum anterior-to-posterior (SLAP) lesions (O'Brien's clinical test).

Answer: **B**
Magee, p. 203
Cailliet, p. 76
Delee, Drez, Miller, pp. 1027, 1055

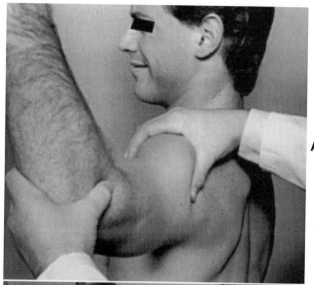

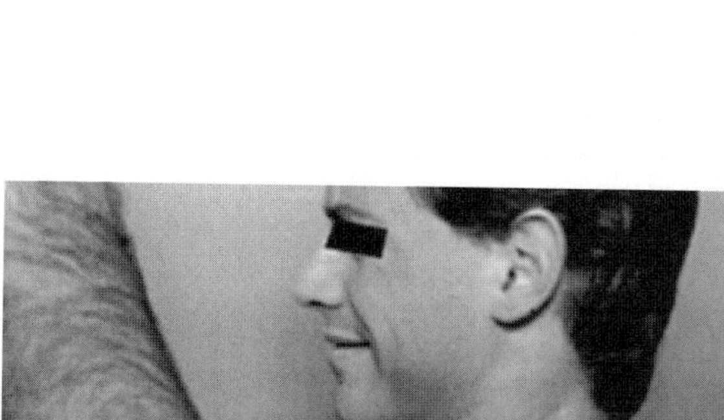

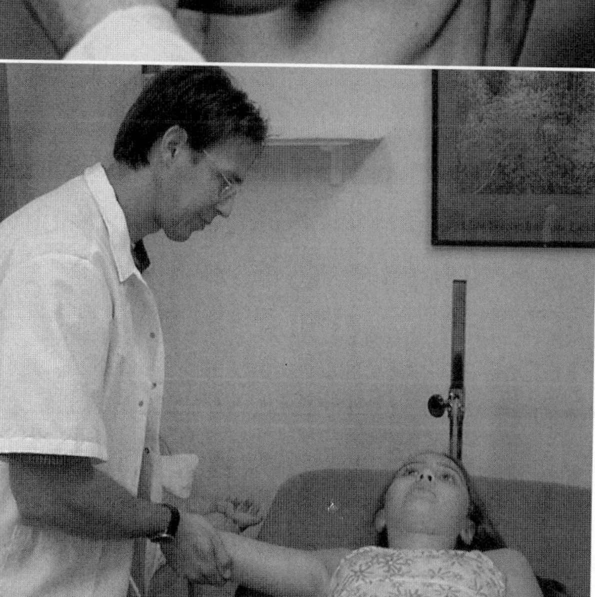

Fig. 10-4 ■ **A,** Apprehension test—sitting (crank test). The examiner's right thumb is applying anterior leverage as the patient's arm is abducted and externally rotated. The examiner's index and middle fingers are positioned on the anterior aspect of the shoulder to protect against any sudden dislocation. **B,** Apprehension test (supine). The patient is positioned with the scapula supported by the edge of the examination table. The patient's arm is positioned in abduction and external rotation. This position elicits a feeling of impending anterior instability, resulting in apprehension by the patient. (**A** From Rockwood CA, Jr, Matsen FA: *The shoulder,* ed 2, Philadelphia, 1998, WB Saunders.)

10 SHOULDER

7. The nerve most commonly injured in fractures around the proximal humerus is which of the following?

A. Musculocutaneous nerve
B. Radial nerve
C. Axillary nerve
D. Suprascapular nerve

The axillary nerve exits the axilla from the brachial plexus and wraps around the posterior aspect of the surgical neck of the humerus, thus innervating the deltoid and teres minor muscles. This nerve is susceptible to trauma from fractures to the proximal humerus.

Answer: **C**
Donatelli, p. 202
Basti, Dionysian, Sherman, pp. 111-112
Refer to Fig. 10-5

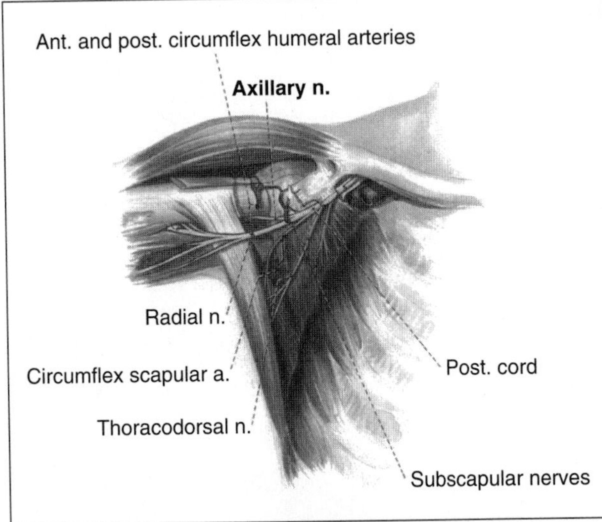

Fig. 10-5 ■ From Mackin EJ, Callahan AD, Skirven TM, et al: *Rehabilitation of the hand and upper extremity,* ed 5, vol 1, St Louis, 2002, Mosby.

8. True or False: The coracoclavicular ligament is the only noncontractile structure suspending the scapula from the clavicle.

The coracoclavicular ligament is the only noncontractile structure that suspends the scapula from the clavicle. The major support of the acromioclavicular (AC) joint is the coracoclavicular ligament. It comprises two parts—the conoid and the trapezoid ligaments—and connects the clavicle and coronoid process. The two parts are oriented differently and resist different forces placed on the scapula and clavicle.

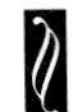
Answer: **True**
Pratt, pp. 66-67
Refer to Fig. 10-6

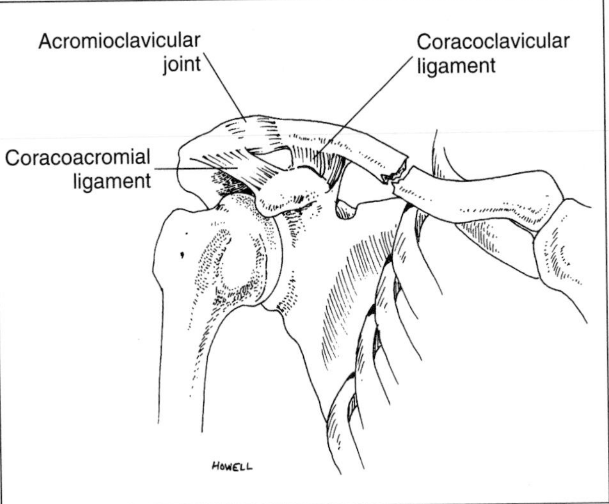

Fig. 10-6 ■ From Hawkins RJ, Bell SB: *Atlas of shoulder surgery,* St Louis, 1996, Mosby.

9. A primary extensor of the shoulder is which of the following?

A. Teres minor
B. Long head of the triceps
C. Latissimus dorsi
D. Trapezius

Primary extensors of the shoulder include the posterior portion of the deltoid, the teres major, and the latissimus dorsi. The teres minor and the long head of the triceps are secondary extensors.

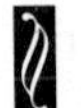
Answer: **C**
Hoppenfeld, p. 26

10. True or False: The three structures that make up the coracoacromial arch are the acromion, the coracoacromial ligament, and the coracoid process.

The coracoacromial arch comprises the acromion, the coracoacromial ligament, and the coracoid process. The arch is anatomically above the rotator cuff. Compression of the rotator cuff, especially the supraspinatus tendon, is believed to lead to rotator cuff degeneration and possibly even biceps tendon rupture. This is because of supraspinatus compression between the humeral head below and the coracoacromial arch above (see Fig. 10-6).

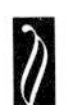

Answer: **True**
Flatow, pp. 20-21

11. True or False: In normal shoulder biomechanics, both the deltoid and the rotator cuff allow elevation of the humerus to occur.

Elevation of the shoulder occurs because of the combined actions of the rotator cuff muscles and the deltoid muscle acting as a "force-couple." As abduction occurs, the action of the deltoid causes the humerus to move into the glenoid fossa. At the end range of motion, the deltoid causes the head of the humerus to translate downward, out of the glenoid cavity. This action is counteracted by the group of muscles known as the *rotator cuff.* The rotator cuff acts to stabilize the humerus in the glenoid fossa.

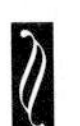

Answer: **True**
Loth, Wadsworth, p. 395

12. What is the difference between a mini-open rotator cuff repair and a standard open rotator cuff repair?

A. A mini repair is used on a smaller tear.
B. Standard rotator cuff repair uses bone tunnels for reattachment.
C. Mini repair involves deltoid split, not detachment.
D. Mini repair is used in smaller patients.

A mini-open rotator cuff repair (Fig. 10-7) involves splitting, not detaching the deltoid. Rehabilitation is more rapid because the deltoid does not need to be protected during postoperative therapy.

Answer: **C**
Fu, Ticker, Imhoff, p. 124

13. What happens to the coracoacromial ligament during subacromial decompression?

A. Nothing
B. It is lengthened.
C. It is detached from the coracoid.
D. It is detached from the acromion.

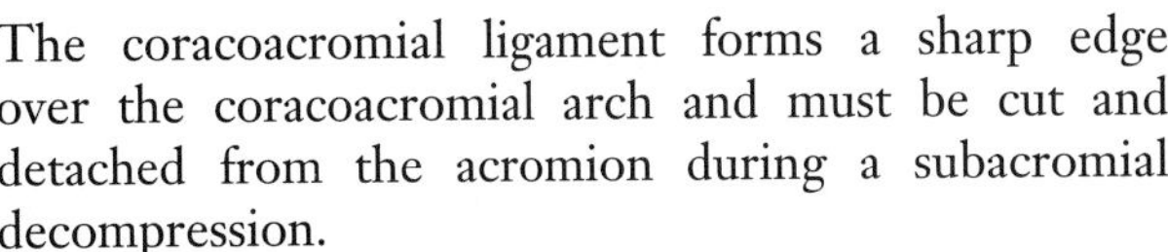

The coracoacromial ligament forms a sharp edge over the coracoacromial arch and must be cut and detached from the acromion during a subacromial decompression.

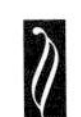

Answer: **D**
Fu, Ticker, Imhoff, p. 155
Refer to Fig. 10-6

14. Match each muscle to the correct innervation.

Muscle

1. Coracobrachialis
2. Subscapularis
3. Levator scapulae
4. Subclavius
5. Latissimus dorsi

Innervation

A. Subscapular nerve
B. Thoracodorsal nerve
C. Musculocutaneous nerve
D. Fifth and sixth cervical nerves
E. Dorsal scapular nerve

Answer: **1, C; 2, A; 3, E; 4, D; 5, B**
Sieg, Adams, pp. 27, 30, 34, 36

15. True or False: When shoulder abduction is measured in the sitting position, the fulcrum of the goniometer is placed over the lateral aspect of the glenohumeral joint.

When shoulder abduction is measured in the sitting position, the fulcrum of the goniometer is placed over the posterior aspect of the acromion process. The proximal stationary arm is aligned parallel to the vertebral body spinous processes. The distal moveable arm is aligned along the lateral midline of the humerus.

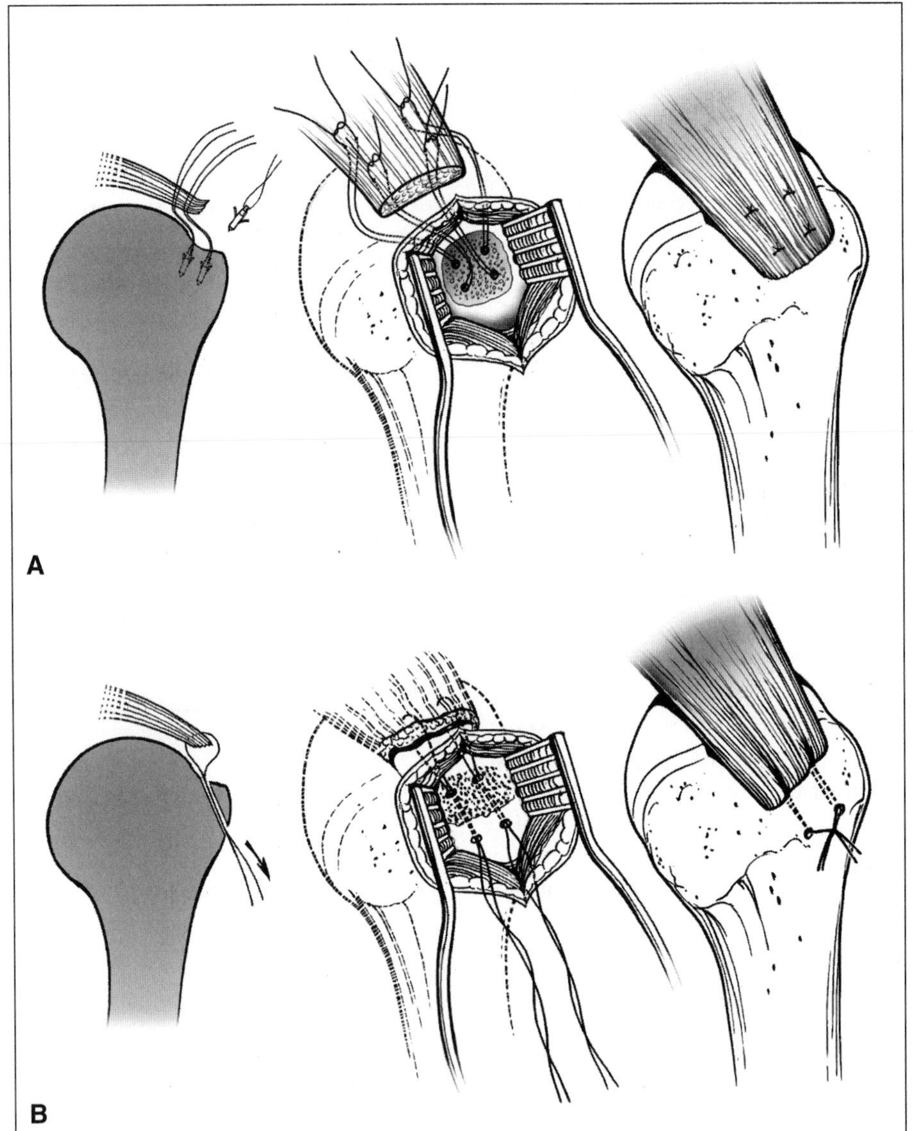

Fig. 10-7 ■ Schematic drawing of **(A)** suture anchor placement and fixation and **(B)** suture tunnel placement and fixation for rotator cuff tear repair with the so-called "mini-open" technique. From Rockwood CA, Jr, Matsen FA: *The shoulder*, ed 2, Philadelphia, 1998, WB Saunders.

Answer: **False**
Norkin, White, p. 61

16. Which of the following muscles comprise the rotator cuff?

A. Supraspinatus, teres minor, teres major, infraspinatus
B. Teres minor, subscapularis, posterior deltoid, infraspinatus
C. Supraspinatus, infraspinatus, teres minor, subscapularis
D. Supraspinatus, teres major, infraspinatus, subscapularis

The four muscles in answer C originate on the scapula and become tendons that fuse with the capsule of the shoulder, thus forming a musculotendinous cuff, which is termed the *rotator cuff.*

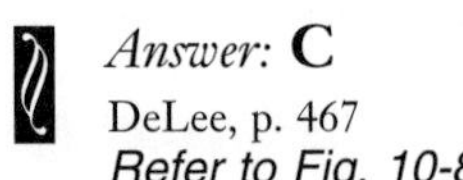

Answer: **C**
DeLee, p. 467
Refer to Fig. 10-8

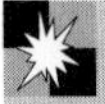

CLINICAL GEM:
One way to remember the muscles of the rotator cuff is to recall that SITS stands for **S**upraspinatus, **I**nfraspinatus, **T**eres minor, and **S**ubscapularis.

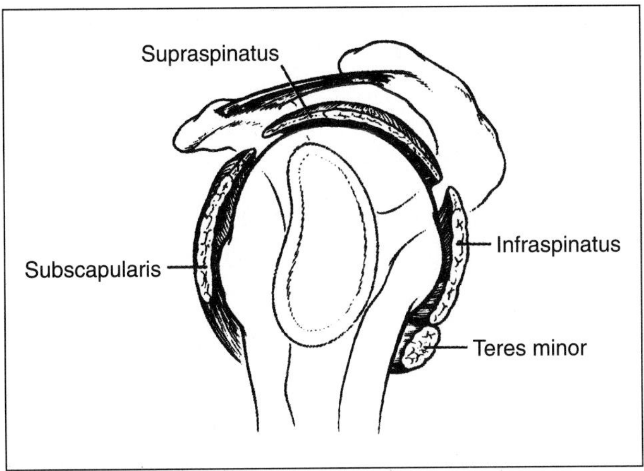

Fig. 10-8 ■ From Rockwood CA, Jr, Matsen FA: *The shoulder*, Philadelphia, 1990, WB Saunders.

17. Which muscle is *not* a horizontal abductor of the shoulder?

A. Infraspinatus
B. Posterior deltoid
C. Teres major
D. Teres minor

The teres major is an internal rotator of the shoulder at 90 degrees of shoulder abduction; it is not a horizontal abductor of the shoulder. It is innervated by the subscapular nerve derived from C_6-C_7.

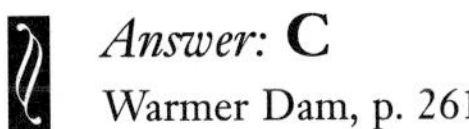

Answer: **C**
Warmer Dam, p. 261

18. True or False: The function of the coracobrachialis muscle is to assist flexion and adduction of the glenohumeral joint.

The coracobrachialis has a flesh and tendinous origin from the coracoid process and distally to the midportion of the humerus. It inserts into the anteromedial surface midhumerus and is bound laterally by the common origin with the biceps. It is innervated by a branch from the lateral cord and the musculocutaneous nerve. Its function or action is flexion and adduction of the glenohumeral joint.

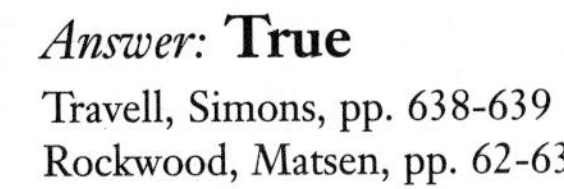

Answer: **True**
Travell, Simons, pp. 638-639
Rockwood, Matsen, pp. 62-63

19. Which of the following is not a suitable treatment technique for thoracic outlet syndrome (TOS)?

A. Strengthening the trapezius, rhomboids, and levator scapulae
B. Strengthening the pectoralis major, pectoralis minor, and subscapularis
C. Postural reeducation
D. Biofeedback

Conservative treatment for TOS consists of modifying aggravating factors (e.g., avoiding overhead activities). Important aspects of rehabilitation for a patient with TOS include strengthening the shoulder girdle and postural reeducation. The muscles to be strengthened include the trapezius, the rhomboids, and the levator scapulae. Other treatments include antiinflammatory medications, ultrasound, transcutaneous electrical nerve stimulation, and biofeedback. Strengthening the pectoralis major, the pectoralis minor, and the subscapularis would cause increased impingement; therefore it is best to stretch these structures.

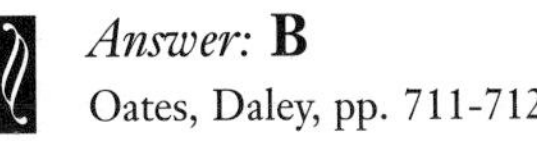

Answer: **B**
Oates, Daley, pp. 711-712

CLINICAL GEM:
If a patient has an arterial obstruction, he or she will report symptoms of coolness, cold sensitivity, numbness in the hand, and exertional fatigue. These symptoms indicate compression at the pectoralis minor loop. If a patient has a venous obstruction, he or she will report symptoms of cyanotic discoloration, arm edema, finger stiffness, and a feeling of heaviness. These symptoms indicate a compression at the first rib.

20. True or False: Rotator cuff pathology almost always occurs with a supraspinatus component.

Because of the rotator cuff's insertion on the greater tuberosity of the humerus, the supraspinatus has a "critical zone" that is prone to calcium deposits and potential rupture. There is constant pressure from the head of the humerus and impingement against the coracoacromial arch during normal joint movements (see Fig. 1-17).

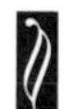
Answer: **True**
Marks, Warner, Irrgang, pp. 91-93

21. During glenohumeral arthroplasty, which is the only muscle transected, then repaired upon closure?

A. Subscapularis
B. Deltoid
C. Supraspinatus
D. Pectoralis major

The subscapularis is sectioned about 1 cm medial to its insertion. It is reattached upon closure and therefore must be protected during postoperative rehabilitation.

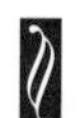
Answer: **A**
Fu, Ticker, Imhoff, p. 196

22. What is the ideal glenohumeral angular position for shoulder arthrodesis (fusion)?

A. Abduction, 30 degrees; flexion, 30 degrees; internal rotation, 30 degrees
B. Abduction, 75 degrees; flexion, 0 degrees; internal rotation, 0 degrees
C. Abduction, 0 degrees; flexion, 45 degrees; internal rotation, 45 degrees
D. Abduction, 30 degrees; flexion, 90 degrees; internal rotation, 0 degrees

The 30 degrees abduction, 30 degrees flexion, and 30 degrees internal rotation position is considered ideal in most instances. In certain situations, depending on the occupation, this position can vary.

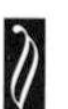
Answer: **A**
Fu, Ticker, Imhoff, p. 216

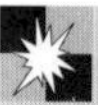
CLINICAL GEM:
Rowe looked at arthrodesis of the shoulder in the adult and recommends the following position: abduction, 20 degrees; flexion, 30 degrees; internal rotation, 40 degrees.

Rockwood, Matsen, p. 881

23. What combination of nerves would have to be damaged to inhibit abduction of the shoulder?

A. Musculocutaneous and upper and lower subscapularis
B. Axillary and suprascapular
C. Suprascapular and long thoracic
D. Axillary and upper and lower subscapular

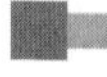

The suprascapular nerve supplies the supraspinatus muscle, which is responsible for abduction initiation. The axillary nerve innervates the deltoid, whose middle portion is a primary abductor. Injuries to both of these nerves inhibit abduction of the shoulder.

Answer: **B**
Hoppenfeld, p. 27
Pratt, p. 73

24. Which of the following actions occurs when the infraspinatus, subscapularis, and teres minor all contract at the same time?

A. Internal rotation
B. Flexion
C. External rotation
D. Depression of the humeral head in the glenoid fossa

The rotator cuff functions to approximate the humeral head to the glenoid fossa. The supraspinatus assists the deltoid in abduction, and the subscapularis, infraspinatus, and teres minor depress the humeral head during elevation of the arm.

Answer: **D**
Marks, Warner, Irrgang, p. 90

25. True or False: The connection of the subscapularis to the humerus is the most anterior attachment of the four muscles that form the rotator cuff.

The subscapularis muscle arises from the subscapular fossa and inserts by a broad tendinous attachment into the lesser tuberosity of the humerus. It is the most anterior portion of the musculotendinous rotator cuff. The other muscles that form the rotator cuff are the supraspinatus, infraspinatus, and teres minor muscles.

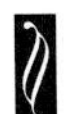

Answer: **True**

Travell, Simons, p. 596
DeLee, Drez, Miller, p. 1125

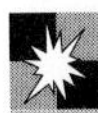

CLINICAL GEM:
Isolated tears of the subscapularis are very rare. Partial ruptures have been documented in association with anterior dislocation of the glenohumeral joint. Subscapularis tendon avulsions are associated with avulsion fractures of the lesser tuberosity.

DeLee, Drez, Miller, p. 1025

26. True or False: The rotator cuff is a vital component of the shoulder in terms of precision and propulsion of the upper limb during throwing activities.

The shoulder is a ball-and-socket joint that connects the axial trunk to the upper extremity. The glenohumeral joint is the most mobile joint in the body. This mobility lends to precise positioning of the hand in space. The shoulder acts as a fulcrum for the lever arm of the upper limb and is important in propulsive action. The rotator cuff is a vital component of the shoulder in terms of precision and propulsion.

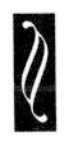

Answer: **True**

Travell, Simons, p. 564
DeLee, Drez, Miller, pp. 1066-1068
Rockwood, Matsen, pp. 58-59

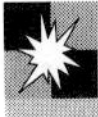

CLINICAL GEM:
The biceps is intimately associated with the rotator cuff and has been called the "fifth" tendon of the cuff.

27. Match each nerve with the muscle that it innervates.

Muscle

1. Anconeus
2. Serratus anterior
3. Teres major
4. Supraspinatus

Nerve

A. Long thoracic nerve
B. Subscapular nerve
C. Radial nerve
D. Suprascapular nerve

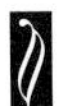

Answer: **1, C; 2, A; 3, B; 4, D**

Magee, p. 177

28. Of the three types of acromion shapes, which two are most often associated with rotator cuff tears?

A. Types one and two
B. Types one and three
C. Types two and three
D. None of the above

There are three types of acromion shapes: type one is flat and has been found in approximately 17% of the population (Fig. 10-9, *A*); type two is curved and has been found in approximately 43% of the population (Fig. 10-9, *B*); and type three is hooked and is believed to be found in approximately 39% of the population (Fig. 10-9, *C*). Types two and three are more often associated with rotator cuff tears because the impingement caused by the anterior curving or hooking leads to degeneration and tearing of the rotator cuff.

Answer: **C**

Flatow, p. 21

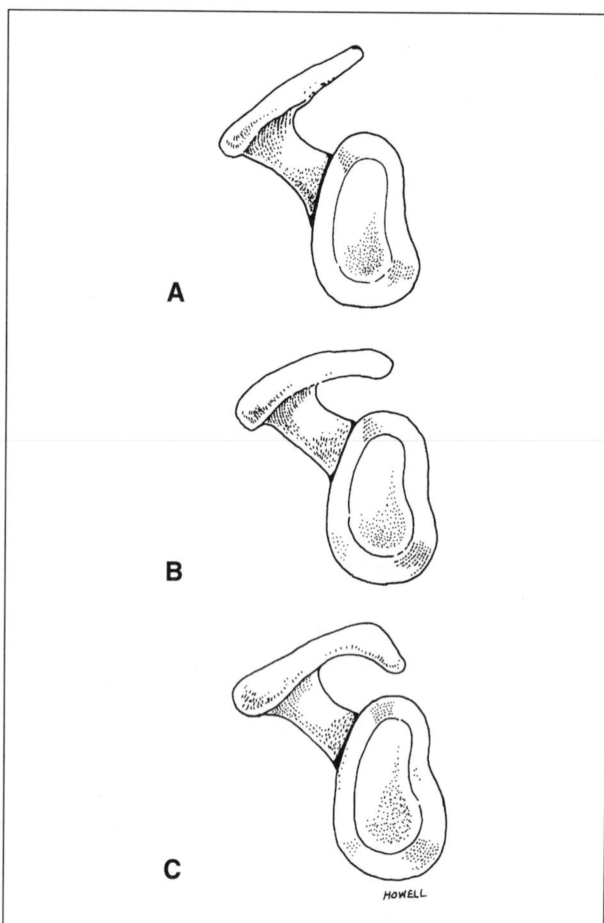

Fig. 10-9 ■ **A** to **C** from Hawkins RJ, Bell RH, Lippitt SB: *Atlas of shoulder surgery,* St Louis, 1996, Mosby.

29. A positive clunk test would indicate which of the following?

A. Rotator cuff tear
B. Labral tear
C. Impingement
D. Frozen shoulder

The clunk test is performed by rotating (internally and externally) the flexed shoulder with the elbow extended. A feeling of a clunk in the joint is believed to indicate that a labral fragment has been caught in the glenohumeral joint.

Answer: **B**
Flatow, p. 45

30. True or False: Generally, postsurgical shoulder rehabilitation can be divided into the following three phases:

Phase I: Passive or assisted exercises to maintain or gain motion
Phase II: Active range of motion
Phase III: Resistive exercises to gain strength

Progression among phases is a balancing act that depends on tissue healing status; therefore timing among phases is crucial. For example, if strict immobilization is required in Phase I to promote tissue healing, active motion (Phase II) commonly is delayed for 6 to 8 weeks, depending on the rate of healing of violated tissues. Resistive exercise (Phase III) is initiated several weeks after Phase II begins.

Answer: **True**
Hawkins, Bell, Lippitt, pp. 309-310

31. Which clinical test can help differentiate cervical pain from primary shoulder pain?

A. Lift-off test
B. Hawkins impingement test
C. Subacromial injection test
D. Spurling's test

A subacromial injection with analgesic and corticosteroid medication can help differentiate pain etiology. Both cervical (referred neural pain) and primary shoulder pain can be located along the deltoid region. Relief of pain with a subacromial injection confirms shoulder pathology as the source of pain. Cervical pain will not be relieved by a subacromial injection.

Answer: **C**
DeLee, Drez, Miller, pp. 1076-1078

32. What is a Hill-Sachs lesion?

A. A complex labral tear
B. An avulsion of the subscapularis
C. A fracture of the glenoid
D. An impaction fracture of the proximal humerus

A Hill-Sachs fracture is an impaction fracture of the humeral head sustained during a glenohumeral dislocation. When large, it may need bone grafting to prevent redislocation.

Answer: **D**
Norris, p. 59
DeLee, Drez, Miller, pp. 613, 900-903
Refer to Fig. 10-10

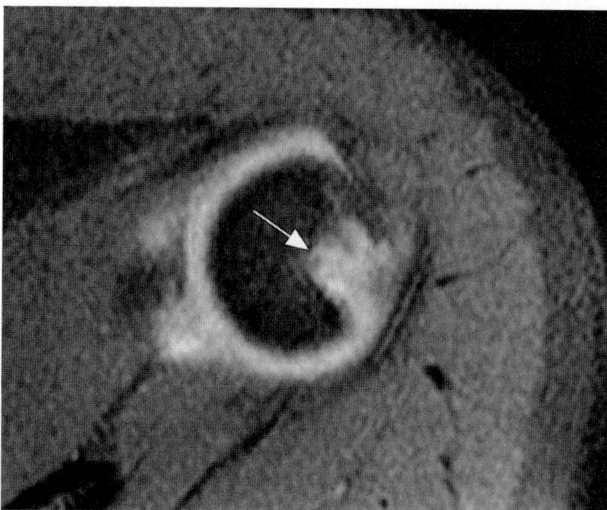

Fig. 10-10 ■ Hill-Sachs defect, magnetic resonance arthrography. Axial T_1-weighted image through the superior aspect of the glenohumeral joint demonstrates a concavity (*arrow*) in the posterosuperior aspect of the humeral head representing a Hill-Sachs deformity, secondary to previous anterior dislocation. (From DeLee JC, Drez D, Miller MD: *DeLee & Drez's Orthopaedic sports medicine: principles and practice*, ed 2, Philadelphia, 2003, Saunders.)

33. Impingement syndrome at the shoulder may be caused by which of the following?

A. Decreased suboccipital space
B. Weakness in the rotator cuff
C. Weakness of deltoid musculature
D. A and B
E. A and C

Weakness of the rotator cuff can cause instability when the deltoid overpowers the cuff muscles, thus allowing the humeral head to "ride up" during deltoid contraction and resulting in impingement. When abduction of the shoulder occurs, the tuberosity approximates the acromion and several structures may become pinched between the tuberosity and the coracoclavicular ligament. If there is repeated trauma, edema results, thus increasing soft tissue volume and decreasing the subacromial space, not the suboccipital space (see Fig. 1-17).

Answer: **B**
Norris, p. 282

34. Rehabilitation of a patient with shoulder impingement should focus primarily on which of the following?

A. Rotator cuff strengthening
B. Scapular rotator strengthening
C. Pectoralis strengthening
D. A and B

In the rehabilitation of a patient with a shoulder impingement problem, it is important to strengthen both the rotator cuff and the scapular rotators. Strengthening the rotator cuff allows for depression of the humeral head into the glenoid fossa and prevents excessive superior movement of the humeral head in shoulder elevation, thus helping to prevent impingement. Strengthening the scapular rotators ensures that the scapula will follow the humerus in shoulder elevation, thus providing proper scapulohumeral rhythm. If the scapulothoracic muscles are weak, abnormal posture of the scapulae exists. This can cause disruption of the normal scapulohumeral rhythm that occurs with arm elevation, thus leading to impingement of the rotator cuff as it passes under the coracoacromial arch. Strengthening of the pectoralis muscles is contraindicated because it can increase impingement; however, stretching of the pectoralis is beneficial in the treatment of impingement syndrome.

Answer: **D**
Brotzman, pp. 93-94

35. True or False: Postural correction exercises, including scapular strengthening, pectoral stretching, and external rotation of the shoulder, can be useful in reducing stage-one impingement of the rotator cuff tendons.

In 1972, when Neer first introduced the concept of rotator cuff impingement, he believed that the majority of rotator cuff lesions were a result of mechanical impingement of the rotator cuff tendons. This impingement is beneath the anteroinferior portions of the acromion, particularly when the shoulder is placed in forward elevation and internal rotation. Therefore if postural correction exercises, including scapular strengthening, pectoral stretching, and external rotation of the shoulder, are used, the impingement should lessen.

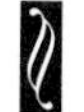
Answer: **True**
Pettrone, p. 143

36. True or False: After arthroscopic surgery for arthroscopic subacromial decompression (ASAD), range of motion exercises should be

delayed for 2 to 4 weeks and resistive exercises should not be attempted for 8 weeks.

After arthroscopic surgery for subacromial decompression, passive range of motion exercises are initiated immediately after surgery and are progressed to active exercise as soon as pain and motion will allow—typically in 4 to 5 days. Resistive exercises may be added at 3 to 4 weeks.

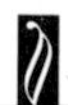
Answer: **False**
Hawkins, Bell, Lippitt, p. 284

37. The term for a tear of the superior labrum and biceps tendon from the glenoid is which of the following?

A. Bankart lesion
B. SLAP lesion
C. Labral tear
D. Rotator cuff tear

The term *SLAP lesion* denotes a tear of the superior labrum anterior to posterior. This area of the labrum also attaches the long head of the biceps tendon to the glenoid. This tear usually is diagnosed with magnetic resonance imaging (MRI), arthrography, or arthroscopy.

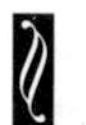
Answer: **B**
Snyder, Karzel, p. 49

38. After a SLAP lesion repair, which motion of the shoulder should be delayed?

A. Shoulder flexion beyond 90 degrees
B. Internal rotation beyond 30 degrees
C. External rotation beyond neutral
D. Shoulder extension
E. C and D

After sling immobilization for the first week, the patient can begin gentle active range of motion with restrictions. The patient should avoid external rotation of the shoulder beyond a neutral position and extension of the arm behind the body with the elbow extended for an additional 4 weeks to prevent stresses to the repaired structures. Patients generally are restricted from activities that place a significant stress on the biceps tendon until 3 to 4 months after surgery.

Answer: **E**
Pettrone, p. 124

39. A Bankart lesion usually results from which of the following?

A. An acromiohumeral impingement
B. A direct blow to the shoulder
C. An anterior dislocation of the shoulder
D. A posterior dislocation of the shoulder

A Bankart lesion results from an anterior dislocation of the shoulder usually results in an avulsion of the attachment of the anteroinferior glenohumeral ligament to the glenoid labrum from the anterior glenoid neck. The anteroinferior glenohumeral ligament is believed to be the key static stabilizer of any anterior dislocation of the shoulder.

Answer: **C**
Snyder, Karzel, p. 57

40. True or False: After a Bankart lesion repair of the shoulder, the earliest recommended time to begin external rotation beyond 0 degrees is 3 weeks.

After a Bankart repair, it is recommended that patients begin external rotation beyond 0 degrees at 6 weeks. Gentle Codman exercises begin at approximately 2 weeks, with a gradual progression of range of motion exercises. Gentle strengthening exercise is initiated at 6 weeks.

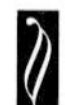
Answer: **False**
Snyder, Karzel, p. 57

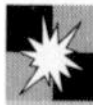
CLINICAL GEM:
Remember that protocol varies depending on the surgeon's preference and the tension on the repair site.

41. True or False: During the first 60 degrees of abduction of the shoulder, the glenohumeral motion is greater than the scapulothoracic motion, with a ratio of 2:1.

When we speak of motion between the scapula and thorax, the scapulothoracic articulation is an integral part of shoulder function. The scapula is mobile in many directions because it is supported by muscle attachments and limited ligament attachments. The relative motion between the scapulothoracic articulation and the glenohumeral joint during abduction is called the *scapulothoracic rhythm*. For the first 30 degrees (not 60 degrees) of abduction, glenohumeral motion is much greater than the scapulothoracic motion; the ratio of motion has been documented in the range of 2:1, 4:1, and up to 7:1. NOTE: the average glenohumeral-to-scapulothoracic motion has been accepted as a 2:1 ratio. After the first 30 degrees, both joints move about the same amount. Therefore when abduction is accomplished, the glenohumeral joint moves more than the scapulothoracic joint, with a noticeable difference at the beginning of abduction and minimal at the end of the motion.

Answer: **False**
DeLee, Drez, Miller, pp. 842-843
Refer to Fig. 10-11

42. A 15-year-old female competitive swimmer complains of diffuse shoulder pain. She notices the problem most when she does the backstroke. She reports that her shoulder sometimes feels unstable when doing this stroke. These symptoms are most likely related to which of the following?

A. Adhesive capsulitis
B. Posterior instability
C. Subacromial bursitis
D. Anterior subluxation

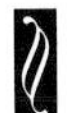

Swimming is a high-demand sport that requires a tremendous amount of repetition. A consistent pattern among swimmers involving shoulder pathologies exists. The major cause of shoulder pain in swimmers is repeated friction of the humeral head and the rotator cuff on the coracoacrominal arch during abduction of the shoulder, thus resulting in an impingement syndrome. The beginning of the pull-through phase of the swimming stroke produces the maximum amount of impingement (Fig. 10-12, *A*). However, during the backstroke, the stress is greatest on the anterior capsule during the pull-through phase (Fig. 10-12, *B*). It is not uncommon for the backstroke swimmer to stretch the capsule, which can result in an anterior subluxation.

Answer: **D**
DeLee, Drez, Miller, pp. 1136-1137
Magee, p. 241

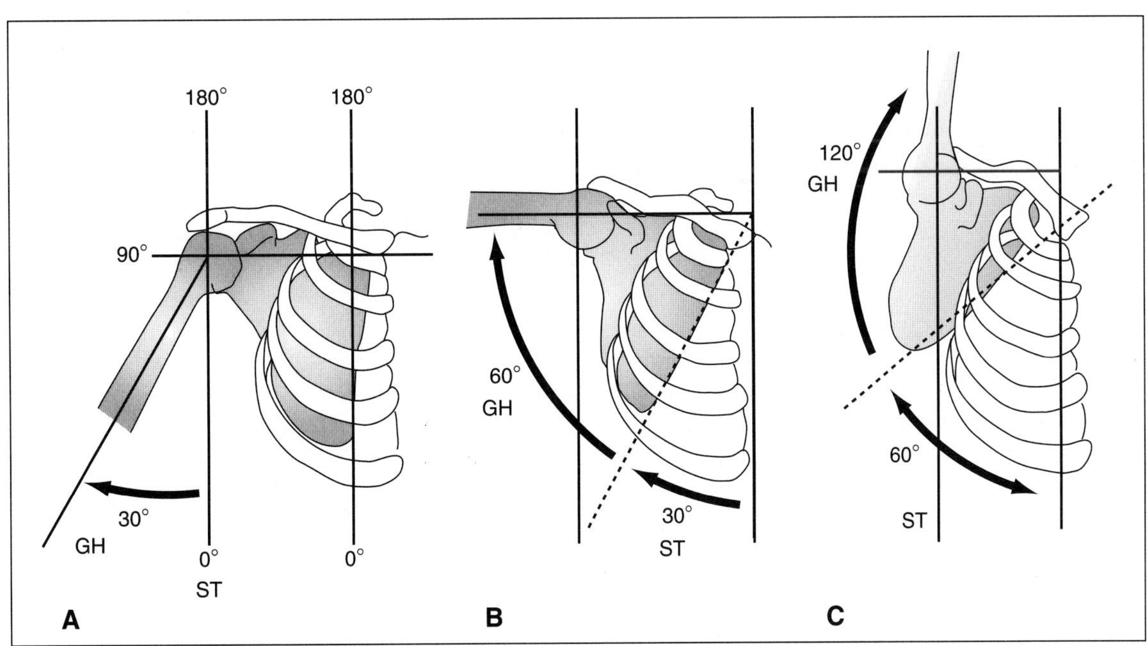

Fig. 10-11 ■ **A** to **C**, The average ratio of glenohumeral (*GH*) to scapulothoracic (*ST*) motion is approximately 2:1. For the first 30 degrees of abduction, it is all glenohumeral motion. In the last 60 degrees of elevation, there is an almost equal contribution between the glenohumeral and the scapulothoracic joints. (From DeLee JC, Drez D, Miller MD: *DeLee & Drez's Orthopaedic sports medicine*, ed 2, Philadelphia, 2003, Saunders.)

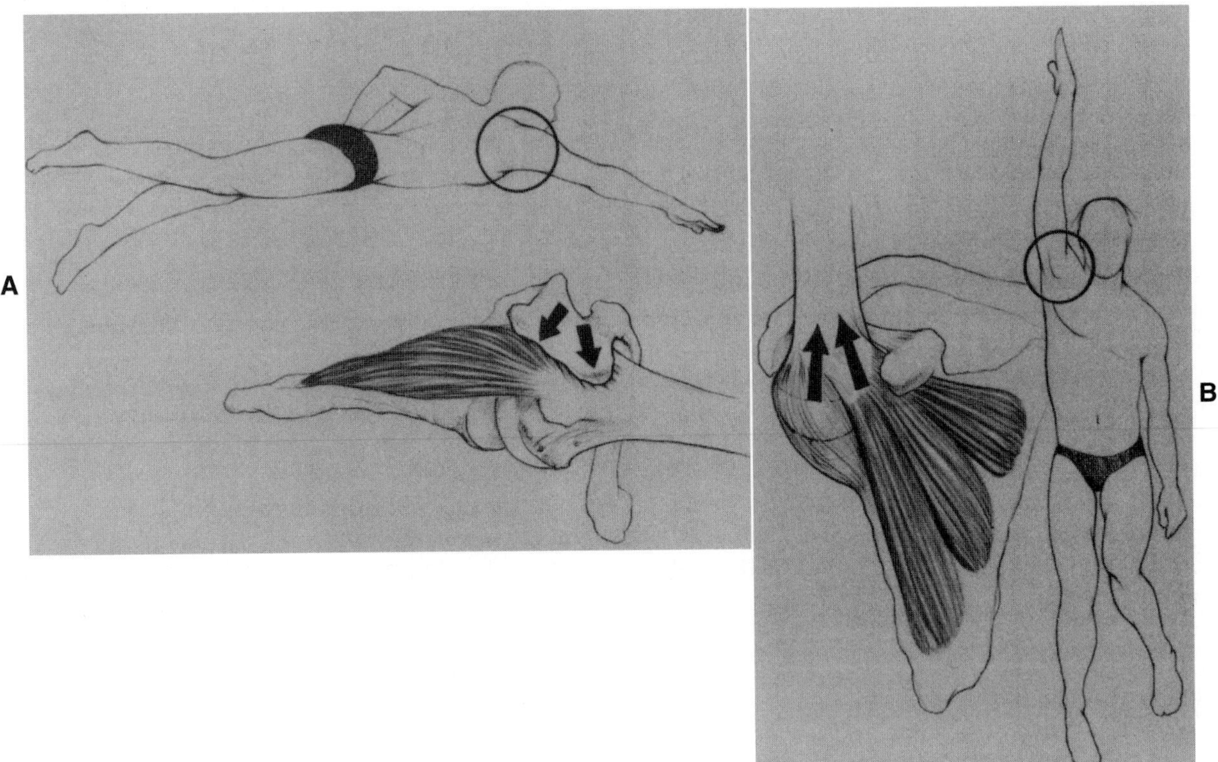

Fig. 10-12 ■ Swimmer's shoulder. **A,** During the beginning of the pull-through phase, the humeral head forces the rotator cuff against the acromion *(arrows),* thus creating an impingement in this area. **B,** In the backstroke, with initiation of the pull-through phase, there is a tendency to place tension on the anterior portion of the glenohumeral capsule *(arrows).* (From DeLee JC, Drez D, Miller MD: *DeLee & Drez's Orthopaedic sports medicine,* ed 2, Philadelphia, 2003, Saunders.)

CLINICAL GEM:

The average male freestyle swimmer has been calculated to perform almost 400,000 strokes per arm per year; women require more strokes to swim the same distance—up to 660,000 strokes per arm per year.

DeLee, Drez, Miller, p. 1136

43. What is the preferred medical term for a "frozen shoulder" when it is not related to any other shoulder problem?

A. Secondary adhesive capsulitis
B. Rotator cuff arthropathy
C. Degenerative arthritis of the glenohumeral joint
D. Primary adhesive capsulitis

Because "frozen shoulder" is a general term for loss of shoulder motion, the use of a more specific term is preferred. Most clinicians refer to idiopathic loss of shoulder motion as *primary adhesive capsulitis*. Certain disease processes are believed to predispose an individual to this condition, including cardiovascular disease, neurologic conditions, and especially diabetes mellitus. The exact cause of the disease is unknown, but possibilities include immunologic, inflammatory, biochemical, and endocrine problems. Secondary frozen shoulder occurs in patients who develop decreased shoulder range of motion after trauma.

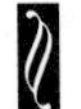

Answer: **D**

Warner, p. 130

44. True or False: The shoulder capsular pattern is as follows: Internal rotation (IR) is more limited than abduction (ABD), which is more limited than external rotation (ER): IR > ABD > ER.

When a joint is injured, a limitation of movement occurs in characteristic proportions. The patterns vary from joint to joint. In the shoulder, the capsular pattern in external rotation is more limited than in abduction, which is more limited than internal rotation: ER > ABD > IR.

Answer: **False**
Cyriax, p. 54

45. True or False: During treatment of adhesive capsulitis of the shoulder with ultrasound, the sound head should be directed toward the anterosuperior portion of the capsule.

Most adhesions occur in the anteroinferior portions of the capsule. This should be the area of focus with mobilizations, modalities, and stretching. When ultrasound is performed, the arm is abducted and externally rotated, and the sound head is directed toward the anteroinferior portion of the capsule.

Answer: **False**
Saunders, p. 161
Michlovitz, p. 203

46. Occupational or physical therapy treatment for primary frozen shoulder would appropriately include all but which of the following?

A. Heat and ultrasound
B. Transcutaneous electrical nerve stimulation or interferential electrical stimulation
C. Massage
D. Aggressive passive stretching
E. Active range of motion exercises

Therapy should include the use of modalities such as heat, ultrasound, and massage of trigger points to increase soft-tissue extensibility. The use of nonsteroidal antiinflammatory agents or subacromial space injection enhances therapy tolerance. This is followed by *gentle* passive and active range of motion exercises. Aggressive passive stretching should be avoided. If significant improvement is not attained after 6 months, manipulation of the shoulder under anesthesia usually is considered.

Answer: **D**
Pettrone, p. 223

47. Which is a critical rehabilitation exercise used for periscapular strengthening and treatment of glenohumeral instability?

A. Push-up plus
B. Pull-ups
C. External rotation isokinetics
D. Shoulder shrugs

The push-up plus is a core strengthening exercise to facilitate dynamic shoulder stabilization.

Answer: **A**
Norris, p. 70
DeLee, Drez, Miller, p. 344
Refer to Fig. 10-13

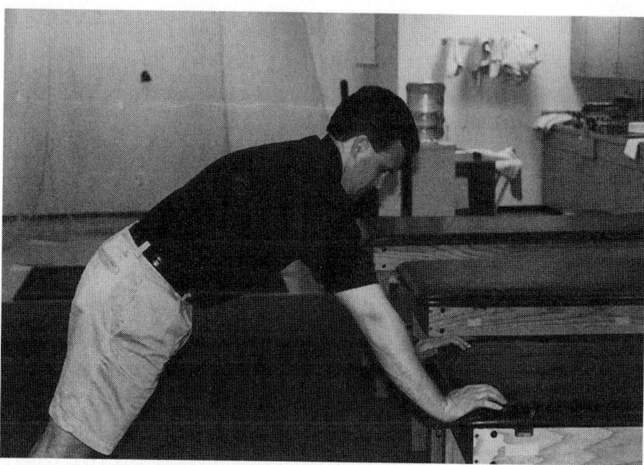

Fig. 10-13 ■ Push-up plus (pectoralis minor and serratus anterior). (From DeLee JC, Drez D, Miller MD: *DeLee & Drez's Orthopaedic sports medicine*, ed 2, Philadelphia, 2003, WB Saunders.)

48. What is the sulcus sign?

A. An indicator of periscapular weakness
B. A hallmark of inferior and multidirectional instability
C. An imbalance of external rotators
D. A sign of supraspinatus weakness

The sulcus sign is a dimple lateral to the acromion seen with caudal distraction of the humerus. It should be ablated with external rotation in a normal shoulder.

Answer: **B**
Norris, p. 86
DeLee, Drez, Miller, p. 1026
Refer to Fig. 10-14

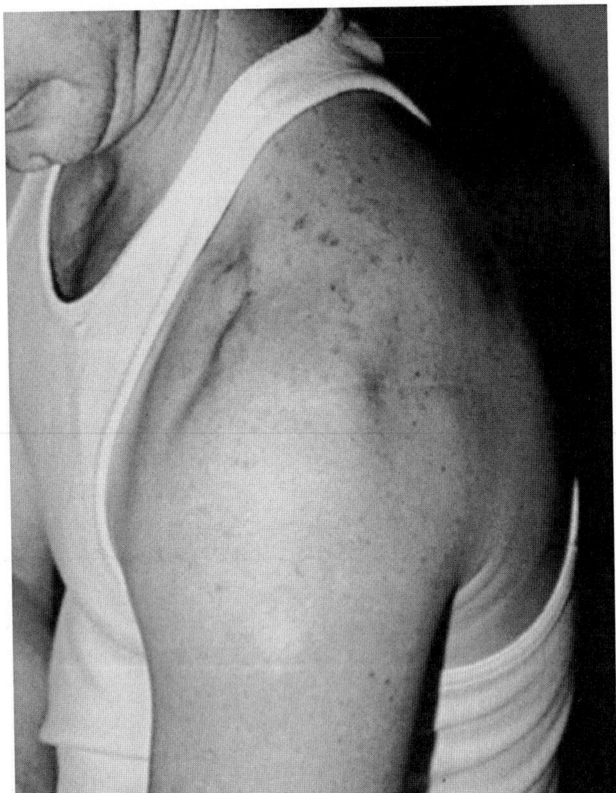

Fig. 10-14 ■ The sulcus sign. This patient had a posterior repair for glenohumeral instability. However, he continues to have inferior instability and demonstrate the sulcus (or hollow) just inferior to the anterior acromion during this sulcus test. (From Rockwood CA, Jr, Matsen FA: *The shoulder*, ed 2, Philadelphia, 1998, WB Saunders.)

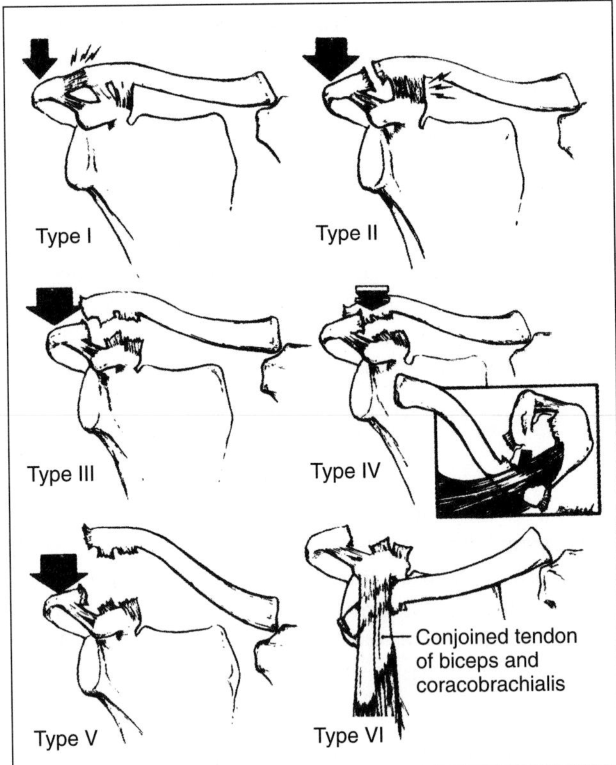

Fig. 10-15 ■ The six types of acromioclavicular disruptions. (From Rockwood CA, Jr, Williams GR, Young DC: Injuries to the acromioclavicular joint. In Rockwood CA, Jr, Green DP, Bucholz RW, eds: *Rockwood and Green's Fractures in adults*, ed 3, Philadelphia, 1991, Lippincott.)

49. True or False: Injury to the AC joint typically is caused by landing on the acromion during a fall or by a blow to the lateral shoulder.

Inferior and sometimes posterior forces to the shoulder stress the AC ligament and the coracoclavicular ligament. If the force is excessive, these ligaments are disrupted sequentially. Rockwood describes six grades/types of injury.

Answer: **True**
Pettrone, p. 167
Hunter, Mackin, Callahan, p. 1652
Refer to Fig. 10-15

50. After a type two AC injury (e.g., AC joint subluxed, AC ligament disrupted), active range of motion should be initiated when acute pain subsides. Which of the following shoulder motions usually is *not* limited?

A. Flexion
B. Abduction
C. Elevation
D. Internal rotation

Shoulder abduction, forward flexion, and elevation are often limited because of injury to the trapezius and deltoid. Internal rotation usually is not limited.

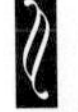

Answer: **D**
Pettrone, p. 171

CLINICAL GEM:
AC injury types one through three, as described by Rockwood, usually can be treated conservatively, but types four through six may require surgical reconstruction.

51. Which of the following is considered a conservative or nonoperative treatment for AC dislocations?

A. Adhesive strapping
B. Sling or bandage
C. Brace or harness
D. All the above are appropriate.

Numerous methods of nonoperative treatment of AC dislocation have been reported in the literature. The two most widely accepted techniques are the following: 1) closed reduction with the use of a brace or harness to maintain reduction of the clavicle; and 2) sling support for a short period followed by early range of motion. Adhesive strapping is also a method used for reduction and immobilization.

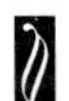

Answer: **D**
Rockwood, Matsen, p. 509

52. True or False: It has been reported that up to 72% of status post cerebrovascular accident (CVA) patients will experience shoulder pain.

The "stroke shoulder" is a painful and stiff shoulder that occurs in up to 72% of stroke patients. The painful shoulder may limit the ultimate goal of independence. Neglect of the symptomatic extremity can cause contractures, resulting in a pain cycle, and even the gentlest maneuvers are often unsuccessful. The overall goal of treatment is to maintain a functional range of motion that will, at least, allow for self-care.

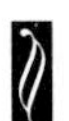

Answer: **True**
Stokes, Stokes, pp. 64-68
Rockwood, Matsen, pp. 986-987

53. Which of the following fractures presents a considerable danger to the surrounding nerves and vessels?

A. Epiphyseal fracture
B. Humeral shaft fracture
C. Proximal humeral fracture
D. Distal humerus fracture

Because of the proximity of the axillary blood vessels and the brachial plexus, a fracture to the proximal humerus may result in severe hemorrhaging or paralysis.

Answer: **C**
Arnheim, p. 763

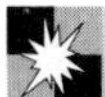

CLINICAL GEM:
Recognizing a fracture of the upper humerus by visual inspection may be difficult; therefore radiographs are mandatory.

54. A 50-year-old patient presents to an orthopedic surgeon with a 6-month history of severe shoulder pain without any history of injury. The range of motion of the shoulder is diminished by approximately 50%, and testing is positive for impingement. The patient also exhibits a positive drop-arm test. The patient refuses any injections or medicines. What should the surgeon do next?

A. Order immediate occupational/physical therapy
B. Instruct the patient in a home exercise program
C. Order an arthrogram
D. Order an MRI

The best choice for this patient would be to order an MRI for evaluation of the rotator cuff. Evaluation of the cuff would be essential before deciding on further treatment. Occupational or physical therapy would likely aggravate the pain at this stage and therefore is not indicated. A home exercise program most likely would be ineffective because this would aggravate the pain. Because the patient refuses injection, an arthrogram would not be possible.

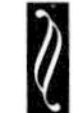

Answer: **D**
Flatow, pp. 43-45

55. The patient in question 54 had an MRI that showed a greater than 50% partial tear of the articular surface of the supraspinatus tendon and anterior acromiohumeral impingement. The patient refuses injection, medication, or therapy and wants something done operatively. The surgeon most likely would do which of the following?

A. Abandon this patient because the patient obviously is uncooperative
B. Perform arthroscopy and debride the tear only
C. Perform arthroscopy with acromioplasty and a mini-open repair
D. Insist that the patient attend occupational or physical therapy

The most appropriate treatment for a greater than 50% partial tear of the rotator cuff would be as follows: first, confirm the presence of the partial tear with arthroscopy; second, perform an arthroscopic acromioplasty; and third, perform a mini-open repair of the partial thickness tear. It has been found that arthroscopy and debridement alone for these types of tears is not as effective.

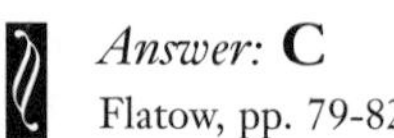
Answer: **C**
Flatow, pp. 79-82

56. The same patient in questions 54 and 55 is seen in the doctor's office 3 days after his mini-open repair. The patient is doing well, and the wounds are healing with no evidence of infection. Pain is controlled with analgesics. What should be done next?

A. Occupational/physical therapy with active range of motion should be ordered.
B. Patient should be kept completely immobilized for 6 weeks.
C. Occupational/physical therapy with passive range of motion only should be ordered.
D. Patient should receive massage therapy.

During the postoperative period after mini-open repair, the patient should be on a passive range of motion program for the first 3 to 6 weeks. If the deltoid was detached and reattached, active range of motion is prohibited for 6 weeks. If the patient had undergone arthroscopic debridement only, gentle active motion may be begun immediately. Specific protocols vary according to surgeon preference and facility guidelines.

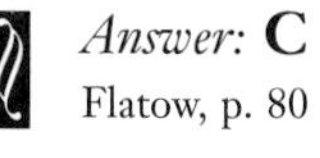
Answer: **C**
Flatow, p. 80

57. What is rotator cuff arthropathy?

A. Diffuse weakness of the rotator cuff
B. A transient pain related to the rotator cuff
C. A combined deficiency of the rotator cuff with glenohumeral arthrosis
D. An advanced case of calcific tendinitis

Rotator cuff arthropathy is a degenerative condition in which a deficient/torn rotator cuff allows the humeral head to migrate superiorly and arthrosis develops.

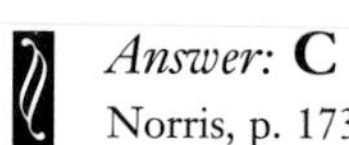
Answer: **C**
Norris, p. 173

58. Which type of lateral third clavicle fractures are typically treated surgically?

A. Comminuted fractures
B. Minimally displaced fractures
C. Fractures with coracoclavicular ligament disruption
D. Oblique fractures

Distal clavicular fractures are classified as types I, II, and III. Type II involves disruption of the coracoclavicular ligaments and leads to symptomatic inferior subluxation of the shoulder girdle. This commonly is treated with surgical repair.

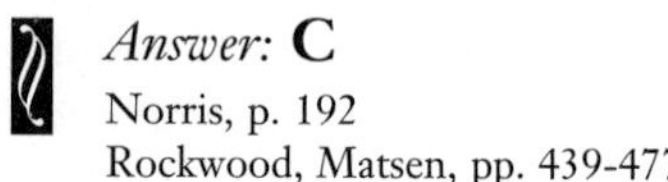
Answer: **C**
Norris, p. 192
Rockwood, Matsen, pp. 439-477

59. True or False: Immediately after shoulder surgery, it is best to assign the patient a complex home exercise program that is performed once a day.

When appropriate in the early days after surgery, it is best to instruct the patient in a short, simple exercise program that is performed frequently. A session should be limited to 10 to 15 minutes and performed 5 to 6 times a day. As healing progresses, the length of the sessions should be expanded, and their frequency should be decreased. After discharge from formal therapy, the patient should be reminded to continue stretching and strengthening once a day.

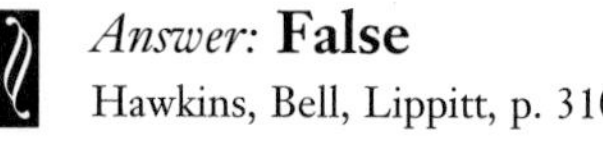
Answer: **False**
Hawkins, Bell, Lippitt, p. 310

60. A 68-year-old female is referred to you with the diagnosis of frozen shoulder. Your treatment includes modalities, joint mobilization, range of motion, strengthening exercises, and functional activities. She reports pain in the posterior deltoid, scapula, and posterior arm and wrist, as well as in the middle deltoid region of the humerus, lateral arm, and lateral epicondyle. She is making slow but steady progress, but you would like to facilitate additional range of motion for the shoulder in all planes and decrease her pain. Which muscle would you assess as a possible source of her pain distribution?

A. Latissimus dorsi
B. Subscapularis
C. Deltoid
D. None of the above

The subscapularis refers pain to the posterior deltoid area, scapula, and posterior arm and wrist. Occasionally it will refer pain to the anterior shoulder and palmar surface of the wrist. The infraspinatus will refer pain to the anterior deltoid region, shoulder joint, and medial border of the scapula and to the front and lateral aspects of the arm and forearm. Because it is the main stabilizer of the scapula, most shoulder injuries involve the subscapularis muscle. Frozen shoulders with limited shoulder abduction may involve the subscapularis muscle. Subscapularis muscle function affects scapular-humeral rhythm, thus causing abnormal shoulder mechanics during movement.

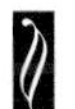
Answer: **B**
Kostopoulos, Rizopoulos, pp. 110, 114

61. A patient presents to the orthopedic surgeon's office with a minimally displaced proximal humeral fracture through the surgical neck. She is quite stoic and does not want any pain medication. What should be done next?

A. The arm and shoulder should be immobilized in a sling for approximately 6 weeks.
B. The arm and shoulder should be immobilized in a sling for approximately 3 weeks.
C. The arm and shoulder should be immobilized in a sling for approximately 7 to 10 days.
D. An open reduction internal fixation should be performed.

Approximately 80% of proximal humeral fractures are slightly displaced. However, most of these fractures are stable. Therefore better results have been seen with early motion—typically as early as 7 to 10 days after injury. When displacement is excessive, various forms of open reduction internal fixation may be considered.

Answer: **C**
Frymoyer, p. 285
Refer to Fig. 10-16

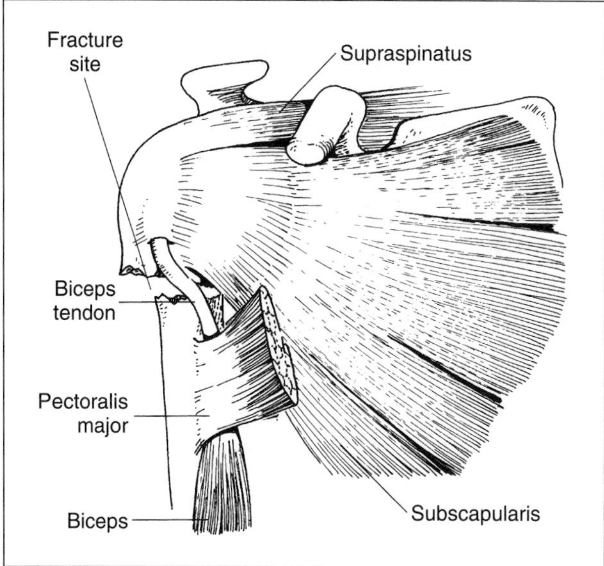

Fig. 10-16 ■ From Hawkins RJ, Bell RH, Lippitt SB: *Atlas of shoulder surgery*, St Louis, 1996, Mosby.

62. Which nerve is most commonly injured with fracture of the humeral shaft?

A. Axillary
B. Musculocutaneous
C. Median
D. Radial

The radial nerve is intimately wrapped around the middle and distal third of the humerus. It may be injured with fractures in this region.

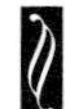
Answer: **D**
Norris, p. 208
Omer, Spinner, Van Beek, pp. 183-184
Refer to Fig. 10-17

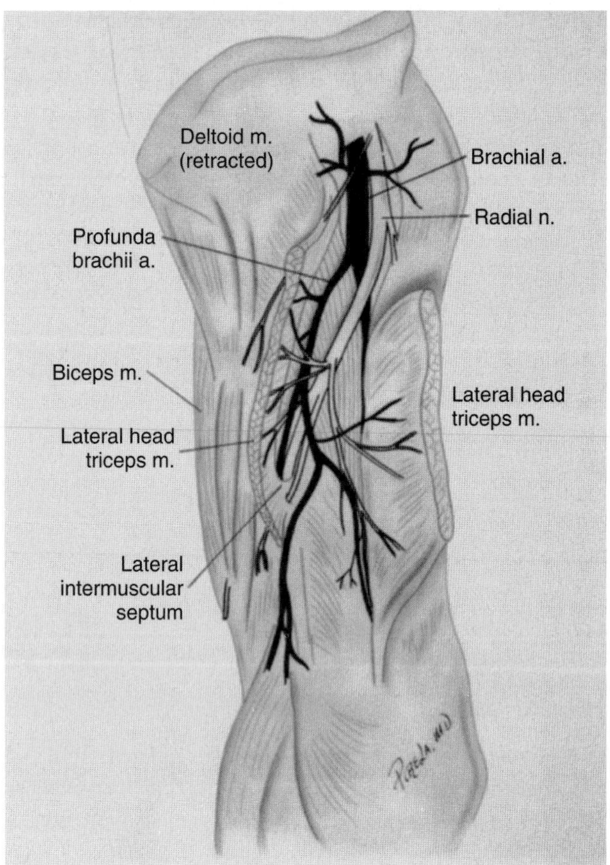

Fig. 10-17 ■ From Omer GE, Jr, Spinner M, Van Beek AL: *Management of peripheral nerve problems*, ed 2, Philadelphia, 1998, WB Saunders.

63. What is internal impingement?

A. Pain from a pinched labrum
B. Biceps subluxation
C. Coracoacromial arch impingement
D. Rotator cuff pain

Internal impingement is pain (typically seen in overhead throwing athletes) in the rotator cuff. The rotator cuff pathology is a consequence of either excessive glenohumeral motion or selective posterior capsular tightness. Internal impingement occurs when the arm is in maximal external rotation—the infraspinatus can be compressed between the posterior superior glenoid rim and the humeral head.

Answer: **D**
Burkhart, Morgan, Kibler, pp. 404-419
DeLee, Drez, Miller, pp. 1238-1240

64. Codman's exercises often are used as postoperative or postfracture exercises for almost all shoulder pathologies. Why are these exercises appropriate?

A. Strengthening of the pectoral girdle occurs without shoulder motion during this exercise.
B. Achieving joint approximation through weight bearing on the extremity occurs rather than muscle contraction.
C. They assist in reduction of the distal postoperative edema while protecting the shoulder joint.
D. Shoulder motion is gained passively by using gravity and body position rather than muscle contraction.

Codman's exercises (Fig. 10-18) are performed by having the patient bend at the waist and allow the arm to dangle away from the body. In this position, gravity alone can achieve up to 90 degrees of shoulder flexion without any muscle contraction. The patient also can use body motion to swing the arm gently clockwise, counterclockwise, forward and back, and side to side. These exercises can be performed with or without a sling to maintain elbow flexion and are easily progressed to an active exercise with minimal use of the shoulder musculature.

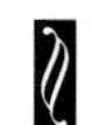

Answer: **D**
Pettrone, p. 214

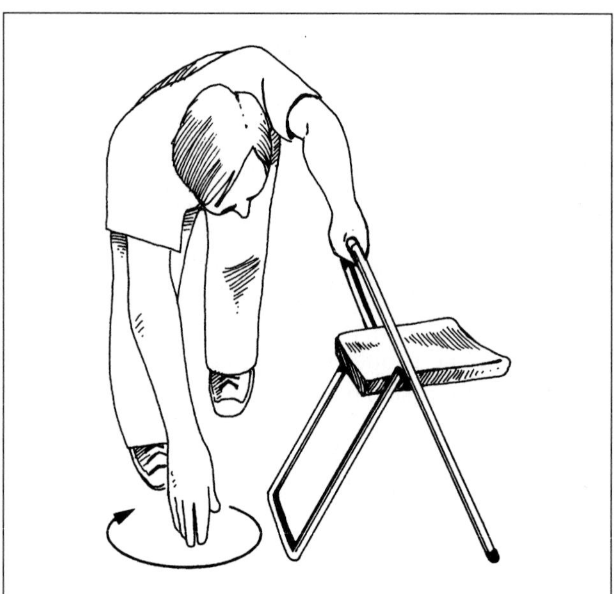

Fig. 10-18 ■ From Hawkins RJ, Bell RH, Lippitt SB: *Atlas of shoulder surgery*, St Louis, 1996, Mosby.

65. Nonoperative treatment for multidirectional instability of the shoulder after acute injury should include which of the following?

A. A prolonged period of immobilization (4 to 6 weeks)
B. Codman's exercises with weights after the acute phase
C. Weighted exercise to create an inferior traction force on the shoulder after the acute phase
D. Strengthening the rotator cuff after the acute phase

After acute dislocation that results in multidirectional instability, an arm sling is worn for a few days to decrease pain. Traction on the shoulder should be avoided. A rehabilitation program that emphasizes rotator cuff and periscapular muscle strengthening is employed after acute pain decreases. Traumatic dislocations respond less favorably to therapy than atraumatic dislocations.

Answer: **D**
Pettrone, p. 132

66. True or False: Osteoarthritis of the glenohumeral joint can be identified by sharp, intermittent pain—often when the joint is at rest.

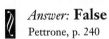

Osteoarthritis of the glenohumeral joint causes a nonlocalizing toothache-like pain that is aggravated by motion and may result in muscle atrophy and contractures. Crepitation is noted with motion. Treatment consists of gentle therapy and pain-relieving measures.

Answer: **False**
Pettrone, p. 240

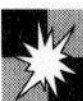
CLINICAL GEM:
Crepitation is a clicking or crackling sound heard during the movement of certain joints; it is caused by irregularities in the articulating surfaces.

67. True or False: After a biceps tenodesis procedure, passive range of motion exercises are started on the second postoperative day for both the shoulder and the elbow.

Biceps pathology is encountered during rotator cuff repair and proximal humeral fractures; occasionally it is caused by acute tears or, rarely, by attritional deterioration. Biceps tenodesis is the fixation of the long biceps tendon in the bicipital groove of the humerus. Passive range of motion exercises are started on the second postoperative day for the elbow and shoulder. The patient is taught to perform progressive elbow extension as pain allows. Full extension may not be achieved for 5 to 6 weeks. The patient is cautioned against active elbow flexion to protect the tenodesis. Active exercise is started for the elbow and shoulder at 2 to 3 weeks, with strengthening at 4 to 6 weeks. Heavy resistance should be avoided for 2 to 3 months.

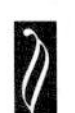
Answer: **True**
Hawkins, Bell, Lippitt, p. 144

68. A 72-year-old woman is seen by an orthopedic surgeon. Her primary complaint is severe pain and a loss of motion in her shoulder during the past 6 months. She was referred to the orthopedic doctor by her primary care physician after 3 months of nonoperative treatment, including occupational/physical therapy, antiinflammatory medications, and steroid injections. Radiographs confirm a superior subluxation of the humeral head with some degenerative changes. The MRI shows a large retracted rotator cuff tear. The patient wants her shoulder to work as well as possible. What is the best option for the surgeon?

A. Explain to the patient that she is too old for surgery
B. Order more occupational/physical therapy
C. Schedule the patient for arthroscopic debridement with no attempt at repair of the tear
D. Schedule the patient for arthroscopy with possible open repair

Rotator cuff tears have been classified as the following: small, less than 1 cm in diameter; medium, 1 to 3 cm; large, 3 to 5 cm; and massive, greater than 5 cm. Many studies have shown that debridement provides satisfactory results for the short term. Long-term studies, however, indicate that for all types of tears a patient is best served by operative repair of the tear.

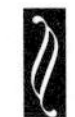
Answer: **D**
Flatow, pp. 117-124

69. Which of the following tests identifies TOS?

A. Halstead maneuver
B. Speed's test
C. Adson maneuver
D. B and C
E. A and C

The Adson maneuver is a common test for identifying TOS. The radial pulse is monitored while the head is rotated toward the involved shoulder. The patient extends his or her head, and the shoulder is placed in extension and external rotation as the patient takes a deep breath and holds it. If the radial pulse decreases or disappears, the test is positive. In some individuals it may be necessary to rotate the head to the opposite side to have an effect on the radial pulse. Therefore both positions must be tested.

The Halstead maneuver is performed by locating the radial pulse and applying a downward traction on the arm while the patient hyperextends the neck and rotates his or her head to the opposite side. A diminished or absent pulse indicates a positive test for TOS.

The two tests just described help determine neurovascular compression within the thoracic outlet; however, they specifically address vascular compression.

Compression at the thoracic outlet can involve the subclavian artery, subclavian vein, or brachial plexus.

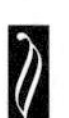

Answer: **E**
DeLee, p. 796
Magee, p. 122

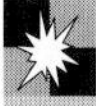

CLINICAL GEM:
TOS presents with vascular and/or neurological symptoms. Controversy surrounds the actual percentage for each category; however, it is accepted that a neurological presentation is more common.

70. Match each shoulder test to the correct interpretation of the test.

Shoulder Test

1. Apprehension test (crank test) (see Fig. 10-4)
2. Hawkins-Kennedy impingement test (Fig. 10-19)
3. Speed's test (Fig. 10-20)
4. Jahnke test (Fig. 10-21)

Test Interpretation

A. Posterior subluxation
B. Bicipital groove tendonitis
C. Anterior instability
D. Supraspinatus tendinitis

Answers: **1, C; 2, D; 3, B; 4, A**
Magee, p. 118

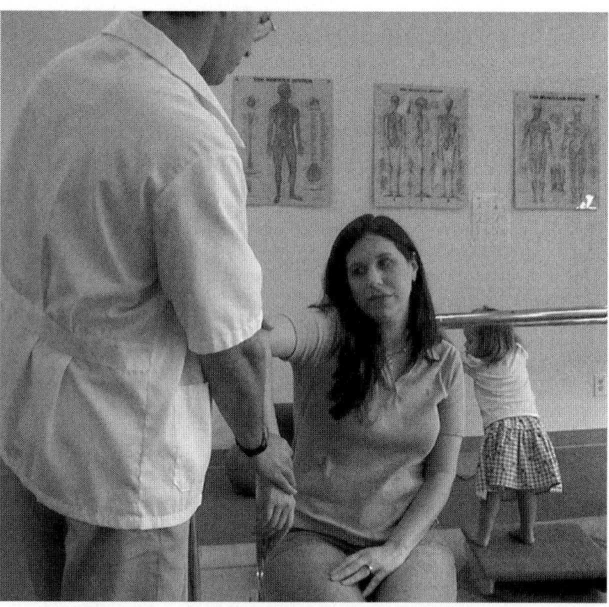

Fig. 10-19 ■ Hawkins-Kennedy impingement test.

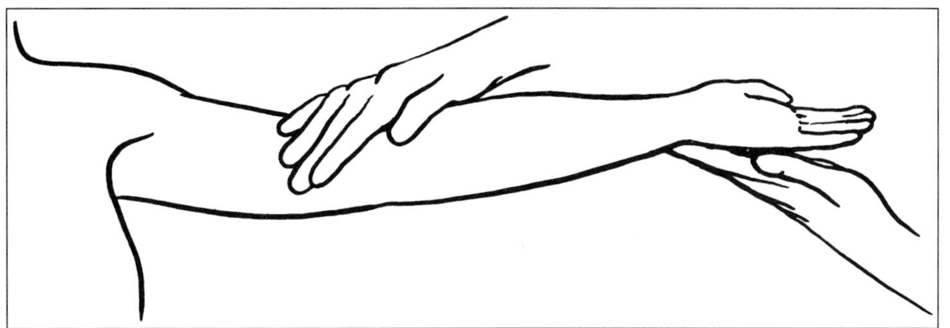

Fig. 10-20 ■ Speed's test. The biceps resistance test is performed with the patient flexing the shoulder against resistance, with the elbow extended and the forearm supinated. Pain referred to the biceps tendon area constitutes a positive result.

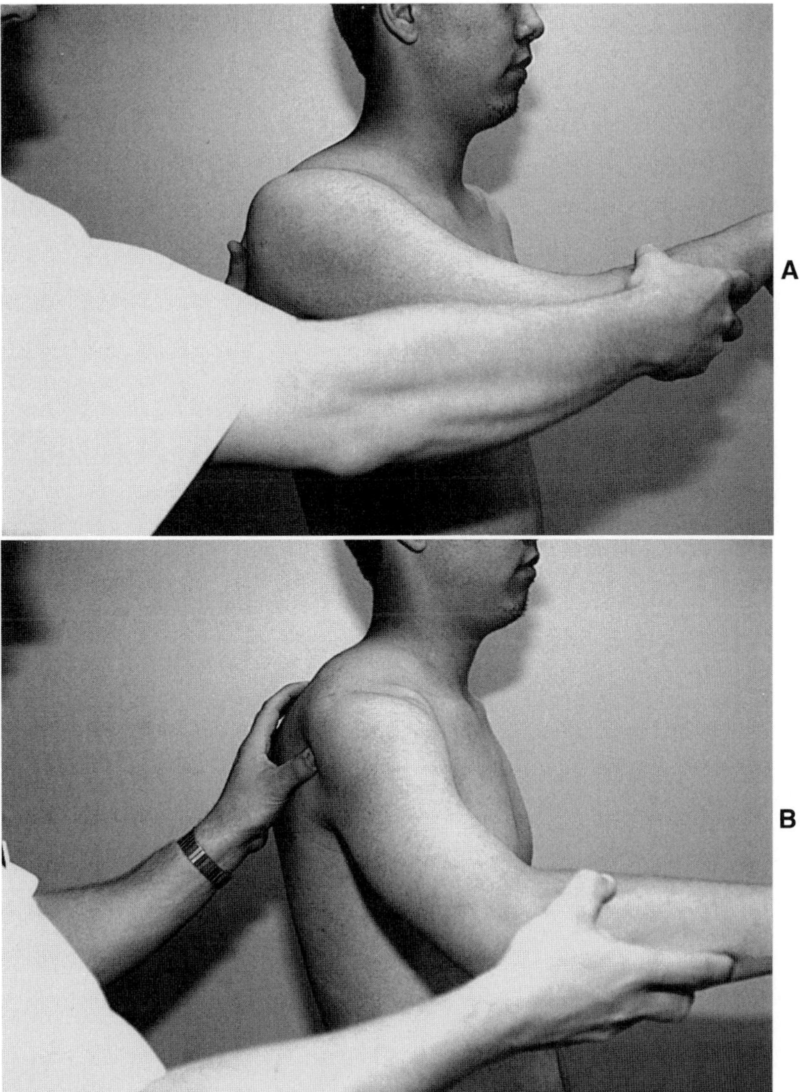

Fig. 10-21 ■ The "Jahnke test" reproduces posterior subluxation by stretching the forward flexed arm posteriorly at 90 degrees of elevation in neutral rotation; the elevated arm is then brought toward the coronal plane and is pushed forward. One can appreciate the reduction. This is a clear feeling of a "clunk" as the shoulder reduces from its subluxed position.

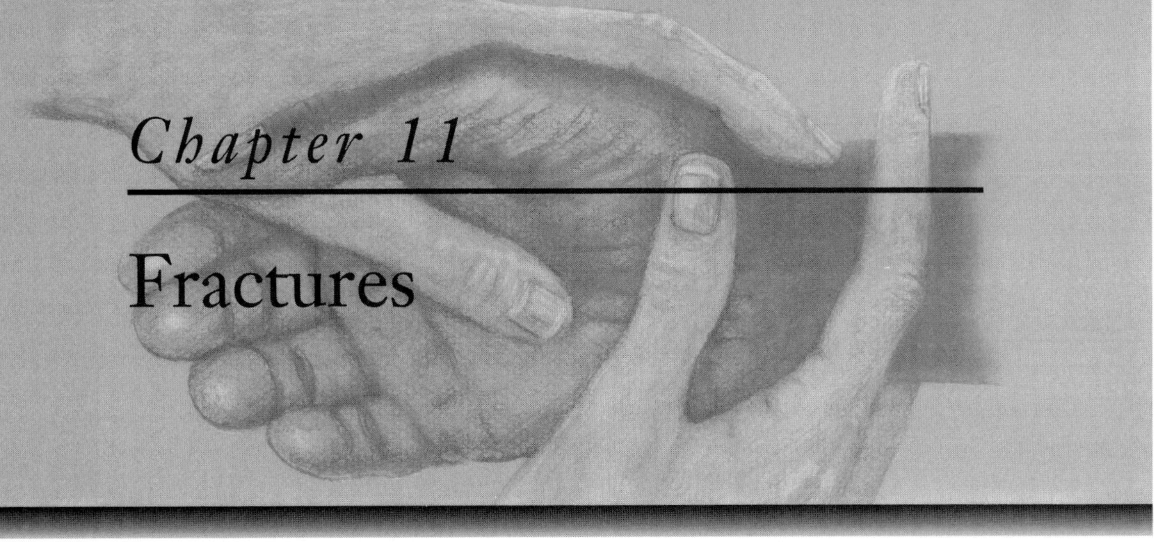

Chapter 11

Fractures

1. The goal of fracture healing is to do which of the following?

A. Regenerate mineralized tissue in the fracture area
B. Restore mechanical strength to the bone
C. Reconstitute normal soft tissue gliding and movement about the fracture site
D. A and C only
E. All of the above

After a fracture, the primary goal of healing is to regenerate mineralized tissue in the fracture area and restore mechanical strength to the bone. In addition, reconstituting normal soft tissue gliding and movement about the fracture site is important.

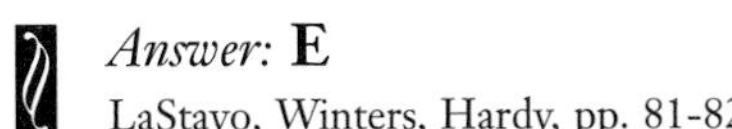

Answer: **E**
LaStayo, Winters, Hardy, pp. 81-82

2. The phases of fracture healing include which of the following?

A. Inflammation, repair, and remodeling phase
B. Inflammation, repair, and revascularization phase
C. Repair, revascularization, and remodeling phase
D. Repair, regeneration, and remodeling phase

The phases of fracture healing include inflammation, repair, and remodeling. In the inflammation phase, the hematoma develops and provides stability at the site and tissue regeneration is initiated. In the repair phase, the callus is formed to stabilize the fracture even more and granulation tissue replaces the hematoma. In the remodeling phase, there is resorption and deposition of bone to restore the strength of the bone.

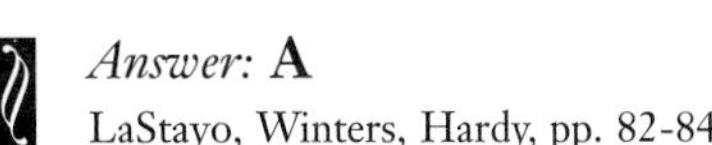

Answer: **A**
LaStayo, Winters, Hardy, pp. 82-84

3. True or False: Secondary healing occurs without a hematoma.

Primary fracture healing occurs without a hematoma. Primary healing is characterized by simultaneous union of fracture ends. It occurs with a mechanically stable environment with motionless fixation such as with plates and screws. In contrast, the process of secondary healing is characterized by three discrete yet overlapping stages: inflammation, repair, and remodeling. The inflammatory stage begins immediately after fracture, initiating cellular and vascular responses to injury that promote fracture stabilization through *early hematoma* clotting. Secondary healing occurs with fractures managed by closed reduction or with semirigid fixation methods (e.g., Kirschner wires, external fixators, intramedullary pins).

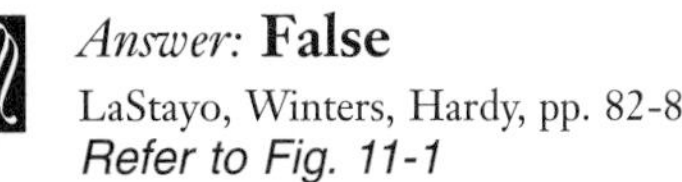

Answer: **False**
LaStayo, Winters, Hardy, pp. 82-83
Refer to Fig. 11-1

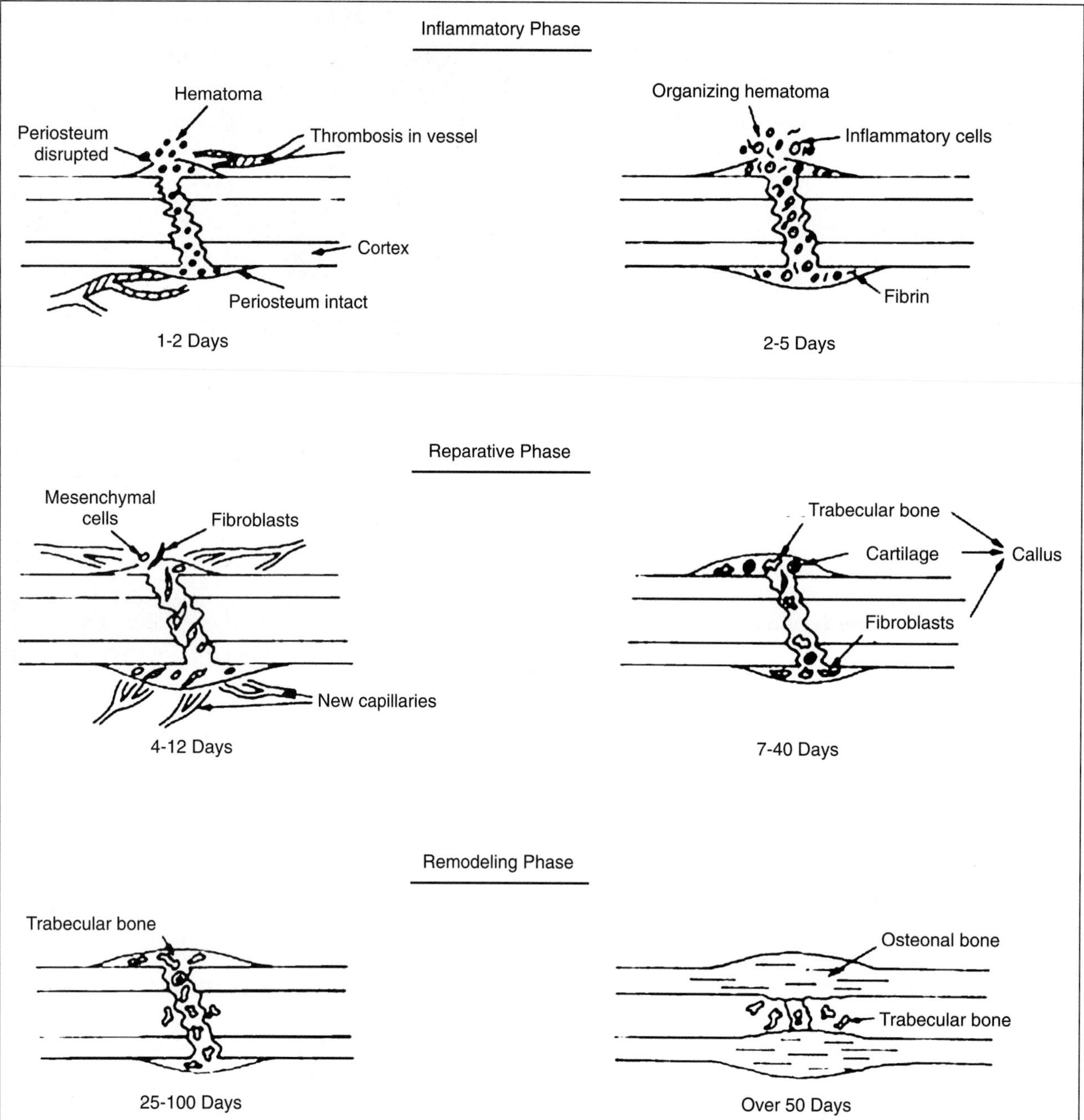

Fig. 11-1 ■ Secondary fracture healing. The three phases of fracture healing with relative time duration are pictured. In the inflammatory phase, the fracture hematoma clots and serves as the initial support. Inflammatory cells invade the hematoma to remove necrosed bone and debris. During the reparative phase, new capillaries are formed, thus providing nutrition for the formation of callus by fibroblasts, chondroblasts, and osteoblasts. The initial soft callus is converted into hard callus, then mineralized into bone during the remodeling phase. Return of medullary and periosteal blood flow also occurs in this final phase. Remodeling of the bone in response to stress to its normal preinjury configuration can take years. (From Brand RA: Fracture healing. In Albright JA, Brand RA: *The scientific basis of orthopaedics*, New York, 1979, McGraw-Hill.)

4. True or False: Stable internal fixation allows the therapist to initiate rehabilitation sooner than closed reduction.

Stable internal fixation provides the rigidity necessary to allow initiation of range of motion (ROM) to the involved extremity earlier than closed reduction. Internal fixation allows the increased stability of bone fragments in proper alignment to allow rapid rehabilitation.

Answer: **True**
Jabaley, Wegener, p. 96
Krop in Mackin, Callahan, Skirven, et al, p. 377

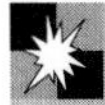

CLINICAL GEM:
Despite stability gained from the procedure, the therapist must respect the soft tissue and the healing process.

5. The term "boxer's fracture" refers to a fracture of which of the following?

A. Shaft of the proximal phalanx
B. Shaft of the middle phalanx
C. Metacarpal neck
D. Metacarpal base
E. Distal interphalangeal (DIP) joint

A boxer's fracture is a fracture involving the metacarpal neck. It usually involves the ring and small fingers and occurs when a clenched metacarpophalangeal (MCP) joint strikes a solid object. Nonunion almost never occurs, but malunion can be a complication. Patients complain of a loss of prominence of the metacarpal head and decreased ROM, and they can palpate the metacarpal head in the palm on occasion. Treatments include closed reduction, closed reduction with percutaneous pin fixation, and/or open reduction (Fig. 11-2).

Answer: **C**
Green, pp. 698-700

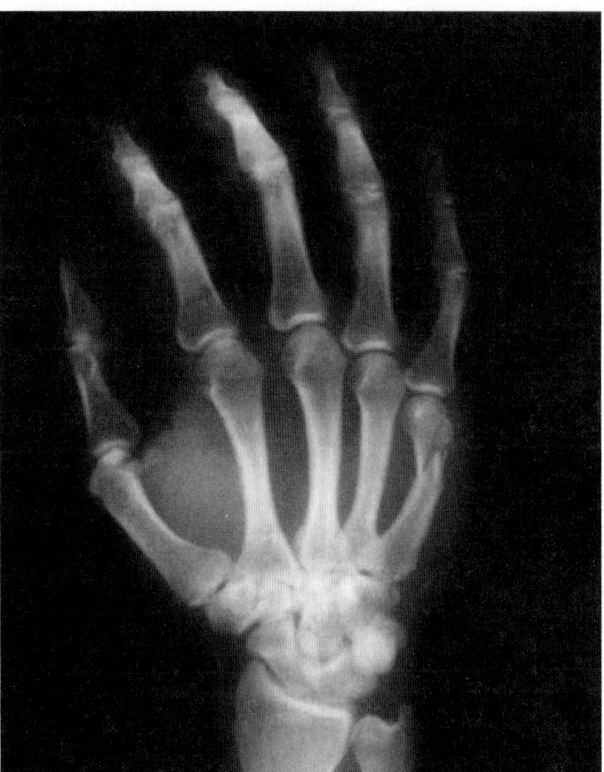

Fig. 11-2 ■ Radiograph of a minimally displaced fracture of the metacarpal neck (boxer's fracture). (From Hunter JM, Mackin EJ, Callahan AD: *Rehabilitation of the hand: surgery and therapy*, ed 4, St Louis, 1995, Mosby.)

6. A boxer's fracture is most commonly seen in which digits?

A. First and second metacarpals
B. Second and third metacarpals
C. Third and fourth metacarpals
D. Fourth and fifth metacarpals

A metacarpal neck fracture, or boxer's fracture, is most commonly seen in the fourth and fifth metacarpals. This fracture occurs when the clenched fist strikes an object at an oblique angle. The boxer's fracture often is treated with a cast or ulnar gutter splint for approximately 3 to 3.5 weeks to allow the fracture pain to subside and sufficient healing to occur. Surgical treatment can be performed for cosmetic reasons and to avoid a palmar metacarpal head deformity, which interferes with high-demand grasping activities.

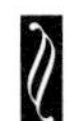

Answer: **D**
Diao, p. 564
Refer to Fig. 11-2

7. True or False: Stable, internal fixation allows fractures to heal faster.

Stable, internal fixation allows for a precise restoration of parts, but it does not make fractures heal faster. It does, however, help them heal more precisely; it also allows for primary bone healing. During primary bone healing, direct deposition of bone in the fracture site occurs without the intermediate phase of cartilage formation and without the formation of an external callus. The major benefit of stable fixation is that early rehabilitation can be initiated. Stable internal fixation also is a deterrent to the development of a chronically painful, swollen, and stiff hand. Although internal fixation does not necessarily speed fracture healing, it may reduce the time required before the patient can return to productive work or leisure.

Answer: **False**
Freeland, Jabaley, Hughes, p. 28

8. Which joint(s) in the hand, after developing stiffness, causes the most serious functional loss?

A. DIP
B. Proximal interphalangeal (PIP)
C. MCP
D. All of the above contribute equally to functional loss

PIP joint stiffness results in the most serious functional loss. The PIP joint is crucial to function, and once it is stiffened, correction is quite difficult. The MCP joint can become stiffened in extension, but typically it can be released. The DIP joint contributes minimally to the flexion arc; therefore loss of motion at this level is not as crucial.

Answer: **B**
McCollister, p. 1297

9. True or False: The stability of a fracture significantly affects the quantity and quality of callus formation.

The stability of a fracture significantly affects the quantity and quality of callus formation. In general, greater amounts of motion at a fracture site result in a greater amount of callus. It is as if the fracture forms an internal splint. In contrast, very stable fixation with accurate reduction results in very small amounts of callus formation. Immobilization and very stable fixation both have advantages and disadvantages.

Answer: **True**
McCollister, p. 105

10. The cylindrical shaft of a long bone is which of the following?

A. Metaphysis
B. Epiphysis
C. Diaphysis
D. None of the above

The diaphysis is the cylindrical shaft of a bone. The metaphysis is the growing portion of a bone; this is the part between the diaphysis and the epiphysis. The epiphysis is the ossification center at each extreme end of the long bones. When bone growth is complete, the diaphysis is fused with the epiphysis by bony synostosis. Fusion of the epiphysis with the diaphysis occurs approximately 1 to 2 years earlier in females than in males. In general, male bone growth is complete by age 20 and female bone growth is complete by age 18. A radiologist can determine the bone age of a person by studying the ossification center.

Answer: **C**
Taber's cyclopedic medical dictionary
Netter, p. 131
Refer to Fig. 11-3

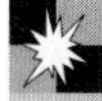
CLINICAL GEM:
The medial epiphysis of the clavicle, which is the last epiphysis of the long bones to appear in the body, develops between the ages of approximately 18 and 20. This epiphysis also is the last to close; closure occurs between the ages of approximately 23 and 25.

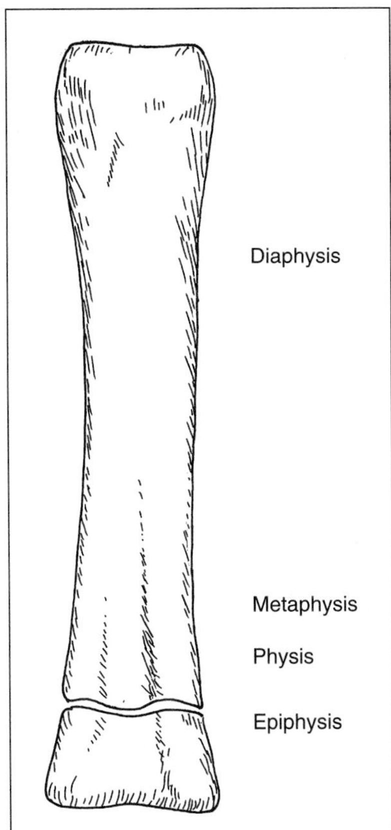

Fig. 11-3 ■ A long bone in a child. (From Mackin EJ, Callahan AD, Skirven TM, et al: *Rehabilitation of the hand and upper extremity*, ed 5, St Louis, 2002, Mosby.)

11. Which of the following fractures is easiest to rehabilitate?

A. Distal phalanx
B. Middle phalanx
C. Proximal phalanx
D. Metacarpal

The distal phalanx is the easiest to rehabilitate because of its anatomic relationship with bone and the surrounding soft tissue. There is only a slight chance of the flexor tendon and the terminal tendon becoming adherent as they insert on the distal phalanx. The primary difficulties noted with rehabilitation of these fractures are pain and hypersensitivity due to the sensory nerve endings surrounding the fingertip. Desensitization of the digit tip is initiated as the site is healed.

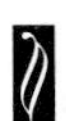
Answer: **A**
Chinchalkar, Gan, p. 118
Purdy, Wilson in Mackin, Callahan, Skirven, et al, p. 385

12. What is the physician's treatment of choice for stable hyperextension and dorsal dislocation injuries of the PIP joint?

A. Open reduction internal fixation (ORIF)
B. Order a dynamic splint
C. K-wire DIP joint in full extension
D. Closed reduction

The physician's treatment of choice for stable hyperextension and dorsal dislocation injuries of the PIP joint is a closed reduction. The patient is often placed in a dorsal block splint with buddy taping to the next digit for approximately 4 to 6 weeks to allow early motion to begin. ROM exercises are performed with focus on active blocking exercises, which also assist with decreasing any tightness in the oblique retinacular ligament.

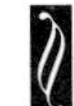
Answer: **D**
Chinchalkar, Gan, p. 121

13. True or False: Pilon fractures can be treated safely using dynamic traction.

A pilon fracture is a comminuted intraarticular fracture of the base of the middle phalanx (Fig. 11-4, *A*). It can be treated with ORIF, external fixation, or dynamic traction (Fig. 11-4, *B*). Schenck has popularized the concept of dynamic traction. Using this method, a K-wire is put through the head of the middle phalanx, and traction is applied to the phalanx with rubber-band traction attached to a hoop mount on a forearm splint. The patient regularly performs passive ROM for both flexion and extension in a specified range. Splinting is continued for 6 to 8 weeks. Studies have shown that the skeletal traction technique can be safer and that it produces results equivalent to those of ORIF.

Answer: **True**
Baratz, Divelbiss, pp. 541-555
Hunter, Mackin, Callahan, p. 384
Campbell, Wilson in Mackin, Callahan, Skirven, et al, p. 401
Jebson, Kasdan, p. 157
Jacobs, Austin, p. 328
Chinchalkar, Gan, p. 125

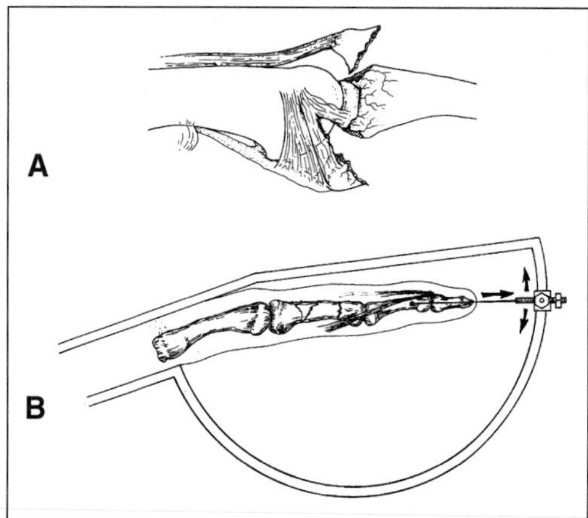

Fig. 11-4 ■ A, Pilon fracture. **B,** Dynamic traction. (From Hunter JM, Mackin EJ, Callahan AD: *Rehabilitation of the hand: surgery and therapy,* ed 4, St Louis, 1995, Mosby.)

14. A 27-year-old male laborer presents with a bullet wound through the MCP joint of his dominant thumb. He works in construction, has three children, and finished the tenth grade in high school. He has intact sensation and intact flexor and extensor tendon function but cannot pinch because of severe posttraumatic arthritis of the MCP joint. The best treatment includes which of the following?

A. Arthrodesis of the first MCP joint
B. MCP joint arthroplasty
C. Short opponens splint
D. Radial thumb spica splint
E. Second metatarsal phalangeal (MTP) toe-to-thumb transplant

A painful unstable MCP joint in a laborer with a need to return to work is best treated by arthrodesis. Arthrodesis will allow the patient to return to work the quickest with the least amount of rehabilitation.

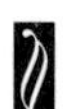
Answer: **A**

15. Which bone in the hand is most commonly fractured?

A. Distal phalanx
B. Middle phalanx
C. Proximal phalanx
D. Metacarpal shaft

The most commonly fractured bone in the hand is the distal phalanx, which accounts for 45% to 50% of all hand fractures. The thumb and middle fingers are most commonly involved. Fractures of the distal phalanx often are the result of crushing injuries. Fortunately, fractures of the distal phalanx usually heal without excessive treatment.

Answer: **A**
Hunter, Mackin, Callahan, p. 360
Purdy, Wilson in Mackin, Callahan, Skirven, et al, p. 384

16. Which of the following is the most serious complication of a proximal phalanx fracture?

A. PIP joint extension contracture
B. MCP joint extension contracture
C. MCP joint flexion contracture
D. PIP joint flexion contracture

After a proximal phalanx fracture, development of a fixed PIP joint flexion contracture is the most serious complication because of the associated functional loss. The most effective way to avoid this complication is to splint the PIP joint in full extension to avoid collateral ligament tightness. A dynamic PIP joint extension splint should be initiated at the first sign of flexion deformity. PIP joint flexion contracture also is a serious complication after middle phalanx fractures.

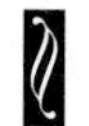
Answer: **D**
Hunter, Mackin, Callahan, p. 367
Purdy, Wilson in Mackin, Callahan, Skirven, et al, p. 389

17. What is considered functional flexion for the MCP, PIP, and DIP joints, respectively?

A. 51 degrees, 39 degrees, 32 degrees
B. 69 degrees, 50 degrees, 21 degrees
C. 61 degrees, 60 degrees, 39 degrees
D. 28 degrees, 42 degrees, 30 degrees

Functional flexion averages 61 degrees at the MCP joint level, 60 degrees at the PIP joint level, and 39 degrees at the DIP joint level. Functional motion for flexion of the thumb is 21 degrees at the MCP joint level and 18 degrees at the interphalangeal (IP) joint level. These measures are based on common activities of daily living. They are not used for addressing individual activities or work skills. They do, however, provide a basic guideline for functional performance of the hand.

Answer: **C**
Hunter, Mackin, Callahan, p. 1185
Cannon in Mackin, Callahan, Skirven, et al, p. 1071

18. Which of the following distal phalanx fractures is inherently unstable because of the pull of the tendons?

A. Tuft fracture
B. Shaft fracture
C. Base fracture
D. All the above

Base fractures usually are unstable because of the pull of the flexor and extensor tendons at the fracture site; they also tend to angulate the fracture with a dorsal apex. Closed fractures usually can be managed with a short Alumafoam splint, which holds the distal phalanx in extension. If the fracture is unstable or open, it is best to treat it with K-wire fixation.

Tuft fractures often are caused by crush injuries and usually are very painful, but they are inherently stable. However, if the disruption of the nail and pulp occur with an open fracture, the fracture is likely to be unstable. Shaft fractures usually have minimal displacement and are stable; they also may be either longitudinal or transverse.

Answer: **C**
Hunter, Mackin, Callahan, pp. 361-362
Refer to Fig. 11-5

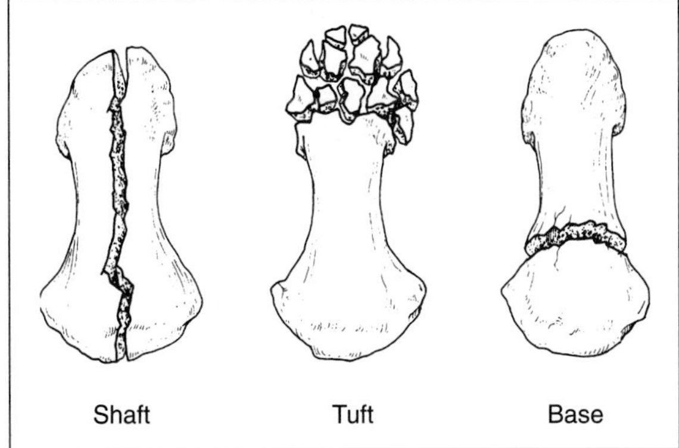

Fig. 11-5 ■ From Hunter JM, Mackin EJ, Callahan AD: *Rehabilitation of the hand: surgery and therapy*, ed 4, St Louis, 1995, Mosby.

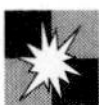

CLINICAL GEM:
The most common problems after distal phalanx fractures, especially crush type injures, are pain and hypersensitivity.

19. If a PIP joint develops a swan-neck deformity and produces an unusual hyperflexion at the MCP, corrective splinting could include which of the following to correct both deformities?

A. Figure 8 splints to maintain PIP in slight flexion
B. Volar MCP joint blocking splint to maximize flexor tendon excursion
C. Dorsal MCP blocking splints
D. A and B only
E. A and C only

A swan-neck deformity is hyperextension of the PIP joint and flexion of the DIP joint. When the PIP joint loses flexion because of the swan-neck deformity, a hyperflexion at the MCP joint may occur. This is increased hyperflexion causes decreased gliding of the flexor digitorum profundus (FDP) tendons because of the overload of forces on the intrinsic musculature. To treat this deformity, splint with figure 8 splints to maintain the PIP joint in slight flexion and a volar MCP joint blocking splint to maximize flexor tendon excursion.

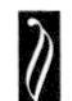

Answer: **D**
Jacobs, Austin, p. 355
Chinchalkar, Gan, pp. 126-127

20. The functional position splint for a nondisplaced fracture of the proximal phalanx at rest should be which of the following?

A. MCPs at 60 to 70 degrees of flexion, PIPs left free
B. MCPs at 60 to 70 degrees of flexion, IPs at 0 degrees of extension
C. MCPs at 60 to 80 degrees of flexion, IPs at 20 to 30 degrees of flexion
D. MCPs at 60 to 80 degrees of flexion, IPs at 40 to 50 degrees of flexion

The functional position of a fractured proximal phalanx in the correct position is imperative for proper healing. The splint should place the MCPs in 60 to 70 degrees of flexion and the IPs at 0 degrees of extension. This position allows the MCP joints to keep the collateral ligaments at their appropriate lengths, thereby preventing MCP extension contractures. Placing the IPs in extension prevents flexion contractures from occurring. This functional position splint allows for fracture healing and also allows for mobilization of the uninvolved joints.

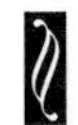

Answer: **B**
Jacobs, Austin, pp. 328-329

21. True or False: Buddy taping is the treatment of choice for a stable nondisplaced or minimally displaced fracture of the PIP.

An excellent treatment for a stable nondisplaced or minimally displaced fracture in a motivated compliant patient is buddy taping to the adjacent digit. Many patients, when instructed in the blocking and gliding exercises, are able to progress well with buddy taping. The active motion exercises compress the fracture site and stimulate callus formation, thus allowing healing to occur.

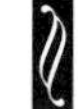

Answer: **True**

Clark, Wilgis, Aiello, p. 323
Freeland, Hardy, Singletary, p. 131
Refer to Fig. 11-6

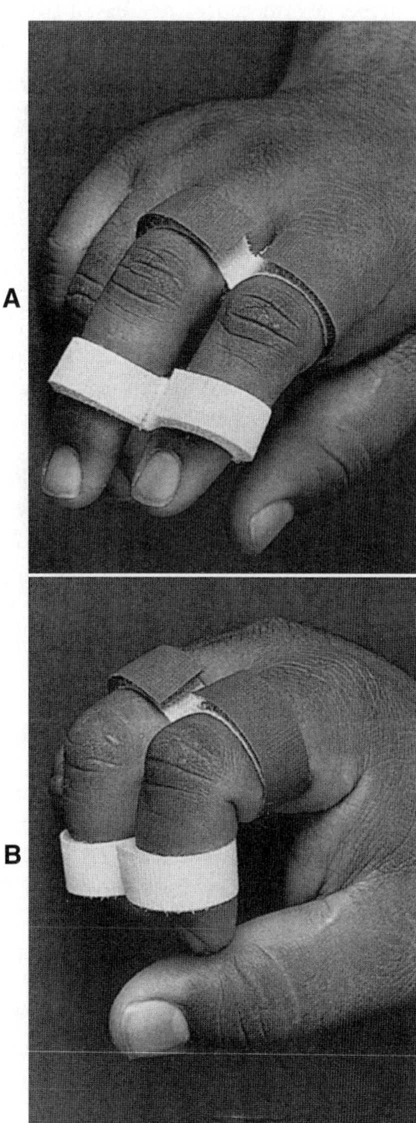

Fig. 11-6 ■ Velcro straps can be fabricated in the clinic and used instead of taping. (From Mackin EJ, Callahan AD, Skirven TM, et al: *Rehabilitation of the hand and upper extremity*, ed 5, St Louis, 2002, Mosby.)

22. A 35-year-old roofer is diagnosed with a boxer's fracture of the fifth metacarpal, with 30 degrees of angulation through the fracture. The patient is anxious to return to work. Which of the following would be the best treatment and splint application?

A. Closed reduction and splint application with the MCP joint flexed at 60 degrees for 3 weeks
B. Closed reduction and splint application with the MCP joint neutral for 3 weeks
C. Application of a static extension splint to the fifth digit with immediate active ROM
D. Application of a hand-based splint with the MCP joint free for 3 weeks, followed by immediate active ROM

Closed reduction, with either a cast application or use of an ulnar gutter splint positioning the fourth and fifth MCP joints at 60 degrees of flexion, has been a successful treatment of the boxer's fracture of the fifth metacarpal. The splint typically is worn for 3 to 6 weeks. Active ROM may be initiated as early as 2 weeks. Immediate motion is contraindicated in patients with boxer's fractures because a loss of reduction may occur. However, immediate ROM may be initiated if the fracture is absolutely stable, as in ORIF.

Answer: **A**

Light, Bednar, pp. 303-314
Hunter, Mackin, Callahan, pp. 370-371
Purdy, Wilson in Mackin, Callahan, Skirven, et al, pp. 388-395
Campbell, Wilson in Mackin, Callahan, Skirven, et al, pp. 396-409

CLINICAL GEM:
The most common complication after a metacarpal fracture is disproportionate dorsal edema.

23. True or False: A patient with osteoporosis has an accelerated loss of bone mass, which leaves the skeleton weakened and more vulnerable to fracture.

Osteoporosis is insidious in nature. It is a progressive disease that causes an accelerated loss of bone mass, thus leaving the skeleton weak and vulnerable to fracture. Fractures of the proximal humerus, pelvis, distal radius, and ribs are present in approximately 20 million osteoporotic individuals in the United States. These fractures cause varying degrees of pain, disability, and loss of independence. Impact activities, such as walking, can increase bone mass before age 35 and maintain bone mass after age 35; therefore it is important that patients with osteoporosis participate in an exercise program that stresses impact exercise.

Answer: **True**
McCollister, p. 177

24. If the elbow is dislocated in a posterolateral direction, which structure is ruptured in nearly all cases?

A. Distal biceps insertion
B. Triceps tendon
C. Medial collateral ligament
D. Posterior interosseous ligament

A complete disruption of the medial collateral ligament of the elbow is seen in nearly all cases of posterolateral dislocation.

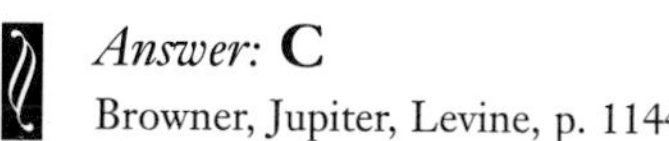

Answer: **C**
Browner, Jupiter, Levine, p. 1144

25. A Galeazzi fracture is which of the following?

A. Fracture of the distal radial shaft with subluxation/dislocation of the distal radioulnar (DRU) joint
B. Fracture of the radius and ulna at the same level
C. Fracture of the ulna shaft with disruption of the radiohumeral joint
D. Fracture of the distal ulna with disruption of the DRU joint

A Galeazzi fracture is a distal radial shaft fracture with subluxation/dislocation of the DRU joint.

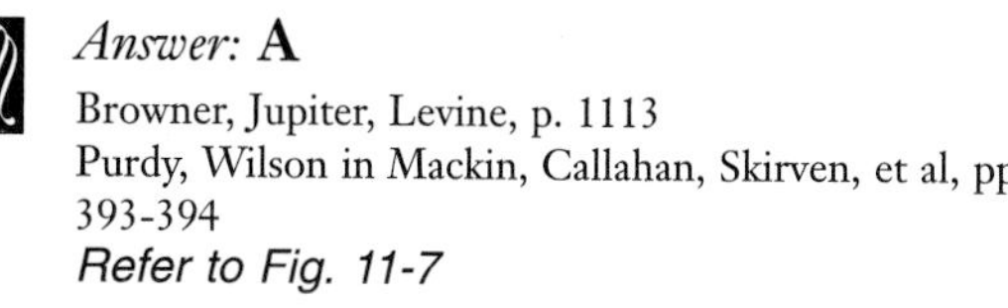

Answer: **A**
Browner, Jupiter, Levine, p. 1113
Purdy, Wilson in Mackin, Callahan, Skirven, et al, pp. 393-394
Refer to Fig. 11-7

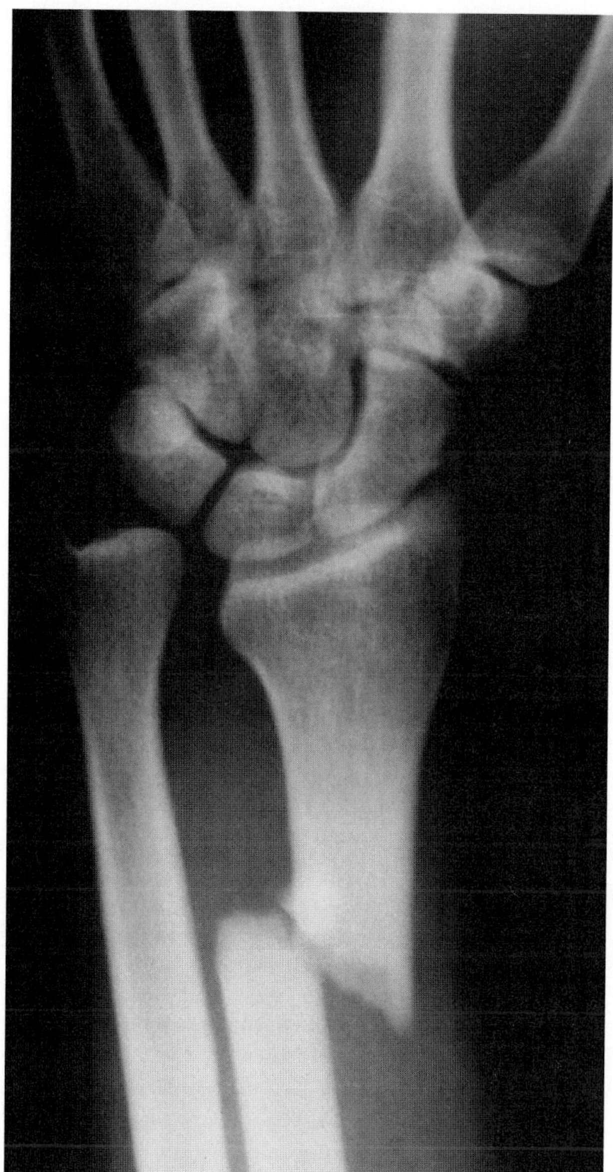

Fig. 11-7 ■ From Cooney WP, Linscheid RL, Dobyns JH: *The wrist: diagnosis and operative treatment*, St Louis, 1998, Mosby.

26. A Monteggia lesion is which of the following?

A. Fracture of the radius and ulna at the same level
B. Fracture of the proximal ulna with dislocation of the radial head
C. Radial head fracture with dislocation
D. Fracture of the distal radius shaft with disruption of the DRU joint

A Monteggia lesion is a fracture of the proximal ulna with dislocation of the radial head (see Fig. 9-10).

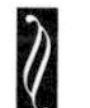

Answer: **B**
Browner, Jupiter, Levine, p. 1117

27. True or False: Boxer's fractures can be treated by the physician with the Jahss maneuver.

A boxer's fracture is a fracture of the metacarpal neck, primarily of the ring and small digits. Metacarpal neck fractures are the most common of all the metacarpal fractures. The Jahss maneuver is used to reduce a fracture of the metacarpal neck. To perform the maneuver, the metaphalangeal (MP) joint is flexed to 90 degrees, and an upward pressure is exerted while using the proximal phalanx on the metacarpal head. Most boxer's fractures are treated with closed reduction and splint immobilization for 3 to 4 weeks.

Answer: **True**

Jebson, Kasdan, pp. 159-160
McNemar, Howell, Chang, pp. 147-148

28. The central slip and the lateral bands work together to do which of the following?

A. Flex the PIP joint
B. Extend the PIP joint
C. Flex and extend the PIP joint
D. Flex the MCP joint

An intricate part of fracture management is tendon gliding. Exercises are performed to prevent adhesions and regain joint motion. After a proximal phalanx fracture, achieving 0 to 40 degrees of motion in the initial 4 weeks after injury is important. When the PIP joint is flexed, the central tendon initiates extension, and the lateral bands work more at the end of PIP joint extension.

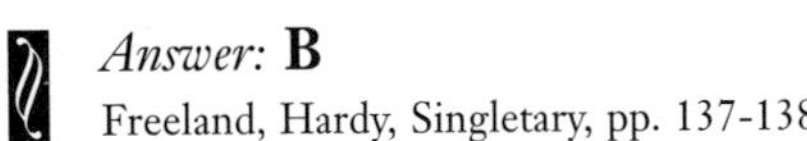

Answer: **B**

Freeland, Hardy, Singletary, pp. 137-138

29. The term *humpback deformity* refers to which of the following?

A. Displacement of the scaphoid and excessive extension at the fracture site
B. Fracture of the distal pole of the scaphoid
C. Displacement of the scaphoid with excessive flexion at the fracture site
D. Fracture of the proximal pole of the scaphoid

The scaphoid is the most commonly fractured carpal bone. A humpback deformity is noted when displacement of the scaphoid with excessive flexion at the fracture site occurs. Surgical intervention is necessary via a dorsal or volar approach to correct this deformity.

Answer: **C**

Brach, Goitz, p. 153

30. The most significant limitation for a patient suffering from a fracture of the hamate is which of the following?

A. Loss of motion
B. Loss of grip strength
C. Loss of pinch strength
D. Loss of sensation

Fractures of the hook of the hamate are the most common of hamate fractures. They occur primarily from direct trauma or crush injuries. Computed tomography (CT) scans are helpful in determining the fracture. Acute nondisplaced fractures are treated in a short arm cast, whereas displaced fractures require surgery with hook excision. Loss of grip strength is the primary limitation that these patients suffer, and this can be addressed with a strengthening program. Hypersensitivity versus loss of sensitivity caused by ulnar nerve irritation is the second most common limitation noted.

Answer: **B**

Dell, Dell in Mackin, Callahan, Skirven, et al, p. 1175
Brach, Goitz, pp. 156-157

31. True or False: Angulation is more disabling than malrotation with respect to metacarpal shaft fractures.

Malrotation can be more disabling than angulation because of the tendency for digits to overlap. Some authors have stated that for every degree of malrotation in the metacarpal there are 5 degrees of malrotation at the fingertip. As little as 5 degrees of rotation produces a 1.5-cm overlap in the fingertips on flexion.

Answer: **False**

Hunter, Mackin, Callahan, p. 368
Purdy, Wilson in Mackin, Callahan, Skirven, et al, pp. 390-391
Smith, p. 69
Refer to Fig. 11-8

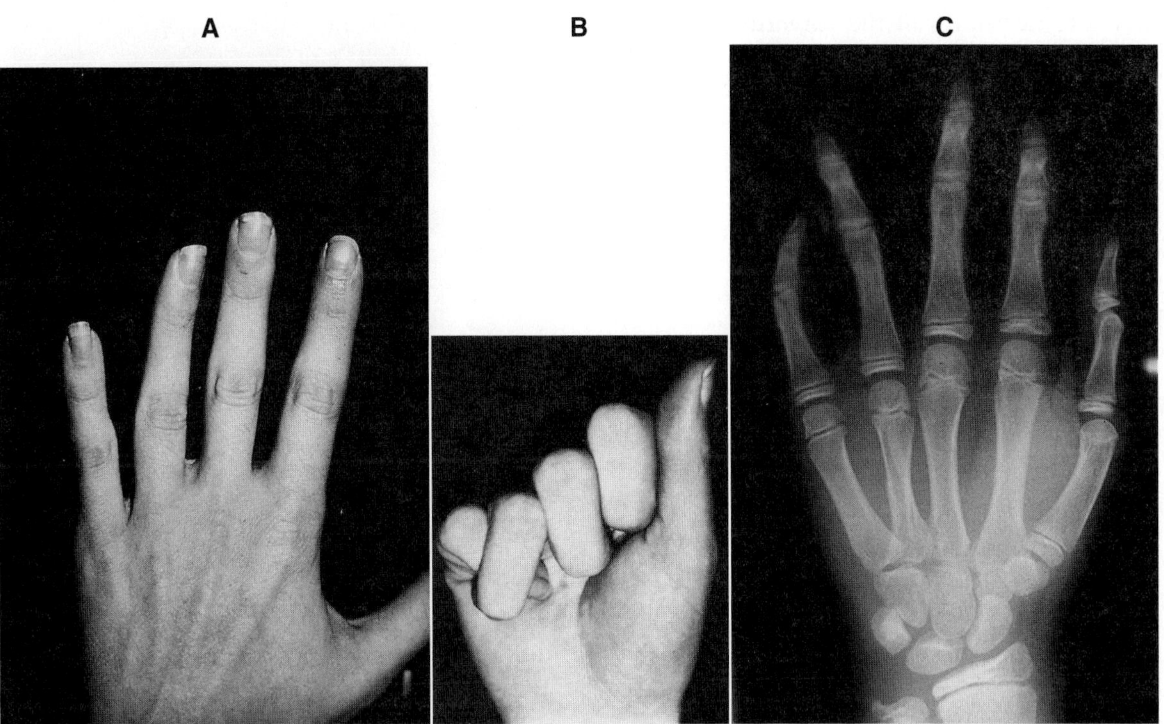

Fig. 11-8 ■ **A** and **B**, This patient had sustained a fracture of the metacarpal of the right ring finger, and insufficient attention was paid to obtaining the correct rotational alignment. This resulted in a deformity functionally and cosmetically unsatisfactory to the patient and embarrassing for the surgeon. **C**, Although the spiral fracture of the fourth metacarpal is not easily seen, the entirely unsatisfactory rotation in the finger can be readily appreciated. This must be corrected. (From Smith P: *Lister's The hand: diagnosis and indications*, ed 4, London, 2003, Churchill Livingstone.)

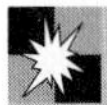

CLINICAL GEM:
When assessing malrotation, examine the patient's nails. If the nail bed is not facing up, malrotation of the digit has occurred.

32. A volar MCP joint capsulectomy is appropriate for all but which of the following diagnoses?

A. Intrinsic muscle contractures
B. Dupuytren's contracture
C. Prolonged immobilization
D. Extension contracture

A capsulectomy is surgical removal of a capsule; a capsulotomy involves cutting into the capsule. Some authors use these terms interchangeably. Volar MCP joint capsulectomies are performed less frequently than dorsal MCP capsulectomies because flexion contractures at the MCP joint level are less common than extensor contractures. Common diagnoses that require volar capsulectomy include long-standing intrinsic muscle contractures, Volkmann's contracture, Dupuytren's contracture, crush injuries, spasticity, prolonged immobilization, soft-tissue contractures along the volar surface of the MCP joints, and burst injuries to the palm. Postoperative therapy—including edema and pain management, ROM exercises, splinting, and therapeutic modalities—should be initiated within 24 hours after surgery. Splinting of choice is with the MCP joints in full extension for 4 to 6 weeks to maintain gains in surgery. Extension contractures are more common and are treated with dorsal MCP joint capsulectomies. Additional common diagnoses that require dorsal MCP joint capsulectomy are metacarpal fractures, proximal phalanx fractures, crush injuries, nerve palsies, Volkmann's contracture, burns, and Colles' fracture with secondary stiffness.

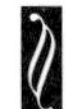

Answer: **D**

Hunter, Mackin, Callahan, pp. 1173-1174, 1185
Cannon in Mackin, Callahan, Skirven, et al, p. 1073

33. After a crush injury of the forearm, a patient develops severe forearm pain, exquisite forearm muscle tenderness, and excruciating pain with passive stretching of the fingers and wrist. The most concerning diagnosis is which of the following?

A. Compartment syndrome
B. Reflex sympathetic dystrophy (RSD)
C. Tendonitis
D. Fictitious lymphedema

Compartment syndrome after crush injury commonly presents with pain during passive stretch, tenderness over involved muscle, sensory deficits, and weakness. Compartment syndromes can be caused by traumatic insults and crush injuries and can occur after postischemic reperfusion (refill of blood to an area previously lacking blood).

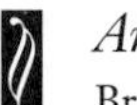

Answer: **A**

Browner, Jupiter, Levine, pp. 289-298
Hunter, Mackin, Callahan, p. 967
Taras, Lemel, Nathan in Mackin, Callahan, Skirven, et al, p. 887

34. The treatment for compartment syndrome is which of the following?

A. Pain medication
B. Evaluation of the extremity
C. Sympathetic block
D. Fasciotomy
E. Custom pressure garments

Fasciotomy, on an urgent basis, is indicated for compartment syndrome. Compartment pressure measurement may be beneficial to determine whether release is warranted, but clinical evaluation often provides enough evidence. Normal tissue pressure is between 8 and 10 mm Hg. Critical pressures are noted at levels of 30 to 45 mm Hg.

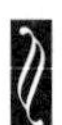

Answer: **D**

Browner, Jupiter, Levine, pp. 285-289, 297-298
Hunter, Mackin, Callahan, p. 967
Taras, Lemel, Nathan in Mackin, Callahan, Skirven, et al, p. 887
Refer to Fig. 11-9

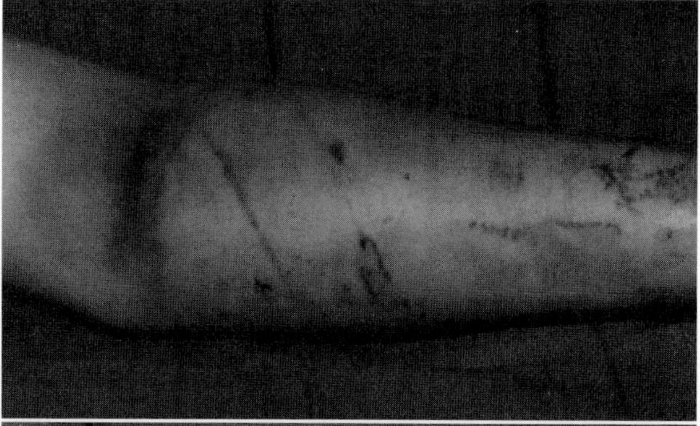

A

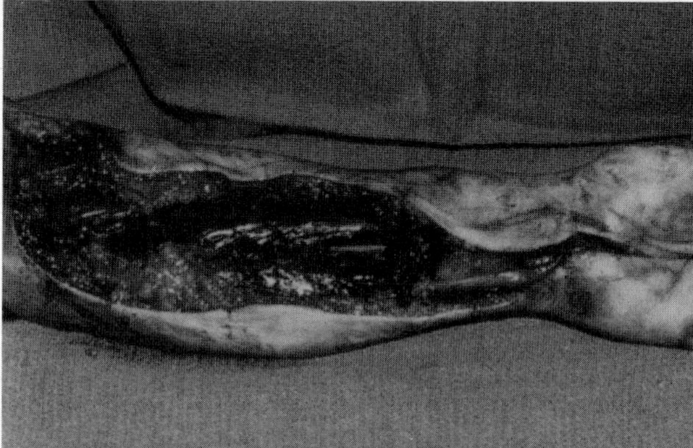

B

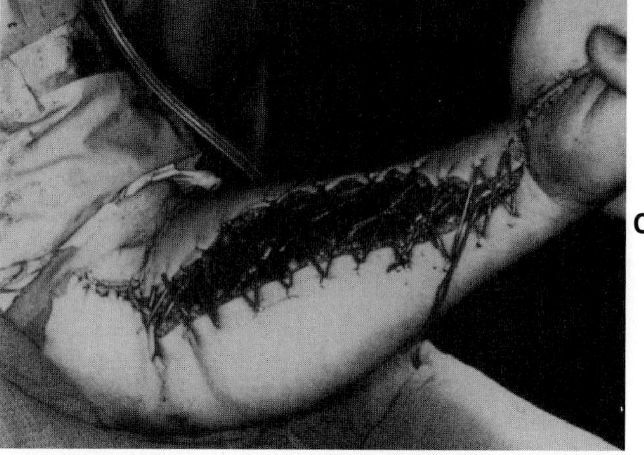

C

Fig. 11-9 ■ **A,** This young woman developed compartment syndrome after an accident in which her car rolled over and pinned her forearm. **B,** Fasciotomy was performed. **C,** After the swelling receded, the wound was approximated by using vessel loops stapled to the skin edges. (From Mackin EJ, Callahan AD, Skirven TM, et al: *Rehabilitation of the hand and upper extremity*, ed 5, St Louis, 2002, Mosby.)

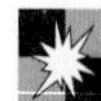

CLINICAL GEM:
The four *P*s for compartment syndrome include *p*ain with passive stretch, *p*aresthesias, *p*allor (pale), and *p*ulselessness.

35. Which structure is most likely to be injured with a dorsal dislocation of the PIP joint?

A. Central slip
B. Volar plate
C. Transverse retinacular ligament
D. Terminal tendon

Dorsal dislocations of the PIP joint usually occur because of hyperextension stress injuries, which result in volar plate damage. These often occur with ball-handling sports. There are three grades of dorsal dislocation injuries.

Answer: **B**
Green, pp. 769-770
Hunter, Mackin, Callahan, p. 383
Smith, Price in Mackin, Callahan, Skirven, et al, p. 339
Purdy, Wilson in Mackin, Callahan, Skirven, et al, pp. 389-399

36. You are treating a patient who is referred to you with a grade two PIP joint dorsal dislocation from a football injury. Orders are to splint, evaluate, and treat. Which splint will you apply to this patient?

A. Dorsal finger splint or figure 8 splint in 20 to 30 degrees of PIP joint flexion
B. Dorsal finger or figure 8 splint in 50 degrees of PIP joint flexion
C. Dorsal finger splint or figure 8 splint in 0 degrees of PIP joint flexion
D. A splint is not indicated for this injury.

Most dorsal dislocations—as well as fracture dislocations of the PIP joint—are treated nonoperatively. For a grade-two injury (Fig. 11-10, *A*), immobilization should be in a dorsal splint (Fig. 11-10, *B*) or a figure 8 splint (Fig. 11-11) with 20 to 30 degrees of PIP joint flexion for approximately 7 to 14 days. It is important not to immobilize the PIP joint in too much flexion because this will predispose the joint to the development of a flexion contracture. After immobilization, the finger can be taped to an adjacent finger (buddy taping) for additional protection while active exercises are initiated. It is not unusual to have stiffness and swelling for months after this injury.

Grade-one injuries can be treated in slight flexion until acute pain subsides. Grade-three injuries are treated conservatively as grade-two injuries, unless reduction is not maintained. Surgery is indicated in irreducible dislocations.

Answer: **A**
Green, p. 771
Hunter, Mackin, Callahan, p. 383
Smith, Price in Mackin, Callahan, Skirven, et al, pp. 339-343
Levin, Moorman, Heller in Mackin, Callahan, Skirven, et al, pp. 344-356
Nathan, Taras in Mackin, Callahan, Skirven, et al, pp. 359-368
Krop in Mackin, Callahan, Skirven, et al, pp. 371-381
Purdy, Wilson in Mackin, Callahan, Skirven, et al, pp. 382-395
Campbell, Wilson in Mackin, Callahan, Skirven, et al, pp. 396-402

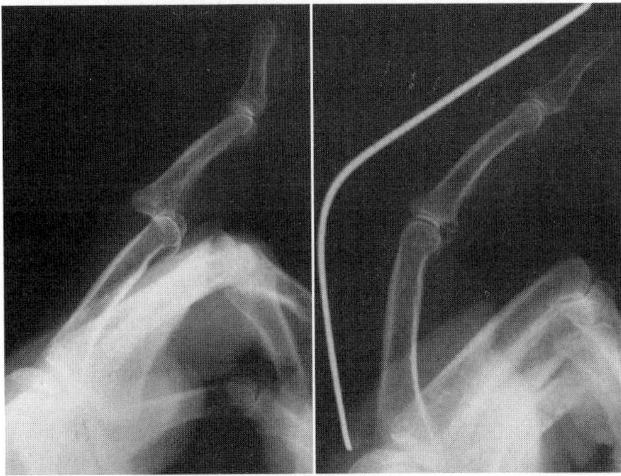

Fig. 11-10 ■ **A** and **B** From Hunter JM, Mackin EJ, Callahan AD: *Rehabilitation of the hand: surgery and therapy,* ed 4, St Louis, 1995, Mosby.

37. True or False: When a patient sustains a stable midshaft metacarpal fracture, it is important to immobilize the MCP joint and the wrist.

Not long ago, immobilization of the joint above and below a fracture was required for treatment of fractures with a closed reduction treatment technique. Currently, whenever possible, we immobilize only the fracture and mobilize the adjacent joints as well as the musculotendinous units. In this case, mobilization of the MCP joint and the wrist is acceptable while protecting the fracture site. This early motion, in addition to maintaining joint function, helps to prevent adhesions between the fracture callus and adjacent tendons. Early motion is an important aspect of fracture care to prevent fracture disease and obtain optimal results.

Answer: **False**
Freeland, Jabaley, Hughes, p. 12

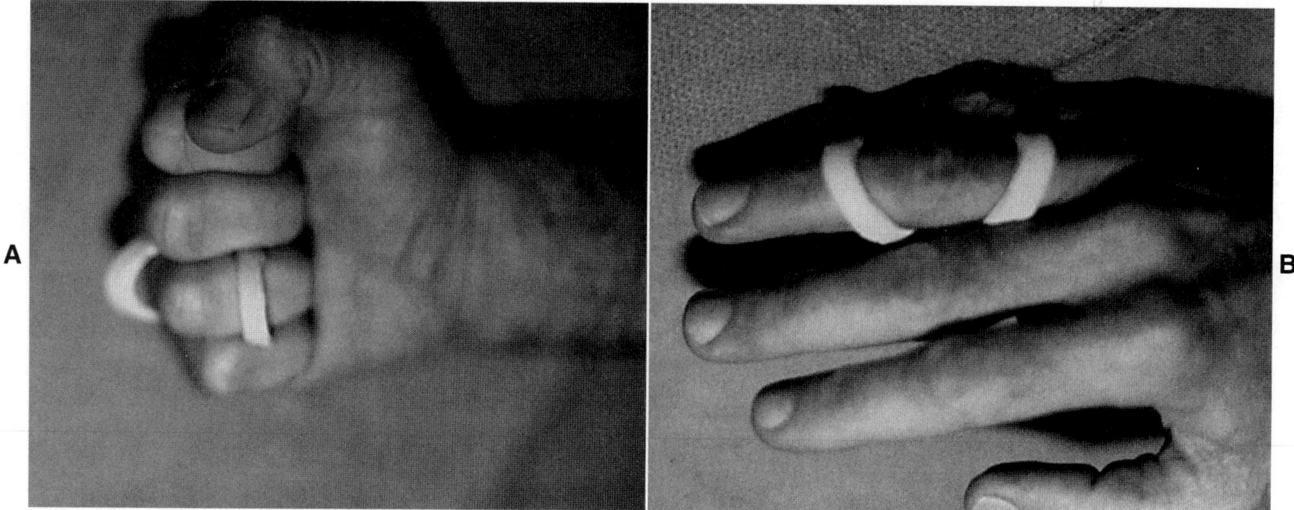

Fig. 11-11 ■ **A** and **B,** This is a figure 8 splint, which positions the finger with 20 to 30 degrees of flexion while allowing full flexion of the digit. (From Mackin EJ, Callahan AD, Skirven TM, et al: *Rehabilitation of the hand and upper extremity*, ed 5, St Louis, 2002, Mosby.)

38. You are treating a patient who is referred to you after a proximal phalanx fracture. The fracture has been fixed internally with mini plates and screws and is considered absolutely stable by the physician. When should ROM begin?

A. In 24 to 72 hours
B. In 7 to 10 days
C. In 2 weeks
D. In 3 to 4 weeks

For a proximal phalanx fracture that has been internally fixed with absolute stability, the patient should be referred to therapy for ROM within 24 to 72 hours after surgery. Of primary concern for the therapist is managing edema, increasing PIP joint mobility, and avoiding PIP joint flexion contracture. Active and passive ROM exercises are performed regularly. A digital extension splint should be worn in between exercise sessions. If absolute fracture stability has not been achieved, active and passive ROM should not be performed immediately. Absolute fracture stability often is not obtained with ORIF. In these cases, ROM can be initiated as soon as 3 to 7 days if sufficient stabilization is obtained; the doctor will give the therapist insight regarding the patient's fracture stability.

Answer: **A**
Hunter, Mackin, Callahan, p. 366
Purdy, Wilson in Mackin, Callahan, Skirven, et al, p. 388

39. Fractures to the _____________ are the second most fractured carpal bone.

A. Triquetrum
B. Capitate
C. Trapezoid
D. Trapezium

The triquetrium is the second most commonly fractured carpal bone. The most commonly fractured carpal bone is the scaphoid. The trapezoid is the least commonly fractured carpal bone. Fractures of the triquetrium usually occur with other fractures of the carpal bones or with distal radius fracture injury. Treatment usually involves cast immobilization for 6 weeks.

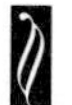
Answer: **A**
Jebson, Kasdan, p. 151
Clark, Wilgis, Aiello, p. 318
Brach, Goitz, p. 157

40. Fifty percent of hand fractures occur in which sport?

A. Men's basketball
B. Men's football
C. Women's basketball
D. Men's wrestling

Sports-related injuries cause many hand fractures. The injuries range from very simple sprains to fractures. Many are treated with splinting and/or return to play with protective devices. The more serious injuries require surgical intervention and reduction in the individual's playing time. Men's football accounts for 50% of all hand injuries in sports-related injuries.

Answer: **B**

Singletary, Freeland, Jarrett, p. 171
Wright, p. 49

41. A volarly comminuted displaced, angulated fracture of the distal radius is known as which of the following?

A. Colles' fracture
B. Smith's fracture
C. Barton's fracture
D. Chauffeur's fracture

A Smith's fracture is a reverse Colles' fracture. It is a volarly displaced, angulated fracture of the distal radius. A Colles' fracture is an extraarticular fracture with dorsal comminution, dorsal displacement, radial shortening, and dorsal angulation of the distal radius. A Barton's fracture is a displaced and unstable fracture subluxation of the distal radius with the carpus. A chauffeur's fracture is a fracture of the radial styloid.

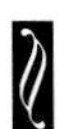

Answer: **B**

Laseter in Mackin, Callahan, Skirven, et al, p. 1137
Jebson, Kasdan, pp. 126-127

42. A 20-year-old who fell while rollerblading suffered a Type II fracture of the radial head. What would be the appropriate care?

A. Long arm cast for 4 weeks and then therapy
B. Long arm splint for two to 3 weeks and then therapy
C. Fragment excision and then long arm cast for 3 weeks
D. Fragment excision and then long arm splint for 3 weeks

There are three types of radial head fractures. Type I is treated nonoperatively with a sling or a long arm splint for 1 to 4 days, and motion is begun as pain decreases and the patient is able to tolerate motion. Type II fractures are also treated nonoperatively with a long arm splint for 2 to 3 weeks, especially if displacement occurred. With the elbow at 90 degrees of flexion and the forearm and wrist in neutral, sometimes range of motion is initiated sooner. Type III is sometimes treated with fragment excision, followed with a long arm cast or splint for up to 3 weeks with the elbow in 90 degrees of flexion, forearm in midpronation, and the wrist in neutral.

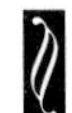

Answer: **B**

Dávila in Mackin, Callahan, Skirven, et al, p. 1237
Morrey, 2000, p. 345
Refer to Fig. 11-12

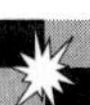

CLINICAL GEM:
Treatment of Type II radial head fractures is controversial.

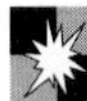

CLINICAL GEM:
The following is a quick reference chart for ROM initiation after fracture fixation:

Fracture fixation	Initiation of ROM
Absolute stability	24 to 72 hours
Sufficient stability	3 to 7 days
Minimal stability	3 to 6 weeks

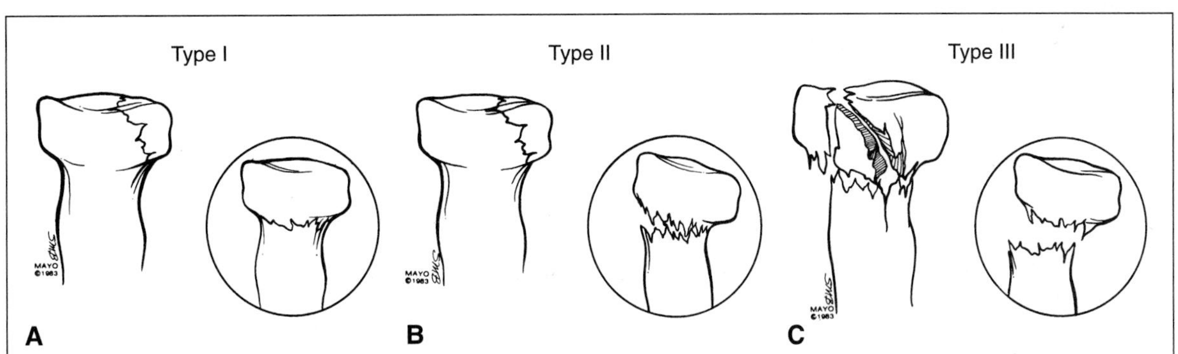

Fig. 11-12 ■ **A** to **C**, Recommended classification of uncomplicated radial head fractures. The exact definition of the Type II fracture is often difficult to determine. Type IV is not included because it represents a complicated fracture. (From Morrey BF: *The elbow and its disorders*, ed 3, Philadelphia, 2000, WB Saunders.)

43. Gamekeeper's thumb involves an injury to which of the following structures?

A. Volar plate of the thumb
B. Radial collateral ligament
C. Ulnar collateral ligament
D. None of the above

Injury to the ulnar collateral ligament occurs when the thumb is forced into radial deviation. This injury has been termed "skier's thumb" and/or "gamekeeper's thumb." If the ulnar collateral ligament is torn completely from the proximal phalanx, it may become situated superficial to the adductor aponeurosis, in which case it would be termed a *Stener's lesion* (Fig. 11-13). When this occurs, no contact between the ligament and its normal insertion exists, and appropriate healing is prevented.

Answer: **C**
Hunter, Mackin, Callahan, pp. 389-390
Campbell, Wilson in Mackin, Callahan, Skirven, et al, pp. 406–407

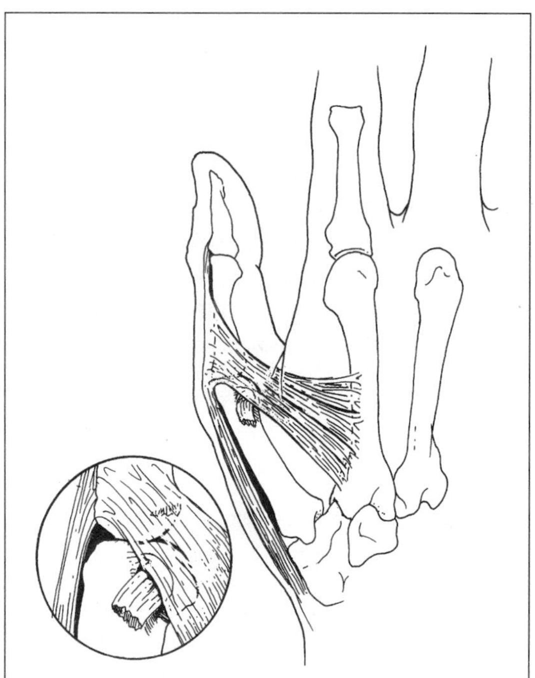

Fig. 11-13 ■ Diagram and enlargement of the Stener's lesion. A hyperabduction force results in complete rupture of the ulnar collateral ligament at its distal insertion, with displacement proximally. The adductor aponeurosis blocks the ligament from returning to its insertion site, thus preventing adequate healing. (From Mackin EJ, Callahan AD, Skirven TM, et al: *Rehabilitation of the hand and upper extremity*, ed 5, St Louis, 2002, Mosby.)

44. Treatment for a Stener's lesion consists of which of the following?

A. Splinting with the thumb in slight flexion for 2 weeks
B. Continuous immobilization of the thumb for 4 weeks
C. Surgical repair by direct attachment of the ligament
D. All of the above

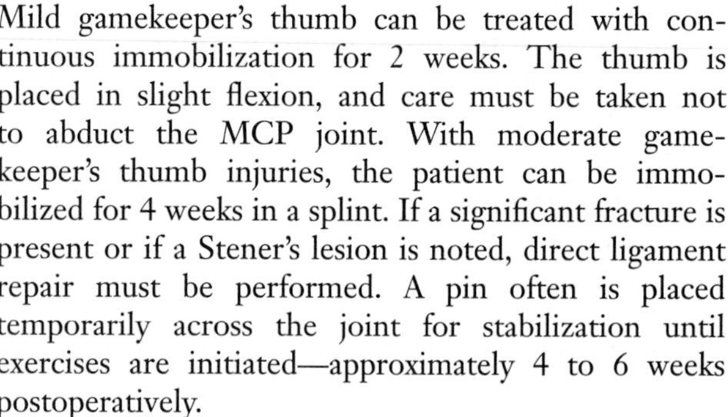

Mild gamekeeper's thumb can be treated with continuous immobilization for 2 weeks. The thumb is placed in slight flexion, and care must be taken not to abduct the MCP joint. With moderate gamekeeper's thumb injuries, the patient can be immobilized for 4 weeks in a splint. If a significant fracture is present or if a Stener's lesion is noted, direct ligament repair must be performed. A pin often is placed temporarily across the joint for stabilization until exercises are initiated—approximately 4 to 6 weeks postoperatively.

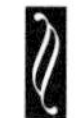

Answer: **C**
Hunter, Mackin, Callahan, p. 390
Campbell, Wilson in Mackin, Callahan, Skirven, et al, p. 407
Refer to Fig. 11-13

CLINICAL GEM:
A tip pinch should be avoided until 8 weeks after gamekeeper's surgery, when progressive resistive exercises are permitted.

45. What thumb fracture occurs through the beak (base) of the metacarpal, with the intact oblique ulnar ligament stabilizing the small fracture fragment? The metacarpal shaft is displaced proximally because of the strong muscle and tendon attached to it.

A. Rolando's
B. Chauffeur's
C. Bennett's
D. None of the above

A Bennett's fracture (Fig. 11-14, *A*) occurs at the beak (base) of the first metacarpal. The result is a bony failure rather than a ligament disruption. The ulnar oblique ligament remains intact while the metacarpal shaft is displaced by the forces of the abductor pollicis longus, extrinsic thumb extensors, and adductor pollicis. Bennett's fractures can be treated with closed reduction and casting for 4 weeks, closed reduction with percutaneous pinning, or ORIF.

A Rolando's fracture is a comminuted intraarticular fracture at the first metacarpal base (Fig. 11-14, *B*). The mechanism of injury is similar to that of a Bennett's fracture. Accurate and anatomic reduction and stable fixation often are impossible because of the many small fragments in this fracture. Treatment options for Rolando's fractures include reduction with cast for 7 to 10 days—followed by early ROM, skeletal traction, or internal fixation for fracture fragments greater than 30% of the articular surface.

Answer: **C**
Hunter, Mackin, Callahan, p. 392
Campbell, Wilson in Mackin, Callahan, Skirven, et al, p. 409

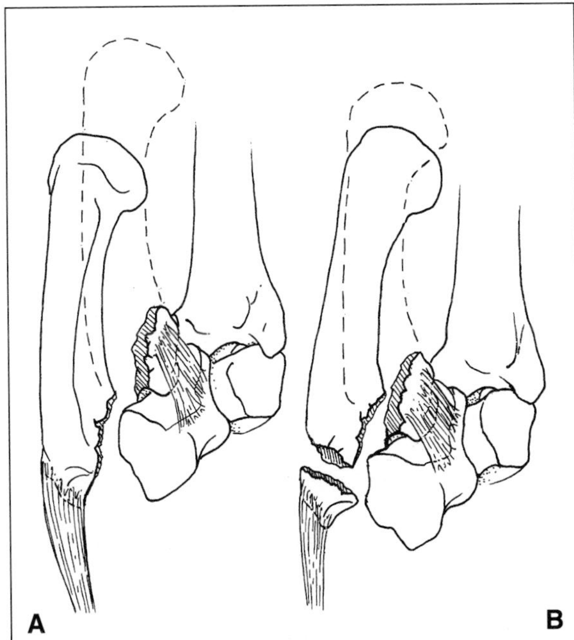

Fig. 11-14 ■ **A**, Bennett's fracture. The fracture occurs through the beak of the metacarpal, with the intact ulnar oblique ligament stabilizing the small fragment. The metacarpal shaft is displaced proximally secondary to the strong muscle and tendon attachments. **B**, Rolando's fracture. This is a T- or Y-shaped intraarticular fracture, which often has even more comminution than is shown here. (From Mackin EJ, Callahan AD, Skirven TM, et al: *Rehabilitation of the hand and upper extremity*, ed 5, St Louis, 2002, Mosby.)

46. A reverse Bennett's fracture describes a fracture at the base of which of the following?

A. First metacarpal
B. Second metacarpal
C. Third metacarpal
D. Fourth metacarpal
E. Fifth metacarpal

A fracture dislocation at the base of the fifth metacarpal is analogous to a Bennett's fracture of the thumb and is termed a *reversed Bennett's fracture*. These fractures tend to be unstable and displace in a manner similar to Bennett's fractures and cause similar functional impairment. The principal dangers of not reducing this fracture dislocation are loss of grip strength and painful arthritis. These fractures often can be managed with closed reduction and percutaneous pinning, but if satisfactory reduction cannot be achieved, open reduction should be performed.

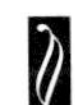
Answer: **E**
Freeland, Jabaley, Hughes, p. 45
Refer to Fig. 11-15

47. Which is the least commonly injured carpal bone?

A. Trapezium
B. Pisiform
C. Hamate
D. Trapezoid

The trapezoid (carpal bone) is tightly positioned between the base of the second metacarpal, capitate, scaphoid, and trapezium; therefore it is the least commonly injured carpal bone; injury of this bone accounts for fewer than 1% of all carpal injuries. When this bone is injured, it typically is from a high-energy, axially directed force through the index metacarpal base.

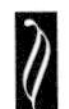
Answer: **D**
Cohen, p. 595
Refer to Fig. 11-16

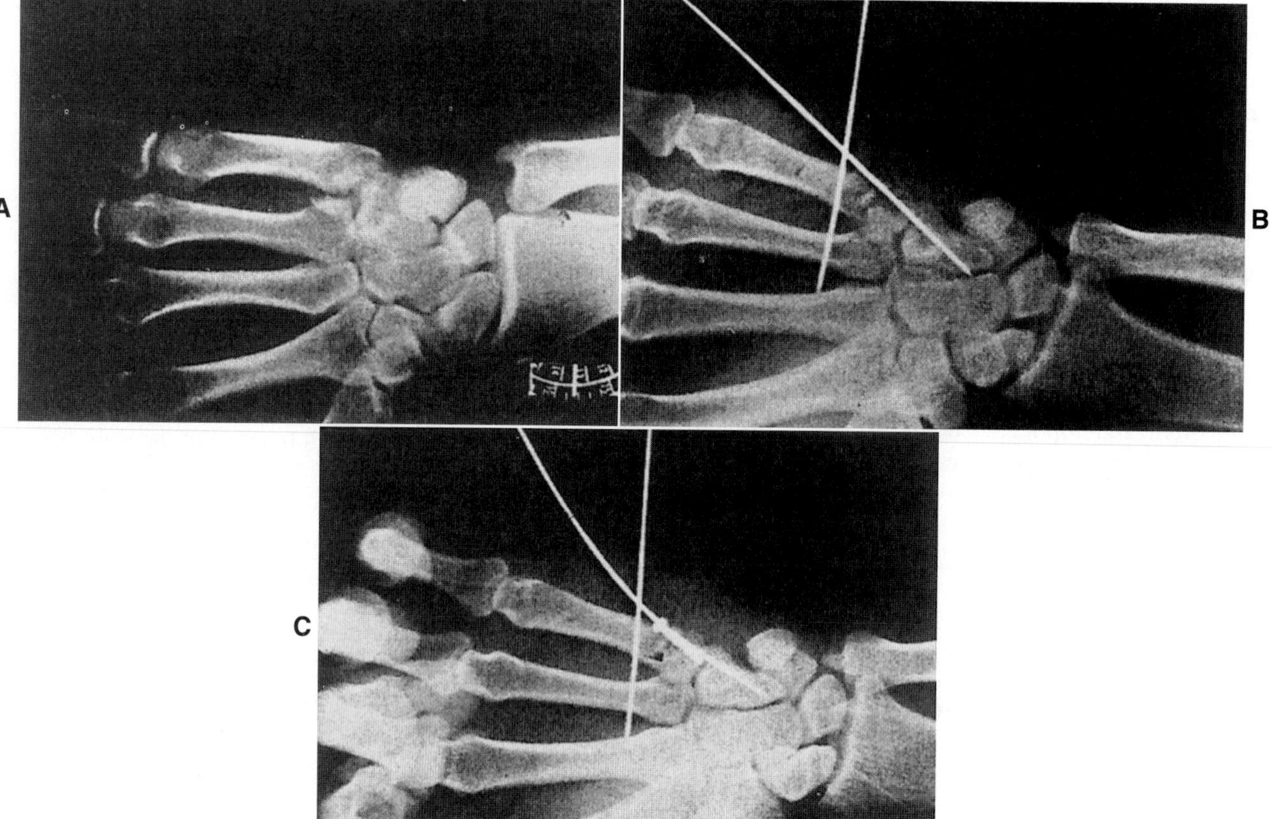

Fig. 11-15 ■ **A,** This is a pronated lateral view of a reverse Bennett's fracture of the base of the fifth metacarpal. **B,** Open reduction and temporary fixation with Kirschner wires were performed. **C,** After ensuring anatomic reduction, the fracture was secured with a 2.0-mm cortical lag screw. (From Freeland AE, Jabaley ME: Management of hand fractures by stable fixation. In Habal MB: *Advances in plastic and reconstructive surgery*, vol 2, Yearbook Medical Publishers, 1986, Chicago.)

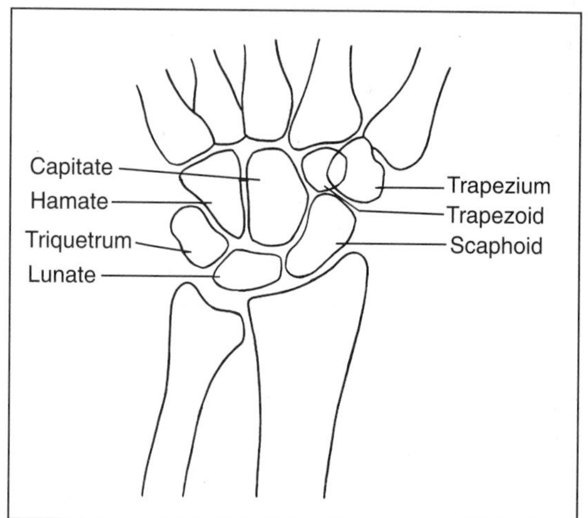

Fig. 11-16 ■ From Hunter JM, Mackin EJ, Callahan AD: *Rehabilitation of the hand: surgery and therapy*, ed 4, St Louis, 1995, Mosby.

48. Which carpal bone fracture is associated with racquet sports?

A. Hamate
B. Capitate
C. Trapezoid
D. Trapezium

The hamate is involved in 2% to 4% of carpal bone fractures. The hook of the hamate protrudes off the hamate into the base of the hypothenar eminence. Hamate hook fractures most commonly occur in people involved in sports that use a racquet or clubs (e.g., golf, baseball, racquetball, tennis). When a forceful swing is performed, the base of the club can impinge against the hook of the hamate, thus causing a fracture. The acute injury often is not recognized; the patient presents late with chronic pain at the base of the hypothenar eminence, weakness of grip, and occasional numbness in the ulnar nerve distribution (see Fig. 11-16).

Answer: **A**
Cohen, p. 591

49. Which of the following is *not* true about Kirschner wires (K wires)?

A. They are easier to use than mini fragment plates and screws.
B. They can be placed with minimal soft-tissue dissection.
C. They can be placed percutaneously (through the skin).
D. They provide compression if applied correctly.

Kirschner wires have many advantages when they are used for fracture fixation. They are readily available, easier to use than mini fragment plates and screws, can be placed with minimal soft-tissue dissection, and can be placed percutaneously. A disadvantage of Kirschner wires is that they do not provide sufficient compression and if applied incorrectly can actually maintain distraction. They also do not provide rigid internal fixation, which can preclude early motion.

Answer: **D**
Hunter, Mackin, Callahan, p. 357
Krop in Mackin, Callahan, Skirven, et al, pp. 377-380
Refer to Fig. 11-17

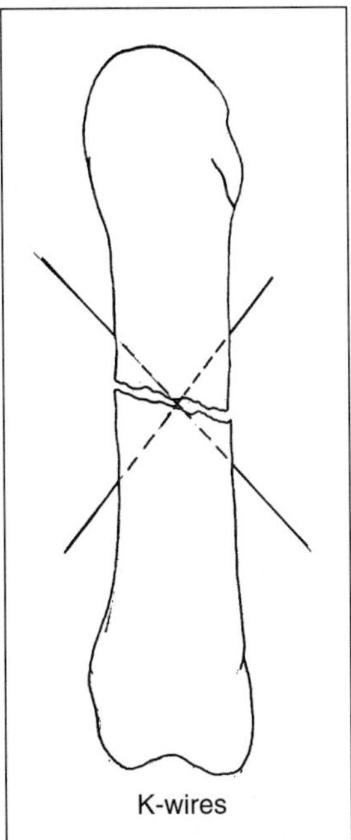

Fig. 11-17 ■ From Mackin EJ, Callahan AD, Skirven TM, et al: *Rehabilitation of the hand and upper extremity*, ed 5, St Louis, 2002, Mosby.

50. Match each of the following fracture stabilization techniques with its advantages:

Stabilization Technique

1. External fixation
2. Plate and screws
3. Intramedullary device
4. Kirschner pins

Advantages

A. Rigid fixation restores and maintains length
B. Readily available, versatile, easy to insert, requires minimal dissection
C. Preserves length and allows access to bone and soft tissue through percutaneous insertion; direct manipulation of the fracture is avoided
D. No special equipment required; easy to insert; no pins protrude; requires minimal dissection

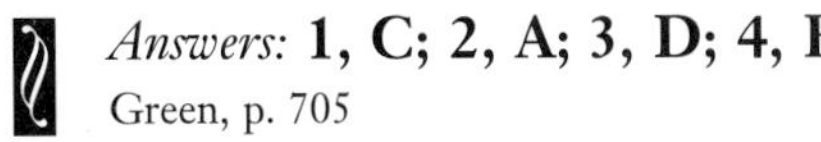

Answers: **1, C; 2, A; 3, D; 4, B**
Green, p. 705

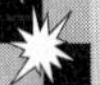

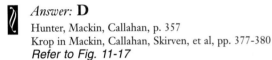

CLINICAL GEM:
Disadvantages and therapeutic management of stabilization techniques include the following:

- Kirschner pins: Lack rigidity, may loosen, may distract the fracture, cause pin tract infections, and require external support. Therapist *cannot* begin immediate active ROM because of lack of absolute stability.
- Intramedullary device: Characterized by rotational instability and rod migration (e.g., rush rod used for humeral fractures). Therapists may begin pendulum exercises within the first week of rush rod fixation.
- Plate and screws: Technically challenging, require special equipment, require extensive exposure, and may require subsequent removal. If absolute stability is obtained, immediate ROM is initiated; however, if sufficient stability is obtained, active ROM commences at 3 to 7 days.
- External fixation: Characterized by pin tract infections, osteomyelitis, overdistraction, nonunion, neurovascular injuries, and loosening of the device. ROM can be initiated immediately to surrounding joints.

51. After a segmental radius shaft fracture is plated through a volar approach, a patient experiences weakened wrist, finger, and thumb extension. The structure most likely involved is which of the following?

A. Anterior interosseous nerve
B. Radial nerve
C. Posterior interosseous nerve
D. Antebrachial cutaneous nerve

The posterior interosseous nerve, a branch of the radial nerve, enters the forearm through the arcade of Frohse and the supinator muscle. This nerve is at risk with volar and dorsal surgical approaches to the forearm. Answer B is incorrect because the radial nerve is called the *posterior interosseous nerve* after it enters the forearm.

Answer: **C**
Hoppenfeld, deBoer, pp. 121, 123, 136

52. After a volar surgical approach for plating of a distal radial shaft fracture, you notice that your patient has no function of the flexor pollicis longus or FDP to the index and long finger, but sensation is normal. The structure most likely involved is which of the following?

A. Posterior interosseous nerve
B. Median nerve
C. Anterior interosseous nerve
D. Common flexor tendon

The anterior interosseous nerve, a branch of the median nerve, is the motor nerve to the flexor pollicis longus, FDP of the index and long fingers, and pronator quadratus. This nerve may be damaged during surgical intervention to stabilize distal radius fractures (see Fig. 18-21, question 44).

Answer: **C**
Hoppenfeld, deBoer, p. 124

53. An elderly patient falls and sustains a nondisplaced humeral neck fracture. What is the most probable course of treatment?

A. Sling use with supervised ROM exercises
B. Sling secured tightly to chest for 14 to 21 days
C. ORIF
D. Intramedullary rods

Fractures of the neck of the humerus commonly are caused by falls onto outstretched arm in elderly people, primarily in women with osteoporosis. Early motion is the most desirable course of treatment, and the length of immobilization will be determined on the severity of the injury. A nondisplaced fracture of the neck of the humerus is treated in a sling with removal for exercise. Displaced fractures require complete immobilization for approximately 14 to 21 days. If surgical intervention were needed, further immobilization would be indicated.

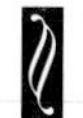
Answer: **A**
Donatelli, p. 451

54. ROM has reached a plateau after working with a patient after a distal radius fracture. Which treatment would you choose?

A. Static splinting
B. Biofeedback
C. Static progressive splinting
D. None of the above; the patient has reached a plateau with therapy

Static progressive splinting should be considered when the loss of motion is related to soft tissue tightness and not to bony blockage. Patient selection is important in determining the splint choice because these splints are time-consuming, may not be covered by insurance, and can be costly to fabricate.

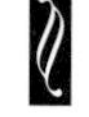
Answer: **C**
Laseter in Mackin, Callahan, Skirven, et al, pp. 1150-1151
Refer to Fig. 11-18

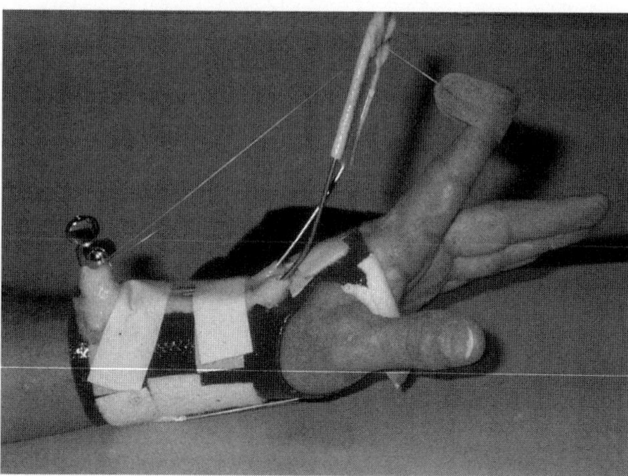

Fig. 11-18 ■ Example of a static progressive splint to gain MCP joint extension.

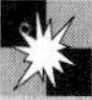

CLINICAL GEM:
Joint Active Systems has an excellent wrist device that works both flexion and extension of the wrist via static progressive splinting (Fig. 11-19).

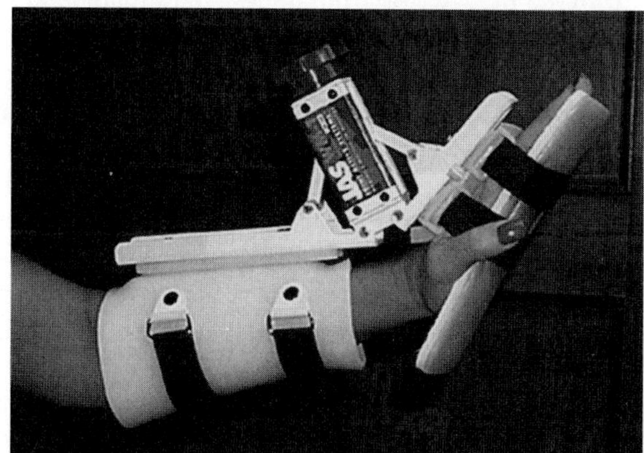

Fig. 11-19 ■ Joint Active Systems static progressive stretch splint facilitating wrist dorsiflexion; also bidirectional. (From Mackin EJ, Callahan AD, Skirven TM, et al: *Rehabilitation of the hand and upper extremity*, ed 5, St Louis, 2002, Mosby.)

55. In the adult, displaced both bone forearm shaft fractures are most often treated by which of the following?

A. Casting
B. Internal fixation with plates and screws
C. Small intramedullary rods
D. External fixation

ORIF with plates and screws is the standard treatment and gives the best results for displaced fractures of both forearm bones (i.e., radius and ulna fractures).

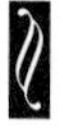

Answer: **B**
Browner, Jupiter, Levine, p. 1095
Refer to Fig. 11-20

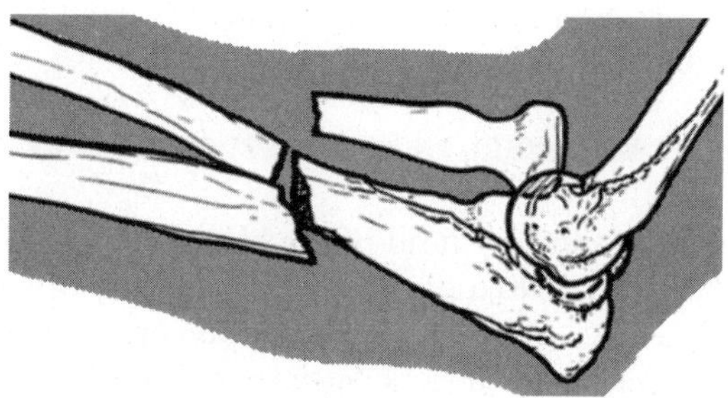

Fig. 11-20 ■ From Reckling FW: Unstable fracture-dislocation of the forearm [Monteggia and Galeazzi lesions], *J Bone Joint Surg* [Am] 64[6]:857, 1982.

56. Six months after severe both bone forearm shaft fractures are treated with ORIF, a patient has complete loss of forearm rotation both actively and passively. Bone growth between the two bones is noted on radiograph. This situation is explained by which of the following?

A. Plating of the wrong bones
B. Neurological injury to the arm
C. Dislocated DRU joint
D. Synostosis

Synostosis is a cross-union between forearm bones, usually in the middle or proximal forearm. Forearm rotation is absent. Incidence of synostosis is low, and its etiology is uncertain, but it may follow severe injury or infection and it can also be congenital.

Answer: **D**
Browner, Jupiter, Levine, p. 1121
Green, p. 488
Ezaki, Kay, Light, et al, in Green, Hotchkiss, Pederson, p. 490
Refer to Fig. 11-21

57. A 35-year-old male carpenter sustains an oblique fracture of the proximal phalanx of his dominant index finger. Methods of fracture fixation commonly employed for this fracture include which of the following?

A. Percutaneous transverse pin fixation
B. Cross K-wires
C. ORIF with mini fragment screws
D. K-wire fixation with supplemental interosseous wiring
E. A, B, and C
F. All of the above

Multiple techniques commonly are employed in the fixation of fractures of phalanges in the hand. All of the above techniques could be used to correct this oblique proximal phalanx fracture. Transverse and short oblique fractures often are treated with ORIF. The fracture pattern and the surgeon's experience with a given technique may determine the choice of fixation used.

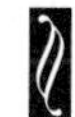

Answer: **F**
McCollister, pp. 350-352

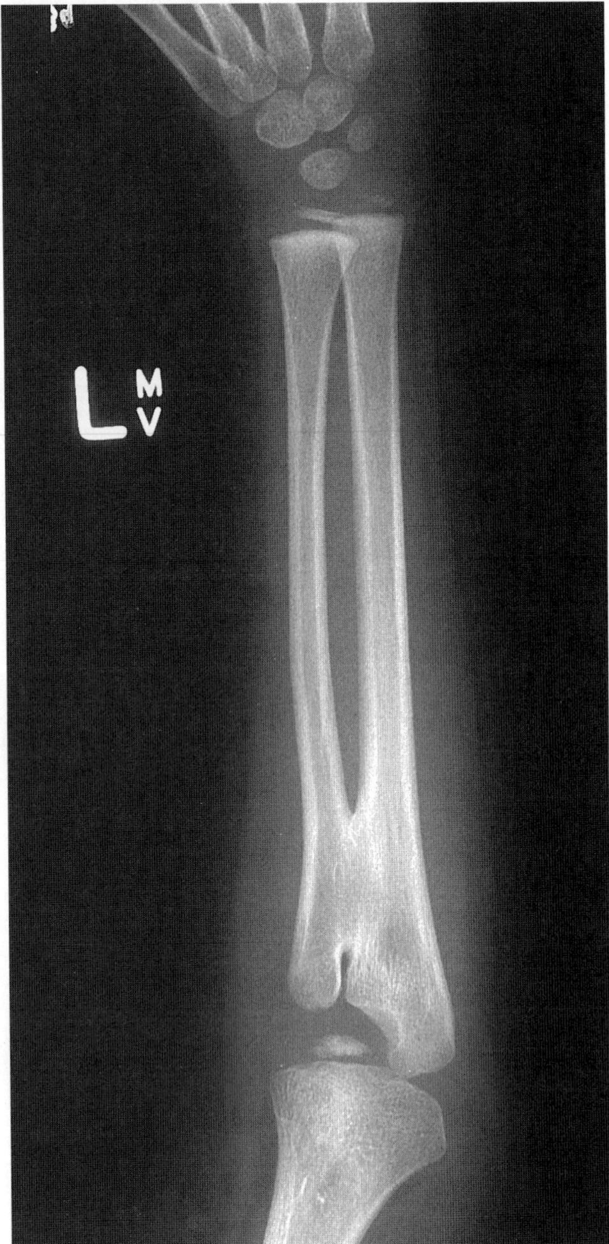

Fig. 11-21 ■ From Green DP, Hotchkiss RN, Pederson WC: *Green's Operative hand surgery*, ed 4, New York, 1999, Churchill Livingstone.

58. A patient you treated 6 months ago and discharged visits your clinic and complains of difficulty with flexing his ring finger fully over the past week. Initially, he underwent ORIF 1 year ago for a comminuted interarticular fracture. When he was discharged from therapy he had excellent ROM. Your quick assessment reveals intact superficial flexors, but absence of DIP joint flexion of the ring finger. The most appropriate treatment is which of the following?

A. Have the patient call his doctor to schedule a follow-up appointment in a few weeks
B. Get an order for a dynamic flexion assist splint of the ring finger DIP joint
C. Get orders to try functional electrical stimulation of the profundus tendons to the hand since he is obviously scarred down
D. Call the patient's treating physician immediately and report the findings

This patient has most likely sustained an attritional rupture resulting from backing out of the screws from a distal radius T-plate. Screw backout from small fragment titanium plates is an extremely common complication. Flexor tendon injuries with acute rupture have a much more favorable prognosis if repaired within the first 10 days. Failure to report a flexor tendon injury in a timely basis may result in secondary tendon reconstruction, the possibility of primary or staged tendon grafting, and lead to otherwise avoidable multiple surgeries and a potentially less-than-favorable outcome.

Answer: **D**
Strickland in Green, Hotchkiss, Pederson, pp. 1855-1890

59. A 50-year-old construction worker presents in the physician's office with a bulge of the muscle of his left upper arm after helping a co-worker move an air conditioner. Physical examination reveals full flexion and extension of the affected arm, mild weakness with elbow flexion, and extreme weakness of supination in the left forearm. X-rays of the elbow and shoulder are normal. He is tender about the proximal shoulder. The most likely diagnosis is which of the following?

A. Radial nerve palsy
B. Axillary nerve injury
C. Rupture of the long head of the biceps proximally
D. Avulsion fracture of the radial tuberosity at the insertion of the distal biceps tendon
E. Pronator syndrome

Rupture of the long head of the biceps can be difficult to diagnose. Weakness of supination is more common than lack of elbow flexion because of normal functioning secondary flexors, such as the brachialis. The biceps tendon is one of the main supinators of the forearm.

Answer: **C**
Netter, p. 35

60. Posterior dislocation of the elbow is most commonly associated with a fracture of which of the following?

A. The coracoid
B. The tip of the olecranon
C. The medial epicondyle
D. The coronoid process
E. A Monteggia fracture

The coronoid process is commonly fractured as the olecranon is driven posteriorly in an elbow dislocation. The radial head is frequently fractured as well.

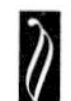
Answer: **D**
Netter, p. 42

61. A 30-year-old male presents with a fracture in the metaphyseal region of the long finger metacarpal from an enchondroma after bumping his finger. The fracture is nondisplaced but is painful. Appropriate physician treatment(s) may include which of the following?

A. Cast immobilization until the fracture heals, followed by curettage and placement of an allograft
B. Immediate injection of hyaluronic acid
C. Application of external fixator with the MCP joint at 30 degrees of flexion
D. Immediate ORIF with a small plate and screw
E. Application of an electrical stimulator

Fractures that occur after minor trauma in patients who have enchondromas will usually heal. However, correction of the enchondroma may require curettage with autogenous or allogenic bone grafting. Although steroid injections in enchondral bone cysts may be successful, most doctors wait until the fracture has healed. Immediate ORIF may be appropriate in many circumstances but requires autogenous or allogenic bone grafting at the time of curettage and internal fixation.

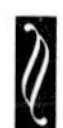
Answer: **A**
Athanasian in Green, Hotchkiss, Pederson, pp. 2233-2234

62. A 21-year-old woman sustains a traumatic mallet finger injury with an avulsion fracture involving 10% of the articular surface of the dorsal distal phalanx. Appropriate initial treatment could include which of the following?

A. Dorsal extension splinting for 2 months
B. ORIF with a longitudinal K-wire transfixing the joint
C. ORIF with indirect K-wire fixation of the fragment involving the distal phalanx
D. Dynamic traction splinting combining early active flexion and extension of the DIP joint
E. A, B, and C
F. All of the above

Treatment of a mallet finger with a bony fragment often is managed with a standard mallet program, using a dorsal extension splint for 6 to 8 weeks and allowing PIP joint ROM. If the fragment is large or substantially displaced, internal fixation often is necessary by either a direct or indirect technique. Postsurgically, the DIP joint is immobilized for 6 weeks, and active ROM is initiated when the pin is removed. Night splinting is continued for 2 to 4 weeks or pending reoccurrence of the extensor lag. Answer D, dynamic traction splinting allowing early flexion and extension, would not promote healing of the dorsal fragment to the distal phalanx and therefore would be contraindicated.

Answer: **E**
Schneider, pp. 267-275
Hunter, Mackin, Callahan, pp. 545-548
Rosenthal in Mackin, Callahan, Skirven, et al, p. 522
Evans in Mackin, Callahan, Skirven, et al, p. 555

63. A 32-year-old hospital employee sustains an intraarticular fracture of the PIP joint with dorsal dislocation of the middle phalanx. Appropriate treatment could include which of the following?

A. Extension block splinting
B. Percutaneous pin fixation in the form of a dynamic force couple
C. Volar plate arthroplasty
D. Dynamic traction and early motion
E. A, B, and C
F. All of the above

All of the above choices are appropriate treatment techniques for the case presented. Percutaneous pin fixation and application of dynamic traction and/or a dynamic force couple are common techniques for treatment of intraarticular fractures involving the PIP joint. Extension block splinting often is employed in fracture dislocations of the PIP joint when the fragment is small and reduction of the joint can be obtained. In late cases or in cases in which extension block splinting alone cannot maintain the reduction, volar plate arthoplasty may be indicated. Active ROM and splinting programs vary depending on the stability gained in surgery.

Answer: **F**

Schenck, pp. 187-209, 327-337

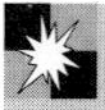

CLINICAL GEM:
PIP joint injuries are difficult to treat and stiffness is a common complication.

64. For a severely comminuted fracture involving the entire base of the proximal phalanx, the appropriate treatment would include which of the following?

A. Dynamic traction
B. Application of a dynamic external fixator with early active ROM
C. Application of a force couple splint
D. A and B only
E. None of the above

In severely comminuted fractures of the base of the proximal phalanx, early motion and dynamic traction (see Fig. 11-4, *B*), such as described by Schenck, can be employed. Application of an external fixator with dynamic traction also has been used successfully. The use of the force couple splint as described by Agee generally is not suitable for such fractures because it does not achieve distraction.

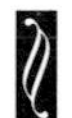

Answer: **D**

Hastings, Ernst, pp. 659-674

65. A 20-year-old male presents with pain at the base of the fourth and fifth metacarpals. A reverse Bennett's fracture is present at the fifth metacarpal and the fourth metacarpal is completely dislocated dorsally. Recommended treatment includes which of the following?

A. ORIF
B. An ulnar gutter splint
C. A long arm splint with the forearm in supination and the wrist in neutral position
D. Dynamic traction splinting
E. Silicone joint replacement arthroplasty

Fractures at the base of the fourth and fifth metacarpals often require percutaneous pinning or ORIF in order to obtain a satisfactory result. None of the alternative answers represents appropriate medical care.

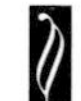

Answer: **A**

Stern in Green, Hotchkiss, Pederson, pp. 727-729

66. A 30-year-old male presents with a crush injury to the hand after he was accidentally run over by the wheel of his father's new car. X-rays are normal; the patient complains of numbness in the thumb, index, and long fingers; he experiences pain with passive stretch of all of his fingers and inability to abduct or adduct his fingers. The hand is swollen and cool to the touch, but pulses are present. The most likely diagnosis is which of the following?

A. Acute carpal tunnel syndrome
B. Posterior interosseus nerve palsy
C. Scaphoid fracture
D. Compartment syndrome of the hand
E. A and D

This patient is presenting with symptoms of acute carpal tunnel syndrome and associated compartment syndrome. The signs of the compartment syndrome include pain with passive stretch and increased pressure in the interosseus spaces, as well as symptoms of acute carpal tunnel syndrome. The most appropriate treatment would be surgical decompression of both the carpal canal as well as release of the interosseus spaces and dorsal compartments.

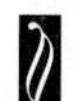

Answer: **E**

Rowland in Green, Hotchkiss, Pederson, pp. 691-697

67. The most common compressive neuropathy of the upper extremity after blunt trauma to the upper extremity is which of the following?

A. Cubital tunnel syndrome
B. Pronator teres syndrome
C. Anterior interosseus nerve syndrome
D. Thoracic outlet syndrome
E. Carpal tunnel syndrome

Carpal tunnel syndrome is a common sequela after multiple blunt trauma to the upper extremity. It often develops after wrist fractures or crush injuries and can occur after any process associated with severe swelling and edema of the arm. Failure to recognize this complication after wrist fractures can lead to a poor clinical outcome.

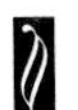
Answer: **E**
Rowland in Green, Hotchkiss, Pederson, pp. 691-697

68. A 60-year-old woman sustains a fall that results in a comminuted interarticular fracture of her distal radius of her dominant hand. The surgeon elects dorsal plating and early active mobilization. Three months after surgery, the patient can not actively extend her IP joint of the thumb past neutral. She has regained active ROM of the wrist to 50 degrees of extension, 70 degrees of flexion, and a 45-degree radioulnar deviation arc. The affected tendon resides in which compartment on the dorsal aspect of the forearm?

A. First compartment
B. Second compartment
C. Third compartment
D. Fourth compartment
E. Fifth compartment

The extensor pollicis longus tendon is entrapped or ruptured because it curves around Lister's tubercle and is often damaged after dorsal plating of distal radius fractures. It is the only tendon of the third compartment and is responsible for extension of the IP joint of the thumb. It also assists in thumb adduction.

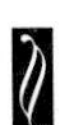
Answer: **C**
Doyle in Green, Hotchkiss, Pederson, pp. 1950-1951
Burton, Melchior in Green, Hotchkiss, Pederson, pp. 1994-1997

69. A 60-year-old jogger falls in a pothole and sustains a fracture dislocation of the PIP joint. He is treated initially with primary arthrodesis because of concomitant arthritis found at the time of surgery. Four months later, the joint is not fused and remains painful, and the finger is pronated 45 degrees. Appropriate treatment would include which of the following?

A. A dorsal splint with the finger taped in the reduced position
B. Arthrodesis with a Herbert-Whipple screw
C. Application of an external fixator with bone graft of the PIP joint
D. Tension band wiring with K-wires
E. Interosseous wiring
F. All of the above

For failed internal fixation with a nonunion of the PIP joint, internal fixation with the techniques described in answers B through E has been performed. Some patients may wish to have the finger splinted for a long period (answer A) and wait for arthrodesis, despite what appears to be an initial nonunion.

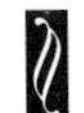
Answer: **F**
Jones, Stern, pp. 267-275

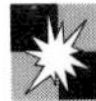
CLINICAL GEM:
Research has indicated that the use of a bone growth stimulator may assist with fracture healing.

70. After olecranon osteotomy for repair of a comminuted distal humerus fracture, a patient experiences intermittent paresthesia in her small and ring fingers. The structure likely to be involved is which of the following?

A. Radial nerve in the arcade of Frohse
B. Ulnar nerve in the cubital tunnel
C. Ulnar nerve in Guyon's canal
D. Ulnar artery

The ulnar nerve is exposed in the posterior approach to the elbow, thus rendering it vulnerable to possible damage at the cubital tunnel (see Fig. 18-2, Question 6).

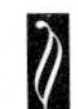
Answer: **B**
Hoppenfeld, deBoer, p. 80

71. A child is referred to you for therapy after a supracondylar fracture of the humerus. While evaluating the patient, you notice that the carrying angle in the injured arm is different from that of the other arm. True or False: This child most likely will present with cubitus valgus.

The carrying angle of the elbow is assessed in the anatomical position. The normal carrying angle measures approximately 5 degrees in males and between 10 and 15 degrees in females. The carrying angle allows the elbow to fit closely to the waist, just superior to the iliac crest. After a medial or lateral supracondylar fracture in a child—in which the distal end of the humerus is subject to either malunion or growth retardation at the epiphyseal plate—the incidence of cubitus varus is more frequent than cubitus valgus. Cubitus valgus is an angle of greater than the normal 5 to 15 degrees described; cubitus varus is a decrease in the carrying angle and is more commonly described as a "gunstock deformity." Cubitus valgus can occur with increased angulation caused by epiphyseal plate damage from a lateral epicondyle fracture.

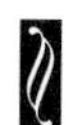

Answer: **False**

Hoppenfeld, pp. 36, 37
Loth, Wadsworth, p. 145
Refer to Fig. 11-22

CLINICAL GEM:
To remember valgus, recall that the *L* in valgus correlates with the *L* in lateral, meaning away from the midline.

72. A 25-year-old male presents 3 months after a skateboarding injury with complaints of persistent ulna-sided wrist pain. Initially, he was treated for 6 weeks in a cast with removal of K-wires, followed by active ROM. He has no tenderness in the radial carpal joint and has full ROM of the wrist. The patient complains of ulna-sided wrist pain when playing tennis and extreme point tenderness distal to his radiographically normal ulnar styloid. The most likely diagnosis is which of the following?

A. Rupture of the DRU joint
B. Ulnar nerve entrapment syndrome
C. Triangular fibrocartilage complex (TFCC) tear
D. Unrecognized reversed Bennett's fracture
E. Pronator quadrata syndrome

A TFCC tear is a common complication of fractures at the wrist. The presentation of the patient described in the question is consistent with a TFCC tear. Appropriate diagnostic tests include arthrogram, magnetic resonance imaging (MRI), and/or wrist arthroscopy.

Answer: **C**

Osterman in Green, Hotchkiss, Pederson, p. 216
Fernandez, Palmer in Green, Hotchkiss, Pederson, pp. 970-972
Refer to Fig. 11-23

73. A 31-year-old carpenter reports a loss of sensation in his small finger and difficulty playing the piano 3 months after a pneumatic nail-gun injury. The nail entered the dorsum of his hand between the capitate and hamate. The nail was then surgically removed. Examination reveals a pulsatile mass the size of a grape in his midpalm. The likely diagnosis is which of the following?

A. Sterile abscess
B. Epidermal inclusion cyst
C. Acute ganglion cyst
D. Pseudoaneurysm associated with Guyon's canal syndrome
E. Aneurysm of a rudimentary interosseus artery

The area in question is near Guyon's canal. The presence of a pulsatile mass and the ulnar nerve symptoms yield suspicion for posttraumatic pseudoaneurysm of the superficial palmar artery compressing the ulnar nerve.

Answer: **D**

Koman, et al, in Green, Hotchkiss, Pederson, pp. 2286-2288

74. Mr. S. complains of a painful clunking sound with weakness that occurs while playing tennis. Six months ago this patient suffered a wrist hyperextension injury. X-rays were normal. The patient has pain when pressure is applied at the base of the thenar region as the patient's hand is passively moved from ulnar to radial

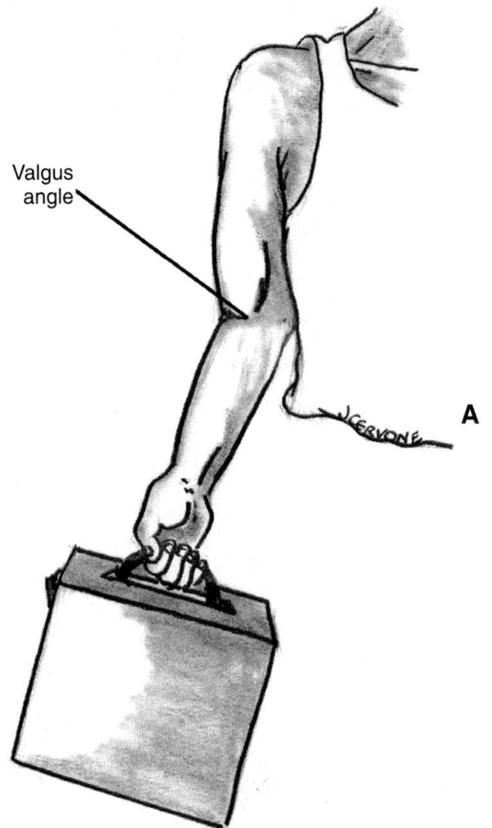

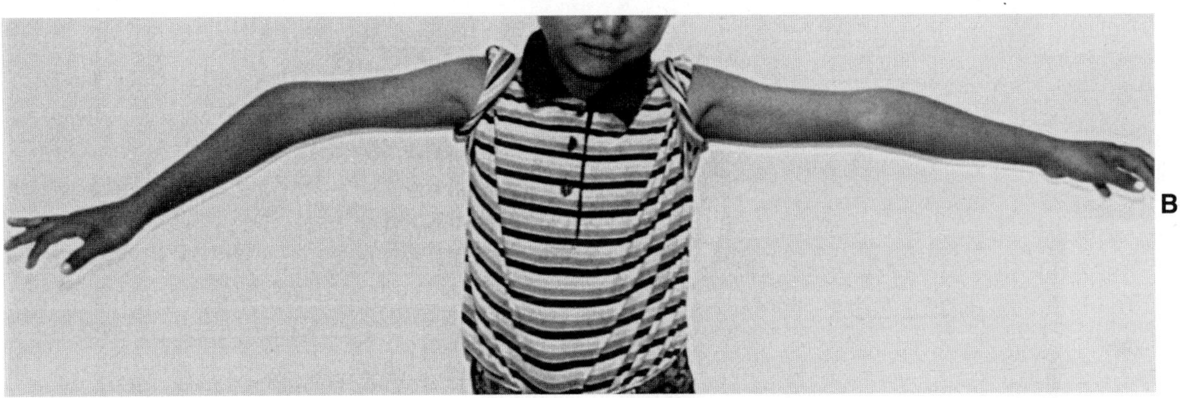

Fig. 11-22 ■ **B,** A 6-year-old boy with a 64-degree cubitus varus of the right elbow following supracondylar fracture (classic "gunstock" deformity). (From Morrey BF: *The elbow and its disorders*, ed 3, Philadelphia, 2000, Saunders.)

deviation. This positive Watson test indicates which of the following?

A. Posttraumatic midcarpal instability
B. De Quervain's tendonitis
C. Scapholunate instability
D. Kienböck's disease
E. Basilar joint arthritis

Watson described this test, in which preventing the scaphoid from palmar flexing from external pressure as the wrist is moved passively from ulnar to radial deviation can be diagnostic for ligamentous injuries of the scapholunate joint.

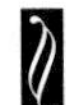

Answer: **C**

Watson, Weinzweig in Green, Hotchkiss, Pederson, pp. 114-115

Refer to Fig. 11-24

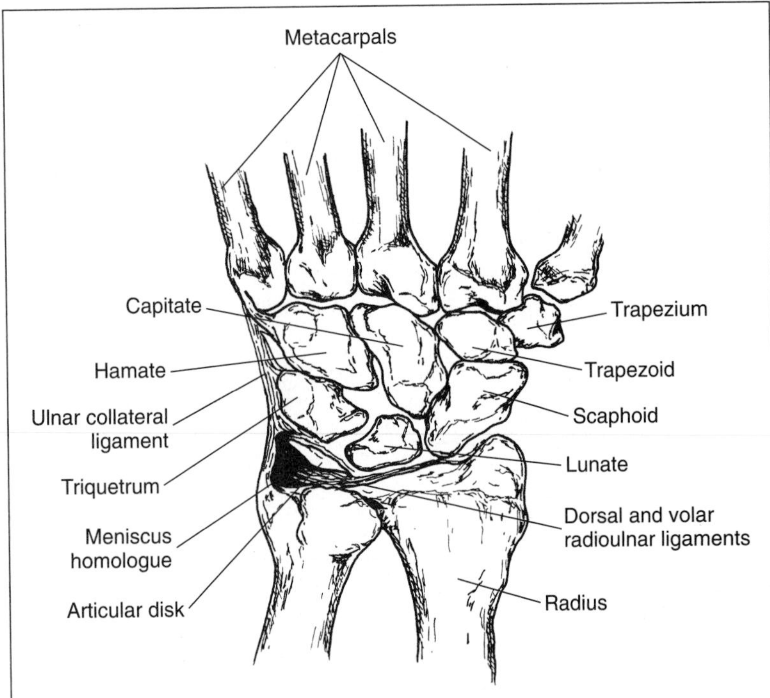

Fig. 11-23 ■ The carpal bones and TFCC (triangular fibrocartilage, ulnar meniscus homologue, ulnar collateral ligament, dorsal and volar radioulnar ligaments, ulnolunate and ulnotriquetral ligaments, and extensor carpi ulnaris tendon sheath). (From Lillegard WA, Butcher JD, Rucker KS: *Handbook of sports medicine: a symptom-oriented approach*, ed 2, Boston, 1998, Butterworth-Heinemann.)

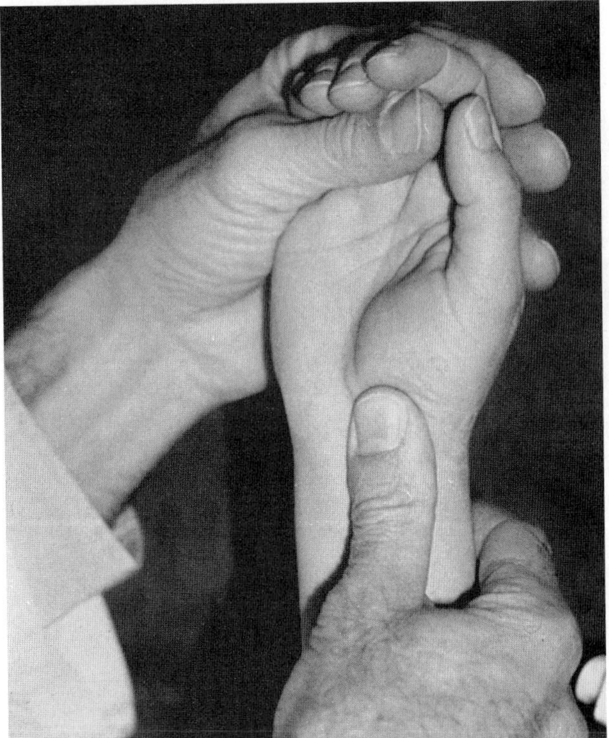

Fig. 11-24 ■ Scaphoid shift maneuver. The examiner grasps the wrist from the radial side and places the thumb on the palmar prominence of the scaphoid while wrapping the fingers around the distal radius. This enables the thumb to push on the scaphoid with counterpressure provided by the fingers. The examiner's other hand grasps the patient's hand at the metacarpal level to control wrist position. Starting in ulnar deviation and slight extension, the wrist is moved radially and slightly flexed with constant thumb pressure on the scaphoid. (From Watson HK, Weinzweig J: Physical examination of the wrist, *Hand Clin* 13[1]:17-34, 1997.)

75. A 20-year-old male sustains a baseball-bat injury to his upper arm and has fractured his right humerus spirally in the distal one third. Which of the following structures is most at risk for injury?

A. Radial artery
B. Median nerve
C. Radial nerve
D. Ulnar nerve
E. Brachial artery

A spiral fracture of the distal humerus is associated with a high frequency of radial nerve injuries. These injuries usually resolve with nonoperative treatment.

Answer: **C**
Green in Green, Hotchkiss, Pederson, pp. 1492-1495

76. Which position is selected most often for an elbow arthrodesis?

A. 30 degrees of flexion
B. 60 degrees of flexion
C. 90 degrees of flexion
D. 120 degrees of flexion

The position of arthrodesis is selected according to a patient's specific needs. In general, 90 degrees of flexion offers the most functional position. However, if special needs require positioning the hand away from the body, a 30- or 60-degree flexion position may be selected.

Answer: **C**
McCollister, pp. 17-34

77. The most significant complication after radial head excision is which of the following?

A. Pain at the wrist
B. Regrowth of the radial head
C. Stiffness of elbow flexion
D. Poor cosmetic result

Pain at the wrist caused by ulnar head impaction because of proximal migration of the radius after excision is a significant complication. This migration occurs over time. Weakness of grip, elbow instability, heterotopic bone, and arthritis also are possible complications.

Answer: **A**
Browner, Jupiter, Levine, p. 1134

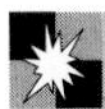

CLINICAL GEM:
The term for this DRU joint disruption with proximal migration of the radius is *Essex-Lopresti fracture.*

78. You are treating a patient after radial head fracture. After extensive therapy, the patient has reached maximum therapeutic improvement, with end ROM 30 degrees shy of full extension to 130 degrees of flexion. How should this patient be managed?

A. Refer back to doctor for surgical release
B. Continue therapy
C. Recommend massage therapy
D. No treatment is indicated.

Functional ROM of the elbow is 30 to 130 degrees of flexion. A lack of the last 30 degrees of full extension does not tend to be a significant functional deficit. Surgical treatment is not indicated because attaining extension beyond 30 degrees is unpredictable. It is recommended that surgery be avoided for flexion contractures that reach a plateau at less than 45 degrees of extension. At this point, because the patient has plateaued, he or she must adjust to the ROM loss.

Answer: **D**
McCollister, p. 1759
Werner, An, p. 359

CLINICAL GEM:
Studies have shown that functional forearm rotation is 50 degrees for both pronation and supination.

79. You are treating a patient after a severe elbow fracture and notice progressive loss of motion after initial ROM gains. The patient describes pain and tenderness throughout the elbow region and increased swelling is noted. What do you suspect occurred during the management of this fracture?

A. You were too aggressive in therapy.
B. The patient obviously fell and refractured the elbow.
C. Heterotopic bone ossification (HO) occurred.
D. The patient was noncompliant with his home program.

The patient exhibits symptoms of HO (Fig. 11-25). HO typically is accompanied by local tissue swelling and hyperemia. Progressive loss of motion can be found after the initial satisfactory achievement of ROM. The manifestation of these symptoms usually occurs within 1 to 4 months, although symptoms have been noted to develop for up to 1 year after insult. Radiographs can reveal the development of HO within the first 4 to 6 weeks. Direct trauma to the elbow and forearm is the most common cause of HO. If surgery for HO is performed, early motion is required. Overaggressive mobilization is contraindicated. Continuous passive motion is advocated to maintain intraoperative gains. A dynamic supination-pronation splint often is indicated in the early postoperative stage.

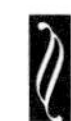

Answer: **C**
Hastings, Graham, pp. 417-421

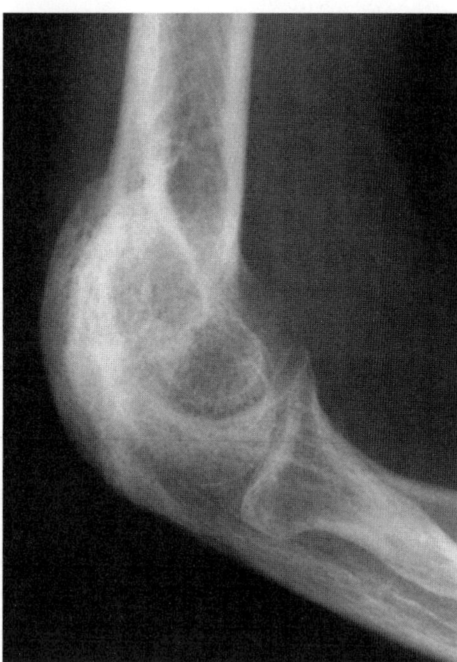

Fig. 11-25 ■ Lateral radiograph of the elbow shows significant posterior heterotopic ossification bridging the humerus and ulna. Additional diagnostic studies to determine the cause of elbow ankylosis are not needed. (From Mackin EJ, Callahan AD, Skirven TM, et al: *Rehabilitation of the hand and upper extremity*, ed 5, St Louis, 2002, Mosby.)

80. After a minimally displaced shoulder fracture, when can passive ROM be initiated?

A. In 7 to 10 days
B. In 14 to 21 days
C. In 6 weeks
D. Therapy is not indicated for patients with shoulder fractures.

With a minimally displaced shoulder fracture, sling immobilization is indicated for the first 7 to 10 days. Humeral fracture bracing also is indicated in shaft fractures. Gentle, passive ROM can be initiated at approximately 7 to 10 days or when the pain has diminished and the patient is less apprehensive. Advancement of the therapy is based on fracture configuration, stability, signs of fracture healing through radiographs, and patient tolerance. Overaggressive rehabilitation can distract a minimally displaced fracture, thus resulting in a malunion or a nonunion.

Answer: **A**
Basti, Dionysian, Sherman, p. 113

81. A 16-year-old girl sustains a closed crush injury to her long finger when she slams it in a car door. X-rays confirm a minimal tuft fracture. After 24 hours of splinting, you see the patient in therapy, and she reports excruciating pain with a blackened nail. Recommended treatment is which of the following?

A. Ice packs to the distal phalanx
B. Refer back to the physician for evacuation of a sublingual hematoma
C. Fluidotherapy to decrease pain
D. Dynamic traction splinting to increase blood flow
E. Cast immobilization with wrist extended and the MCPs flexed to 90 degrees and the IP joints in full extension

This patient is developing a sublingual hematoma. Under sterile preparation, either an 18-gauge needle or an ophthalmic cautery can be used to decompress the hematoma by drilling through the tuft base of the nail. The hole that is created must be large enough to allow prolonged drainage. Sublingual hematomas can be extremely painful and may develop progressively as late as 72 hours after the initial fracture.

Answer: **B**
Green, p. 1356
Fleegler in Green, Hotchkiss, Pederson, p. 2198
Refer to Fig. 11-26

82. A 20-year-old male sustains a crushing injury to his nondominant index finger. Despite ORIF, digital nerve and flexor tendon repair, and 6 months of hand therapy, his index finger remains numb, stiff, painful and deformed. His surgeon recommends ray resection of the index finger; the patient wishes to discuss this with you, his trusted hand therapist. You advise which of the following?

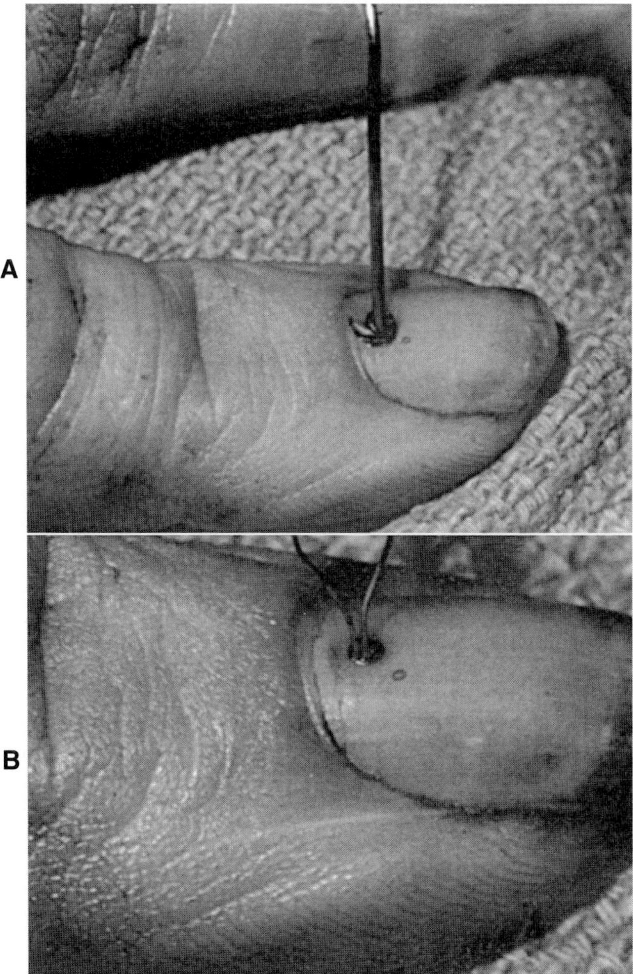

Fig. 11-26 ■ A, A time-honored method of burning a hole through the nail is with a heated paper clip. B, The authors' preferred method of burning a hole through the nail is with an ophthalmic battery-powered cautery. (From Green DP, Hotchkiss RN, Pederson WC: *Green's Operative hand surgery*, ed 4, New York, 1999, Churchill Livingstone.)

A. That the surgeon's recommendations seem reasonable and that an index ray resection usually results in both a good cosmetic and functional result
B. That he see another hand surgeon for a second opinion; the index finger is critically important for fine motor work and all efforts should be made to save it
C. That he seek another opinion because narrowing of the breadth of the hand with ray resection will lead to extreme weakness and the amputation should be further distal
D. That he seek another opinion because toe-to-finger transplant could be more effective
E. That the surgeon's recommendations seem reasonable but that you believe he has reflex sympathetic dystrophy which should be treated first

A numb, painful, stiff index finger, especially in the nondominant hand may best be treated by ray resection. Excellent cosmetic and functional results can be obtained in the vast majority of cases.

Answer: **A**
Louis, Jebson, Graham in Green, Hotchkiss, Pederson, pp. 60-62
Refer to Fig. 11-27

83. An 18-year-old male who was noncompliant and removed his cast after closed treatment of a distal radius fracture complains of pain in the wrist and altered motion. Radiographs reveal a malunion of the distal radius with an ulnar positive variance. Reasonable treatment includes which of the following?

A. Aggressive hand therapy to break down adhesions
B. Functional electrical stimulation to increase ROM
C. Ulnar shortening osteotomy with no other treatment
D. Biplanar corrective radial osteotomy
E. Application of an electrical stimulator

This patient has a fixed malunion of the distal radius with an ulnar positive variance. It may be corrected by a single biplanar osteotomy of the distal radius but in severe cases may also require ulnar shortening. Hand therapy would be of little benefit initially in this setting.

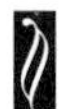

Answer: **D**
Fernandez, Palmer in Green, Hotchkiss, Pederson, pp. 973-977

84. An extraarticular fracture through the base of the thumb metacarpal with 15 degrees of dorsal angulation is best treated by which of the following?

A. Dynamic traction splint
B. ORIF
C. Percutaneous K-wire fixation
D. A closed reduction in a short arm cast for 3 weeks
E. Closed reduction in a short arm cast for 7 weeks

Extraarticular metaphyseal fractures of the thumb metacarpal are extremely forgiving because of the mobility of the thumb. Three weeks of immobilization is usually adequate for most fractures. Although most intraarticular fractures require ORIF—or at least an

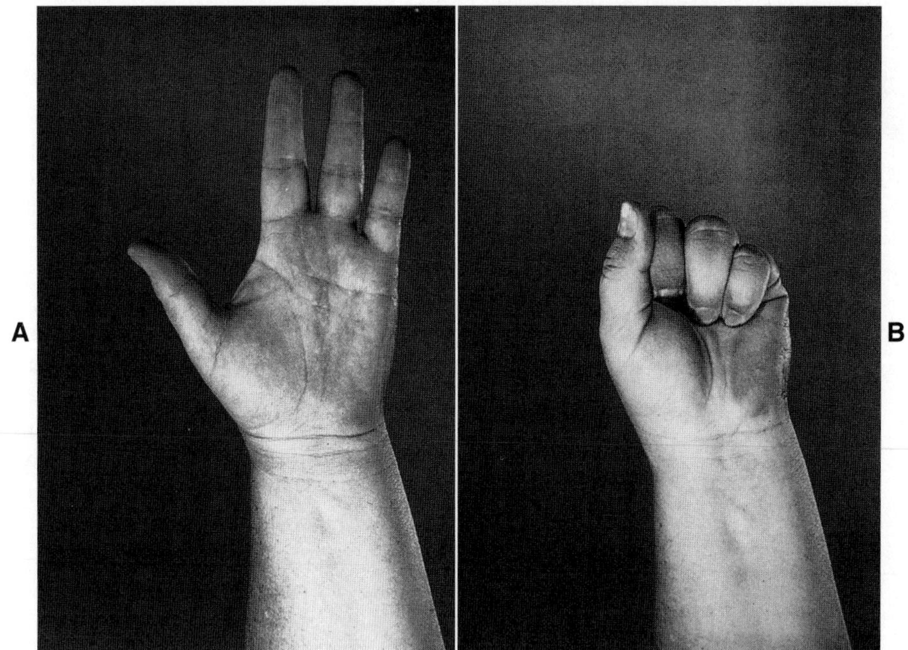

Fig. 11-27 ■ From Smith P: *Lister's The hand: diagnosis and indications*, ed 4, London, 2003, Churchill Livingstone.

anatomic alignment and percutaneous pinning—extraarticular fractures can usually be treated by closed means.

Answer: **D**
Stern in Green, Hotchkiss, Pederson, p. 759

85. Which bone of the hand is the least often fractured?

A. Distal phalanx
B. Proximal phalanx
C. Middle phalanx
D. Metacarpal

The middle phalanx is the least fractured of all hand bones. Most of the fractures that occur here are avulsion fractures of the PIP joint in sports-related and work accidents. The distal phalanx is the most common finger fracture.

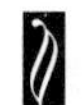
Answer: **C**
Cannon, p. 105

Chapter 12

Sports Injuries of the Upper Extremity

1. What percentage of all athletic injuries are of the hand and wrist?

A. Less than 1%
B. 3% to 25%
C. 40% to 70%
D. More than 80%

The incidence of hand and wrist injuries in all athletic injuries is 3% to 25%. Hand and wrist injuries in athletic participation are common and usually involve athletes younger than 16 years. The more severe injuries such as fractures can be seen with greater contact sports such as football.

Answer: **B**
DeHaven, Linter, pp. 218-224
Rettig, Ryan, Stone, pp. 37-48

2. Cindy, a 23-year-old soccer player, fell and sustained a displaced, noncomminuted olecranon fracture (Type IIA). The patient underwent surgery with placement of a compression AO screw. When would you begin active range of motion (ROM)?

A. Same day of surgery
B. 3 to 7 days postoperatively
C. 4 weeks postoperatively
D. 6 to 8 weeks postoperatively

When a postoperative compression AO screw is used to stabilize an olecranon fracture, gentle active ROM should begin when postoperative pain has subsided, which is usually between 3 to 7 days after surgery. You should avoid extremes of motion, primarily flexion, for 4 weeks postoperatively. Begin strengthening around 8 weeks postoperatively.

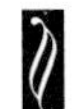

Answer: **B**
Morrey, pp. 374-375
Refer to Fig. 12-1

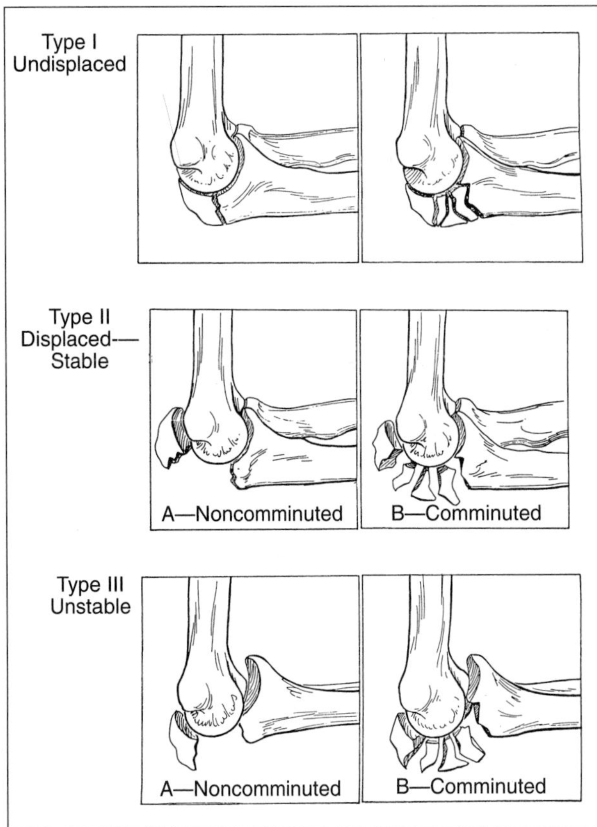

Fig. 12-1 ■ Mayo classification for olecranon fractures. Types IIB, IIIA, and IIIB are at risk for developing nonunions. (From Morrey BF: *The elbow and its disorders*, ed 3, Philadelphia, 2000, WB Saunders. By permission of the Mayo Foundation for Medical Education and Research. All rights reserved.)

CLINICAL GEM:
After an olecranon fracture, ROM is generally indicated within 3 to 7 days, regardless of treatment technique.

3. What is the most difficult functional activity to recover after a successful hemiarthroplasty reconstruction of a four-part fracture of the proximal humerus?

A. Positioning the arm at the side comfortably
B. Strength to carry a gallon of milk at the side
C. Strength to hold the arm rotated against the body
D. Reaching overhead and behind the back to the shoulder blade
E. Ability to reach the hand to the face

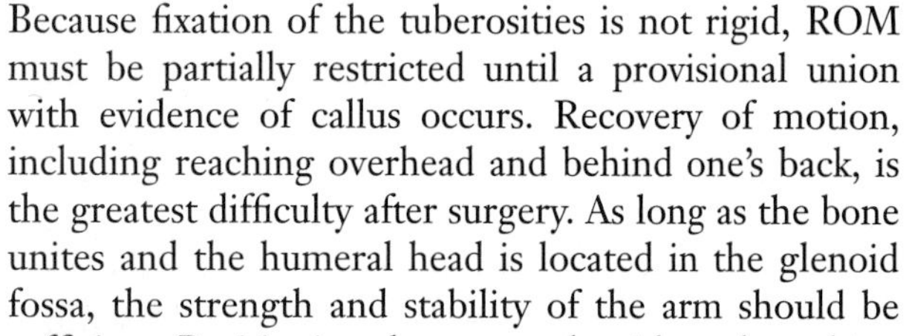

Because fixation of the tuberosities is not rigid, ROM must be partially restricted until a provisional union with evidence of callus occurs. Recovery of motion, including reaching overhead and behind one's back, is the greatest difficulty after surgery. As long as the bone unites and the humeral head is located in the glenoid fossa, the strength and stability of the arm should be sufficient. Positioning the arm at the side and reaching the hand to the face is easily performed after hemiarthroplasty for four-part fractures.

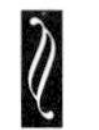

Answer: **D**
Zyto, Kronberg, Brostrom, pp. 331-336

4. A 24-year-old man dislocates his elbow as a result of a fall but sustains no other injuries. The elbow is reduced and is stable. How long should the elbow be immobilized in a splint before motion can begin?

A. 3 to 10 days
B. 2 to 3 weeks
C. 4 weeks
D. 6 weeks
E. 8 weeks

Flexion contractures are the most common complication of dislocations of the elbow, and approximately 15% of patients lose more than 30 degrees of flexion. The risk of contracture is proportional to the duration of immobilization. The elbow is immobilized for protection and comfort and should be moved within the first few days after reduction.

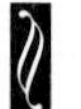

Answer: **A**
Mehlhoff, Noble, Bennett, pp. 244-249

5. Mr. B, a 49-year-old retired football coach, underwent two previous shoulder stabilization procedures for recurrent dislocations. He now has advanced arthritis with continuous pain and severe restrictions of motion. Although shoulder replacement relieved his pain, he now has increased passive external rotation, weakness when using his arm in front of his body, and instability to lift the back of his hand away from his back. Which of the following muscles is related to the weakness in his arm?

A. Deltoid
B. Infraspinatus
C. Supraspinatus
D. Subscapularis
E. Pectoralis major

Patients with subscapularis tears have an increase in passive external rotation and weakness of internal rotation. The patient's inability to move the dorsum of the hand from the lumbar spine (the lift-off test, Fig. 12-2) indicates that the subscapularis muscle is incompetent.

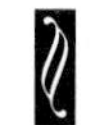

Answer: **D**
Gerber, Hersche, Farron, pp. 1015-1023
Rockwood, Matsen, pp. 191-192

A

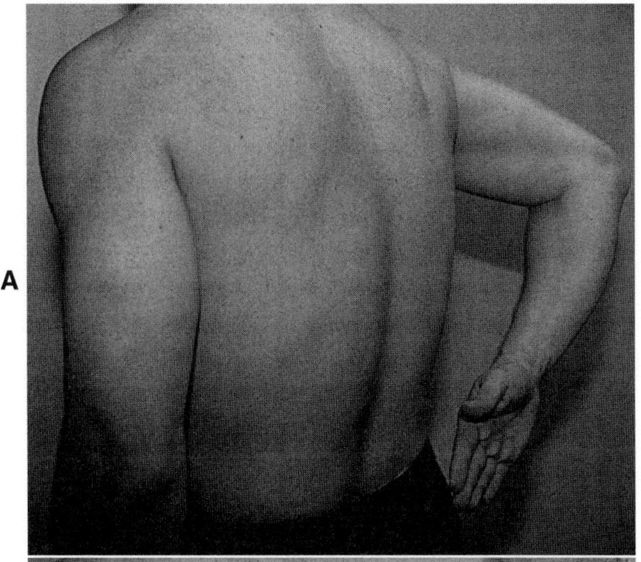

B

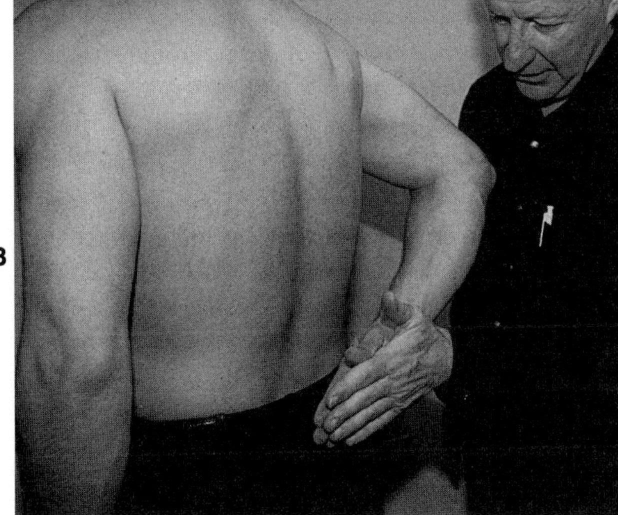

Fig. 12-2 ■ **A,** The lift-off test is performed by having the patient lift the palm of the hand backwards, away from the small of the back. The patient must have sufficient internal rotation to allow this test to be performed. It is suggestive of a subscapularis rupture if the patient cannot lift off. **B,** The same lift-off test can be further refined by having the patient resist in the lifted-off position to provide a quantitated estimate of subscapularis strength. This could be called a *lift-off test with resistance.* (From Rockwood C, Matsen F: *The shoulder,* ed 2, Philadelphia, 1998, WB Saunders.)

6. A 15-year-old girl who participates in high school gymnastics reports pain in the right shoulder with frequent numbness and paresthesias that began 1 week ago in the arm and hand. The left shoulder is normal. Examination reveals marked hyperlaxity of the elbows and metacarpophalangeal (MCP) joints, and her patellae are hypermobile. Stress X-rays in the clinic reveal inferior subluxation of the glenohumeral joint. Initial treatment should consist of which of the following?

A. Physical/occupational therapy
B. Laser capsulorraphy
C. Inferior capsular shift
D. Bankart repair
E. Arthroscopic capsular repair

Shoulder pain and paresthesias in a young female gymnast suggest the diagnosis of instability. Because of the recent onset, a nonsurgical approach of physical therapy for muscle strengthening should be undertaken. Surgery of any type should be performed only on those patients who have participated in a therapy program for at least 6 months without success.

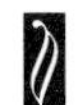

Answer: **A**
Burkhead, Rockwood, pp. 890-896

7. A 44-year-old woman reports persistent aching pain, a recurrent pop in the right shoulder when raising her arm in front of her, and weakness with pushing. She was injured in an automobile accident in which she braced herself before impact with her elbows locked and her arms holding the steering wheel. Examination reveals pain on internal rotation and forward elevation of the arm when a posterior directed force is applied along the humeral shaft. A sudden pop is noted on horizontal abduction to the coronal plane with the arm internally rotated. What is the most likely diagnosis?

A. Biceps tendon tear
B. Subscapularis tear
C. Posterior labral tear
D. Supraspinatus tendon tear
E. Internal impingement syndrome

The patient has a traumatic posterior labral tear and posterior instability. The jerk test (Fig. 12-3) is described here, and symptomatic pathologic posterior translation is produced when the humeral head is translated posteriorly in forward elevation and relocated as the arm is forced into coronal plane abduction.

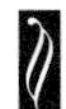

Answer: **C**
Matsen, Lippitt, Sidles, pp. 19-109
Rockwood, Matsen, pp. 680-681

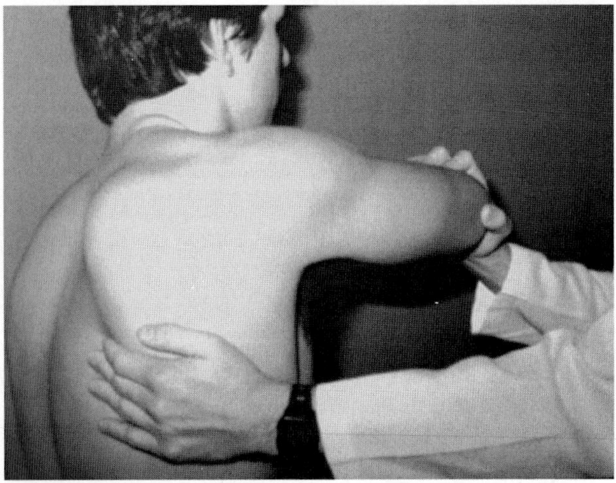

Fig. 12-3 ■ The jerk test. The patient's arm is abducted to 90 degrees and internally rotated. The examiner axially loads the humerus while the arm is moved horizontally across the body. The left hand stabilizes the scapula. A patient with a recurrent posterior instability may demonstrate a sudden jerk as the humeral head slides off the back of the glenoid or when it is reduced by moving the arm back to the starting position. (From Rockwood C, Matsen F: *The shoulder*, ed 2, Philadelphia, 1998, WB Saunders.)

8. A 35-year-old woman sustains an isolated, minimally displaced fracture of the radial head as a result of a fall on the ice. Initial treatment includes immobilization in a posterior splint with a sling. The next step of treatment should consist of which of the following?

A. Application of a cast in 7 to 10 days
B. Application of a hinged elbow brace in 3 weeks
C. Beginning an active ROM program within 1 week
D. Continued use of the splint and sling at all times for the next 6 weeks
E. Continued use of the splint and sling for 4 weeks, followed by use of the sling only until radiographic union occurs

A minimally displaced radial head fracture should be immobilized for only 1 week to minimize long-term stiffness; then an active ROM program should begin. Begin to wean the patient from the sling when you begin active ROM.

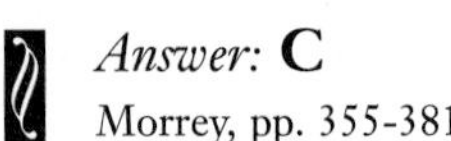
Answer: **C**
Morrey, pp. 355-381

9. A 20-year-old woman who exercises her arms regularly has multidirectional instability (MDI) and ligamentous laxity. She wishes to have shoulders that "stay in place." Results from Cybex testing reveal that her external rotators are only 40% as strong as her internal rotators. Why would specific exercises for MDI be effective?

A. External rotation strength should be at least 60% of internal rotation, and increasing muscular strength should help stabilize up to 80% of shoulders with MDI.
B. External rotation strength should be at least 80% of internal rotation, and increasing muscular tone improves glenohumeral stability in up to 80% of patients with MDI.
C. An external rotation strength of 30% of internal rotation is normal, but the scapular forces need to be trained to position the scapula and align the joint reaction forces in patients with MDI.
D. The ratio of external to internal rotation strength does not matter because the essential lesion is excessive capsuloligamentous laxity in patients with MDI.
E. The ratio of external to internal rotation strength is unimportant because the scapular stabilizers must be the primary focus of rehabilitation.

The essential lesion of MDI appears to multifactorial, and patients with MDI often exhibit rotator cuff weakness, diminished proprioception, lack of coordinated scapular motion, ligamentous laxity, and excessive capsular redundancy. External rotation strength is typically 60% of internal rotation strength in women. Burkhead and Rockwood report that MDI will improve with exercises in up to 80% of patients with MDI. Strengthening exercises should include rotator cuff, deltoid, and scapular stabilizers to align the glenohumeral joint reaction force. Scapular exercises alone would be insufficient for adequate stabilization of the glenohumeral joint.

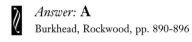

Answer: **A**
Burkhead, Rockwood, pp. 890-896

10. A 30-year-old man participating in recreational hockey dislocates his right shoulder and stiffness develops in the elbow after he is immobilized in a sling for 4 weeks. Nine months after the arm was immobilized, the shoulder has healed, but the patient lacks 30 degrees of elbow extension, which equates to a residual flexion contracture. Management should now include which of the following?

A. An open elbow capsular release through a lateral approach
B. An open elbow capsular release through an anterior approach
C. Arthroscopic elbow capsular release of the anterior capsule
D. Observation
E. Stretching exercises, a static progressive splint, and adjustable static night splints

A flexion contracture from an injury that occurred less than 1 year ago should be treated conservatively with stretching and splints. Results from a surgical release for a flexion contracture of 30 degrees or less are unpredictable. Most surgeons will not perform a surgical or arthroscopic release in patients with an elbow flexion contracture of 30 degrees or less.

Answer: **E**
Cooney, pp. 433-451

11. What are the three primary constraints that are necessary and sufficient for stability of the elbow?

A. Coronoid, lateral ulnar collateral ligament, capsule
B. Coronoid, lateral ulnar collateral ligament, anterior band of the medial collateral ligament
C. Coronoid, anterior band of the medial collateral ligament, radial head
D. Capsule, anterior band of the medial collateral ligament, radial head
E. Capsule, lateral ulnar collateral ligament, radial head

The three primary constraints necessary for stability of the elbow are the lateral ulnar collateral ligament (Fig. 12-4, *A*), the anterior band of the medial collateral ligament (Fig. 12-4, *B*), and the coronoid (Fig. 12-4, *C*). The radial head and the capsule are secondary constraints and are very important if a primary constraint is deficient; however, elbow stability is not acutely compromised if a secondary constraint is lost and the primary constraint is intact.

Answer: **B**
King, Morrey, An, pp. 165-174
Morrey, p. 47

12. A 17-year-old boy who plays volleyball has had pain in the left nondominant shoulder for the past 6 weeks. The athletic trainer instructs him to work harder on bench press and push-up exercises; however, the shoulder becomes more symptomatic, and he reports numbness in his hand. On physical examination, he has a supple neck, painless cross-chest adduction, and symmetric wrist pulses in all positions. What is the most likely diagnosis?

A. Cervical disk disease
B. Impingement syndrome
C. Thoracic outlet syndrome
D. Anterior shoulder instability
E. Acromioclavicular joint arthrosis

Shoulder pain associated with paresthesias in an athlete usually establishes a diagnosis of instability, and anterior shoulder instability is commonly aggravated by bench press activity. A supple neck and symmetric wrist pulses are not associated with cervical disk disease or thoracic outlet syndrome. Impingement may be a symptom in this patient, but instability is the most likely diagnosis.

Answer: **D**
Rowe, Zarins, pp. 863-872

13. The largest single component of the total force generated during a tennis serve is derived from which of the following?

A. Wrist flexion
B. Shoulder flexion
C. Shoulder eccentric contraction
D. Scapular stabilization
E. Hip and trunk rotation

Maximum velocity of the tennis serve is achieved through efficient generation and transmission of force through all segments of the kinetic chain. Because of their mass and their location at the base of the chain, the hip and trunk generate 50% to 55% of the total force or energy of the serve. Lower extremity strength measures are more highly correlated with throwing velocity than are upper extremity strength measures.

Answer: **E**
Kibler, pp. 79-85

14. An 18-year-old basketball player sustains a direct blow to the tip of the long finger of the right dominant hand, resulting in a 45-degree

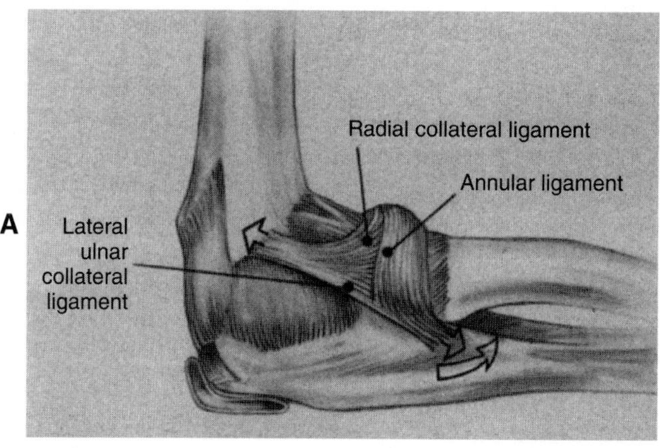

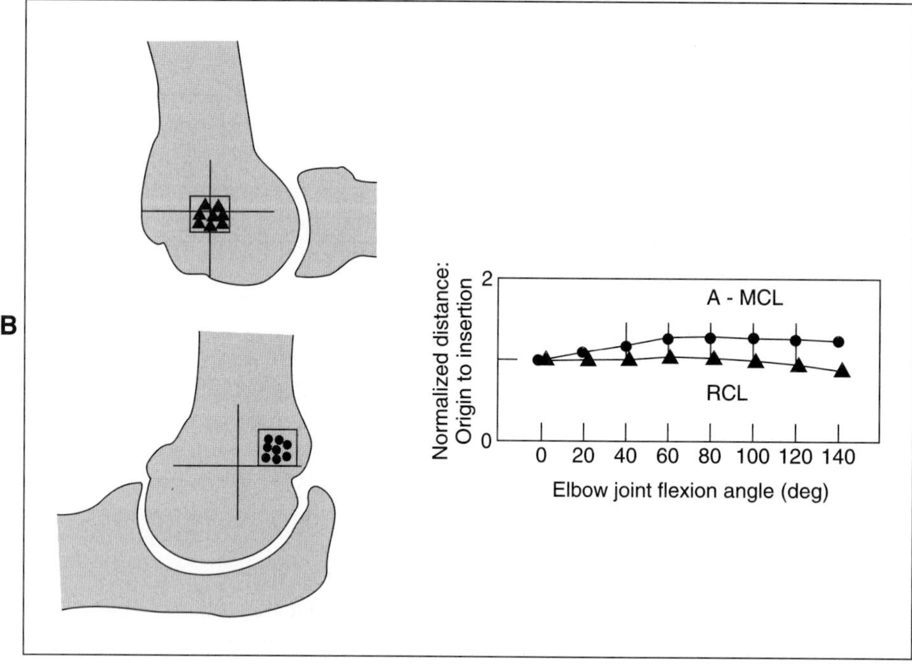

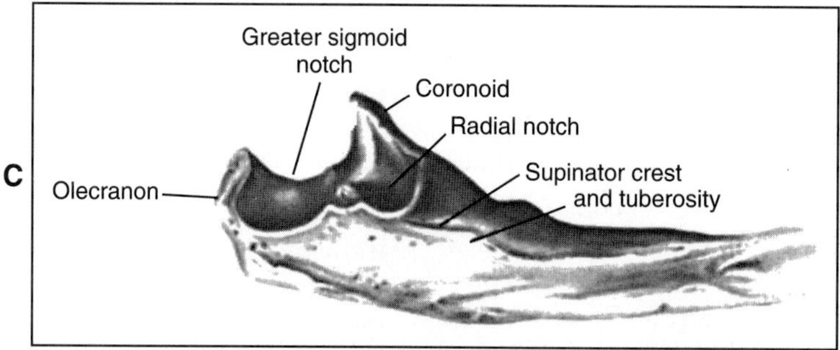

Fig. 12-4 ■ **A,** The anterior medial collateral ligament remains more taut during elbow flexion than does the posterior segment of the ligament. The radial collateral ligament originates at the axis of rotation for elbow flexion; hence the ligament has little length variation during flexion and extension. **B,** The classic orientation of the medial collateral ligament, including the anterior and posterior bundles, and the transverse ligament. This last structure contributes relatively little to elbow stability. (From Morrey BF: *The elbow and its disorders*, ed 3, Philadelphia, 2000, WB Saunders. By permission of the Mayo Foundation for Medical Education and Research. All rights reserved.)

flexion deformity of the distal interphalangeal (DIP) joint. Passive extension is maintained, but he cannot actively extend the joint. Treatment should consist of which of the following?

A. Active extension exercises with dynamic splinting
B. Percutaneous pinning of the DIP joint in extension
C. Continuous splinting of the DIP joint in extension
D. Continuous splinting of the DIP and proximal interphalangeal (PIP) joints in extension

This patient has a mallet finger deformity with avulsion of the extensor mechanism from the base of the distal phalanx. The proper treatment is continuous splinting of the DIP joint in maximal extension for 6 to 8 weeks. The PIP joint does not require splinting. Percutaneous pinning or primary repair is not often indicated, and research has shown nonoperative treatment of even large articular fractures of the distal phalanx respond well to splinting. Splinting decreases the postoperative complications such as decreased flexion of the DIP joint from scar tenodesis over the PIP joint, wound infection, thinning of the dorsal skin, joint injury, nail-bed injury, pain, pulp fibrosis, and dysesthesias. Dynamic splinting is contraindicated because the DIP joint must be maintained in extension for the extensor tendon to heal.

Answer: **C**
Rosenthal in Mackin, Callahan, Skirven, et al, pp. 518-520
DeLee, Drez, Miller pp. 1396-1398

15. A 28-year-old softball player has chronic right shoulder pain that developed gradually and that worsens with the throwing motion (Fig. 12-5). The patient reports a feeling of popping and catching but no "dead arm" or giving way symptoms. Rotator cuff strengthening exercises have exacerbated the symptoms. Examination shows a drooping posture of the involved shoulder, a positive impingement sign with abduction and internal rotation, crepitus in the subacromial space, and no crepitus with scapular motion. She also exhibits scapular winging. There is no neurologic deficit. At this point, management should consist of which of the following?

A. A scapular stabilization program
B. A series of subacromial injections
C. An arthroscopic subacromial decompression
D. A magnetic resonance imaging (MRI) scan to check for rotator cuff function
E. Continuation of previous rotator cuff program

This patient has secondary impingement or impingement due to factors outside the subacromial arch. Scapular dyskinesias, as noted by abnormal static and dynamic posture and winging, produce acromial depression due to loss of scapular protraction. They also produce loss of the scapular anchor for rotator cuff function. Exercises to stabilize this anchor and elevate the acromion should be instituted before surgical management.

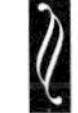

Answer: **A**
Pink, Screnar, Tollefson, pp. 3-15
DeLee, Drez, Miller, p. 1271

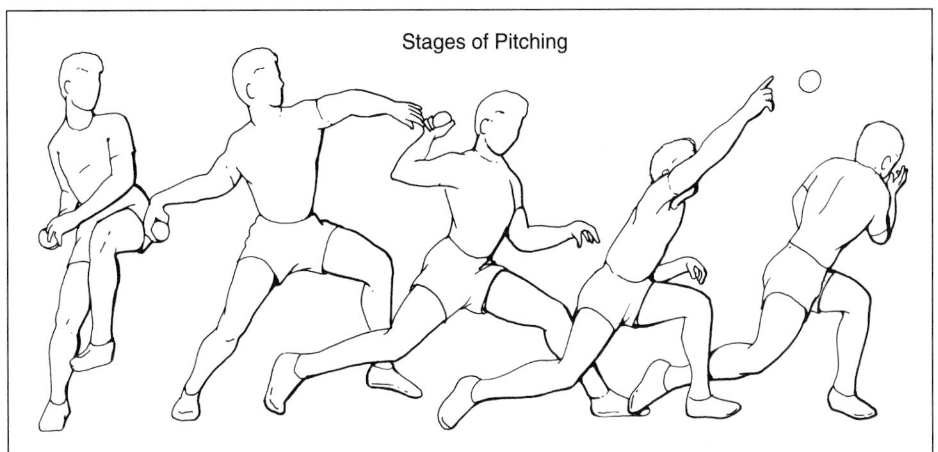

Fig. 12-5 ■ The four phases of throwing: cocking, wind-up, acceleration, and follow-through. (From DeLee JC, Drez D, Miller MD: *DeLee & Drez's Orthopaedic sports medicine: principles and practice*, ed 2, Philadelphia, 2003, WB Saunders.)

16. Which of the following muscular rehabilitation exercises would be most effective in helping a patient regain normal shoulder "concavity compression," or dynamic stabilization of the humeral head within the glenoid socket?

A. Trapezius shoulder shrugs
B. Rotator cuff co-contractions at 90 degrees of abduction
C. Internal rotation strengthening at 0 degrees of abduction
D. Serratus anterior strengthening at 45 degrees of abduction
E. Eccentric external rotation strengthening through full ROMs

Concavity compression refers to the biomechanical result of anatomy and muscular forces to compress and stabilize the humeral head in the glenoid cavity upon motion. Muscular activity to help accomplish this result would require co-contraction force couples acting along the axis of the arm in a position of function. Therefore it is best accomplished by rotator cuff exercises at 90 degrees of abduction. None of the other muscular activities or joint positions allows compression of the joint surfaces.

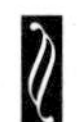

Answer: **B**
Lippitt, Vanderhooft, Harris, pp. 27-35

17. A throwing athlete sustains a rupture of the ulnar collateral ligament of the elbow and elects to undergo reconstruction. The reconstructive graft is placed in an attempt to recreate which of the following?

A. Anterior capsule
B. Anterior band
C. Posterior band
D. Transverse ligament
E. Accessory collateral ligament

The medial stabilizing ligaments of the elbow are thickenings within the medial capsule. Attempts to recreate stability after rupture of the ulnar collateral ligament are directed toward reconstructing the anterior band (Fig. 12-6) of the ulnar collateral ligament. The anterior band provides most of the stability, whereas the posterior and transverse ligaments contribute much less. The anterior capsule does not play a significant role in elbow stability. The accessory collateral ligament is a lateral stabilizer.

Answer: **B**
Andrew, Jelsma, Joyce, pp. 109-113
Jobe, p. 404

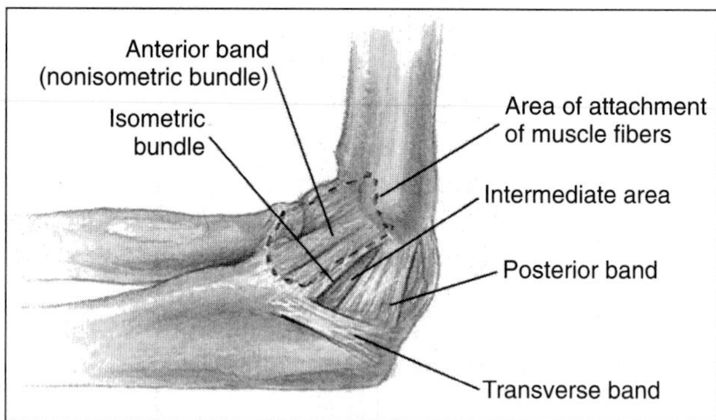

Fig. 12-6 ■ Medial capsuloligamentous complex. Bony anatomy, anterior band: isometric bundle, nonisometric bundle. (From Jobe FW: *Operative techniques in upper extremity sports injuries,* St Louis, 1996, Mosby.)

18. Tearing of the rotator cuff due to tensile failure occurs during what phase of the pitching act?

A. Windup
B. Cocking
C. Acceleration
D. Deceleration
E. Follow-through

Deceleration is the most violent phase of pitching (Fig. 12-7). The rotator cuff is the principal decelerator and is susceptible to tensile failure from eccentric loading. Windup is variable, but most muscle groups are relaxed. The anterior muscles are extrinsically loaded by extreme external rotation during the cocking phase. Maximal firing of the anterior musculature occurs during the acceleration phase. Follow-through allows the pitcher to regain balance.

Answer: **D**
Fleisig, Dillman, Andrews, pp. 151-170
DeLee, Drez, Miller, pp. 1070-1075

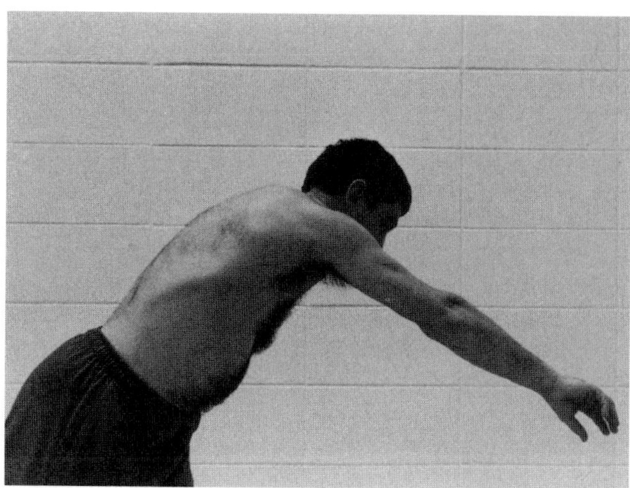

Fig. 12-7 ■ Deceleration or follow-through phase of throwing motion. (From DeLee JC, Drez D, Miller MD: *DeLee & Drez's Orthopaedic sports medicine: principles and practice*, ed 2, Philadelphia, 2003, WB Saunders.)

19. Internal impingement of the shoulder is defined as which of the following?

A. Partial rotator cuff tear on the undersurface
B. Rotator cuff impingement against the posterior glenoid labrum
C. Rotator cuff impingement on the anterior glenoid labrum
D. Rotator cuff impingement from a loose body
E. Rotator cuff impingement from intrasubstance degeneration

With anterior instability of the shoulder, the posterior aspect of the rotator cuff impinges against the posterior aspect of the glenoid labrum with the shoulder in external rotation and anteriorly translated. A positive relocation test occurs when this discomfort is relieved by posterior translation of the humeral head, relieving the impingement. This phenomenon can be viewed via arthroscope.

Answer: **B**
Walch, Boileau, Noel, pp. 238-245

20. Why are plyometric exercises important in conditioning programs?

A. They improve aerobic endurance.
B. They reduce joint reactive forces.
C. They allow exercise through limited arcs of motion.
D. They create more powerful concentric contractions.
E. They can be performed on conventional weight-training machines.

By definition, plyometrics are brief, explosive exercises that involve an eccentric (lengthening) muscle by a concentric (shortening) contraction. Plyometric exercises are free-form exercises that consist of a stretching cycle followed closely by a rapid shortening cycle—a quick changeover from eccentric to concentric muscle action. They are designed to be used through a full range of functional motion. Plyometrics are important in conditioning programs because they reduce joint reactive forces. These exercises are not performed on conventional weight-training machines and do not affect aerobic endurance.

In the upper extremity, different-sized balls can be used to create a plyometric exercise. These exercises can be initiated safely as long as motion and heavy loads through the joint are limited.

Answer: **B**
Wilk, Voight, Keirns, pp. 225-239
DeLee, Drez, Miller, pp. 343-344, 422-425
Refer to Fig. 12-8

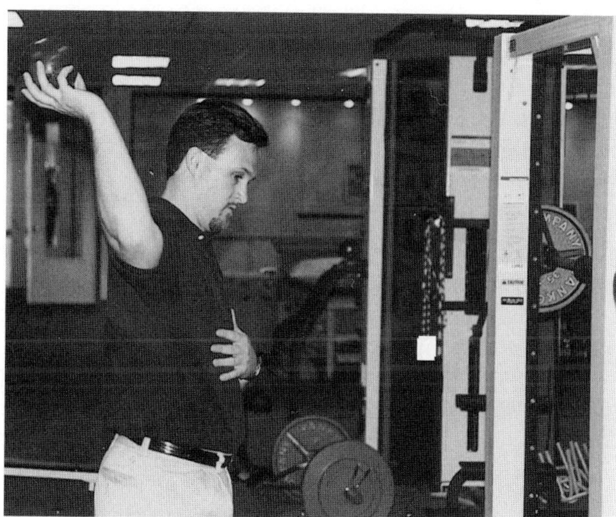

Fig. 12-8 ■ Upper extremity plyometric activity. (From DeLee JC, Drez D, Miller MD: *DeLee & Drez's Orthopaedic sports medicine: principles and practice*, ed 2, Philadelphia, 2003, WB Saunders.)

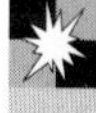

CLINICAL GEM:
The easiest way to think of this quick changeover from eccentric to concentric muscle action is to imagine a spring coiling and uncoiling.

21. Mr. X, a 30-year-old recreational athlete, sustains a posterior shoulder dislocation to his nondominant arm from a fall on an outstretched hand. After reduction, radiographs are normal. This is a recurrent injury for Mr. X. Management should include which of the following?

A. Arthoscopic stabilization
B. Posterior opening wedge osteotomy
C. Posterior bone block reconstruction
D. A structured strengthening program
E. Immobilization of the shoulder for 6 weeks

Although no consensus on the treatment of recurrent posterior glenohumeral instability exists, most authors feel that initial management should be nonoperative. Structured strengthening programs appear to be helpful in reducing recurrent posterior instability. There are no data to support prolonged immobilization as a treatment.

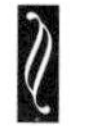
Answer: **D**
Schwartz, Warren, O'Brien, pp. 409-419

22. Which of the following is not part of the "terrible triad of the shoulder" in a patient over 40 years of age?

A. Anterior shoulder dislocation
B. Bankart labral tear
C. Rotator cuff tear
D. Neurologic injury

The "terrible triad of the shoulder" is a rare combination of anterior shoulder dislocation, rotator cuff tear, and neurologic injury. This diagnosis should be considered in any patient over 35 years who reports persistent pain and weakness after shoulder dislocation. This can be evaluated with an MRI to assess the rotator cuff and electromyography (EMG) to assess neurologic injury. The Bankart labral tear is not part of the "terrible triad."

Answer: **B**
Simonich, Wright, pp. 566-568

23. A 17-year-old girl who has had bilateral shoulder instability for the past 5 years now wants to play volleyball, but her dominant shoulder slips in a wide variety of positions. Treatment of the (hyperflexibility) instability with rotator cuff strengthening exercises has not been successful. A capsular shift procedure to correct the problem will likely make the shoulder more stable. Which pair of primary mechanisms of glenohumeral stability is enhanced by these treatment methods?

A. Capsular constraint and adhesion-cohesion
B. Capsular constraint and glenolabral depth
C. Concavity-compression and capsular constraint
D. Concavity-compression and adhesion-cohesion
E. Concavity-compression and glenolabral suction cup (negative pressure)

The patient described above has atraumatic MDI, often associated with a patulous capsule. Therefore capsular shift is the mainstay of operative treatment in patients for whom rehabilitation has been unsuccessful. The primary mechanism enhanced by a capsular shift procedure is capsular constraint. Concavity-compression, which is the maintenance of the humeral head in the concave glenoid fossa by the compressive force generated by the surrounding muscles, is the primary mechanism enhanced by strengthening rehabilitation. The mechanism of glenolabral depth is typically a problem associated with unilateral, traumatic shoulder instability in which a Bankart labral tear has occurred.

Answer: **C**
Lazarus, Sidles, Harryman, pp. 94-102

24. True or False: The MCP joint is more stable than the PIP joint.

The MCP joint is a condyloid joint, whereas the PIP joint is a bicondylar joint. The MCP joint has a greater freedom of movement and therefore is less stable, which makes it more susceptible to injury.

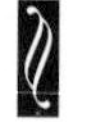
Answer: **False**
DeLee, Drez, Miller, p. 1383
Refer to Fig. 12-9

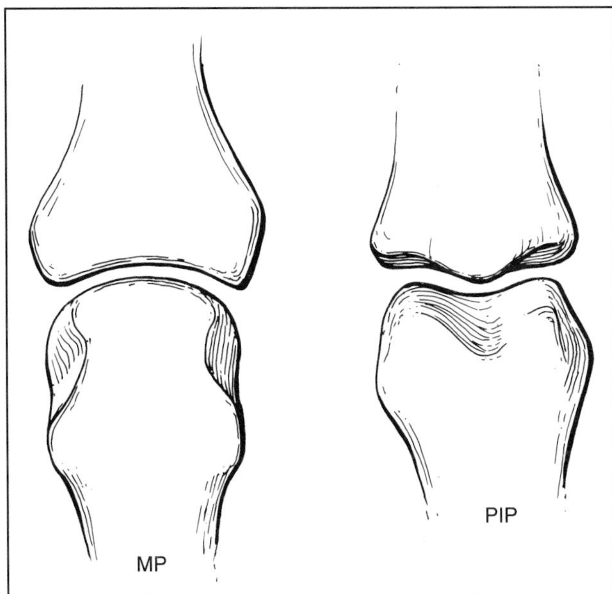

Fig. 12-9 ■ The MCP and PIP joints are structurally quite different. The PIP joint has a bicondylar configuration, thus making it inherently more stable than the globular MCP joint. (From DeLee JC, Drez D, Miller MD: *DeLee & Drez's Orthopaedic sports medicine: principles and practice*, ed 2, Philadelphia, 2003, WB Saunders.)

25. A 41-year-old male softball athlete sustained a volar dislocation of the PIP joint as he slid into home plate. What is the recommended safe position for splinting of the PIP joint for volar dislocation?

A. Extension
B. 30 degrees of flexion
C. 60 degrees of flexion
D. 90 degrees of flexion
E. More than 100 degrees of flexion

A volar dislocation is rare and usually occurs when an extended digit is forcibly flexed at the PIP joint, such as when sliding into home plate with extended arms. A stable closed reduction should be maintained in a position of PIP joint extension for 4 weeks. The safe position for splinting of the PIP joint is extension to protect the central slip. If splinting is used and the PIP joint is stable the athlete may return to full practice sports.

Answer: **A**
DeLee, Drez, Miller, pp. 1384-1385, 1391-1393
Refer to Fig. 12-10

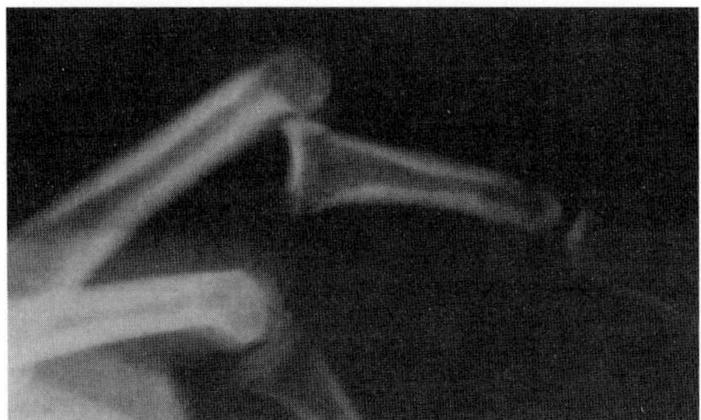

Fig. 12-10 ■ Volar dislocation of the PIP joint is a relatively uncommon injury. It should be obvious from this radiograph that the central slip must be torn for this injury to occur; therefore these patients should be treated in the same manner as those with a boutonnière injury. (From DeLee JC, Drez D, Miller MD: *DeLee & Drez's Orthopaedic sports medicine: principles and practice*, ed 2, Philadelphia, 2003, WB Saunders.)

CLINICAL GEM:
If the PIP joint has difficulty maintaining stability in a splint or if the patient is noncompliant, joint pinning may be used to assist in achieving a stable joint.

26. A 17-year-old high school football player sustained a dorsal MCP joint dislocation. What soft tissue structure is most commonly associated with an irreducible dorsal MCP joint dislocation?

A. Extensor tendon
B. Flexor digitorum superficialis tendon
C. Volar plate
D. Flexor digitorum profundus (FDP) tendon

The volar plate is the most common structure to prevent reduction of a dorsal MCP joint dislocation. When dislocations occur, the volar plate usually remains attached to the volar aspect of the proximal phalanx and is interpositioned between the metacarpal (MC) head and the base of the proximal phalanx.

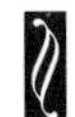
Answer: **C**
McLaughlin, pp. 683-688
DeLee, Drez, Miller, pp. 1385-1387
Refer to Fig. 12-11

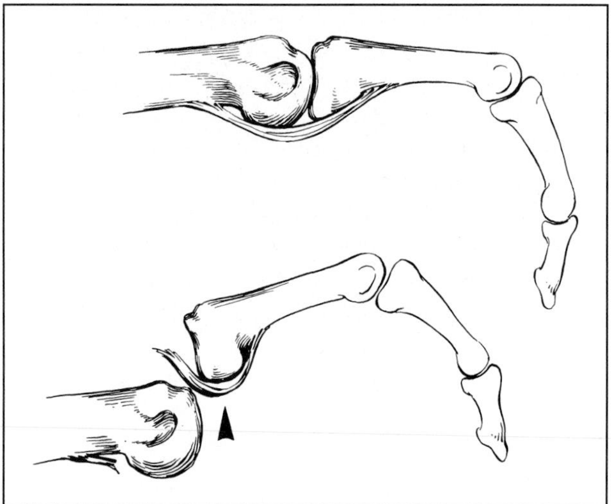

Fig. 12-11 ■ The single most important element in preventing reduction of a complex MCP dislocation is interposition of the volar plate between the base of the middle phalanx and the MC head. (From DeLee JC, Drez D, Miller MD: *DeLee & Drez's Orthopaedic sports medicine: principles and practice*, ed 2, Philadelphia, 2003, WB Saunders.)

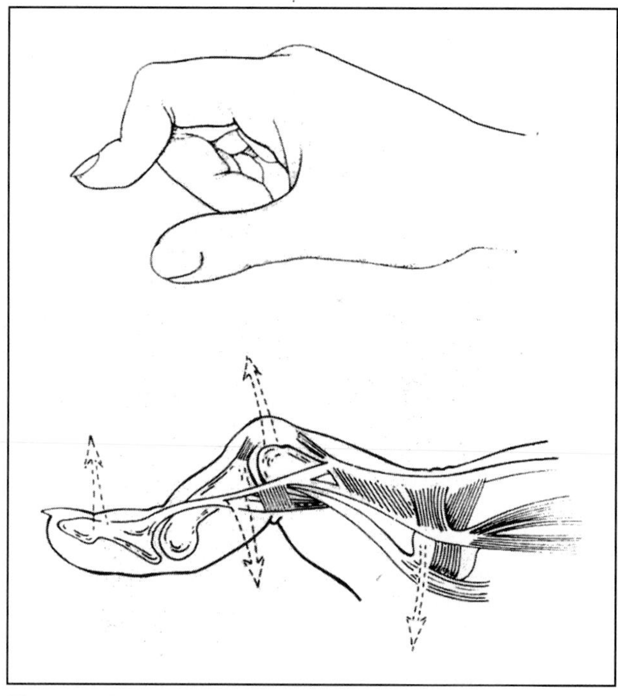

Fig. 12-12 ■ From DeLee JC, Drez D, Miller MD: *DeLee & Drez's Orthopaedic sports medicine: principles and practice*, ed 2, Philadelphia, 2003, WB Saunders.

27. True or False: A boutonnière deformity results from injury to the flexor mechanism of the finger.

Boutonnière deformity (Fig. 12-12) results from injury to the central slip insertion on the epiphysis of the middle phalanx. This is part of the extensor mechanism. The lateral bands move volar to the axis of rotation at the PIP joint. This results in hyperflexion of the PIP joint with hyperextension of the DIP joint.

Answer: **False**

Imatami, Hashizume, Wake, pp. 107-109
DeLee, Drez, Miller, p. 1394

28. Ms. S, a 26-year-old professional softball player, sustained an acute boutonnière deformity while playing the final game of the season. What is the treatment protocol of an acute boutonnière deformity?

A. Immobilization of both PIP and DIP joints in extension
B. Immobilization of both PIP and DIP joints in flexion
C. Immobilization with the PIP joint in extension with passive flexion of the DIP joint
D. Immobilization of the DIP joint in extension with passive flexion of the PIP joint

Acute boutonnière deformity may be treated with nonoperative measures up to 6 weeks after the injury. The PIP joint should be immobilized in extension for 6 weeks while the DIP joint is actively and passively stretched into flexion.

Answer: **C**

DeLee, Drez, Miller, p. 1395
Coons, Green, pp. 387-402

29. A 23-year-old lacrosse athlete sustained an injury to his left middle finger, thus resulting in a disruption of the terminal extension mechanism at the distal phalanx. What is this type of injury is known as?

A. Boxer's knuckle
B. Central slip disruption
C. Jersey finger
D. Mallet finger

Mallet finger, or disruption of the terminal extension at the distal phalanx, is common in sports and results from a hyperflexion force on an external DIP joint.

The basic diagnosis is made by asking the patient to extend the tip of his finger. The inability to extend the DIP joint actively strongly indicates a disruption of the terminal extensor tendon. Additional clinical findings may be an extensor lag, swelling, and tenderness at the site of injury. Most surgeons recommend radiographs to confirm the diagnosis but also to determine whether a fracture and/or joint subluxation has occurred. The mallet finger is almost always treated with splinting of the DIP joint in extension for 6 to 8 weeks. You can choose to use a stack splint or customized thermoplastic splinting (either volar or dorsal). Nearly every study indicates splinting achieves the best results and minimal complications.

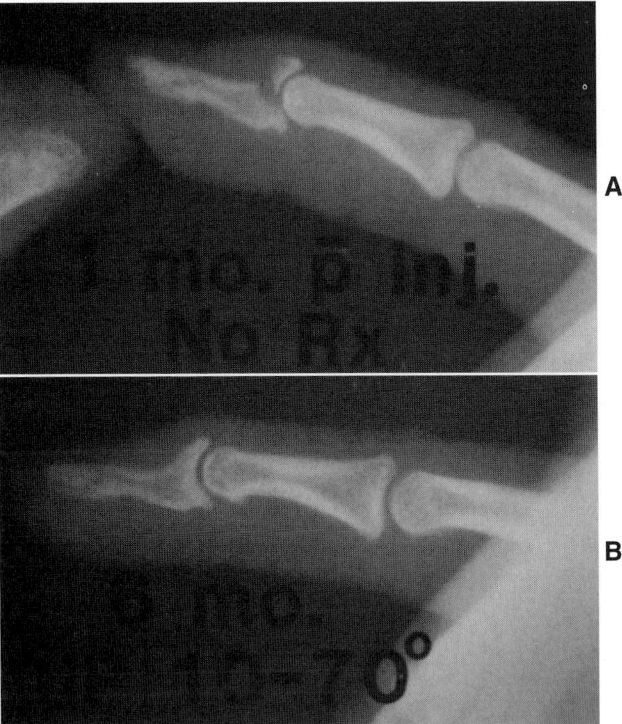

Fig. 12-13 ■ Most mallet fractures should be treated nonoperatively. **A,** This patient, who had received no treatment, was seen 1 month after injury. He was then treated with simple splint immobilization of the DIP joint for 6 weeks. **B,** Six months later, there is excellent remodeling of the articular surface. ROM in the DIP joint is 10 to 70 degrees. (From DeLee JC, Drez D, Miller MD: *DeLee & Drez's Orthopaedic sports medicine: principles and practice*, ed 2, Philadelphia, 2003, WB Saunders.)

Answer: **D**

DeLee Drez, Miller, pp. 1396-1397
Rosenthal in Mackin, Callahan, Skirven, et al, pp. 521-522
Wright, Rettig in Mackin, Callahan, Skirven, et al, pp. 2091, 2097
Refer to Fig. 12-13

CLINICAL GEM:
If splinting is the method of treatment, the athlete may return to full practice immediately.

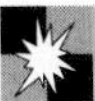

CLINICAL GEM:
Classic mallet finger splinting, as proposed by Smillie, immobilized the PIP joint in flexion and the DIP joint in hyperextension. This is *no longer* advocated. The PIP joint is left free, and the DIP joint is splinted in extension or neutral. Hyperextension can produce dorsal skin blanching with cutaneous and terminal tendon ischemia.

30. A 16-year-old high school football player sustained an injury to the tip of his ring finger, thus resulting in an avulsion of FDP tendon from its insertion at the distal phalanx. This injury is known as which of the following?

A. Mallet finger
B. Jersey finger
C. Bennett's fracture
D. Jones fracture

Jersey finger, or avulsion of the FDP tendon at the distal phalanx resulting from forced extension of a flexed DIP joint, occurs as one player grabs another player and the tip of the finger becomes caught in the opponent's jersey or equipment. The ring finger is the most commonly injured digit because the ring profundus tendon shares a common muscle belly with the long and small fingers. As the athlete grabs another player, the eccentric load placed on the DIP joint is believed to rupture the ring finger FDP.

Clinical findings include DIP joint pain or discomfort and swelling. The examiner must test both the FDP and flexor digitorum superficialis (FDS) for integrity because simultaneous rupture of the superficialis and profundus in athletes is not uncommon.

Treatment for a Jersey finger depends on the athlete's age, level of play, and future plans. In a high school athlete with a ruptured profundus, surgical intervention is often recommended and best treated within 2 weeks of injury.

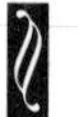

Answer: **B**
Leddy, Packer, pp. 66-69
Wright, Rettig in Mackin, Callahan, Skirven, et al, p. 2091

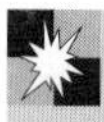

Clinical Gem:
The DIP joint represents approximately 15% of the function of the digit.

31. David, a 15-year-old travel hockey player, was skating from the opposite side of the rink with significant speed. He collided with the side boards, creating enough shear force to produce a Bennett's fracture. What is the primary deforming force in a Bennett's fracture of the thumb?

A. Extension pollicis longus
B. Abductor pollicis longus
C. Abductor pollicis
D. Flexor pollicis longus
E. Flexor pollicis brevis

A Bennett's fracture is an intraarticular fracture at the base of the thumb. The shear force transmits to the trapeziometacarpal joint at the volar ulnar quadrant of the proximal metacarpal surface, thus creating instability at the base of the thumb. The abductor pollicis longus acts as the primary deforming force. It draws the MC shaft proximally and dorsally away from the volar-ulnar lip of the MC's articular surface, thus causing the thumb to adduct. Because the thumb is strenuously used, the deformity is usually corrected surgically, especially with a young individual.

Answer: **B**
Stener, pp. 869-879
Freeland, p. 167
Refer to Fig. 11-14, A

32. Mr. Bill, a 36-year-old nurse, plays on a coed softball league. He was running to third base and collided with the baseman, resulting in a torn ulnar collateral ligament to the thumb. True or False: Ulnar collateral ligament injuries associated with a Stener's lesion are best treated nonoperatively.

A Stener's lesion refers to the interposition of the abductor tendon between the torn end of the ulnar collateral ligament and its insertion site. Operative intervention is required to reposition the ends of the ulnar collateral ligament.

Answer: **False**
Stener, pp. 869-879
DeLee, Drez, Miller, p. 1413
Refer to Fig. 11-13

33. A 21-year-old football player collided with his opponent's helmet and suffered a mallet thumb. A mallet thumb is a disruption of which of the following?

A. Extensor pollicis brevis
B. Extensor pollicis longus
C. Abductor pollicis
D. Extensor digitorum communis

A mallet thumb is a disruption of the extensor pollicis longus. In general, it is an uncommon injury. Primary repair is usually recommended in the athletic population and requires thumb immobilization.

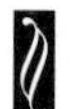

Answer: **B**
DeLee, Drez, Miller, pp. 1416-1417

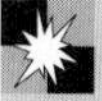

Clinical Gem:
Splinting or taping the thumb does not provide enough protection to return to athletic participation. Regardless of treatment plan, one should expect a 5- to 6-week period without play.

34. Which of the following is not a vascular syndrome associated with athletics?

A. Digital ischemia
B. Hypothenar hammer syndrome
C. Mallet thumb
D. Ulnar artery thrombosis

Vascular syndromes are rarely seen with athletes. However, athletes who participate in hand impact sports (martial arts, baseball, lacrosse, handball, and all racquet sports) are at higher risk of sustaining a vascular injury. Hypothenar hammer syndrome or ulnar artery thrombosis results from damage to the ulnar artery at the level of the wrist. Digital ischemia occurs secondarily to repetitive microtrauma to the palm just distal to the wrist. Mallet thumb is not a vascular injury; it involves the extensor pollicis longus tendon.

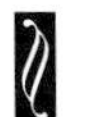
Answer: **C**
DeLee, Drez, Miller, pp. 1417-1419

35. All but which of the following are associated with nerve compression injuries?

A. Bowler's thumb
B. Bowler's finger
C. Handlebar palsy
D. Hypothenar hammer syndrome

Hypothenar hammer syndrome is a vascular syndrome associated with ulnar artery damage at the wrist level. It is not associated with nerve compression injuries. Bowler's thumb is a perineural fibrosis of the ulnar digit nerve of the thumb due to repetitive microtrauma during gripping of the ball. Bowler's finger is a similar involvement of the dorsal branch of the radial digital nerve of the ring finger. Handlebar palsy is an entrapment of the motor branch of the ulnar nerve seen in cyclists.

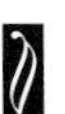
Answer: **D**
DeLee, Drez, Miller, p. 1423
Kornberg, Aulicino, Du Puy, pp. 25-33
Eversmann, pp. 759-766

36. True or False: The National Federation of State High School Associations (NFSHSA) prohibits the use of orthotics made of sole leather, plaster, metal, or other hard substances regardless of any soft padded covering.

The NFSHSA prohibits the use of orthotics made of sole leather, plaster, metal, or other hard substances regardless of any soft padded covering. The NCAA (National Collegiate Athletic Association), unlike the NFSHSA, will allow the use of orthotics covered by ½-inch closed-cell, slow-recovery foam padding. Most state high schools abide by the NFSHSA rules; a few follow the NCAA rules.

Answer: **True**
DeLee, Drez, Miller, p. 1424
National Collegiate Athletic Association
National Federation Football Rules Committee

37. A 19-year-old college volleyball player injured her long finger while spiking the ball. Her medical doctor and athletic trainer opted for buddy taping via adhesive tape. True or False: Adhesive taping in the form of budding taping is effective for functional injuries to the digits.

Although athletic trainers are masters with taping hand, wrist, ankle, and other sport injury areas, adhesive tape alone does not provide adequate support for most injuries. However, adhesive taping is most effective when used to securely buddy tape an injured digit to the adjacent uninjured digit for functional use and ROM.

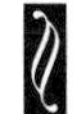
Answer: **True**
DeLee, Drez, Miller, p. 1424

38. A 59-year-old squash player is complaining of aching pain in the flexor musculature at the medial elbow. Weakness of grip strength in the symptomatic hand is noted. Pain is increased with flexing and pronating the wrist against resistance (Fig. 12-14). The patient is diagnosed with medial epicondylitis or golfer's elbow. Medial epicondylitis is usually exacerbated by what motions?

A. Repetitive or forceful pronation and/or resisted wrist extension
B. Repetitive or forceful supination and/or resisted elbow flexion
C. Resisted and forceful wrist flexion and repetitive supination
D. Repetitive or forceful pronation and/or resisted wrist flexion

Injuries to the medial common flexor tendon generally result from repetitive valgus and forearm stress. Medial epicondylitis is primarily exacerbated by activities that use repetitive or forceful pronation and/or resisted wrist flexion. The patient usually complains of point tenderness over the common anterior aspect of the medial epicondyle. Medial epicondylitis usually involves the flexor carpi ulnaris and pronator teres. It is much less common than lateral epicondylitis. Medial epicondylitis is often treated conservatively with rest, activity modification, stretching, nonsteroidal antiinflammatory drugs (NSAIDs), splinting, and steroid injection.

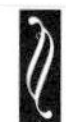

Answer: **D**

Canale, p. 1324
DeLee, Drez, Miller, pp. 591, 1226-1228
Wadsworth in Mackin, Callahan, Skirven, et al, p. 1269
Fedorczyk in Mackin, Callahan, Skirven, et al, pp. 1279-1280

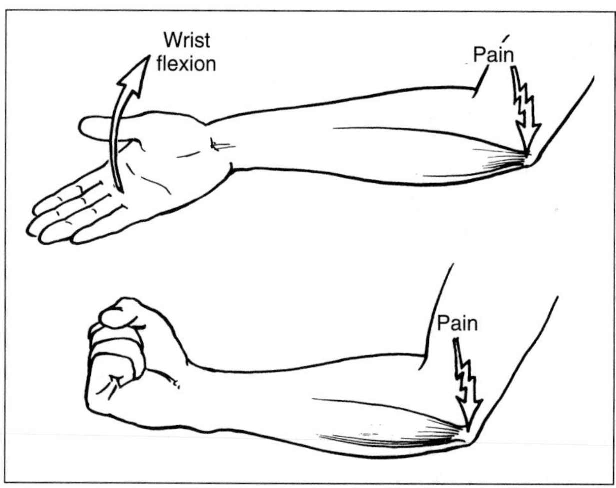

Fig. 12-14 ■ Medial epicondylitis may be diagnosed clinically from pain localized to the medial epicondyle during wrist flexion and pronation against resistance. Pain is often elicited after a tight fist is made, and grip strength is usually diminished on the affected side. (From Morrey BF: *The elbow and its disorders*, Philadelphia, 1985, WB Saunders.)

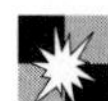

CLINICAL GEM:
Sporting activities that produce medial epicondylitis include squash, racquetball, tennis, golf, and most racquet sports.

Chapter 13

Arthritis

1. If in rheumatoid arthritis (RA) a swan-neck deformity is caused by intrinsic tightness, which of the following treatments would be beneficial?

A. Hand exercises that encourage full proximal interphalangeal (PIP) flexion and metacarpophalangeal (MCP) joint extension
B. A dorsal orthotic to keep the MCP joints in full extension for intrinsic stretching to be used at night only
C. Avoidance of prolonged intrinsic plus positions (resting chin on dorsum of fingers, prolonged holding of a book, hand activities such as knitting and crocheting)
D. A and C
E. All of the above

A swan-neck deformity (Fig. 13-1) is usually caused by synovitis of the flexor tendon sheaths with resulting loss of PIP flexion. This transfers the flexor forces to the MCP joint. This position creates intrinsic muscle pull on the central tendon, with resulting stretch on the palmar plate of the PIP joint. Eventually hyperextension of the PIP joint and flexion of the distal interphalangeal (DIP) joint is created. It is important to do exercises to the hand that encourage full PIP joint flexion and MCP extension to stretch tight intrinsics (Fig. 13-2, *A*). Avoiding prolonged intrinsic plus positions will also reduce contributions to deforming forces (Fig. 13-2, *B*).

Answer: **D**

Melvin, pp. 284-287, 427
Hunter, Mackin, Callahan, pp. 1318-1319
Alter, Feldon, Terrono in Mackin, Callahan, Skirven, et al, p. 1551
Biese in Mackin, Callahan, Skirven, et al, pp. 1576-1580
Refer to Figs. 13-1 and 13-2

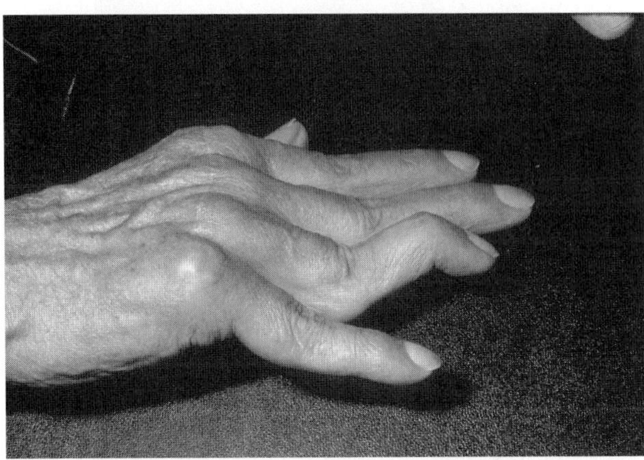

Fig. 13-1 ■ From Mackin EJ, Callahan AD, Skirven TM, et al: *Rehabilitation of the hand and upper extremity*, ed 5, vol 2, St Louis, 2002, Mosby.

CLINICAL GEM:
Swan-neck deformities can originate from abnormalities at the DIP, PIP, or MCP joints.

CLINICAL GEM:
A splint that prevents PIP joint hyperextension will often improve function during ADLs (Fig. 13-3).

2. Which medications are used in the treatment of osteoarthritis?

A. Celebrex
B. Vioxx
C. Mobic
D. Enbrel
E. A, B, and C
F. All of the above

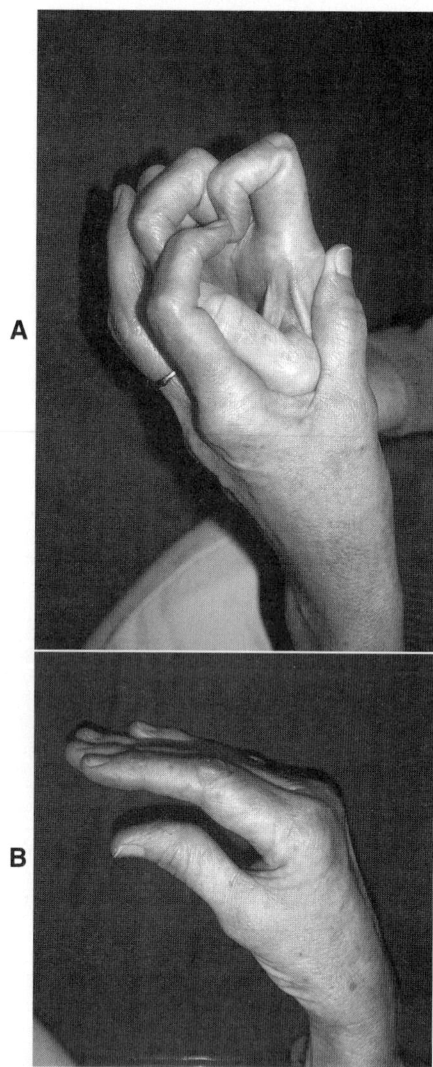

Fig. 13-2 ■ From Mackin EJ, Callahan AD, Skirven TM, et al: *Rehabilitation of the hand and upper extremity*, ed 5, vol 2, St Louis, 2002, Mosby.

Celebrex, Vioxx, Mobic, and all nonsteroidal antiinflammatory drugs (NSAIDs) are used to treat both osteoarthritis and RA. Enbrel, Humira, and Remicade are used to treat RA. The medications used to treat osteoarthritis are NSAIDs and analgesics.

The NSAIDs provide relief of pain, swelling, and stiffness. As a group the primary side effect of NSAIDs is their ability to cause peptic ulcer disease. The DMARDs, anti-TNFs and anti–Il 1 (interleukin 1) receptor antagonists provide all of the relief of the analgesics and NSAIDs but also prevent disease progression and heal the bone damage (erosions) of RA. DMARDs have various potential side effects, the most common of which is bone marrow suppression. The anti-TNFs and anti–Il 1 receptor antagonists increase susceptibility to infection. The current thinking is to use DMARDs and anti-TNF (or anti–Il 1 receptor antagonists) early in the course of the disease in an attempt to prevent joint damage.

A spectrum of medication that ranges from milder to more aggressive therapy is available for the treatment of RA. In order from mildest to strongest are analgesics, NSAIDs (which include the Cox-2 agents), disease-modifying antirheumatic drugs (DMARDs), anti–tumor necrosis factors (TNFs), and anti–Il one receptor antagonists. The analgesics provide pain relief only.

Answer: **E**

Package Inserts: Celebrex, Pfizer, Inc., New York, NY; Vioxx, Merck and Co. Inc., West Point, PA; Mobic, Boehringer Ingelheim Pharmaceuticals, Inc., Ridgefield, CT; Enbrel, Immunex Corp, Seattle, WA; Humira, Abbott Laboratories, Abbott Park, IL; Remicade, Centocor, Inc., Malvern, PA

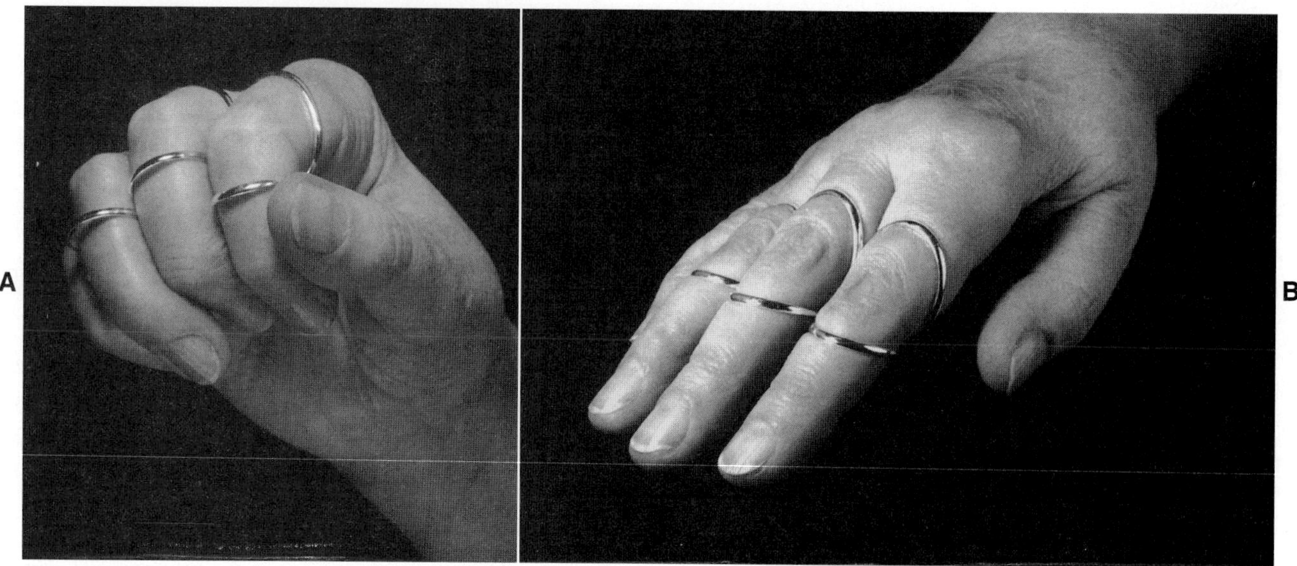

Fig. 13-3 ■ Courtesy of Silver Ring Splint Company, Charlottesville, VA.

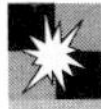

CLINICAL GEM:
The following drugs are DMARDs: methotrexate, gold, Sulfasalazine, Avara, and Plaquenil. Kinaret is a receptor antagonist. Humira, Enbrel, and Remicade are anti-TNF medications.

3. Which of these antiinflammatory medications are considered Cox-2 inhibitors?

A. Vioxx
B. Celebrex
C. Bextra
D. All of the above

Vioxx, Celebrex, and Bextra are Cox-2 inhibitors. The importance of this concept is that these *new* Cox-2 inhibitors are associated with less frequent ulcer and kidney disease than the older antiinflammatory medications (which were Cox-1 inhibitors).

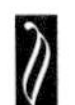

Answer: **D**
Package Inserts: Vioxx, Merck and Co, Inc., West Point, PA; Celebrex, Pfizer, Inc., New York, NY; Indocin, Merck and Co., Inc., West Point, PA; Voltaren, Novartis Pharmaceuticals Corp, East Hanover, NJ; Bextra, Pfizer Inc., New York, NY

4. How often may a joint be injected with a steroid preparation?

A. Monthly
B. One time per year
C. Three to four times per year
D. Never

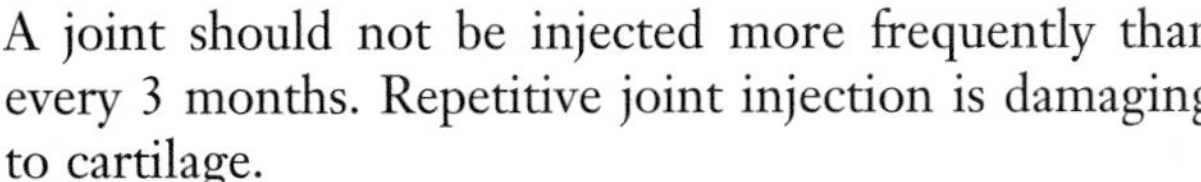

A joint should not be injected more frequently than every 3 months. Repetitive joint injection is damaging to cartilage.

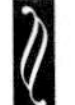

Answer: **C**
Owen, p. 55

5. True or False: RA is primarily a disease of the articular cartilage.

RA is a generalized disease that primarily affects the synovium. RA affects approximately 3% of the population. Osteoarthritis is a disease that typically affects the articular cartilage. Women are more often affected than men. Adult onset usually occurs between the ages of 20 and 60 years. Osteoarthritis is common in adults. Approximately 8% of all adults are estimated to have some degree of osteoarthritis in their hands and feet. Nearly 85% of all people between the ages of 75 and 79 demonstrate evidence of osteoarthritis.

Answer: **False**
Hunter, Mackin, Callahan, p. 1307
Alter, Feldon, Terrono in Mackin, Callahan, Skirven, et al, p. 1545

6. Stenosing tenosynovitis of the digits is common in RA and can include the following signs and symptoms?

A. Trigger finger due to granulomatous plaques (nodules) catching on the pulleys (annular ligaments)
B. Numbness and paresthesias
C. Swelling on the volar aspect of the digit
D. A and C
E. All of above

The tendons of the hand pass through a synovium-lined sheath. The sheath's purpose is to facilitate lubrication and gliding of the tendons. Inflammation in the synovial tissue results in excessive fluid on the volar aspects of digits and when chronic, synovial tissue will proliferate, causing nodules and swelling. The nodules can get caught on any of the pulleys of the finger during active flexion of the digits. It most commonly occurs at the A1 pulley. This is commonly referred to as *trigger finger.*

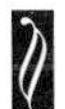

Answer: **D**
Melvin, pp. 295-302
Alter, Feldon, Terrono in Mackin, Callahan, Skirven, et al, pp. 1545-1550
Biese in Mackin, Callahan, Skirven, et al, p. 1578

7. Tenosynovitis with trigger finger and the resulting loss of tendon excursion is most effectively treated with which of the following?

A. Heat, gradual active and passive range of motion (ROM) exercises, static orthotic immobilization at night
B. Ice, MCP blocking orthotic, iontophoresis, and/or cortisone injection
C. Heat, gradual active ROM exercises with emphasis on tendon excursion, and orthotic immobilization of digit only
D. All of the above are appropriate.

Steroid injections along with ice compresses are the recommended conservative treatment. A hand- or finger-based (when only one digit is involved) MCP blocking orthotic is very helpful is preventing maximal PIP/MCP flexion. This splint allows for partial tendon excursion and performance of light activity of daily living (ADL) tasks while preventing the triggering at the digit. When worn full time for up to 3 months, the triggering usually stops.

Answer: **B**

Melvin, pp. 299, 302

8. The most common collapse deformity in the rheumatoid thumb is which of the following?

A. Boutonnière deformity
B. Swan-neck deformity
C. Adducted retropositioned thumb
D. All of the above are equally common.

The most common collapse deformity of the rheumatoid thumb is a boutonnière deformity (Fig. 13-4). In this deformity, the joint capsule and the extensor apparatus around the MCP joint are stretched by synovitis. The extensor pollicis longus and adductor expansion are displaced ulnarly. The attachment of the extensor pollicis brevis to the proximal phalanx is lengthened and becomes ineffective. The long extensor tendons and extensor insertions of the intrinsics apply their power to the distal joint, thus producing a hyperextension deformity of this joint. Pinching further accentuates this deformity and a vicious cycle develops; eventually the deformity becomes fixed.

Answer: **A**

Hunter, Mackin, Callahan, pp. 1322-1323
Alter, Feldon, Terrono in Mackin, Callahan, Skirven, et al, pp. 1545, 1553
Terrono, Nalebuff, Philips in Mackin, Callahan, Skirven, et al, p. 1555

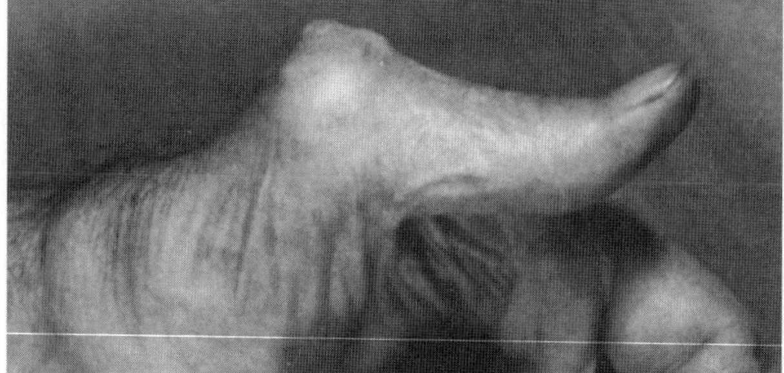

Fig. 13-4 ■ From Hunter JM, Mackin EJ, Callahan AD: *Rehabilitation of the hand: surgery and therapy,* ed 4, St Louis, 1995, Mosby.

CLINICAL GEM:
The second most common thumb deformity is the swan-neck.

9. A patient with RA should avoid staying in one position for a prolonged period. How often should this patient change positions?

A. Every 10 minutes
B. Every 20 to 30 minutes
C. Hourly
D. Three times a day

Maintaining a static position can put undue stress on underlying structures and lead to joint dysfunction. It is recommended that the patient change his or her position every 20 to 30 minutes. Activities can be alternated to facilitate positional changes; for example, if a patient is reading, a break should be taken after 20 minutes and a stretch should be performed, or the patient should switch to another task, such as folding the laundry.

Answer: **B**

Hunter, Mackin, Callahan, p. 1345
Melvin in Mackin, Callahan, Skirven, et al, p. 1657

10. True or False: RA is a painful disease and a patient with RA should expect to have pain for several hours after any activity.

A patient with RA often has a high tolerance for pain. It is important for the patient, however, to monitor his or her activities and to stop when pain or fatigue begins. If discomfort lasts for longer than an hour after an activity, the activity should be modified. In contrast, some patients have a fear of pain, which leads to needless inactivity. A careful balance between rest and use must be employed to allow for maximal function.

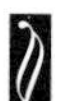

Answer: **False**

Hunter, Mackin, Callahan, p. 1348
Biese in Mackin, Callahan, Skirven, et al, pp. 1573, 1579

11. Which of the following is *not* a principle of joint protection?

A. Maintain muscle strength and joint ROM
B. Avoid positions of deformity
C. Use the weakest joint available for a job
D. Respect pain
E. Avoid prolonged static positions

All the above are principles of joint protection with the exception of using the weakest joint available for a job. It is important to use the strongest joint available to perform a job.

Answer: **C**

Hunter, Mackin, Callahan, pp. 1377-1378
Biese in Mackin, Callahan, Skirven, et al, p. 1579
Refer to Table 13-1

12. During an acute stage of RA, how much sleep is recommended in a 24-hour period?

A. 6 to 8 hours
B. 8 to 10 hours
C. 10 to 12 hours
D. 12 to 14 hours

When a patient has a systemic disease, the entire body must be rested—not only the part that hurts. During an acute stage of RA, 10 to 12 hours of sleep every 24 hours is recommended. The patient also must be encouraged to balance activity with daytime rest to avoid fatigue. The therapist is responsible for educating the patient to help relieve symptoms in the hand and/or other parts of the body.

Table 13-1

Overview of Protection Principles

Principle	Recommendation
Respect pain.	1. Stop activities before the point of discomfort. 2. Decrease activities that cause pain that lasts more than 2 hours. 3. Avoid activities that put strain on painful or stiff joints.
Balance rest and activity.	1. Rest before exhaustion. 2. Take frequent, short breaks. 3. Avoid activities that cannot be stopped. 4. Avoid staying in one position for a long time. 5. Alternate heavy and light activities. 6. Take more breaks when inflammation is active. 7. Allow extra time for activities—avoid rushing. 8. Plan your day ahead of time. 9. Eliminate unnecessary activities.
Exercise in a pain-free range.	1. Initiate warm-water pool exercise programs. 2. Exercises should be specific to each deformity.
Reduce the effort.	1. Avoid excessive loads with carts, get help; use appliances. 2. Keep items near where they are used. 3. Use prepared foods. 4. Avoid low chairs. 5. Maintain proper body weight. 6. Freeze leftovers for easy meals later. 7. Try to eliminate trips up and down stairs by completing work on each floor. 8. Sit to work when possible.
Avoid positions of deformity.	1. Avoid bent elbows, knees, hips, and back while sleeping. 2. Practice good posture during the day. 3. Use workstation evaluation for proper posture.
Use the larger joints.	1. Slide heavy objects on kitchen counters. 2. Use palms, rather than fingers, to lift or push. 3. Carry a backpack, instead of a handheld purse. 4. Keep packages close to the body—use two hands. 5. Push swinging doors open with side of body instead of the hands.
Use adaptive equipment.	Use jar openers, button hooks, etc. that are specific to each patient's needs.
Distribute pressure.	Use both hands, leverage, carts, etc.

From Mackin EJ, Callahan AD, Skirven TM, et al: *Rehabilitation of the hand and upper extremity*, ed 5, vol 2, St Louis, 2002, Mosby.

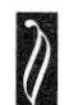

Answer: **C**
Hunter, Mackin, Callahan, p. 1378

13. CREST syndrome is a variant of which of the following?

A. RA
B. Osteoarthritis
C. Scleroderma
D. Ollier's disease

Scleroderma is an umbrella term for disorders in which sclerosis of the skin is a predominant feature. Under the general category of scleroderma, there are many classifications. One classification is generalized scleroderma, which includes subcategories of diffuse scleroderma and limited scleroderma. CREST syndrome belongs to the limited scleroderma category. CREST is an acronym that stands for *c*alcinosis, *R*aynaud's phenomenon, *e*sophageal hypomotility, *s*clerodactyly, and *t*elangiectasia.

Answer: **C**
Hunter, Mackin, Callahan, p. 1385
Melvin in Mackin, Callahan, Skirven, et al, pp. 1677-1678

14. Maintaining which of the following is important during treatment for scleroderma?

A. PIP joint flexion
B. MCP joint flexion
C. DIP joint flexion
D. Carpometacarpal (CMC) joint flexion

A patient with scleroderma typically presents with the following deformities: MCP joint extension contractures, PIP joint flexion contractures, thumb adduction contractures, and contracture of the wrist in the neutral position. DIP joints often become fixed in mid-range. Therapy must focus on preserving MCP joint flexion and PIP joint extension as primary goals. It also is important to prevent thumb CMC adduction contractures, and from a functional standpoint, preserving lateral pinch is extremely crucial. Lateral pinch is maintained by preserving MCP joint flexion. Loss of lateral pinch represents a tremendous loss of hand function.

Answer: **B**
Hunter, Mackin, Callahan, p. 1387
Melvin in Mackin, Callahan, Skirven, et al, p. 1679
Melvin, pp. 106-117
Refer to Fig. 13-5

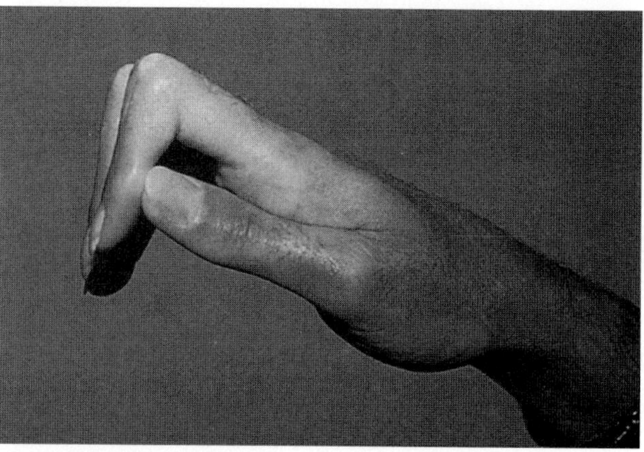

Fig. 13-5 ■ This patient can barely pinch and is unable to do a true lateral pinch. Therapy that would increase index MCP flexion 15 to 20 degrees would significantly improve her ability for pinch and hand function. (From Mackin EJ, Callahan AD, Skirven TM, et al: *Rehabilitation of the hand and upper extremity*, ed 5, vol 2, St Louis, 2002, Mosby.)

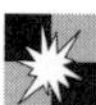

CLINICAL GEM:
If a patient can have only one type of pinch, lateral pinch is the most functional.

Melvin, pp. 106-117

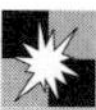

CLINICAL GEM:
Hand therapy goals with scleroderma include the following:

- Maintain maximal ROM (don't expect to increase ROM)
- Prevent unnecessary contractures by providing daily ROM
- Maintain MCP flexion and thumb abduction
- Maintain lateral pinch
- Use assistive devices to improve function
- Encourage optimal skin care

15. Which of the following is not a risk factor in osteoarthritis?

A. Trauma
B. Obesity
C. Genetic factors
D. All of the above are risk factors in osteoarthritis.

All of the above are risk factors in osteoarthritis. It is important to recognize these risk factors in order to reduce the ones that can be modified. Both trauma and repetitive stress have been implicated as causes of osteoarthritis. Previous vocational or avocational activities also can contribute to symptoms of osteoarthritis. An increased body mass, as in the obese patient, is associated with an increase in the prevalence of osteoarthritis, especially in the knees. Genetic factors have been shown to be noncoincidental in osteoarthritis; these include an autosomal dominant transmission in females and a recessive inheritance in males.

Answer: **D**
Brandt, pp. 25-30
Bozentka in Mackin, Callahan, Skirven, et al, pp. 1642-1643

16. True or False: In the early stages of osteoarthritis, the cartilage is thicker than normal.

Most descriptions of the pathology of osteoarthritis focus on the progressive loss of articular cartilage that occurs in the disease. However, in the early stages of osteoarthritis, the cartilage is thicker than normal. This is caused by an increase in water content, which reflects damage to the collagen network of the tissue and results in swelling of the cartilage. Cartilage thickening is associated with an increase in the net rate of synthesis of proteoglycans. With the progression of osteoarthritis, the joint surface thins, and the proteoglycan concentration diminishes, thus softening the cartilage. This loss of articular cartilage is the pathologic hallmark of osteoarthritis.

Answer: **True**
Brandt, pp. 35-36
Bozentka in Mackin, Callahan, Skirven, et al, p. 1637

17. True or False: Joint pain from osteoarthritis arises from the articular cartilage.

The articular cartilage is aneural. Therefore the joint pain in osteoarthritis must arise from other structures. Joint pain in osteoarthritis can occur from stretching of the nerve endings in the periosteum covering osteophytes, microfractures in subchondral bone, medullary hypertension from the distortion of blood flow by thickened subchondral trabeculae, or synovitis.

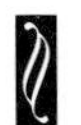

Answer: **False**
Brandt, p. 56

18. Bony enlargements of the DIP joint are known as which of the following?

A. Heberden's nodes
B. Bouchard's nodes
C. Synovial effusions
D. All of the above

Bony enlargements of the DIP joints are called *Heberden's nodes.* Bony enlargements of the PIP joints are called *Bouchard's nodes.* In some joints, gross deformity is obvious. The incidence of these nodes increases with age, and they are more common in women than men.

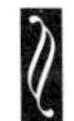

Answer: **A**
Brandt, p. 61
Bozentka in Mackin, Callahan, Skirven, et al, pp. 1640-1641
Refer to Fig. 13-6

19. True or False: Joint protection should be issued as a last resort when the patient cannot perform the activity in any other manner.

In the presence of arthritis, it is important to protect joints prior to the presence of deformity, not just for a compensation for loss of function. The goal of joint protection is to reduce pain and stress in the involved tissues or joints and consequently reduce inflammation and preserve the integrity of the joint structures.

Answer: **False**
Melvin, p. 420
Biese in Mackin, Callahan, Skirven, et al, p. 1579

20. Which of the following statements is true about arthritis?

A. Activities and equipment involving strong, full grasp are contraindicated for patients with MCP involvement.
B. Lower extremity dressing aids sometimes do more harm than good.
C. Equipment needs in the morning may differ from those in the afternoon.
D. A and C
E. All of the above

All of the statements are true. With active MCP involvement, hand tasks should be performed with the MCPs in extension or not at all if hand stress is too great. In the patient with ankylosing spondylitis, the movements

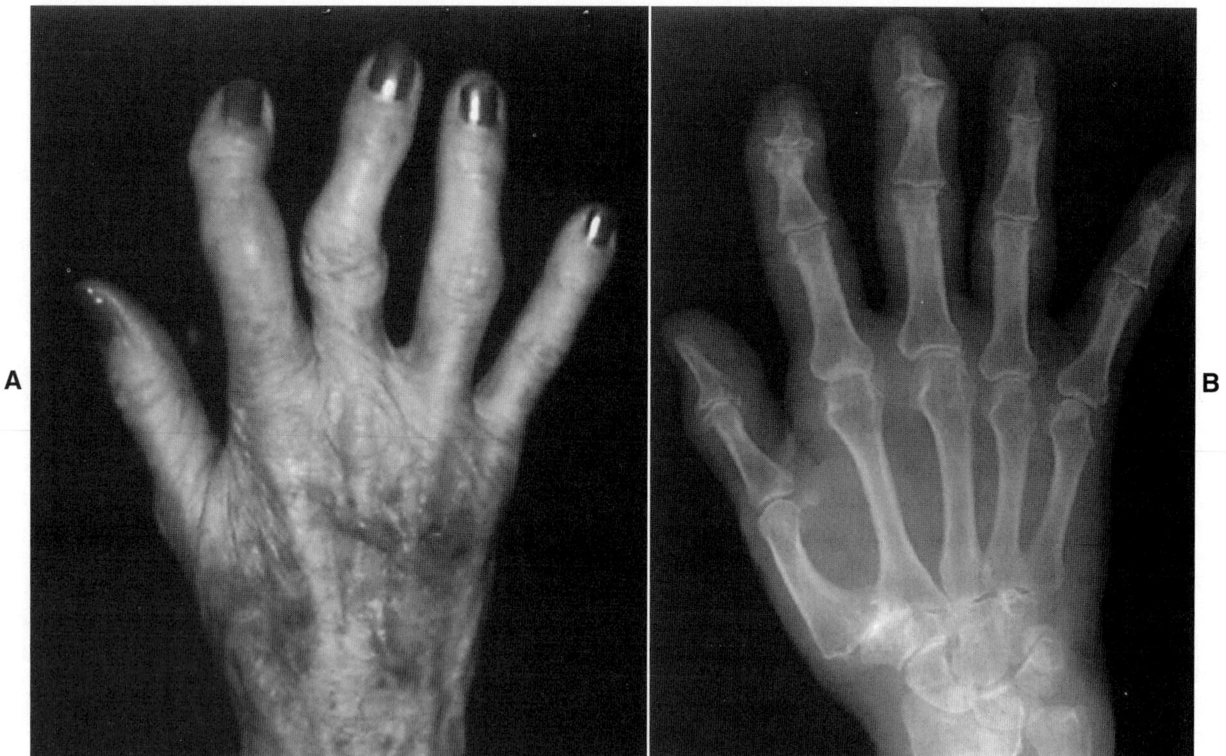

Fig. 13-6 ■ **A,** Osteoarthritis of the hand. Heberden's nodes are noted at the DIP joints, and Bouchard's nodes are noted at the PIP joints. **B,** Radiograph of hand with osteoarthritis. Asymmetric narrowing of the joint space, subchondral sclerosis, osteophytes, and cyst formation are noted. The MCP joints are typically not involved in osteoarthritis. (From Mackin EJ, Callahan AD, Skirven TM, et al: *Rehabilitation of the hand and upper extremity,* ed 5, vol 2, St Louis, 2002, Mosby.)

required to put on socks and shoes helps maintain hip and spinal motion. Unless there is acute pain or muscle spasm, using lower extremity aids may contribute to increased loss of active ROM. Finally, many patients' needs for assistive equipment differ greatly in the morning in the presence of morning stiffness.

Answer: **E**
Melvin, p. 438
Biese in Mackin, Callahan, Skirven, et al, p. 1579
Melvin in Mackin, Callahan, Skirven, et al, pp. 1656-1658

21. Which of the following pharmacological management techniques is not indicated in the treatment of osteoarthritis?

A. Acetaminophen
B. NSAIDs
C. Capsaicin
D. Systemic corticosteroid treatments

Systemic corticosteroid treatments are not indicated in the treatment of osteoarthritis. Prolonged systemic use of corticosteroids has significant side effects, which greatly outweigh any possible benefits. However, intraarticular injections of corticosteroids may be beneficial.

The use of NSAIDs has reduced joint pain and improved mobility for millions of people with osteoarthritis. However, some studies have indicated that a simple analgesic, such as acetaminophen, may be as effective as an NSAID in the treatment of patients with osteoarthritis. Capsaicin is a cream that is applied locally to a painful area. This substance may be useful in symptomatic management of osteoarthritis.

Answer: **D**
Brandt, pp. 135-160

22. True or False: Subluxation occurs when joint surfaces are no longer in contact with each other and no potential for normal joint motion exists.

A subluxation of a joint indicates that the articular surfaces are still in contact but that the joint surfaces are no longer in their normal alignment. A joint that is subluxed often can be manually reduced to its anatomical position but is unable to maintain the position without support. A dislocation occurs when joint surfaces are no longer in contact with each other and there is no potential for normal joint motion. In an arthritic dislocation, the articular surfaces usually are obliterated and the joint cannot be manually reduced. Attempting to splint a dislocation often increases the patient's pain and discomfort. Surgical intervention is indicated for dislocated arthritic joints.

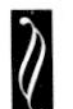

Answer: **False**

Malick, Kasch, p. 118

23. Which medication is not a cortisone derivative and can be injected into joints?

A. Indocin
B. Naproxen
C. Hyalgan
D. Synvisc
E. C and D

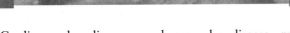

Hyalgan and Synvisc are not cortisone derivatives that can be injected into a joint. Hyalgan and Synvisc are examples of viscosupplementation. These medications chemically simulate synovial fluid in composition and may provide many months of relief. An ideal patient to receive these medications is one with osteoarthritis of the knee who attains only short-term benefit from a cortisone injection. A patient may receive up to 8 months of relief from Synvisc or Hyalgan. These two medications are only Food and Drug Administration (FDA) approved for use in osteoarthritis, specifically, osteoarthritis of the knee. Their intent is to reduce the need for total knee replacement.

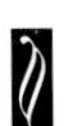

Answer: **E**

Pritchard, Sripada, Bankes, pp. 197-205

24. True or False: RA can shorten a person's lifespan.

Cardiovascular disease, cerebrovascular disease, pulmonary disease, malignancy, and infection are leading causes of premature death in the RA population.

Answer: **True**

Doran, Pond, Crowson, pp. 625-631

25. Research tests have shown that __________ pounds of grip and __________ pounds of pinch are necessary to accomplish most ADLs.

A. 10; 1 to 2
B. 15; 8 to 10
C. 20; 5 to 7
D. 5; 1 to 2

Research has shown that a grip strength of 20 pounds allows patients to perform most ADLs. It also has been shown that a pinch strength of 5 to 7 pounds is useful in accomplishing most daily living tasks. However, it must be remembered that patients with RA have strength far below these functional levels; it is therefore understandable that they encounter difficulties in accomplishing many daily living tasks.

Answer: **C**

Hunter, Mackin, Callahan, p. 1333
Terrono, Nalebuff, Philips in Mackin, Callahan, Skirven, et al, p. 1559

26. A patient is referred to you by his primary care doctor for treatment of his hand pain. During your evaluation you note a scaly, erythematous skin rash. You also note severe nail changes. The patient has flexion deformities of the PIP joints without DIP joint hyperextension. He also reports difficulty with grasping activities and intermittent swelling. What might this patient have?

A. Osteoarthritis
B. Boutonnière deformities
C. Psoriatic arthritis
D. None of the above

Psoriatic arthritis, an uncommon form of arthritis, is described in this case. There are similarities between this form of arthritis and RA or degenerative arthritis. The classic finding in psoriatic arthritis is a scaly, erythematous skin rash. Patients with psoriatic arthritis also have characteristic changes of the nails. These patients tend to present with asymmetric involvement of the hands; asymmetry also can be present unilaterally. The most common deformities seen with this type of arthritis are flexion deformities of the PIP joints without the corresponding DIP joint hyperextension that would be seen in a patient with a boutonnière deformity.

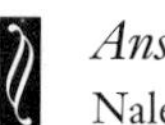

Answer: **C**
Nalebuff, pp. 603-610

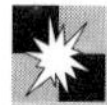

CLINICAL GEM:
Patients with psoriatic arthritis have a negative rheumatoid factor on serology testing.

27. What is the most commonly ruptured flexor tendon in a patient with RA?

A. Flexor pollicis longus
B. Flexor pollicis brevis
C. Flexor digitorum profundus to the index finger
D. Flexor digitorum profundus to the small finger
E. Flexor digitorum superficialis to the ring finger

The most commonly ruptured flexor tendon in patients with RA is the flexor pollicis longus. When this flexor tendon ruptures, the patient loses active flexion of the interphalangeal (IP) joint of the thumb. Rupture results when the tendon is worn away by a volar osteophyte on the scaphoid that penetrates through the volar wrist capsule. Rupture of the flexor pollicis longus also is known as a "Mannerfelt lesion." Functional loss is variable with this injury. The flexor digitorum profundus to the index and middle fingers may also be involved.

Answer: **A**
Green, p. 1612
Alter, Feldon, Terrono in Mackin, Callahan, Skirven, et al, pp. 1547, 1598
Refer to Fig. 13-7

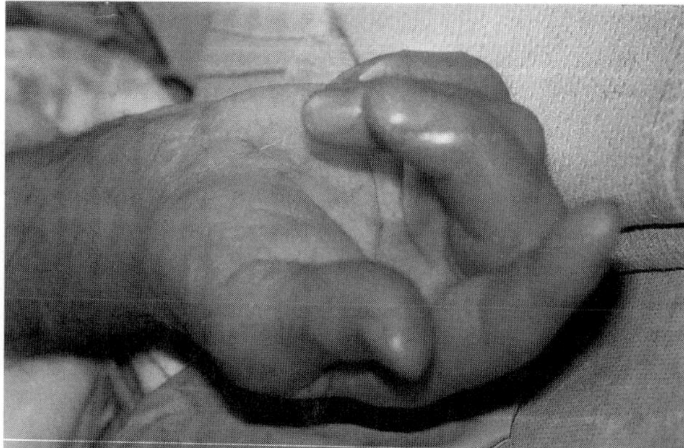

Fig. 13-7 ■ The posture of a hand with rupture of the flexor pollicis longus and profundus tendons to the index and middle fingers. (From Mackin EJ, Callahan AD, Skirven TM, et al: *Rehabilitation of the hand and upper extremity*, ed 5, vol 2, St Louis, 2002, Mosby.)

28. Which finger is most commonly involved in single extensor tendon ruptures in RA?

A. Index finger
B. Middle finger
C. Ring finger
D. Small finger

The small finger is most commonly involved in single extensor tendon ruptures in RA. With an isolated rupture of a single tendon, surgical intervention is advised because of the danger that additional ruptures may occur. Surgical treatment of an isolated rupture is relatively easy; surgical repair of multiple tendons is more complicated. Rupture of the extensor pollicis longus also is common in RA.

Answer: **D**
Green, pp. 1612-1614
Alter, Feldon, Terrono in Mackin, Callahan, Skirven, et al, p. 1547
Lubahn, Wolfe in Mackin, Callahan, Skirven, et al, p. 1599

CLINICAL GEM:
Two types of tendon ruptures are as follows:

1. Attrition rupture: A tendon moving across a roughened bone (most commonly the distal ulna or Lister's tubercle) will cause a rupture.
2. Ischemic rupture: Tenosynovitis that causes tendon compression, weakens the tendon, and decreases the blood supply results in a rupture.

29. The caput ulnae syndrome includes all but which of the following?

A. Weakness of the wrist and hand
B. Pain with rotation of the distal radioulnar (DRU) joint
C. Decreased ROM of the DRU joint
D. Dorsal prominence of the distal ulna
E. All of the above are findings associated with the caput ulnae syndrome.

The caput ulnae syndrome is described as an end-stage presentation of rheumatoid destruction of the DRU joint. Findings associated with this syndrome include weakness of the wrist and hand, pain with rotation of the DRU joint, decreased ROM of the DRU joint, dorsal prominence of the distal ulna, bulging of the synovial bursae of the long extensors and extensor carpi ulnaris, and rupture of one or more extensor tendons.

Answer: **E**

Blank, Cassidy, p. 500
Lubahn, Wolfe in Mackin, Callahan, Skirven, et al, p. 1598

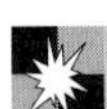

CLINICAL GEM:
Vaughn-Jackson syndrome occurs with a caput ulnae and is a rupturing of the tendons of the fourth, fifth, and occasionally the sixth extensor compartment.

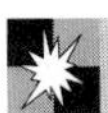

CLINICAL GEM:
A prominent ulnar head is easily recognized. One way to evaluate caput ulnae syndrome is to manually reduce the ulnar head, which resembles the up-and-down action of a piano key; this finding has been termed the *piano-key sign.*

30. True or False: An ulnar drift of the fingers is commonly seen in RA. This disease also causes the metacarpals to shift into ulnar deviation.

The typical zig-zag or Z pattern of deformity in RA is a palmar subluxation of the radius and the carpus in relation to the ulnar head. The ulnar half of the carpus droops in a palmar direction and the metacarpals shift into radial deviation; this is followed by a shift of the digits into ulnar deviation.

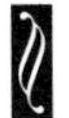

Answer: **False**

Taleisnik, p. 345
Biese in Mackin, Callahan, Skirven, et al, pp. 1570-1571
Refer to Fig. 13-8

CLINICAL GEM:
The typical pattern of deformity in RA is known as a zig-zag deformity of the wrist. Carpal supination occurs with a secondary radial shift of the metacarpals followed by an ulnar deviation of the digits. A patient with RA often requires management of the wrist, via fusion or ligament stabilization, before management of the MCP joints.

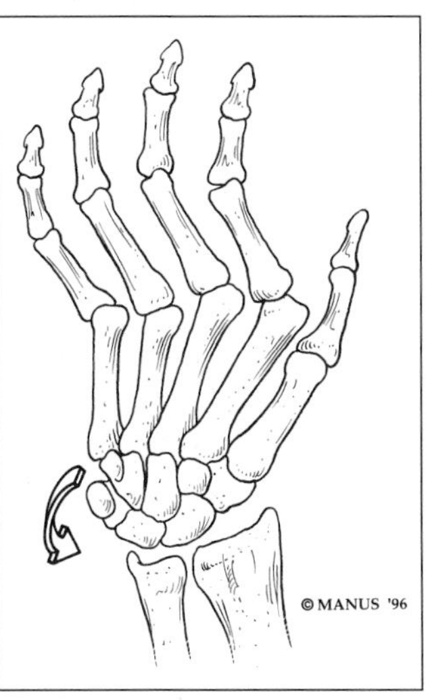

Fig. 13-8 ■ Characteristic Z deformity of the hand and wrist in RA. The wrist translates ulnarly, the metacarpals angle radially, and the fingers deviate ulnarly at the metaphalangeal joints. (Reprinted with permission from the Indiana Hand Center.)

31. You are evaluating a patient with RA. The patient has severe joint deformity and ulnar drift of the fingers and cannot extend his small and ring fingers. What might have occurred?

A. Rupture of the extensor tendons to the small finger
B. A radial nerve palsy
C. Subluxation of the extensor tendons to the ulnar aspect of the MCP joint
D. Subluxation of the extensor tendons to the radial aspect of the MCP joint
E. A, B, and C
F. All of the above

The inability to extend the small and ring fingers has many possible causes. Radial nerve palsy is an uncommon etiology but it may be the cause if the rheumatoid deformity is around the elbow joint. Rupture of the extensor tendons is not uncommon and occurs at the level of the distal ulna in the condition known as *caput ulnae syndrome*. Patients with RA often have subluxation of the extensor tendons, which can preclude extension. Subluxation of the extensor tendons occurs in the ulnar direction at the MCP joint. It is extremely rare for the extensor tendons to sublux to the radial aspect of the MCP joint; therefore answer D is incorrect.

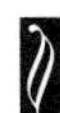

Answer: **E**

McCollister, pp. 1098-1103
Lubahn, Wolfe in Mackin, Callahan, Skirven, et al, p. 1585
Refer to Fig. 13-9

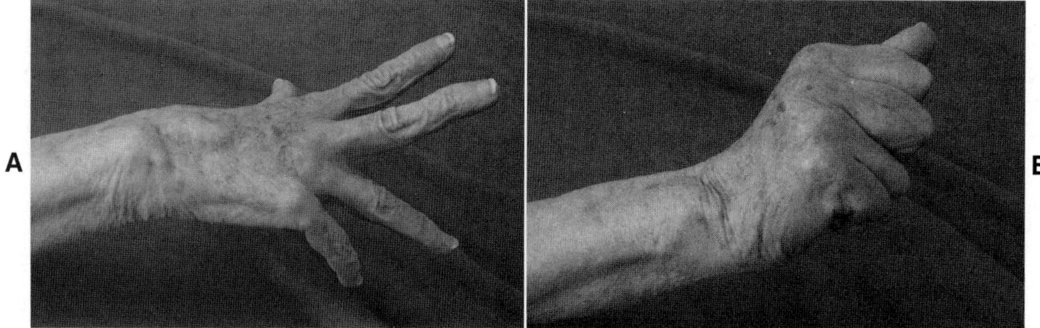

Fig. 13-9 ■ **A,** A patient with extensor tendon ruptures is not able to actively extend the involved digits; in this case, the ring and small fingers. **B,** With extension of the wrist, the fingers easily flex. There should be a symmetrical cascade from index to small fingers. This patient has normal active flexion of all fingers. (From Mackin EJ, Callahan AD, Skirven TM, et al: *Rehabilitation of the hand and upper extremity*, ed 5, vol 2, St Louis, 2002, Mosby.)

32. You are treating a patient who has had MCP joint reconstruction. The following statements are included in the operative note:

The intrinsic tendons are exposed and released. The extensor expansion is opened on the radial side to expose the collateral ligament. The intrinsic tendon is sutured to the radial collateral ligament at its phalangeal attachment, using 4-0 sutures.

What type of surgical repair did this patient undergo?

A. MCP joint synovectomy
B. Extensor tendon relocation
C. Crossed-intrinsic transfer
D. MCP joint arthroplasty

Crossed-intrinsic transfers are used as an additional means of restoring finger alignment and preventing recurrent ulnar drift. The intrinsics are released from the ulnar side of the index, long, and ring fingers and transferred to the radial aspect of the adjacent fingers to provide additional radial stability. Some authors have found that this provides effective, long-term correction of ulnar drift in early RA. For treating a patient with crossed-intrinsic transfers, it is recommended that the fingers be splinted for 3 weeks before exercises are begun. A dynamic splint may be applied afterward and used for an additional 3 weeks.

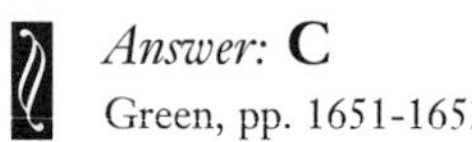
Answer: **C**
Green, pp. 1651-1652

33. The primary treatment of the MCP joints during stage one of RA is which of the following?

A. MCP joint arthroplasty
B. Wrist fusion followed by MCP joint arthroplasty
C. Splinting
D. Strengthening the intrinsics

Splinting is the main treatment used in stage one of the diseased MCP joint. Patients wear night splints that hold the fingers in relative extension and correct ulnar deviation with finger separators. A resting hand splint also can be used during the day during periods of inflammation. The therapist is responsible for providing the patient with joint protection, adaptive equipment, and general exercise instructions. During stage two of RA, decisions regarding hand surgery become more important. In stage two or stage three, synovectomies and soft-tissue reconstructions become options. In stage three and stage four, implant arthroplasty is the procedure of choice.

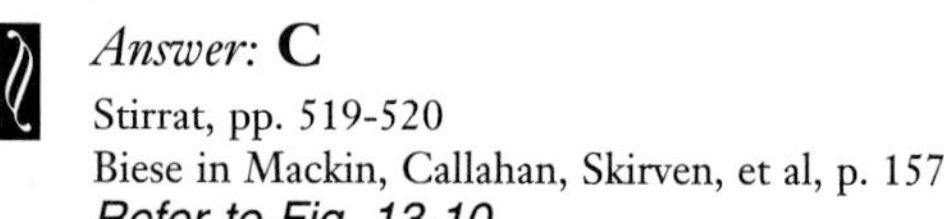
Answer: **C**
Stirrat, pp. 519-520
Biese in Mackin, Callahan, Skirven, et al, p. 1574
Refer to Fig. 13-10

34. Indications for silastic arthroplasty of the MCP joints include which of the following?

A. Deformity
B. Pain
C. Desire for cosmetic improvement
D. Joint dislocation
E. All of the above

Pain and severe deformity, which commonly are associated with joint dislocation, are the predominant indications for implant arthroplasties. Secondarily, patients

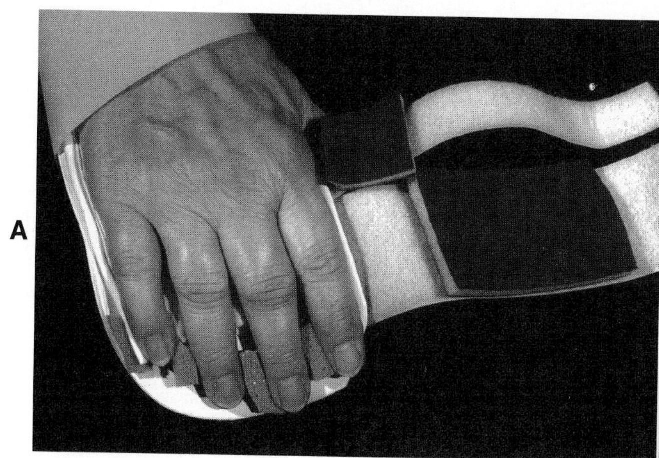

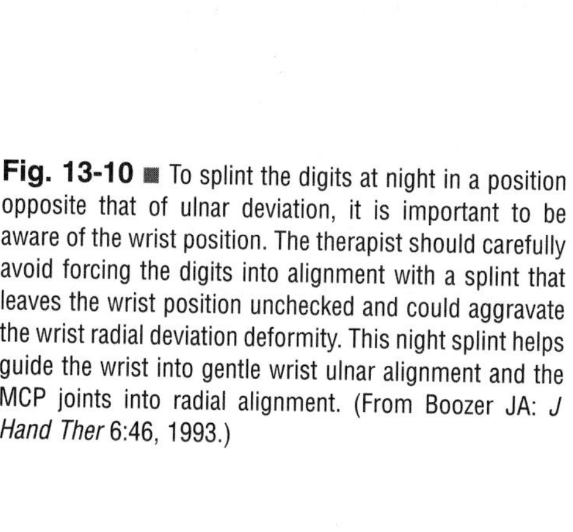

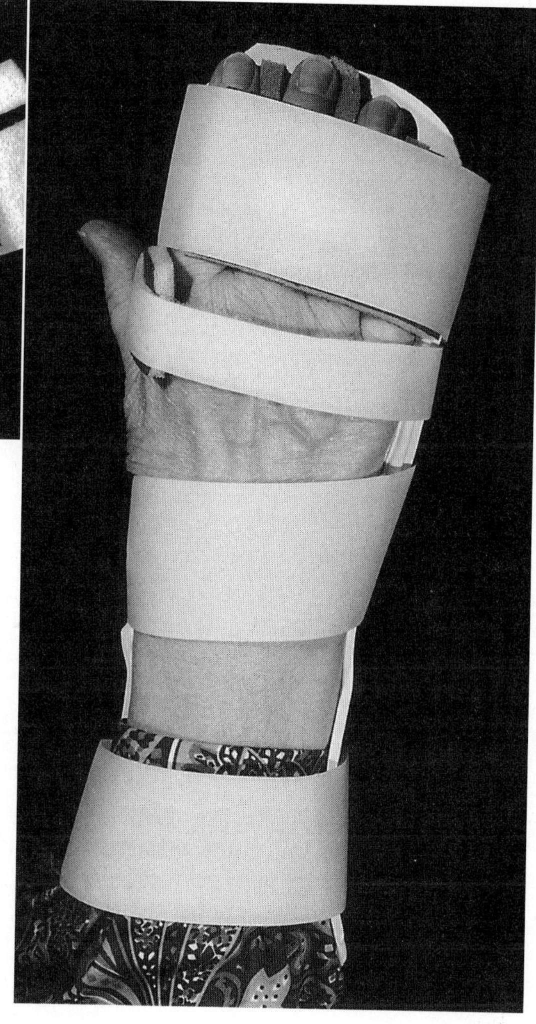

Fig. 13-10 ■ To splint the digits at night in a position opposite that of ulnar deviation, it is important to be aware of the wrist position. The therapist should carefully avoid forcing the digits into alignment with a splint that leaves the wrist position unchecked and could aggravate the wrist radial deviation deformity. This night splint helps guide the wrist into gentle wrist ulnar alignment and the MCP joints into radial alignment. (From Boozer JA: *J Hand Ther* 6:46, 1993.)

are often unhappy with the cosmetic appearance of the hand preoperatively and want to improve the appearance of the hand and its function.

Answer: **E**
McCollister, pp. 1118-1126

35. True or False: Patients who have swan-neck deformities with end-stage arthritic changes of the MCP joints should have the swan-neck deformities corrected before the MCP arthoplasty, but surgery would be performed during, or ater MCP correction.

The swan-neck deformity should not be surgically corrected before the MCP joint imbalance is corrected. Treatment options vary depending on the stage of the swan-neck deformity, but surgery would be performed during or after MCP correction.

Answer: **False**
McCollister, pp. 1126-1129

36. A 21-year-old model is injured in a volleyball accident while on vacation in the Caribbean. When she is seen 3 weeks later, the PIP joint of her ring finger shows a fracture with a dorsal dislocation of the proximal phalanx. Which of the following is an appropriate surgical treatment?

A. Open reduction internal fixation
B. Volar plate arthroplasty
C. PIP joint arthroplasty
D. Arthrodesis of the PIP joint
E. All of the above are appropriate surgical treatments.

All of the above surgical treatments could be employed for this patient. Fractures with substantial comminution or displacement of the joint space commonly require open reduction internal fixation. When the volar plate has been avulsed at its insertion site with comminution, a volar plate arthroplasty may be the only means of restoring stability. In late dislocations of the joint, an arthrodesis or arthroplasty may be necessary to restore a stable, pain-free joint and reduce the risk of persistent arthritis.

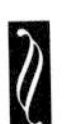

Answer: **E**

Eaton, Malerich, pp. 260-268
McCollister, pp. 372-377

CLINICAL GEM:
A quick reference for the treatment of PIP joint arthroplasty follows:

- A digit extension splint is applied at 3 to 5 days postoperatively
- Active ROM exercises are initiated 3 to 5 days postoperatively (avoiding lateral forces)
- Passive ROM is initiated at 3 weeks
- Light strengthening is initiated at 6 weeks
- Use of the extension splint is reduced to nighttime only at 6 weeks

37. A 65-year-old woman is involved in a motor vehicle accident and sustains a severe fracture dislocation of the MCP joint of the index finger, which leads to posttraumatic arthritis. She is treated with MCP arthoplasty of the index MCP joint. Her postoperative therapy program should include which of the following?

A. Application of a bulky hand dressing for 3 to 7 days
B. Active MCP joint flexion and extension exercises
C. Splinting, both dynamic and static, of the index finger
D. Splinting of the hand with MCP joints in 90 degrees of flexion for the first 2 weeks
E. A, B, and C
F. All of the above

The postoperative program for silastic arthroplasty of the MCP joint involves application of a bulky hand dressing or cast for the first 3 to 7 days, followed by a splinting and exercise program. Active and passive MCP joint flexion and extension exercises are performed hourly in the dynamic splint. Both dynamic and static splints are essential for an excellent postoperative result. A static splint is applied at night and a dynamic splint is applied during the day. Initial splinting should be with the fingers in extension, not in flexion, as described in answer D.

Answer: **E**

McCollister, pp. 1120-1126
Hunter, Mackin, Callahan, pp. 1366-1368
Lubahn, Wolfe in Mackin, Callahan, Skirven, et al, pp. 1592-1595

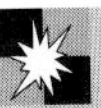

CLINICAL GEM:
After MCP joint arthroplasty, watch digits carefully for pronation or supination deformities and add additional outriggers to the distal phalanx if these develop.

38. True or False: It is acceptable for a patient to begin writing 2 weeks after an MCP arthroplasty.

After an MCP joint arthroplasty, lateral pinch should be avoided because it pushes the fingers in an ulnar direction. In selective cases a working splint can be fabricated in the early postsurgical stage to allow the individual to resume pinch activities earlier than the usual postoperative date of 6 to 8 weeks (Fig. 13-11). A protective writing splint reduces the risk of recurring ulnar drift after reconstruction.

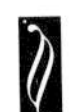

Answer: **False**

Hunter, Mackin, Callahan, pp. 1378-1379
Lubahn, Wolfe in Mackin, Callahan, Skirven, et al, pp. 1592-1595

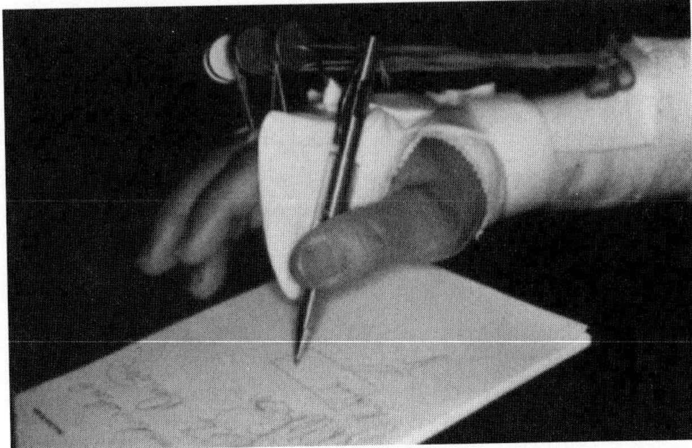

Fig. 13-11 ■ Courtesy Judy Colditz, OTR/L.

39. You are treating a patient after an MCP joint arthroplasty. What is your ROM goal per MCP joint?

A. Index through small fingers: 90 degrees of flexion
B. Index and middle fingers: 45 to 60 degrees of flexion; ring and small fingers: 70 degrees of flexion
C. Index and middle fingers: 75 to 80 degrees of flexion; ring and small fingers: 60 to 70 degrees of flexion
D. Index and middle fingers: 30 to 40 degrees of flexion; ring and small fingers: 50 to 60 degrees of flexion

ROM goals after MCP joint arthroplasty vary from author to author. In general, a goal of 45 to 60 degrees of flexion in the index and middle fingers and 70 degrees of flexion for the ring and small fingers is acceptable. Remember, more mobility yields less stability; therefore it is less important to have extensive motion in the index and middle fingers. More motion should be obtained in the ring and small fingers to allow for grasp; limited motion of the index and middle fingers allows for dexterity and stable pinch. The desired result after MCP arthroplasty is an arc of motion that is functional for the patient.

Answer: **B**
Hunter, Mackin, Callahan, pp. 1367-1368
Lubahn, Wolfe in Mackin, Callahan, Skirven, et al, p. 1595

40. You are treating a patient with an MCP joint arthroplasty. When can a flexion outrigger be added to the splint postoperatively on this patient?

A. 1 week
B. 3 weeks
C. 6 weeks
D. 10 weeks

A flexion outrigger can be applied 3 weeks after surgery. It is recommended that the flexion outrigger be worn approximately five times a day for 20- to 30-minute intervals to passively stretch the MCP joints. This is done in conjunction with active flexion exercises. Some authors recommend initiating flexion splinting to the MCP joints as early as 2 weeks postoperatively to prevent scar formation that will limit motion. The reconstructed joints begin to get tight during the second postoperative week and are very tight by the end of the third week. If ROM has not been obtained by the end of the third week, it will be difficult to gain further improvement.

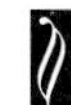

Answer: **B**
Hunter, Mackin, Callahan, p. 1368
Lubahn, Wolfe in Mackin, Callahan, Skirven, et al, p. 1595

41. Which patients with osteoarthritis should receive DMARD or anti-TNF therapy?

A. Osteoarthritis patients with very severe disease
B. Osteoarthritis patients who are becoming disabled
C. Osteoarthritis patients with very good insurance
D. No osteoarthritis patients
E. Patients with inflammatory osteoarthritis

No osteoarthritis patients should receive DMARD or anti-TNF therapy. DMARDs are reserved for the treatment of RA and psoriatic arthritis.

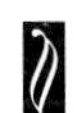

Answer: **D**
Brandt, p. 1397

42. When should an anti-TNF such as Enbrel, Humira, or Remicade be given to a patient with RA?

A. When there is X-ray or MRI evidence of disease progression
B. When functional status is worsening
C. When DMARD therapy has failed
D. All of the above

The anti-TNF agents used alone or in combination with a DMARD may arrest the disease (thereby lessening pain stiffness and swelling), improve function, and prevent disease progression.

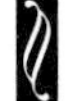

Answer: **D**
Weinblatt, Keystone, Furst, pp. 35-45

43. In ligament reconstruction tendon interposition arthroplasty of the thumb, the tendon most commonly used to reconstruct the palmar oblique ligament is which of the following?

A. Abductor pollicis longus
B. Extensor pollicis brevis
C. Extensor pollicis longus
D. Flexor carpi radialis
E. Flexor carpi ulnaris

During reconstruction of the thumb basal joint (first CMC joint), the flexor carpi radialis is the preferred tendon for reconstructing the palmar oblique ligament when instability exists. This technique is known as *ligament reconstruction tendon interposition arthroplasty of the basal joint of the thumb.*

Answer: **D**
Burton, Pellegrini, pp. 324-332

44. Which of the following procedures commonly is used for treating a patient with pantrapezial arthritis at the base of the thumb?

A. Excision of the trapezium and ligament reconstruction tendon interposition arthroplasty
B. Hemiresection of the trapezium and use of a metacarpal resurfacing silicone implant
C. Arthrodesis of the trapezial first metacarpal joint
D. All of the above

Pantrapezial arthritis refers to all joints surrounding the trapezium. All of the above techniques are used to reconstruct the basal joint when arthritis involves the first metacarpal joint and trapezium. However, when arthritis also exists between the scaphoid and trapezium and between the trapezium and trapezoid, hemiresection of the trapezium or arthrodesis of the trapezial first metacarpal joint alone may not adequately relieve the patient's pain. Therefore, a complete trapezium excision is indicated in this situation.

Answer: **A**
McCollister, pp. 1134-1149

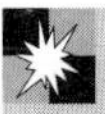
CLINICAL GEM:
Some surgeons use silicone implant arthroplasty to reconstruct the basal joint. The silicone implant arthroplasty technique is not used as commonly as other reconstructive procedures.

45. Which orthotic is most commonly selected for fabrication for treatment of osteoarthritis of the CMC joint in the thumb?

A. Wrist-thumb orthotic
B. CMC-MCP stabilization orthotic
C. Circumferential wrist-thumb orthotic
D. None of the above

The CMC-MCP stabilization orthotic made from highly contourable material is best of the above choices. The most important part of the orthotic is the C-Bar, which maintains thumb abduction and restricts CMC joint mobility. Care should be taken to fit the orthotic while the patient touches the thumb to the middle finger so that functional pinch and writing (with the dominant hand, Fig. 13-12) are maintained. Often the MCP can be left out of the splint if the patient has good stability at the MCP joint (Fig. 13-13). The wrist only needs to be included when patients have wrist combined problems.

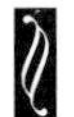
Answer: **B**
Melvin, pp. 412-413
Mackin, Callahan, Skirven, et al, p. 1653

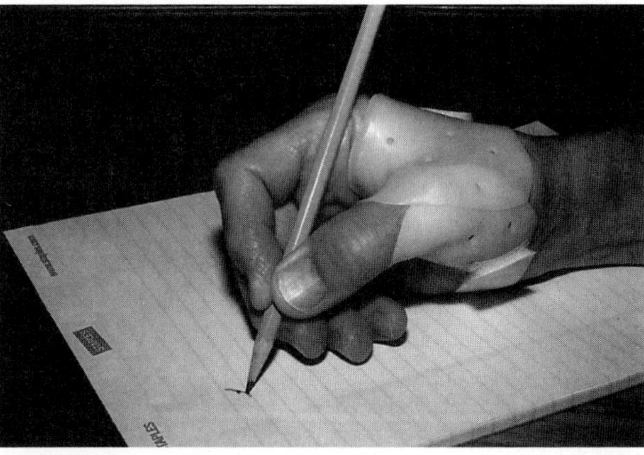

Fig. 13-12 ■ From Mackin EJ, Callahan AD, Skirven TM, et al: *Rehabilitation of the hand and upper extremity,* ed 5, vol 2, St Louis, 2002, Mosby.

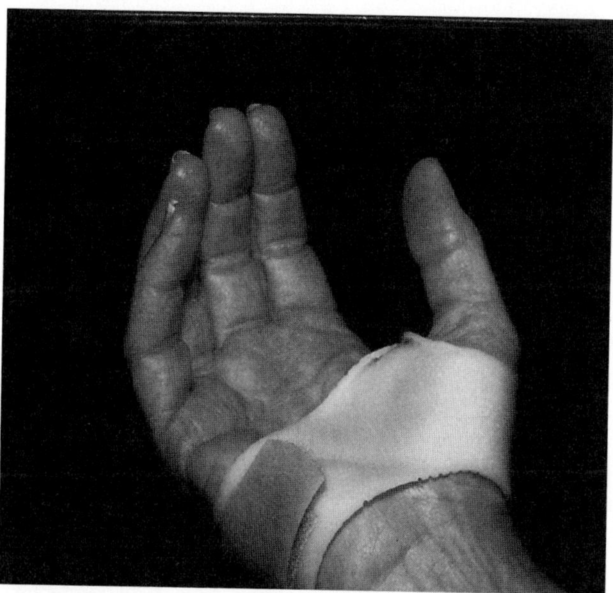

Fig. 13-13 ■ A hand-based CMC joint splint fitted to stabilize the CMC joint in extension. It encourages MCP joint flexion and unloads the CMC joint. (From Mackin EJ, Callahan AD, Skirven TM, et al: *Rehabilitation of the hand and upper extremity*, ed 5, vol 2, St Louis, 2002, Mosby.)

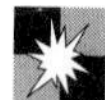

CLINICAL GEM:
A hand-based CMC joint splint fitted to stabilize the CMC joint only is an excellent choice for CMC joint osteoarthritis (Fig. 13-13).

46. The most effective wearing schedule for the CMC/MCP orthotic in acute CMC osteoarthritis is which of the following?

A. Full-time wear for 2 to 3 weeks
B. At night only
C. 3 weeks continual wear, 1 week of 75%, 1 week of 50%, and then 1 week of 25% wearing time
D. Full-time wear until patient has minimal pain

To create maximal joint rest, the orthotic should be worn day and night until the thumb is pain-free or has only minimal pain in severe cases. This period should be followed by a gradual weaning process (1 to 2 weeks) so that the patient is able to resume functional activity without re-creating a painful thumb. Joint protection and activity modification play key roles in decreasing aggravating forces of repetitive pinch, grasp, and wringing prehension activities. Ultimately, to return to some functional activities, it may be necessary to wear the orthotic as a preventative measure (i.e. gardening, counting money as a bank teller).

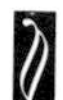

Answer: **D**
Melvin, pp. 413-414
Melvin in Mackin, Callahan, Skirven, et al, p. 1652

47. The most common procedure associated with ligament reconstruction tendon interposition arthroplasty of the thumb for basal joint arthritis is which of the following?

A. Arthrodesis of the first MCP joint
B. Arthrodesis of the IP joint of the thumb
C. de Quervain release
D. Trigger finger release
E. None of the above

De Quervain tenosynovitis commonly occurs in patients who have basal joint arthritis. However, instability of the first MCP joint is the most common associated condition, and it requires either stabilization or arthrodesis, depending on the degree of instability. When instability and arthritis are both present in the MCP joint, arthrodesis is the treatment of choice.

Answer: **A**
Burton, Pellegrini, pp. 324-332
Melvin in Mackin, Callahan, Skirven, et al, p. 1659

48. Appropriate rehabilitation of the thumb after CMC joint implant arthroplasty includes which of the following?

A. Immediate mobilization of the joint
B. Immobilization of the thumb for 1 week followed by active ROM exercises
C. Cast immobilization of the thumb for 3 to 4 weeks, followed by use of a protective splint for 2 weeks
D. Cast immobilization of the thumb and index finger for 6 weeks
E. None of the above

After most implant arthroplasties of the thumb, cast immobilization is recommended for 3 to 4 weeks, followed by the use of thumb spica splinting for an additional 2 weeks. Active ROM exercises are initiated 3 to 4 weeks postoperatively when the cast is removed.

Answer: **C**
McCollister, pp. 1134-1145
Melvin in Mackin, Callahan, Skirven, et al, pp. 1658-1659

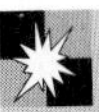

CLINICAL GEM:
A quick reference for rehabilitation after ligament reconstruction tendon interposition arthroplasty follows:

- A cast is applied for the initial 3 to 4 weeks.
- A thumb spica splint is applied after cast removal.
- Active ROM of the thumb and wrist is initiated at 3 to 4 weeks.
- Gentle passive ROM of the CMC joint is initiated at 6 weeks.
- The splint is discontinued at 6 weeks (and used as needed).
- Light resistance is initiated at 8 weeks.

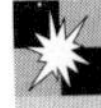

CLINICAL GEM:
Ensure your patients that discomfort for 6 to 12 months after ligament reconstruction tendon interposition surgery is not uncommon.

49. A 65-year-old patient presents with an acute onset of swelling, redness, and severe pain in the wrist. The differential diagnosis includes pseudogout, RA, infectious arthritis and gout. If the wrist joint was aspirated, what kind of crystal would be seen in pseudogout?

A. Monosodium urate
B. Calcium pyrophosphate
C. Hydroxy apatite
D. None of the above

The acute onset of an inflammatory arthritis at the wrist commonly is caused by pseudogout, which is an inflammatory arthritis caused by the deposition of calcium pyrophosphate in cartilage adjacent to the involved joint. Calcium pyrophosphate breaks free from the cartilage and precipitates in the synovial space. Crystals within the joint space trigger an inflammatory reaction. White blood cells attempt to phagocytose (engulf) the crystals. The white blood cells are unable to contain the crystals and lyse (break apart). When the white blood cells break apart, they release enzymes that inflame the synovium, thus resulting in joint swelling, stiffness, pain, and redness. The crystals of calcium pyrophosphate can be seen in the joint fluid when it is examined using a polarizing microscope. An X-ray of the wrist and hand may demonstrate calcification at the triangular cartilage at the wrist. It is important to exclude the possibility of infection. This is done by sending joint fluid to the laboratory for culture.

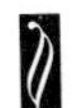
Answer: **B**
Reginato, Hoffman, pp. 1941-1944

50. Which of the following is an acceptable treatment(s) for an acute attack of gout?

A. Colchicine
B. NSAIDs
C. Tapering course of prednisone
D. None of the above
E. All of the above

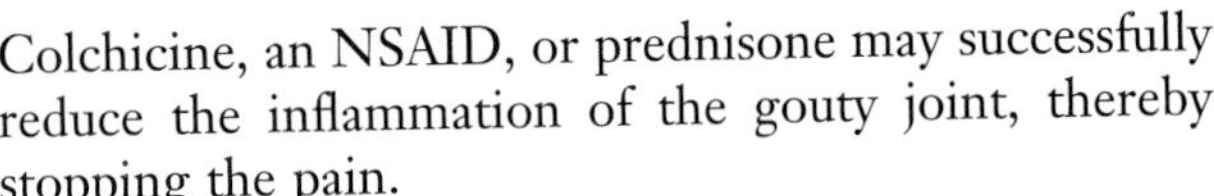

Colchicine, an NSAID, or prednisone may successfully reduce the inflammation of the gouty joint, thereby stopping the pain.

Answer: **E**
Kelley, Wortmann, pp. 1342-1343

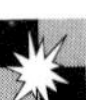

CLINICAL GEM:
Allopurinol or Probenecid may worsen and prolong an attack of gout. Both Allopurinol and Probenecid reduce the uric acid level and are indicated for chronic gouty arthritis and uric acid nephrolithiasis (kidney stones). Allopurinol prevents the body from producing uric acid, which is a breakdown product of deoxyribonucleic acid (DNA) and ribonucleic acid (RNA). Probenecid prevents the excretion of uric acid by the kidney. Any agent that raises or lowers the serum uric acid level may worsen the attack.

51. What factors are most likely to increase susceptibility to gouty arthritis?

A. Alcohol
B. Burger with fries
C. Diuretics
D. Aspirin
E. A, C, and D
F. All of the above

Alcohol, diuretics, and aspirin decrease the kidney's ability to secrete uric acid. The effects of alcohol, aspirin, and diuretics are more important factors than diet in the causation of gouty arthritis.

Answer: **E**
Kelley, Wortmann, pp. 1313-1351

52. Ligaments in the rheumatoid wrist typically loosen on the ulnar aspect of the radiocarpal joint, thus allowing a radial displacement of the proximal carpal row. True or False: When this occurs, the result is ulnar deviation of the hand on the forearm.

When ligaments loosen on the radial aspect of the radiocarpal joint, ulnar displacement of the proximal carpal row will occur. Radial deviation of the hand occurs secondarily on the forearm. An associated subluxation of the DRU joint often occurs, thus causing a loss of stability on the ulnar aspect of the wrist. A palmar subluxation of the proximal row on the radius also is commonly seen (see Figs. 13-8 and 13-14).

Answer: **False**
Hunter, Mackin, Callahan, pp. 1325-1326

53. True or False: A total wrist arthrodesis is an excellent procedure for a patient with RA and is used often.

A total wrist arthrodesis is not often performed on a patient with RA for several reasons. First, patients with RA maintain relatively good function in a relatively pain-free range after synovectomy and ligament stabilization. Second, maintenance of wrist motion allows for tendon excursion in patients who require tendon transfers or repairs. Third, the involvement of other joints, including the elbow, shoulder, and contralateral hand and wrist, hampers function of these patients significantly with a fusion of one wrist. Total wrist arthrodesis is reserved for the completely destroyed, painful wrist in young, vigorous patients—particularly in those who have less involvement of other joints.

Answer: **False**
Taleisnik, p. 387

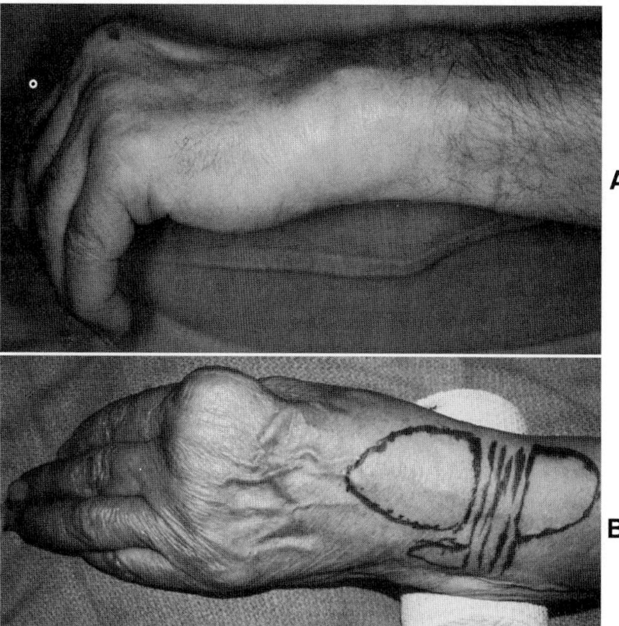

Fig. 13-14 ■ **A,** Ulnar aspect of the hand and carpus, palmarly subluxed and supinated relative to the forearm bones. **B,** Apparent radial deviation of the wrist as a result of ulnar translation of the carpus relative to the radius. The *outlined area* illustrates soft-tissue swelling, which is characteristic of extensor tenosynovitis. (From Cooney WP, Linscheid RL, Dobyns JH: *The wrist: diagnosis and operative treatment,* St Louis, 1998, Mosby.)

54. Postoperative treatment of a 61-year-old woman who has undergone silastic implant arthroplasty of the wrist should include which of the following?

A. Cast immobilization for 2 to 4 weeks
B. Cast immobilization for 3 to 5 days
C. Nighttime splinting for 3 years to prevent a recurrence of deformity
D. Bulky dressing with immediate active ROM exercises

After a wrist implant arthroplasty, immobilization in a bulky hand dressing or plaster shell cast for 2 to 4 weeks postoperatively is applied to ensure that the ligaments and the capsule have time to heal. Depending on stability of the prosthesis, gentle active ROM for the wrist may be started as early as 2 weeks. A custom splint, with the wrist at 20 to 30 degrees of extension, is used for an additional 3 to 4 weeks after cast removal. Long-term nighttime splinting often is performed for MCP joint arthroplasty but is rarely necessary for wrist arthoplasty;

it certainly is not indicated for a 3-year period. Under ideal circumstances, a 40- to 60-degree arc of total active flexion and extension of the wrist may be obtained.

Answer: **A**

McCollister, pp. 1106-1112
Lubahn, Wolfe in Mackin, Callahan, Skirven, et al, p. 1589

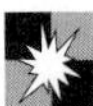

CLINICAL GEM:
A quick reference for rehabilitation of wrist arthroplasties follows:

- Cast immobilization for 3 to 4 weeks
- Wrist support splint applied after cast removal
- Active ROM to the wrist at 3 to 4 weeks
- Gentle passive ROM to the wrist at 6 weeks
- Light strengthening at 8 weeks
- Splint used as needed at 6 to 8 weeks

55. A 65-year-old woman with a 5-year history of RA and chronic wrist synovitis presents to the therapy clinic with numbness and tingling in the thumb, index, and middle fingers at night. Her therapy program should include which of the following elements?

A. Orthotic positioning in 0 to 10 degrees of wrist extension
B. Grip and pinch strengthening
C. Median nerve and/or upper limb neural gliding program
D. Sensory reeducation
E. A and C
F. All of the above

Wrist pain and paresthesias in the fingers at night are attributed to prolonged positioning in wrist flexion or extension as well as nocturnal swelling. With chronic wrist synovitis, there may also be swelling in the tendon sheaths and thickening of tendons or bones that can lead to compression of the superficial median nerve at the wrist. The goal of a median nerve–gliding program is to alter the formation of motion-limiting adhesions between the median nerve and the surrounding tissue in the face of chronic wrist synovitis. Grip and pinch strengthening and sensory reeducation are not indicated at this time.

Answer: **E**

Melvin, pp. 308-310
Butler, pp. 195-198
Evans in Mackin, Callahan, Skirven, et al, p. 660

56. When we test for osteoporosis we measure the bone mineral density and calculate the fracture risk. The "T-score" is a comparison of the subject's bone density to that of a young adult population. What factor(s) or medication(s) will increase the bone density or bone strength and thereby reduce the risk of fracture?

A. Fosamax
B. Actonel
C. Miacalcin
D. Hormone replacement therapy
E. Parathyroid hormone
F. Calcium (dietary or supplementation)
G. Exercise, including walking and weight-lifting
H. All of the above

All of the above are approved medications and factors that, when effective, increase bone density and decrease the risk of fracture. Calcium (both dietary and supplemental) and exercise are effective ways to increase bone strength.

Answer: **H**

Orwoll, Bliziotes

57. Scleroderma may cause all but which of the following?

A. Tightening of the skin
B. Mouth ulceration
C. Dryness of the eyes and mouth
D. Difficulty swallowing
E. Calcification of soft tissues
F. Dilated blood vessels just below the surface of the skin (telangiectasia)
G. Hypertension
H. Inflammation of the pleura and pericardium
I. Kidney disease
J. Calcinosis (calcium deposits in soft tissue)
K. Raynaud's phenomenon
L. Hand contracture

The word *scleroderma* means "hard skin." It is a connective tissue disease in which there is fibrosis of the skin and internal organs. The above choices represent some of the clinical manifestations that result from the connective tissue inflammation and subsequent fibrosis that are caused by scleroderma. Scleroderma does not cause mouth ulceration.

Answer: **B**
Seibold, pp. 1133-1162
Melvin in Mackin, Callahan, Skirven, et al, pp. 1677-1681

58. Systemic lupus erythematosus is an autoimmune disease (a disease in which the body's own tissue is treated as if it is foreign) that has many manifestations. These include a sun-sensitive skin rash, hair loss, mouth and nasal ulcers, Raynaud's phenomenon, sicca syndrome (mouth and eye dryness), arthritis, fever, pleuropericarditis, nephritis, seizures, and lowering of blood counts (anemia, neutropenia, thrombocytopenia). Lupus may be mild and not life-threatening. Lupus severity varies from one patient to the next. Obviously, when there is internal organ involvement the disease is more severe and may reduce survival. Which of the treatments below is *not* used to treat systemic lupus erythematosus?

A. Prednisone
B. NSAIDs
C. Cyclophosphamide
D. Sunscreens
E. Plaquenil

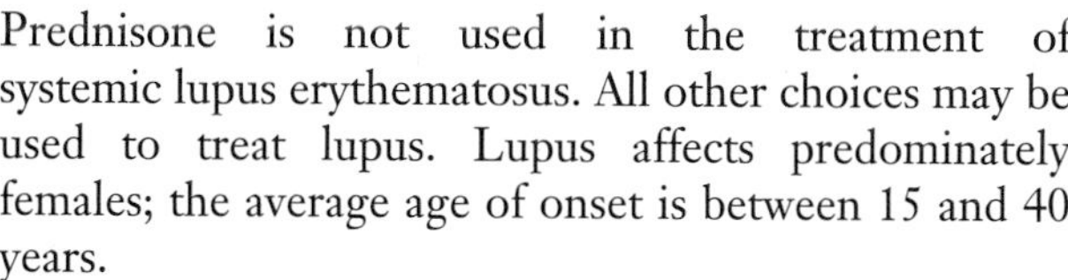

Prednisone is not used in the treatment of systemic lupus erythematosus. All other choices may be used to treat lupus. Lupus affects predominately females; the average age of onset is between 15 and 40 years.

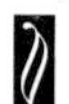

Answer: **A**
Hahn, pp. 1015-1054
Melvin in Mackin, Callahan, Skirven, et al, pp. 1667-1665

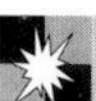

CLINICAL GEM:
Deformities in the lupus hand are generally passively correctable, and the initial treatment of passively correctable deformities should be joint protection, splinting, and exercise.

59. De Quervain's tenosynovitis involves the first dorsal wrist compartment, which includes which of the following?

A. Extensor pollicis longus and extensor digitorum communis
B. Flexor pollicis longus and flexor digitorum profundus
C. Abductor pollicis longus and the extensor pollicis longus
D. Abductor pollicis longus and the extensor pollicis brevis

De Quervain's tenosynovitis involves the abductor pollicis longus and extensor pollicis brevis tendons. Repetitive lateral pinch with the wrist in ulnar deviation is the most common cause for aggravation of these tendons. It is characterized by pain over the first dorsal compartment with active or passive thumb motion, swelling, and occasional warmth.

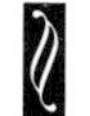

Answer: **D**
Melvin, p. 302

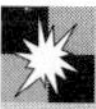

CLINICAL GEM:
When testing de Quervain's tenosynovitis with a RA patient, passively flex the patient's thumb and gently deviate the wrist ulnarly, while asking the patient to identify areas of pain. A positive test elicits pain over the first compartment with possible radiation to the first metacarpal bone or up the forearm along the radial border. Do *not* make a fist over the thumb, as traditionally performed; this will be too painful for the RA patient.

60. Which type of joint replacement has shown the highest complication rate?

A. Basal joint
B. MCP joint
C. Elbow joint
D. Knee joint

Of all major total joint arthroplasties, elbow arthroplasty has the highest complication rate. Complications include infection, dislocation, loosening of components, malalignment, nonunion, delayed union, and instability. In the future, elbow arthroplasty designs may include smaller components that save bone stock, provide alternatives to cement fixation, or allow for a biological implant such as an allograft. As a therapist you must be aware of this and keep a keen eye for complications.

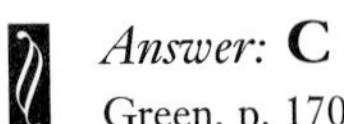

Answer: **C**
Green, p. 1706

61. The patient in Fig. 13-15 presents primarily with what pathology?

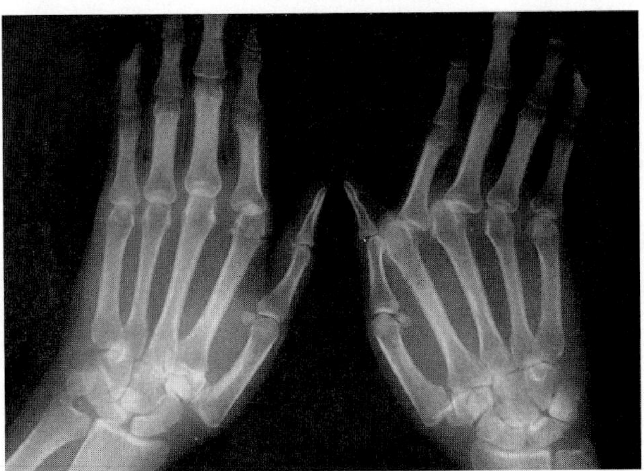

Fig. 13-15 ■ From Jebson PJL, Kasdan ML: *Hand secrets,* ed 2, Philadelphia, 2002, Hanley & Belfus.

A. RA
B. Systemic lupus erythematosus
C. Generalized osteoarthritis
D. It could be any of the above.

The patient in Fig. 13-15 has systemic lupus erythematosus. The deformities resemble RA, but note that the patient has *no* erosive changes or joint space narrowing as are seen with RA. Refer to question 58 for lupus manifestations.

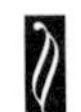

Answer: **B**
Jebson, Kasdan, p. 67
Melvin in Mackin, Callahan, Skirven, et al, pp. 1667-1675

Chapter 14

Complex Regional Pain Syndrome/Reflex Sympathetic Dystrophy

1. Which term was introduced to replace *reflex sympathetic dystrophy*?

A. Causalgia
B. Sympathetic maintained pain
C. Complex regional pain syndrome
D. Sympathetically independent pain

In 1995, the International American Pain Society (IAPS) determined the need for a revision of the taxonomic system. The new nomenclature, *complex regional pain syndrome* (CRPS), was developed to replace the terms *reflex sympathetic dystrophy* (RSD) and *causalgia*, because the IAPS felt the latter poorly described the complex condition. This term provides a descriptive terminology based on clinical features, location, and specifics of an injury, without implying mechanism, cause, or sympathetic maintenance.

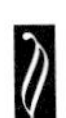
Answer: **C**
Wong, Wilson, pp. 319-325
Koman, Smith, Smith in Mackin, Callahan, Skirven, et al, p. 1695
Walsh, Muntzer in Mackin, Callahan, Skirven, et al, p. 1705
Kirkpatrick

2. True or False: CRPS is subdivided into two types.

The International Association for the Study of Pain (IASP) subcommittee on taxonomy renamed RSD to CRPS. This is subdivided into two types. The first is CRPS 1, a complex disorder that may develop as a consequence of trauma affecting the limb(s), with or without an obvious nerve lesion. This type corresponds to classic RSD. The second is CRPS 2, which is the same as CRPS 1, but with a well-defined peripheral nerve injury. CRPS 2, or causalgia, demonstrates more objective information such as numbness and weakness due to the neurological changes.

CRPS types 1 and 2 can be either sympathetic maintained pain (SMP) or sympathetic independent pain (SIP). *SMP* is defined as pain occurring with relief or improvement of symptoms during or after sympathetic medications or blocks. With SIP symptoms have spread to the central nervous system (CNS), whereas with SMP it is localized within the sympathetic system. CRPS is not synonymous with SMP, as was RSD; it is a significant departure from classic literature.

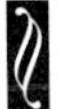
Answer: **True**
Tan, p. 109
Koman, Smith, Smith in Mackin, Callahan, Skirven, et al, pp. 1695-1696
Koman, Poehling, Smith in Green, Hotchkiss, Pederson, pp. 637-640

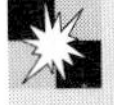
CLINICAL GEM:
Patients who have SIP generally have a poorer prognosis and do not respond as well to sympatholytic modalities and are more likely to progress to chronic pain and disability.

3. True or False: Pain is the hallmark of CRPS/RSD.

Pain is considered the hallmark for the diagnosis of CRPS/RSD. Pain has been described as severe, constant, burning, deep aching, palpable tenderness in muscles, sharp jabs, and/or lancinating (sharp cutting pain). Other symptoms of CRPS/RSD may include swelling, hyperhydrosis, decreased range of motion (ROM), contractures, stiffness, dystonia, and/or trophic changes.

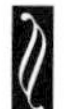

Answer: **True**

Koman, Smith, Smith in Mackin, Callahan, Skirven, et al, pp. 1695–1700
Kirkpatrick

4. In reference to pediatric RSD/CRPS, which of the following statements is true?

A. Often occurs with a preceding traumatic event
B. Predominantly occurs in the arm/hand
C. Consistent findings on bone scan
D. Good outcome in majority of cases

RSD/CRPS in children tends to have the following characteristics: often no preceding traumatic event; occurs more often in the lower extremities than the upper limbs; osteoporosis is rare; has a more favorable prognosis than adults; and bone scan results are more variable (inconsistent) with decreased uptake when the study is positive.

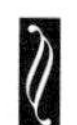

Answer: **D**

O'Young, Young, Stiens, p. 362

5. Match the word with its correct definition.

Word

A. Hyperalgesia
B. Hypoesthesia
C. Hyperpathia
D. Allodynia
E. Dysesthesia

Definition

1. Pain arising from a nonnoxious stimuli
2. Decreased sensitivity to stimulation
3. Excessive reaction to stimuli that outlasts the initiating stimulus and spreads beyond normal dermatomal borders
4. Increased sensitivity to stimulation with a lower threshold to pain
5. An unpleasant abnormal sensation

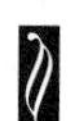

Answer: **A, 4; B, 2; C, 3; D, 1; E, 5**

Abram, Haddox, pp. 13, 467
Koman, Smith, Smith in Mackin, Callahan, Skirven, et al, p. 1696
Koman, Poehling, Smith in Green, Hotchkiss, Pederson, p. 640
Kirkpatrick

6. True or False: According to the IAPS, CRPS/RSD has clear, definitive stages that help the clinician establish a plan of care.

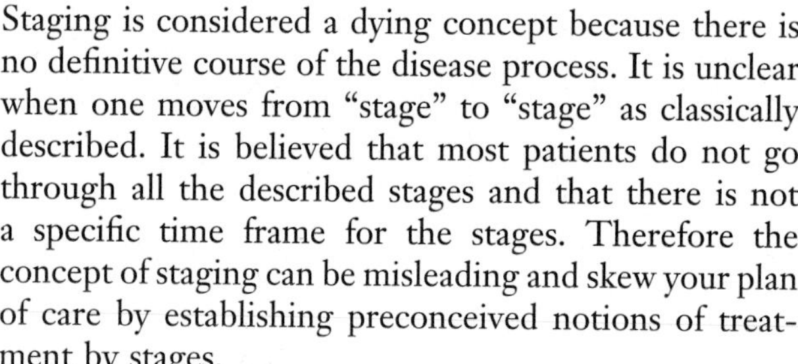

Staging is considered a dying concept because there is no definitive course of the disease process. It is unclear when one moves from "stage" to "stage" as classically described. It is believed that most patients do not go through all the described stages and that there is not a specific time frame for the stages. Therefore the concept of staging can be misleading and skew your plan of care by establishing preconceived notions of treatment by stages.

Answer: **False**

Kirkpatrick

CLINICAL GEM:
For simplicity, we can attempt to show progression of the disease process via stages/phases. Keep in mind time frames of the stages/phases are unclear:
Acute = stage/phase 1
Dystrophic = stage/phase 2
Atrophic = stage/phase 3

7. Match the phases with the symptoms.

Phases

1. Phase 1: Acute
2. Phase 2: Dystrophic
3. Phase 3: Atrophic

Characteristics

A. Diffuse pain; trophic skin changes (pale, gray, or cyanotic) and widespread osteoporosis or osteopenia; brawny edema; increased stiffness
B. Skin atrophy; severe joint stiffness (ankylosed); muscle wasting
C. Disproportionate severe pain; fusiform or pitting edema; joint stiffness; accelerated growth of hyperhydrosis, hyperesthesia, pain that limits motion

Answers: **1, C; 2, A; 3, B**

Hunter, Mackin, Callahan, pp. 782-784
Walsh, Muntzer in Mackin, Callahan, Skirven, et al, p. 1713
Wong, Wilson, pp. 319-341
Kirkpatrick
Refer to Fig. 14-1

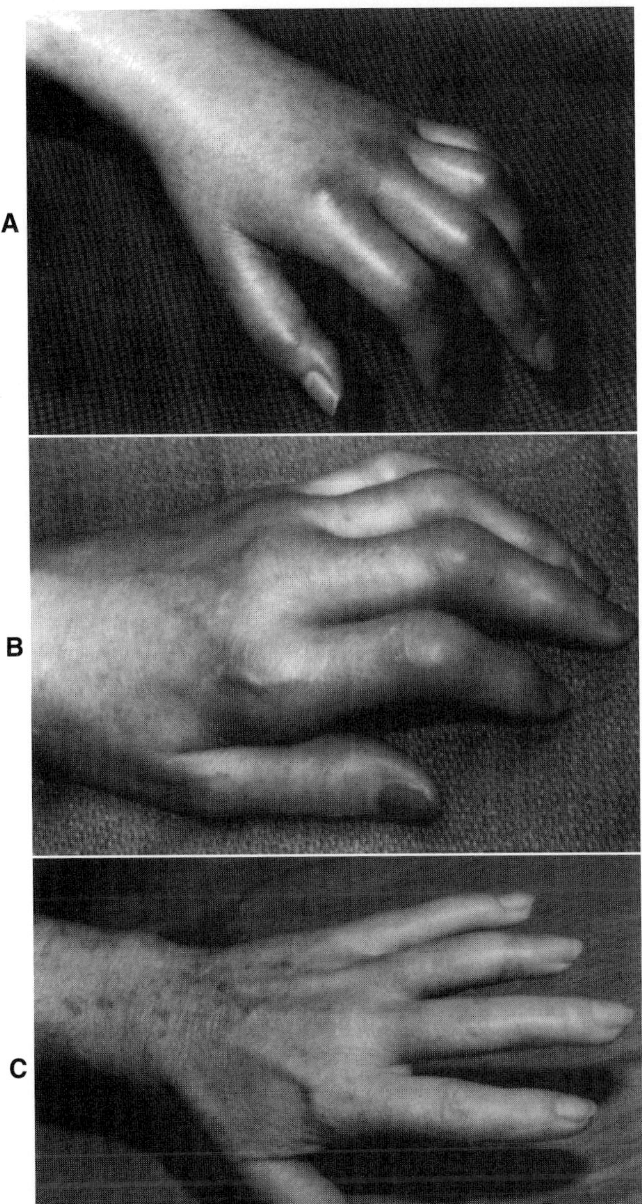

Fig. 14-1 ■ **A,** Acute. **B,** Dystrophic. **C,** Atrophic. (From Lankford LL, Thompson JE: Reflex sympathetic dystrophy, upper and lower extremity: diagnosis and management. In *American Academy of Orthopaedic Surgeons: instructional course lectures,* vol 26, St Louis, 1977, Mosby.)

CLINICAL GEM:
If CRPS/RSD is treated within the first year of injury, 80% of patients will show significant improvement, but only 50% of those treated after the first year will improve.

8. Which of the following conditions is associated with CRPS/RSD?

A. Fracture
B. Cerebrovascular accident
C. Soft tissue injury
D. Immobilization
E. All of the above

Conditions associated with CRPS/RSD can be grouped into the following three categories: 1) peripheral; 2) central; and 3) other. In the peripheral category, abnormalities include fracture, malignancy, immobilization, infection, dislocation, or myocardial infarction. In the central category, problems include cerebrovascular accident, cerebral tumor, head injury, or spinal cord injury. In the other category, associations include diabetes, genetic and idiopathic conditions, and/or medication.

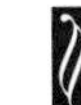

Answer: **E**
Dumitru, p. 91

CLINICAL GEM:
Fracture of the distal radius and ulna is the most common injury that results in CRPS/RSD.

9. The diagnosis of CRPS/RSD depends primarily on which of the following?

A. Triple-phase bone scan
B. Sweat test
C. Thermography
D. History and physical exam

In the evaluation of patients with CRPS/RSD, the patient's history and the physical examination usually provide the diagnosis; the laboratory data often are normal. A few nonspecific diagnostic tests may aid in the diagnosis and rule out other disease states. A triple-phase bone scan may be helpful, especially in the third phase. The sweat test is not diagnostic and may vary from patient to patient. Thermography can indicate various temperatures but is nonspecific and is of questionable prognostic significance. Many conditions can show skin temperature changes; therefore thermography is not considered a reliable test.

Answer: **D**

Dumitru, pp. 95-96
Hunter, Mackin, Callahan, p. 789
Koman, Smith, Smith in Mackin, Callahan, Skirven, et al, p. 1699
Koman, Poehling, Smith in Green, Hotchkiss, Pederson, pp. 646-648
Kirkpatrick

10. Which of the following are classic findings of upper-extremity CRPS/RSD on electrodiagnostic studies?

A. Prolonged nerve conduction velocities of the upper extremity
B. Generalized decreased SNAP amplitudes
C. Fibrillation potentials and positive sharp waves on the electromyogram of the hand muscles
D. Prolonged median and ulnar F waves
E. Electrical findings typically are normal, unless there is a concomitant nerve injury.

Electrodiagnostics essentially are normal in CRPS/RSD, except when there is damage to the peripheral nervous system during the initial injury.

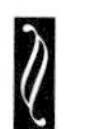
Answer: **E**

Dumitru, p. 96

11. The *test* that is considered the gold standard to diagnose CRPS/RSD is which of the following?

A. Intravenous injection
B. Quantitative sudomotor axon reflex test (QSART)
C. Thermography
D. Triple phase bone scan (TPBS)

The diagnosis of CRPS/RSD is based primarily on the physician's examination. No laboratory test can stand alone as proof of CRPS/RSD. However, the TPBS can be useful in providing evidence for CRPS/RSD. The TPBS is considered the gold standard test to diagnose CRPS/RSD. It has three phases: 1) early blood flow phase—shows a diffuse increase in perfusion; 2) blood pool or tissue phase—demonstrates increased juxtaarticular activity in all joints; and 3) delayed metabolic phase—monitors uptake 2 to 4 hours after injection.

Phase 3 is the most diagnostically important for the detection of CRPS/RSD, with a sensitivity of 96% and specificity of 98%. However, a positive phase 3 scan is not a prerequisite for the diagnosis of CRPS/RSD.

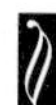
Answer: **D**

Abram, Haddox, p. 180
Raj, p. 476
Jebson, Kasdan, p. 110
Koman, Smith, Smith in Mackin, Callahan, Skirven, et al, pp. 1697-1698
Kirkpatrick
Refer to Fig. 14-2

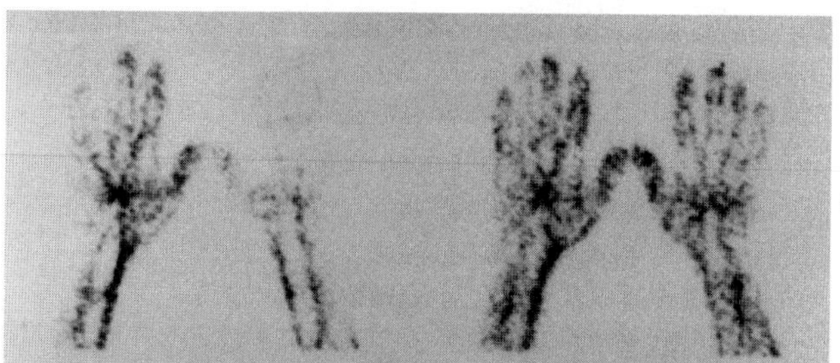

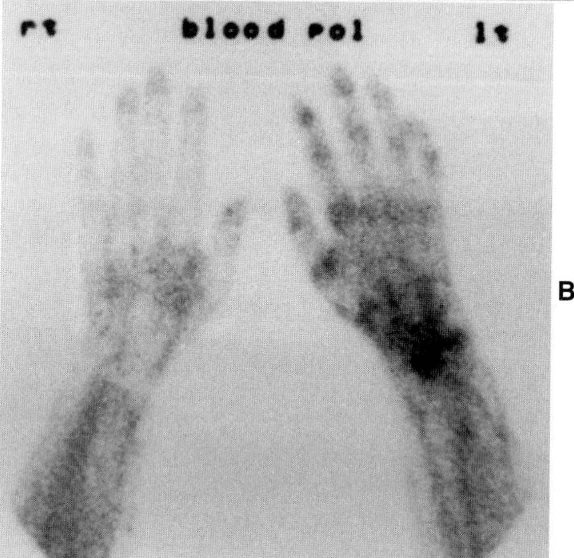

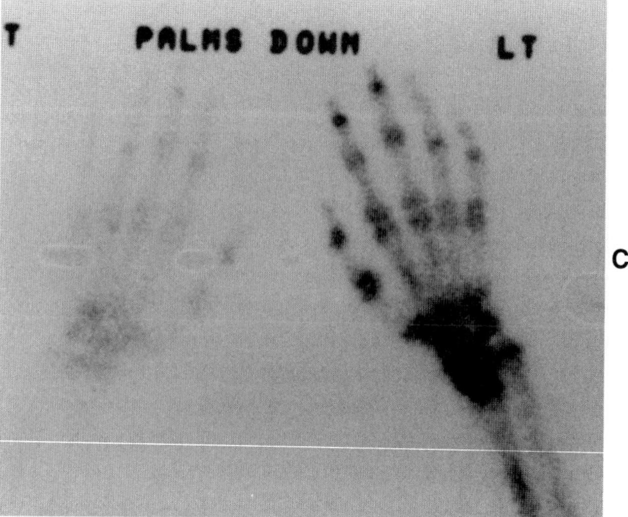

Fig. 14-2 ■ From Koman LA: *Department of orthopaedic surgery, Wake Forest University orthopaedic manual,* Winston-Salem, NC, 1998, Orthopaedic Press.

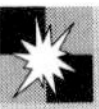

CLINICAL GEM:
Other helpful tests to diagnose CRPS/RSD include the following: bilateral radiographs to look for osteoporosis; isolated cold stress test, which is highly sensitive to vasomotor disturbances; and laser Doppler velocimetry, which will provide information about total blood flow.

12. Match the test to its description.

Test

1. Phentolamine
2. Thermography
3. Stellate ganglion block
4. QSART

Description

A. Mixed alpha 1–/alpha 2–adrenergic antagonist; blocks the sympathetic receptors from receiving circulating norepinephrine and epinephrine; specific for SMP
B. Measurement of stimulated sweat output; greater and prolonged with a hyperfunctioning sympathetic nervous system
C. Successful blockade of the upper extremity based on the presence of Horner's syndrome after the injection
D. Temperature differential of +/− 1° C; noninvasive

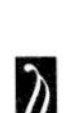

Answer: **1, A; 2, D; 3, C; 4, B**
Abram, Haddox, pp. 180-181
Raj, p. 476

13. According to the IASP, what is not a criterion for the diagnosis of CRPS/RSD?

A. Continuing pain
B. Allodynia
C. Edema
D. All of the above are criteria.

All the above are criteria recognized by the IASP for establishing a diagnosis of CRPS/RSD. Evaluation is an ongoing process. The criteria for CRPS diagnosis are listed in Box 14-1.

Answer: **D**
Koman, Poehling, Smith in Green, Hotchkiss, Pederson, p. 638
Walsh, Muntzer in Mackin, Callahan, Skirven, et al, p. 1708
Kirkpatrick

BOX 14-1
International Association for the Study of Pain (IASP) criteria for the presence of CRPS/RSD

1. An inciting noxious event or an immobilization
2. Continuing pain, allodynia (a painful response to nonnoxious stimuli), or hyperalgesia (pain disproportionate to any inciting event)
3. Evidence at some time of edema, changes in skin blood flow, or abnormal sudomotor activity in the region of pain

From Mackin EJ, Callahan AD, Skirven TM, et al: *Rehabilitation of the hand and upper extremity,* ed 5, St Louis, 2002, Mosby.

CLINICAL GEM:
CRPS signs and symptoms are dynamic (**complex**), extend beyond the area of injury (**regional**), always include disproportionate continuing **pain**, and occur in variable combinations (**syndrome**).

14. True or False: Neuromuscular electrical stimulation may be used to help gain ROM in patients with CRPS/RSD.

The goals of neuromuscular electrical stimulation (NMES) with patients who have CRPS/RSD are to decrease pain, increase ROM, increase strength, and improve blood flow. It is recommended that NMES be avoided until a good rapport with the patient has been established. To avoid adverse effects, the patient should be taught electrode placement, and mastery of the device should be ensured before a home unit is issued.

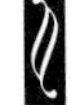

Answer: **True**
Hareau, p. 368

15. Which of the following is *not* indicated when the patient is in a state of vasoconstriction?

A. Massage
B. Thermal agents
C. High-intensity (burst) transcutaneous electrical nerve stimulation (TENS)
D. All of the above are appropriate

When the patient is in a state of vasoconstriction, the hand may present as cool and pale. The goal is to increase circulation in the hand by creating vasodilation. Massage, thermal agents (including ultrasound), and high-intensity (burst) TENS have all been reported to assist with increasing blood flow.

On the other hand, if the patient presents with a vasodilated hand, modalities may be used to create vasodilation. Brief, intense TENS can reduce vasodilation when applied for 10- to 15-minute intervals. CAUTION: Cold modalities should be avoided because they can cause an exacerbation of pain.

Finally, temperature biofeedback has been advocated to assist with vasodilation and/or vasoconstriction. It alters sympathetic activity, thereby increasing or decreasing blood flow.

Answer: **D**

Walsh, Muntzer in Mackin, Callahan, Skirven, et al, p. 1719

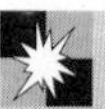

CLINICAL GEM:
CRPS/RSD is a dynamic process and vasomotor status may change day to day or hour to hour. Avoid getting into a rut in treatment.

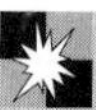

CLINICAL GEM:
Nontraditional treatment interventions may be useful to control pain and regain function. Some of the nontraditional treatments may include acupuncture, spirituality, and/or meditation.

16. True or False: The conventional mode is recommended during TENS for patients with RSD.

TENS has been used for pain control to treat CRPS and is theorized to modulate pain based on the gate-control theory. Conventional TENS is recommended as a first choice for treatment because it allows the patient to adjust to the stimulus sensation and gain confidence in the unit's operation. After failure, the other parameters can be used. The other two modes require the patient to tolerate a more intense stimulation and accompanying muscle contraction. Table 14-1 gives the settings used for each of the TENS applications.

Answer: **True**

Hareau, p. 378
Hunter, Mackin, Callahan, p. 821
Walsh, Muntzer in Mackin, Callahan, Skirven, et al, p. 1713

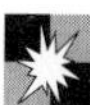

CLINICAL GEM:
Because the patient often cannot tolerate direct placement over the area of greatest discomfort, some helpful guidelines for electrode placement are the following:

- Proximal to pain/hyperesthesia
- Anatomic site
- Peripheral or cutaneous nerve
- Motor/trigger/acupuncture points
- Posterior primary ramus
- Dermatomal distribution
- Contralateral versus ipsilateral

From Mackin EJ, Callahan AD, Skirven TM, et al: *Rehabilitation of the hand and upper extremity*, ed 5, St Louis, 2002, Mosby.

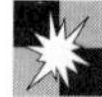

CLINICAL GEM:
High-voltage galvanic stimulation is helpful in managing edema in patients with CRPS/RSD. It also provides a residual TENS effect.

17. Which of the following statements is true with regard to choosing static progressive and/or dynamic splinting to increase ROM in a stiff joint for a patient with CRPS/RSD?

A. Do not use splints for CRPS/RSD patients.
B. Use low force or to patient tolerance to avoid exacerbation of pain.
C. Use moderate force or above patient tolerance to overcome contractures.
D. Use high force tension above patient's tolerance.

Dynamic and/or static progressive splinting may be a helpful adjunct in the treatment of CRPS/RSD as long as it is used with a low force or to patient's tolerance to avoid pain exacerbation while mobilizing stiff joints. Mobilization splinting is a useful tool if it does not sacrifice the active functional use of the extremity and therefore is best used for short durations (30-minute intervals) throughout the day.

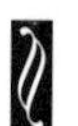

Answer: **B**

Hunter, Mackin, Callahan, p. 827
Walsh, Muntzer in Mackin, Callahan, Skirven, et al, p. 1717
Refer to Fig. 14-3

Table 14-1

TENS Stimulus Parameters, Reported Effect, and Duration for Treatment of CRPS/RSD

	Conventional TENS	Brief-intense TENS	High-intensity train (burst) TENS
Frequency	50-100 Hz	100-250 Hz	70-100 Hz (modulated)
Width	40-75 μsec	150-250 μsec	100-200 μsec
Amplitude	10-30 mA Perceptible paresthesia	30-80 mA Tetanic/nonrhythmic contraction	30-60 mA Strong rhythmic contraction: background paresthesia
Effect	Pain modulation	Vasoconstriction, pain modulation	Vasodilation, pain modulation
Duration	Continuous or until pain relief	10-15 minutes/treatment	25-45 minutes

CRPS, Complex regional pain syndrome; *TENS*, transcutaneous electrical nerve stimulation.

From Mackin EJ, Callahan AD, Skirven TM, et al: *Rehabilitation of the hand and upper extremity*, ed 5, St Louis, 2002, Mosby.

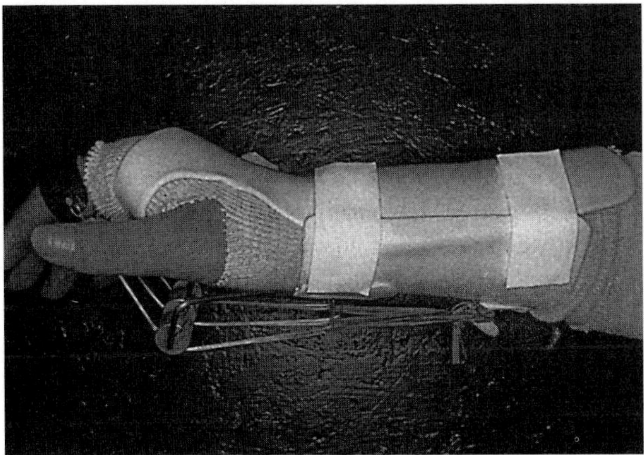

Fig. 14-3 ■ From Mackin EJ, Callahan AD, Skirven TM, et al: *Rehabilitation of the hand and upper extremity*, ed 5, St Louis, 2002, Mosby.

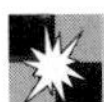

Clinical Gem:

Static splints are indicated to position the hand properly for functional use if the patient has difficulty maintaining positions such as wrist extension or for nighttime use. Caution: Daytime splinting may increase stiffness and decrease functional use if overused.

18. True or False: A therapist may cause pain through gentle, light touch in patients with CRPS/RSD.

A firm touch is recommended for a patient with CRPS/RSD because light touch or gentle stimuli can increase temporal summation of pain.

Temporal summation can occur with 3-second interval tactile stimulation or with monofilament testing performed at 3-second intervals. To avoid causing this phenomenon, do not repetitively remove hands from the surface of the skin during massage or tactile stimulation. During CRPS/RSD treatment, the patient should remain in control of all movements to help reduce anxiety and pain. Minimal manipulation of the symptomatic extremity is important. To avoid touching the patient's painful extremity during passive ROM exercises, a self-inflatable splint (long-arm air cast) allows continuous pressure over the extremity and avoids direct hand contact.

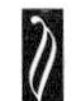

Answer: **True**

Hardy, Hardy, pp. 143-145
Hareau, p. 379
Hunter, Mackin, Callahan, p. 825

19. You have a patient who has difficulty grooming and washing her face because of CRPS/RSD. All but which of the following should be included in your initial plan of care?

A. Instructing the patient to walk daily
B. ROM exercises with proximal joints, progressing distally
C. Informing the patient that intense pain is expected during ROM exercises
D. Stress-loading program

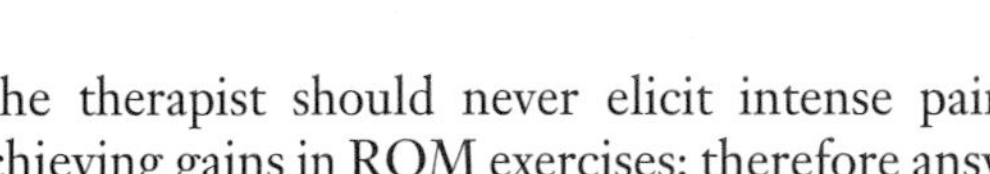

The therapist should never elicit intense pain while achieving gains in ROM exercises; therefore answer C is incorrect. Initial goals are to teach relaxation techniques and gain the patient's trust. Next, gentle ROM exercises, proximal to distal, are begun. A walking protocol should

be incorporated to help increase ROM and circulatory flow because this is necessary for muscle performance. Muscles deprived of oxygen fatigue easily and eventually do not contract. A stress-loading program is appropriate for treatment of patients with CRPS/RSD.

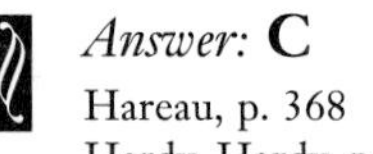

Answer: **C**
Hareau, p. 368
Hardy, Hardy, p. 145

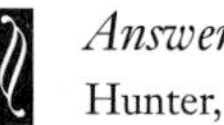

CLINICAL GEM:
It is important for the clinician to realize that "hurt is not harmful" but "pain is disastrous."
Kirkpatrick

20. True or False: In patients with CRPS/RSD, it is helpful to treat edema preventatively because interstitial fluid volume can increase 30% to 50% above normal before it is visibly noted.

It is helpful to begin edema control in a preventative fashion because interstitial fluid volume can increase 30% to 50% before visual detection. Edema should be controlled early and management should be continuous, with the use of various pressure techniques. Edema management techniques include elevation, active exercise, retrograde massage (in patients with CRPS/RSD, it is important to maintain continuous contact to avoid temporal summation of pain), manual edema mobilization, intermittent compression, and edema control garments.

Answer: **True**
Hunter, Mackin, Callahan, p. 824
Walsh, Muntzer in Mackin, Callahan, Skirven, et al, p. 1716

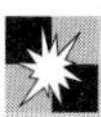

CLINICAL GEM:
Swelling may be caused by vasomotor instability and lack of ROM, causing inflammation rather than edema. See Chapter 18, question 58 for more information.

21. True or False: Continuous passive motion is contraindicated in patients with CRPS/RSD.

Continuous passive motion can be used safely in patients with CRPS/RSD as long as it is used in a pain-free range. It is helpful in reducing pain through stimulation of large-diameter fibers.

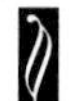

Answer: **False**
Hunter, Mackin, Callahan, p. 828
Walsh, Muntzer in Mackin, Callahan, Skirven, et al, pp. 1717-1718

22. In reference to shoulder-hand syndrome (SHS), all but which of the following are applicable?

A. Poststroke complication
B. Metacarpal and digital edema
C. Pain with wrist flexion
D. All of the above are applicable.

SHS can be a poststroke complication. The clinical presentation of SHS includes pain with active and passive ROM at the shoulder, wrist extension, and passive flexion of the metacarpophalangeal (MCP) and proximal interphalangeal (PIP) joints. Other causes of SHS include proximal trauma to the shoulder, neck, or rib cage; visceral organ pathology; stomach ulcers; and Pancoast tumors in the lung. Usually there is little or no pain with wrist flexion because the patient's wrist often rests in flexion.

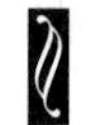

Answer: **C**
Garrison, p. 404
Hunter, Mackin, Callahan, pp. 784-786, 797

23. Which of the following is true with regard to the stress-loading program for patients with CRPS/RSD?

A. It should be avoided during the early stages because it can increase the patient's pain.
B. It is a passive program directed and administered by the therapist.
C. It consists of active exercises that require stress to tissues with minimal joint motion.
D. It uses exercises such as scrubbing, carrying, and aggressive passive stretching.

Stress loading is a program that consists of active exercises that provide stress to tissue with minimal joint motion. It uses scrubbing (Fig. 14-4, *A*) and carrying (Fig. 14-4, *B*) activities. It is not a passive program and is best used early in the rehabilitation of patients with

CRPS/RSD. According to Watson and Carlson, this is the treatment of choice; however, pain and swelling may increase before effectiveness is noted.

Answer: **C**

Carlson, Watson, pp. 149-153
Walsh, Muntzer in Mackin, Callahan, Skirven, et al, p. 1721

A

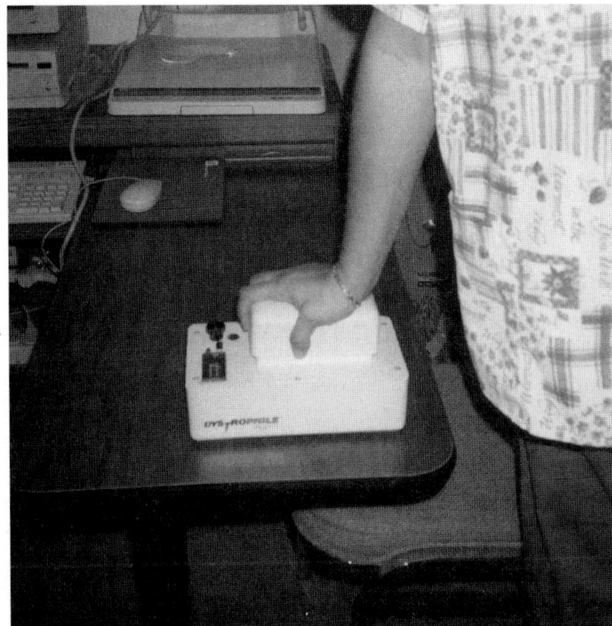

B

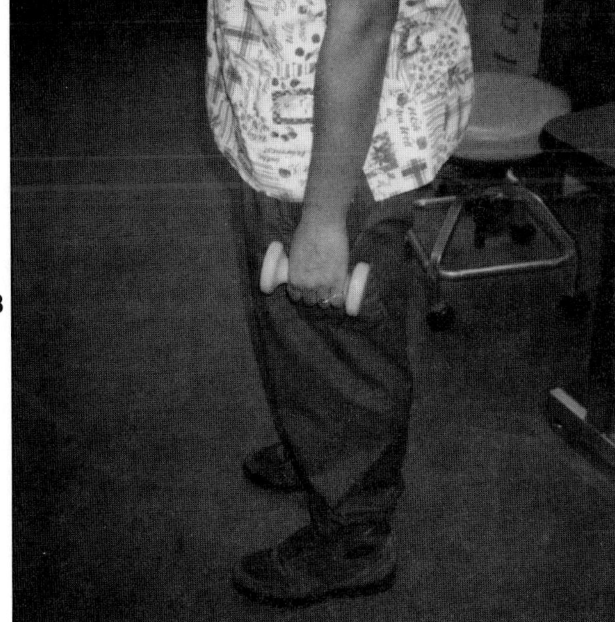

Fig. 14-4

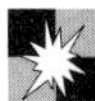

CLINICAL GEM:
Protocol: Begin scrubbing 3 to 5 minutes a day and work up to 10 minutes three times a day. Follow this by carrying 1 to 5 pounds for 3 to 5 minutes and working up to 10 minutes three times per day.

24. Which of the following statements applies to sympathetic blockade in the cervical/thoracic region?

A. It is also called a *stellate ganglion block.*
B. Patients notice an immediate change in the condition of their hands or extremities.
C. The development of a Horner's syndrome is a sign of a successful block.
D. All of the above

After sympathetic blockade (stellate ganglion block), patients notice immediate changes in the condition of their hands or extremities. A patient should be observed for 1 hour after injection to monitor vital signs for complications and to assess the block outcome. Successful sympathetic blockade is indicated by the development of an ipsilateral Horner's syndrome (Fig. 14-5), nasal congestion, facial anhidrosis, increase in temperature (greater than 2° F) of the extremity, venous engorgement of the hand veins, dry skin, and/or changes in skin color.

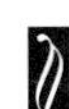

Answer: **D**

Lennard, pp. 254-259
Hunter, Mackin, Callahan, p. 797
Koman, Poehling, Smith in Green, Hotchkiss, Pederson, p. 646
Koman, Smith, Smith in Mackin, Callahan, Skirven, et al, pp. 1699-1700

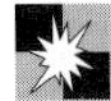

CLINICAL GEM:
Patients with SMP will respond to the blockade because the CNS is not involved. In patients with SIP, stellate ganglion blocks will be ineffective.

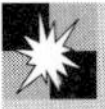

CLINICAL GEM:
Effective stellate ganglion blocks, even when administered by experienced anesthesiologists, occur in only 70% to 75% of cases.

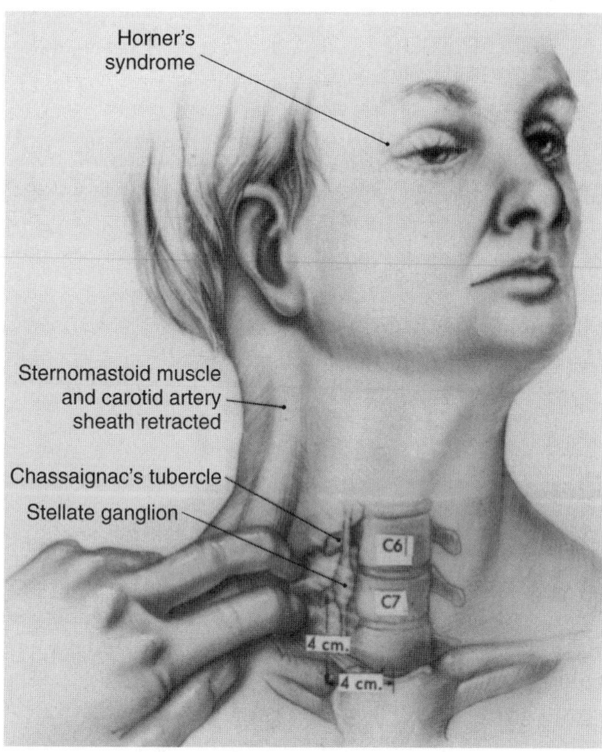

Fig. 14-5 ■ Modified from Lankford LL, Thompson JE: *Reflex sympathetic dystrophy, upper and lower extremity: diagnosis and management.* In *American Academy of Orthopaedic Surgeons: instructional course lectures,* vol 26, St Louis, 1977, Mosby.

25. After a stellate ganglion nerve block, when should therapy be initiated?

A. Immediately
B. 24 hours later
C. 3 to 5 days later
D. Therapy is not indicated; the block will resolve the symptoms.

Therapy should begin immediately after the block is administered (Fig. 14-6). During this pain-free state, gentle passive exercises can be performed as long as they do not exacerbate symptoms. Active functional use of the hand is emphasized during this time.

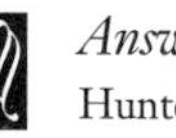

Answer: **A**

Hunter, Mackin, Callahan, p. 831
Walsh, Muntzer in Mackin, Callahan, Skirven, et al, p.1722

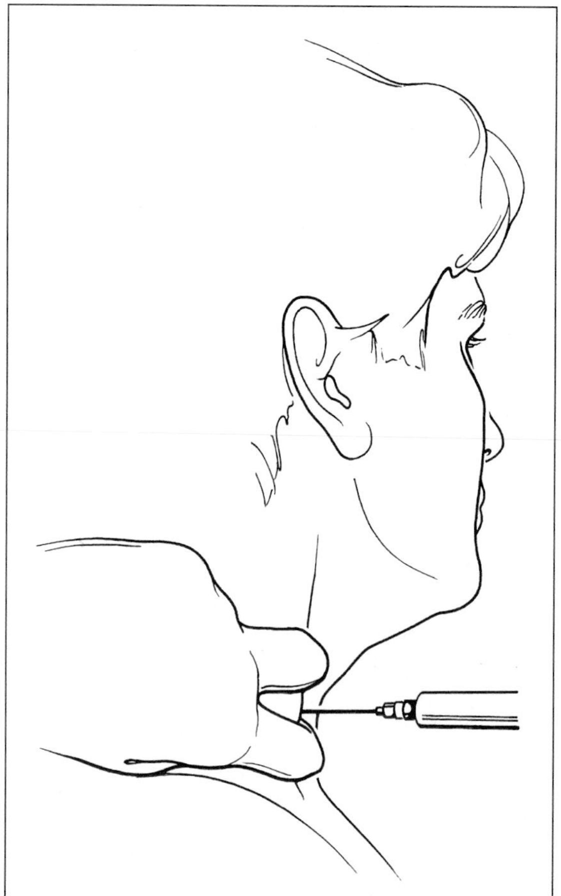

Fig. 14-6 ■ From Mackin EJ, Callahan AD, Skirven TM, et al: *Rehabilitation of the hand and upper extremity,* ed 5, St Louis, 2002, Mosby.

26. What is the average recommended number of blocks needed to assist in the reversal of an abnormal sympathetic reflex?

A. One to two
B. Four to five
C. 10 to 15
D. More than 20

It is rare for a patient to have a complete reversal after only one block. The average number of blocks needed for a reversal of an abnormal sympathetic reflex is approximately four or five. Occasionally more blocks are needed to reverse the disease process. Sympathetic blockade is most effective when the diagnosis is detected early, such as within the first 3 to 4 months of onset.

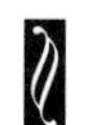

Answer: **B**

Hunter, Mackin, Callahan, p. 797
Koman, Smith, Smith in Mackin, Callahan, Skirven, et al, pp. 1699-1700

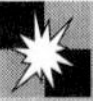

CLINICAL GEM:
Patients with SMP who have a favorable response to the nerve blocks may have more than the recommended number of nerve blocks.

27. After a sympathetic block, the hand should be examined for signs of all but which of the following?

A. Pain relief
B. Functional gains
C. Objective testing
D. Autonomic dysreflexia

Autonomic dysreflexia is a medical emergency that is seen in patients with spinal cord lesions above T6 because of noxious afferent input and in whom the vasculature above the level has reduced sympathetic tone, which results in sudden onset of headache and high blood pressure. All the other choices are correct.

Answer: **D**
Braddom, p. 1159

28. A 33-year-old female presents with a 6-month history of left wrist pain after a motor vehicle accident. She sustained a distal radioulnar fracture that required surgical repair and postoperative casting. She reports a burning, dysesthetic pain that is exacerbated by loading the hand. The injection of choice is which of the following?

A. Placebo saline block
B. Paravertebral somatic block
C. Differential stellate block
D. Brachial plexus block

The differential blockade is based on the principle of using low concentrations of local anesthetics to select out the sympathetic fibers, specifically the C and A-delta, which are smaller and thinner with less myelin sheath covering of the nerve. Higher concentrated solutions of anesthetic will produce a spillover effect and block predominantly the somatic nerve fibers. A placebo block will rule out a psychogenic mechanism of pain. The brachial plexus is the injection site for a patient with upper extremity pain, whereas the cervical plexus is more specific for neck pain, and the C2 spinal root/trigeminal nerve—branches I, II, III—is indicated for head pain of sympathetic origin.

Answer: **C**
Raj, p. 89

CLINICAL GEM:
CRPS/RSD is *not* a psychogenic condition. However, chronic pain is known to play a role in psychological well-being.

29. All but which of the following are theories that explain CRPS/RSD?

A. Artificial synapse
B. Gate control
C. Spontaneous discharge
D. Wide dynamic range
E. All of the above

All of the above are theories to explain CRPS/RSD. The next question will elaborate on the theories.

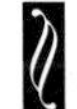

Answer: **E**
O'Young, Young, Stiens, pp. 360-364

30. Match the theory to its mechanism.

Theory

1. Wide dynamic range
2. Gate control
3. Spontaneous discharge
4. Artificial synapse

Mechanism

A. Central perception of pain with peripheral release of pain-sensitizing substances
B. Input from large-diameter fibers inhibit small, thinly unmyelinated nociceptive fibers (in CRPS/RSD, the large fibers are injured, thus sparing the small fibers so that the pain input is unmodulated).
C. Regenerating axons result in excessive calcium and sodium channels as well as alpha-adrenergic receptors that are sensitized by circulating catecholamines.
D. Large type-A myelinated fibers are abnormally augmented by type-C unmyelinated fibers and excited by sympathetic activity.

Answers: **1, D; 2, B; 3, C; 4, A**
O'Young, Young, Stiens, p. 361

31. A patient presents in your clinic with pain, tenderness, swelling, stiffness, and discoloration in the hand after a Colles' fracture. During a radiograph, osseous demineralization is noted. The patient is sent for a sympathetic blockade and afterward has a significant reduction in pain. What is the diagnosis for this patient?

A. Carpal tunnel syndrome
B. Fictitious lymphedema
C. CPRS with SIP
D. CRPS with SMP

If a patient has a significant resolution of signs and symptoms after a sympathetic blockade, the diagnosis of CRPS with SMP is confirmed. Symptom resolution may not be long-lasting, and more than one block often is needed. A stellate ganglion block is a reliable, specific test for CRPS with SMP.

Answer: **D**
Hunter, Mackin, Callahan, pp. 788-790
Koman, Poehling, Smith in Green, Hotchkiss, Pederson, p. 645

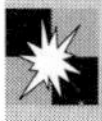
CLINICAL GEM:
The theory of using blocks is to interrupt sympathetic outflow to the painful area. After each block, therapy is recommended. Begin immediately to achieve maximal functional improvements.

32. A 66-year-old male is employed as a factory worker on an assembly line doing repetitive activity. He sustained an on-the-job soft-tissue injury to his right upper extremity (UE) that was complicated by compartment syndrome, which required surgical repair via a decompressive fasciotomy. Postoperative complications included lancinating pain in the entire hand, digit numbness, and atrophy in the thenar eminence. Electromyographic (EMG) nerve conduction velocity (NCV) studies showed evidence of a sensorimotor median neuropathy at the wrist. Based on the above information, what is the most likely clinical diagnosis?

A. CRPS 1
B. CRPS 2
C. Cubital tunnel syndrome
D. Posterior interosseous nerve (PIN) syndrome

CRPS 1 and CRPS 2 are both characterized by spontaneous pain with associated hyperalgesia to stimuli. However, only the second type has a specific involved peripheral nerve injury.

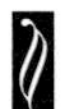
Answer: **B**
Koman, Smith, Smith in Mackin, Callahan, Skirven, et al, p. 1695

33. Therapeutic modalities for hand rehabilitation in the CRPS/RSD patient include which of the following?

A. Desensitization
B. Edema reduction
C. Graded activity
D. TENS unit
E. All of the above

All of the above have been shown to benefit by reducing pain and improving sympathetic symptoms in the early stages of this condition. The overall goal is functional gains documented by the therapist.

Accurate assessment by the therapist is crucial; otherwise, the therapist becomes a "pain terrorist." The therapist must have clinical reasoning, observational skills, and ongoing knowledge concerning pain and CRPS/RSD to develop an appropriate treatment plan. No recipe for treating CRPS/RSD exists.

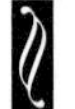
Answer: **E**
Braddom, p. 781
Walsh, Muntzer in Mackin, Callahan, Skirven, et al, p. 1713

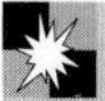
CLINICAL GEM:
CRPS/RSD patients and their treating therapists can find more information at www.rsds.org.

34. Which of the following applies to CRPS/RSD in children?

A. It involves females more often than males.
B. It can be treated with conservative treatment, including cognitive and behavioral treatments, TENS, tricyclic antidepressants, and/or neural blockade.
C. It is best treated with corticosteroids.
D. B and C
E. A and B

The mean age of children who have CRPS/RSD was found to be 12.5 years, and 84% were females. Therapy has been reported by many to be the mainstay of treatment. TENS has been described as a highly effective treatment. Sympathetic blocks are appropriate when the patient has a clear clinical diagnosis of CRPS/RSD. Some patients respond to a multidisciplinary program that includes therapy and behavioral management. Most children with CRPS/RSD do not benefit from the use of corticosteroids.

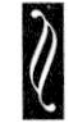

Answer: **E**
Wilder, Berde, Wolohan, pp. 910-919

35. Select the terms that are synonymous with CRPS/RSD.

A. Causalgia
B. Algodystrophy
C. Posttraumatic dystrophy
D. Sudeck's atrophy
E. Pourfour del petit syndrome
F. SHS
G. Postinfarctional sclerodactyly

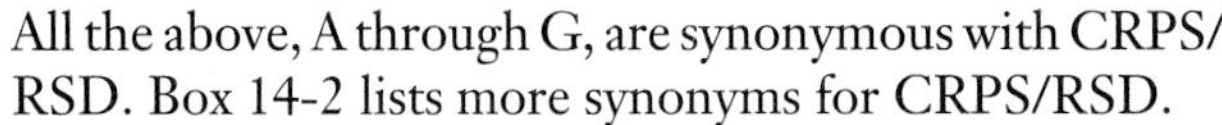

All the above, A through G, are synonymous with CRPS/RSD. Box 14-2 lists more synonyms for CRPS/RSD.

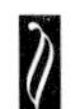

Answer: **A through G**
van der Laan, Goris, p. 379
Koman, Smith, Smith in Mackin, Callahan, Skirven, et al, p. 1696

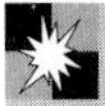

CLINICAL GEM:
Some common misdiagnoses of CRPS/RSD include diabetic neuropathy, spinal cord disease, traumatic arthropathy, psychogenic problems, hypertrophic arthritis, epilepsy, stiff/frozen hand, and peripheral vascular disease.

BOX 14-2
Synonyms for CRPS/RSD

Acute atrophy of bone
Algodystrophy
Algoneurodystrophy
Causalgia state/syndrome
Chronic traumatic edema
Complex regional pain syndrome (CRPS)
Major causalgia
Major traumatic dystrophy
Mimocausalgia
Minor causalgia
Minor traumatic dystrophy
Neurodystrophy
Neurovascular dystrophy
Osteoneurodystrophy
Pain dysfunction syndrome
Painful posttraumatic osteoporosis
Peripheral trophoneurosis
Postinfarctional sclerodactyly
Posttraumatic pain syndrome
Posttraumatic sympathetic dystrophy
Posttraumatic vasomotor abnormality
Posttraumatic vasomotor instability
Reflex nervous dystrophy
Reflex neurovascular dystrophy
Reflex sympathetic dystrophy (RSD)
Shoulder-hand syndrome (SHS)
Shoulder-hand-finger syndrome
Sudeck's atrophy
Sympathalgia
Sympathetic algodystrophy
Sympathetic-mediated pain
Sympathetic neurovascular dystrophy
Sympathetic overdrive syndrome
Traumatic angiospasm

From Mackin EJ, Callahan AD, Skirven TM, et al: *Rehabilitation of the hand and upper extremity,* ed 5, St Louis, 2002, Mosby.

36. True or False: Desensitization is recommended to be performed with one or two separate modalities for a 20-minute period five times a day.

Desensitization programs for the CRPS/RSD patient should be used for 20-minute periods five times daily while using one or two separate modalities. Encourage patients to stick with their programs because inadequate time spent on desensitization will not produce sensory accommodation to the stimulus and will thus result in continued hypersensitivity. Desensitization should be part of the active ROM and functional activity program.

Keep the program simple, and use everyday objects and surfaces to desensitize. For example, rub the sensitive area on the upholstery in the car while driving and/or on the couch when sitting in front of the television. Remember that retrograde massage is part of the desensitization program.

Answer: **True**

Walsh, Muntzer in Mackin, Callahan, Skirven, et al, p. 1715

37. True or False: Antidepressants are frequently used in the management of CRPS/RSD.

Antidepressants are used to manage chronic pain such as CRPS/RSD. They were originally used to relieve posttraumatic depression but also provide analgesia and modulate sympathetic hyperactivity in the peripheral nervous system and CNS.

Answer: **True**

Koman, Poehling, Smith in Green, Hotchkiss, Pederson, p. 650

38. Which of the following drugs is *not* used to manage CRPS/RSD?

A. Adrenergic compounds
B. Calcium channel blockers
C. Corticosteroids
D. All of the above can be used.

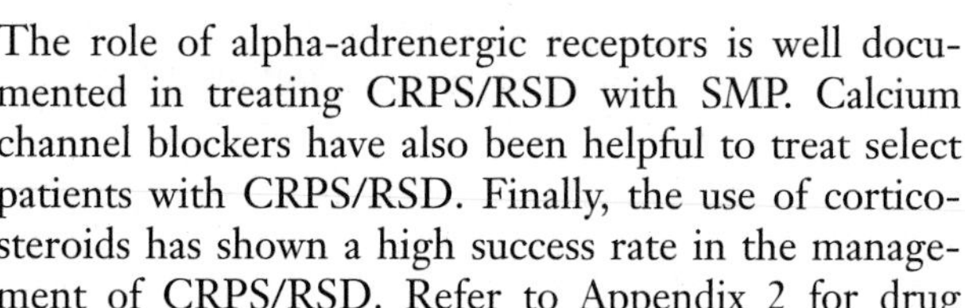

The role of alpha-adrenergic receptors is well documented in treating CRPS/RSD with SMP. Calcium channel blockers have also been helpful to treat select patients with CRPS/RSD. Finally, the use of corticosteroids has shown a high success rate in the management of CRPS/RSD. Refer to Appendix 2 for drug categories.

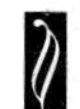

Answer: **D**

Koman, Poehling, Smith in Green, Hotchkiss, Pederson, pp. 653-654

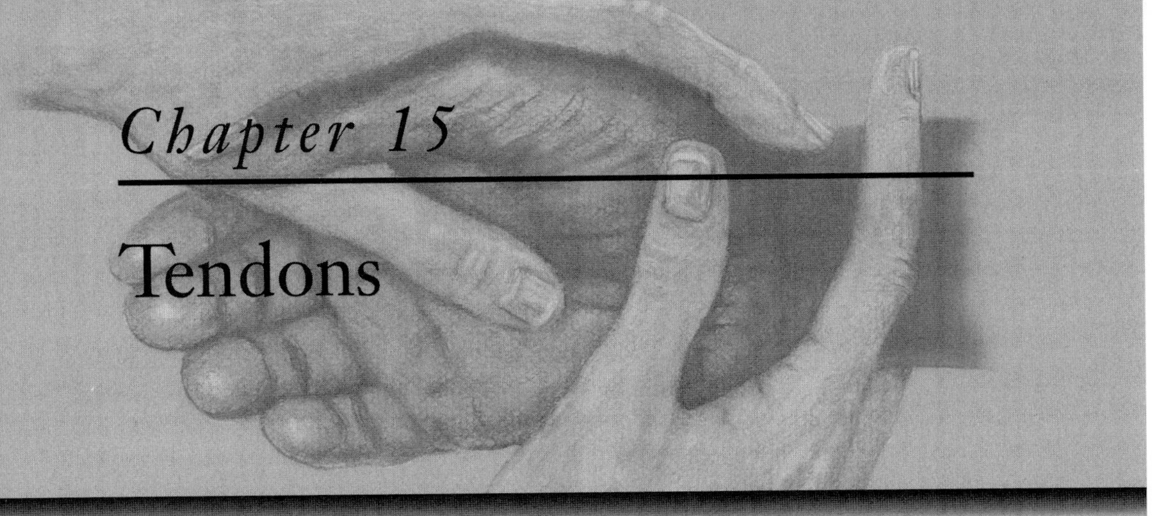

Chapter 15

Tendons

1. Match each statement to the correct flexor tendon zone:

Zone

1. Zone I
2. Zone II
3. Zone III
4. Zone IV
5. Zone V

Statement

A. The zone that contains "Camper's Chiasma," where the two slips of the flexor digitorum superficialis (FDS) merge deep to the flexor digitorum profundus (FDP) and insert at the mid-portion of the middle phalanx
B. A cut in this zone will result in an isolated FDP laceration.
C. The zone that contains the flexors' musculotendinous junction
D. The zone in which the digital synovial sheath ends for digits 2, 3, and 4 and in which the lumbrical muscles take their origin from the FDP tendons
E. The zone in which the flexor tendons pass under the flexor retinaculum (carpal canal)

Answers: **1, B; 2, A; 3, D; 4, E; 5, C**

Culp, Taras in Mackin, Callahan, Skirven, et al, pp. 418, 432-433
Strickland in Green, Hotchkiss, Pederson, p. 1857
Boyer, Strickland, Engles, p. 1684
Refer to Fig. 15-1

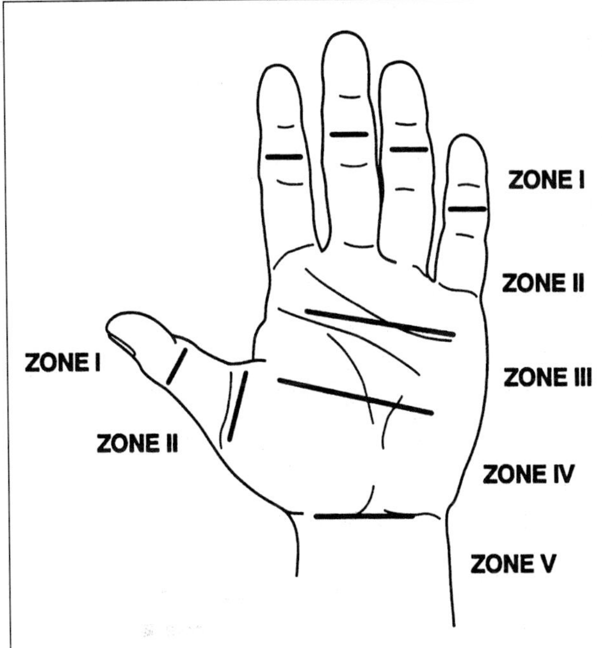

Fig. 15-1 ■ From Mackin EJ, Callahan AD, Skirven TM: *Rehabilitation of the hand and upper extremity,* ed 5, St Louis, 2002, Mosby.

2. You are preparing to see a patient 3½ weeks after zone II FDP and FDS repair. Which of the following modifications in treatment is appropriate after an early passive mobilization tendon protocol at this time?

A. Adjust the dorsal block splint to neutral (0 degrees of wrist extension)
B. Initiate neuromuscular electrical stimulation (NMES) to provoke a strong muscle contraction and enhance tendon excursion
C. Begin differential tendon glides actively
D. Begin aggressive blocking exercises
E. Both A and C

At 3½ weeks after flexor tendon repair (intermediate stage) following an early passive mobilization protocol, the splint is modified to bring the wrist to neutral. The patient is taught to remove the splint hourly for exercise. With the wrist at 10 degrees of extension, the patient performs 10 repetitions of active differential tendon gliding exercises. These exercises elicit maximum total and differential flexor tendon glide at the wrist/palm level. The straight fist elicits maximum glide to the FDS in relation to the surrounding tissues. The full fist does the same for the FDP tendon. In the hook fist, maximum differential gliding between the two tendons is achieved (Fig. 15-2).

Gentle blocking exercises for isolated FDP and FDS glide are not started until the late stage, between 4 to 6 weeks. Blocking exercises can be dangerous for a newly healed tendon if not performed correctly. This is particularly true in the case of isolated distal interphalangeal (DIP) joint flexion. Patient education includes the danger of rupture with overzealous blocking exercise. Some patients may not be appropriate candidates for blocking exercises for 2 to 3 additional weeks, when the tendon repair is stronger.

NMES should not be used until later to provoke a stronger muscle contraction; this would not be appropriate until approximately 1 week after initiating resisted exercise.

Answer: **E**

Pettengill, van Strien in Mackin, Callahan, Skirven, et al, pp. 440-444

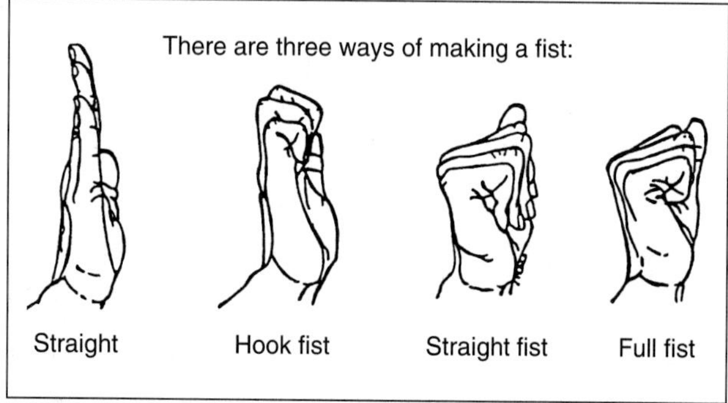

Fig. 15-2 ■ From Mackin EJ, Callahan AD, Skirven TM: *Rehabilitation of the hand and upper extremity*, ed 5, St Louis, 2002, Mosby.

3. Duran and Houser determined through clinical and experimental observation that controlled stress through early mobilization prevents adhesion formation. According to their work, how much tendon glide is needed?

A. 5 to 6 mm
B. 3 to 5 mm
C. 2 to 3 mm
D. 1 to 2 mm

Duran and Houser popularized the technique of controlled passive motion in which a posterior splint was applied immediately after surgery and specific limited passive exercises were then permitted at the PIP and DIP joints in an effort to impart 3 to 5 mm of excursion to the repaired tendons. Additionally, Gelberman indicates that 3 to 4 mm of tendon glide decreases gap formation in flexor tendon repairs.

Answer: **B**

Strickland in Green, Hotchkiss, Pederson, p. 1864
Pettengill, van Strien in Mackin, Callahan, Skirven, et al, p. 443
Evans in Mackin, Callahan, Skirven, et al, p. 546
Hunter, Schneider, Mackin, p. 335
Boyer, Strickland, Engles, p. 1688
Refer to Fig. 15-3

4. True or False: Total active motion (TAM) is calculated by taking the sum of the metacarpophalangeal (MCP), PIP, and DIP joint flexion (measured goniometrically in degrees) and subtracting the sum of the MCP, PIP, and DIP joint extension of the digit.

TAM is a calculation rather than a measurement. Total motion of a digit is described by a single number that represents the summation of the joint flexion measurements minus the summation of the joint extension deficits. Total motion measurements may be computed to facilitate comparison of data by providing a composite statement of the integrated motion of a digit. This calculation may not be valid in cases where hyperextension exists.

Answer: **True**

Adams, Greene, Topoozian, p. 68
Pettengill, van Strien in Mackin, Callahan, Skirven, et al, p. 439

5. Match each extensor zone with its correct definition.

Zone

1. Zone I
2. Zone II
3. Zone III
4. Zone IV
5. Zone V

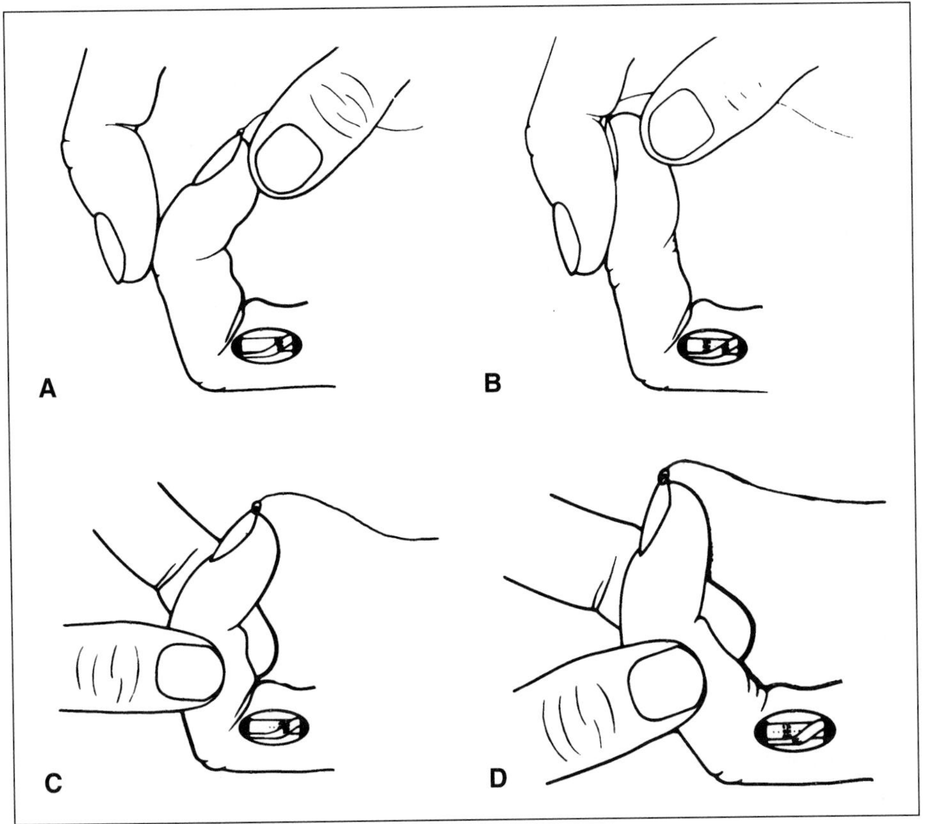

Fig. 15-3 ■ Duran and Houser's exercises for passive flexor tendon gliding. With the MCP and PIP joints flexed, **A**, the DIP joint is passively extended, **B**, thus moving the FDP repair distally, away from an FDS repair. Then, with the DIP and MCP flexed, **C**, the PIP is extended, **D**; both repairs glide distally away from the site of repair and any surrounding tissues to which they might otherwise form adhesions. (From Mackin EJ, Callahan AD, Skirven TM: *Rehabilitation of the hand and upper extremity*, ed 5, St Louis, 2002, Mosby.)

6. Zone VI
7. Zone VII
8. Zone VIII

Definition

A. Extensor retinaculum
B. Central slip
C. Distal to extensor retinaculum to just proximal to the MCP joint
D. Terminal tendon
E. Proximal to the extensor retinaculum
F. Triangular tendon (middle phalanx)
G. Sagittal bands
H. Distal to the sagittal bands and proximal to the central slip

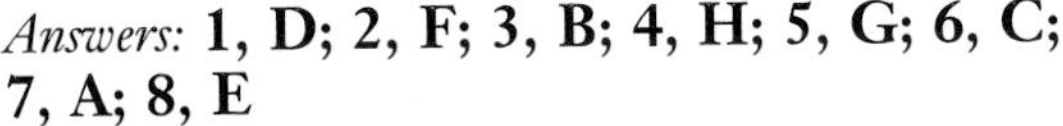

Answers: **1, D; 2, F; 3, B; 4, H; 5, G; 6, C; 7, A; 8, E**

Thomas, Moutet, Guinard, p. 309
Hunter, Schneider, Mackin, p. 547
Culp, Taras in Mackin, Callahan, Skirven, et al, p. 418
Pettengill, van Strien in Mackin, Callahan, Skirven, et al, pp. 432–433
Refer to Fig. 15-4

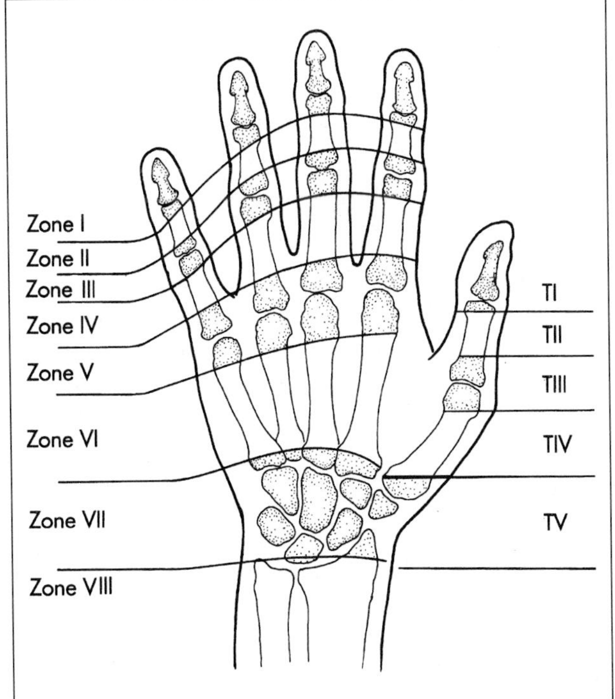

Fig. 15-4 ■ From Wilson RL: Management of acute extensor tendon injuries. In Hunter JM, Schneider LH, Mackin EJ, editors: *Tendon surgery in the hand,* St Louis, 1987, Mosby.

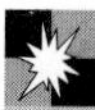

CLINICAL GEM:
Clinical Gem: Zones I, III, V, and VII (excluding the thumb) all correspond with joints, as follows:

Zone I—DIP joint
Zone III—PIP joint
Zone V—MCP joint
Zone VII—wrist joint

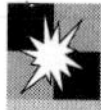

CLINICAL GEM:
The thumb generally is classified into five extensor zones (TI, TII, TIII, TIV, and TV; see Fig. 15-4).

6. The largest amount of gap formation acceptable in healing tendon repairs is which of the following?

A. 0 mm; no amount of gap is acceptable
B. 1 to 3 mm
C. 4 to 5 mm
D. 5 to 6 mm

Gapping at the repair site becomes the weakest part of the tendon, unfavorably alters tendon mechanics, and may attract adhesions, resulting in decreased tendon excursion. Most surgeons believe that gapping above 1 to 3 mm is incompatible with a good result. Tendons without a gap or gaps less than 3 mm in length have been shown to have a significant increase in repair site tensile strength between 3 and 6 weeks postoperatively, whereas those with a gap of more than 3 mm did not have significant accrual of repair site strength; the latter may pose a greater risk of rupture as motion rehabilitation progresses after 3 weeks. The importance of the addition of a peripheral circumferential epitendinous suture to the core suture of a tendon repair may provide anywhere from a 10% to 30% increase in flexor tendon repair strength and a significant reduction in gapping between the tendon ends.

Answer: **B**
Evans in Mackin, Callahan, Skirven, et al, p. 551
Strickland in Green, Hotchkiss, Pederson, p. 1860
Boyer, Strickland, Engles, p. 1687

7. All but which of the following statements are true regarding tenolysis?

A. The degree of circulatory sufficiency of the digit is important to assess before surgery to determine whether this procedure is appropriate.
B. A tenolysis is recommended for **all** patients who do not obtain full range of motion (ROM) after flexor tendon repair.
C. The earliest that tenolysis is generally considered to be appropriate is between 3 to 6 months after tendon repair to allow adequate healing and to lengthen adhesions as much as possible through hand therapy intervention
D. The best candidate for tenolysis is a patient whose repaired tendon has localized adhesions that limit glide and who has full passive motion of that digit
E. The patient must be prepared to undergo two-stage reconstruction of the tendon at the time of tenolysis if tendon quality is found to be poor

Many factors need to be taken into account before proceeding to a tenolysis. A cold insensate finger will not be improved even if full ROM could be regained. All fractures should be healed, and wounds must have soft, pliable skin and subcutaneous tissues. Joint contractures must have been mobilized, and there must be a normal or nearly normal passive range of digital motion. The patient must be carefully informed about the objectives, surgical techniques, postoperative course, and pitfalls of the procedure. Many patients will be content with less-than-normal active digital motion and might choose not to undergo the procedure. When a patient elects to undergo tenolysis, he or she must understand that if the findings at surgery preclude the possibility of regaining satisfactory function, it may be necessary to proceed with the implantation of a silicone rod as the first step of a staged flexor reconstruction. It is generally accepted that tenolysis may be considered as early as 3 months after repair, provided that the other criteria for the procedure have been satisfied and there has been no measurable improvement in active motion during the preceding 4 to 8 weeks.

Answer: **B**
Boyer, Strickland, Engles, p. 1695
Schneider in Green, Hotchkiss, Pederson, pp. 1921-1922
Schneider, Feldscher in Mackin, Callahan, Skirven, et al, p. 457

8. Which of the following statements is true regarding early controlled active motion rehabilitation following tendon repair?

A. A two-strand core suture provides adequate tensile strength to tolerate early active motion.
B. In the minimal active muscle-tendon tension (MAMTT) program, proposed by Evans, flexors are worked with the wrist in slight flexion, and extensors are worked with the wrist in slight extension.
C. The early controlled active motion protocols suggest beginning active differential tendon gliding through *full* ROM for *all* early active motion protocols at day 3.
D. According to Evans, a certain amount of active muscle-tendon tension is required to create proximal migration of a healing tendon and that passive motion may only cause the tendon to buckle, fold, or roll up at the repair site.

Four- and six-strand repairs with strong peripheral epitendinous sutures should permit repair strength to tolerate passive and light composite grip during the entire healing period, whereas two-strand repairs may be vulnerable from 1 to 3 weeks after repair.

MAMTT is defined as the minimal tension required to overcome the viscoelastic resistance of the antagonistic muscle-tendon unit. Tendon forces are the sum of the muscle contraction and the resistance of viscoelastic drag imposed on the repair site by the swollen tendon, periarticular soft tissues, edema, tension in the antagonistic muscle-tendon unit, and bandaging. To apply MAMTT to the healing tendon, the hand therapist must have a working knowledge of the tensile strength of the repairs employed and must understand the effects of the variables of timing, healing, and drag on these measurements.

Wrist position influences tension in the extrinsic tendons of the digits because of the viscoelasticity of the antagonistic muscle-tendon unit. In the MAMTT program, digit *flexors* are worked with the wrist in slight *extension*, and digit *extensors* are worked with the wrist in slight *flexion*.

Full active digital motion is not recommended in many of the early active motion protocols. Evans has demonstrated that moderate digit flexion angles with an applied fingertip pressure of <50 g produce internal tendon forces that are fairly low. However, after the flexion angles become greater, even though the external force is the same, tendon forces rise dramatically and are felt to be incompatible with traditional two-strand epitendous repair techniques.

Studies on early active motion have been pursued since stronger suture techniques have been developed. The studies are based on the presumption that a certain amount of active muscle-tendon tension may be required to create proximal migration of a healing tendon and that passive motion may only cause the tendon to buckle, fold, or roll up at the repair site.

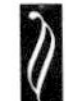

Answer: **D**
Evans, pp. 266-267
Strickland in Green, Hotchkiss, Pederson, pp. 1862-1863

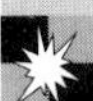

CLINICAL GEM:
Not every tendon injury can be treated with an identical protocol. Choice of protocol must take into account the needs and requirements of the patient. Implementation of early active motion protocols requires an experienced hand therapist who has good communication with the physician regarding the quality and strength of repair. It is better for an inexperienced therapist to take a more conservative approach to tendon rehabilitation.

9. Match the following extensor tendons to the correct corresponding dorsal compartments:

Compartment

1. First dorsal compartment
2. Second dorsal compartment
3. Third dorsal compartment
4. Fourth dorsal compartment
5. Fifth dorsal compartment
6. Sixth dorsal compartment

Extensor Tendon

A. Extensor pollicis longus
B. Extensor carpi ulnaris
C. Extensor digitorum communis
D. Extensor carpi radialis longus
E. Extensor digiti minimi
F. Abductor pollicis longus

Answers: **1, F; 2, D; 3, A; 4, C; 5, E; 6, B**
Netter, p. 443

10. How many pulleys are in the thumb?

A. Two
B. Three
C. Four
D. Five

The thumb has one oblique pulley overlying the proximal phalanx and two annular pulleys. The A1 pulley is just proximal to the MCP joint, and the A2 pulley is at the volar plate of the DIP joint. The most important pulley in the thumb is the oblique pulley.

Answer: **B**

Hunter, Schneider, Mackin, p. 269
Hunter, Mackin, Callahan, pp. 418-419
Culp, Taras in Mackin, Callahan, Skirven, et al, p. 416
Refer to Fig. 15-5

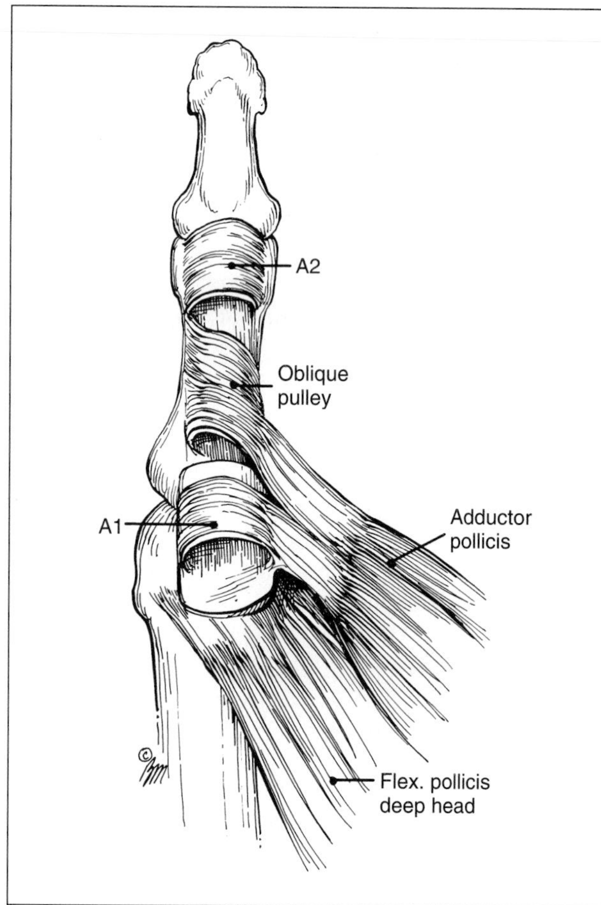

Fig. 15-5 ■ Copyright Elizabeth Roselius. Modified from Doyle JR, Blythe WF: Anatomy of the flexor tendon sheath and pulleys of the thumb, *J Hand Surg* [Am] 2(2):149-51, 1977.

11. Which pulley in the thumb is the most important in the prevention of bowstringing?

A. A1 pulley
B. Oblique pulley
C. A2 pulley
D. All of the above are equally important.

The pulley system in the thumb is distinct from that of the digits. One oblique and two annular pulleys have been identified. The first annular pulley of the thumb arises from the palmar plate of the MCP joint, and the second annular pulley arises from the palmar plate of the interphalangeal (IP) joint. The oblique pulley originates and inserts on the proximal phalanx in close association with the insertion of the adductor pollicis tendon. The oblique pulley is the most important. Its loss results in decreased IP joint motion. Incompetence of both the A1 and oblique pulleys of the thumb leads to a 30% loss of IP joint motion (see Fig. 15-5).

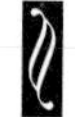

Answer: **B**

Culp, Taras in Mackin, Callahan, Skirven, et al, p. 416
Schneider in Green, Hotchkiss, Pederson, p. 1934

12. Which of the following statements regarding tendon healing is false?

A. Tendons heal by intrinsic and extrinsic means; the more intrinsic the healing, the fewer the adhesions.
B. If tendon repair is not stressed, the healing process may take up to 8 weeks and the tendons will have minimal tensile strength.
C. Stressed tendons heal and gain tensile strength faster and have fewer adhesions than unstressed tendons.
D. Repair strength usually decreases by 30% to 50% between 1 and 2 days after repair.
E. None of the above

Statement D is incorrect. Repair strength in the unstressed tendon usually decreases by 10% to 50% between 3 and 5 days after repair. From days 5-21, tensile strength begins to increase as the collagen matures.

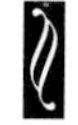

Answer: **D**

Hunter, Schneider, Mackin, p. 354
Pettengill, van Strien in Mackin, Callahan, Skirven, et al, p. 435

13. Which statement is true regarding the intrinsic healing process?

A. It occurs through a fibroblastic response from surrounding tissue.
B. It requires peritendinous adhesions to allow complete healing of the tendon.
C. It occurs in the absence of cells and tissue extrinsic to the tendon.
D. It is the dominant healing process when a delayed mobilization protocol is used.

Intrinsic healing suggests that healing of the tendon is possible in the absence of cells and tissue extrinsic to the tendon. Controlled mobilization of repaired tendons to allow healing but prevent adhesions was the stated advantage of this theory of healing. Extrinsic healing suggests that healing occurs though cells extrinsic to the tendon through a fibroblastic response from surrounding tissue. This presupposes the necessity of surrounding peritendinous adhesions to allow complete healing of the tendon; thus immobilization after flexor tendon repair was encouraged. Almost all investigators now believe that tendons have both an intrinsic and extrinsic capability of healing.

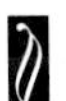
Answer: **C**

Culp, Taras in Mackin, Callahan, Skirven, et al, pp. 417-418
Pettengill, van Strien in Mackin, Callahan, Skirven, et al, p. 436
Strickland in Green, Hotchkiss, Pederson, p.1854
Gelberman, Woo, p. 66

14. Match each flexor zone with its correct description.

Zone

1. Zone I
2. Zone II
3. Zone III
4. Zone IV
5. Zone V

Description

A. The A1 pulley to the insertion of the FDS
B. Proximal to the carpal tunnel
C. From the insertion of the FDS at the middle phalanx to the FDP at the distal phalanx
D. From the distal end of the carpal tunnel to the first annular ligament
E. The carpal tunnel

Answers: **1, C; 2, A; 3, D; 4, E; 5, B**

Hunter, Mackin, Callahan, p. 420
Culp, Taras in Mackin, Callahan, Skirven, et al, p. 418
Pettengill, van Strien in Mackin, Callahan, Skirven, et al, pp. 432–433
Refer to Fig. 15-1

15. True or False: Intrinsic tendon healing suggests that surrounding peritendinous adhesions allow healing of the tendon.

The **extrinsic** healing theory suggests that peritendinous adhesions allow healing of the tendon. The sequence of healing by extrinsic means is through the ingrowth of capillaries and fibroblasts during the first 4 days after the injury, followed by the formation of collagen at 4 to 21 days, and scar remodeling after 21 days. The theory of **intrinsic** healing suggests that healing occurs in the absence of cells and tissue extrinsic to the tendon. **Intrinsic healing** occurs between the **tendon ends**. Tendon healing probably is a combination of extrinsic and intrinsic cellular activity. Theoretically, if more intrinsic healing occurs, fewer adhesions are formed.

Answer: **False**

Hunter, Mackin, Callahan, p. 419
Culp, Taras in Mackin, Callahan, Skirven, et al, pp. 417-418
Pettengill, van Strien in Mackin, Callahan, Skirven, et al, p. 436

16. What is the major nutritional pathway for extensor tendons underneath the extensor retinaculum?

A. Vascular perfusion
B. Synovial diffusion
C. Vincula
D. All of the above are equally involved.

Synovial diffusion is the major nutritional pathway for the extensor tendons beneath the extensor retinaculum. Extensor tendons also receive their blood supply through vascular mesenteries or mesotendons. Vascular perfusion through the mesotendons provides 30% of nutrition, and synovial diffusion, the major nutritional pathway, provides 70%.

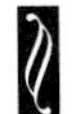
Answer: **B**

Hunter, Mackin, Callahan, pp. 520-521
Rosenthal in Mackin, Callahan, Skirven, et al, p. 499

17. Which flexor zone did Bunnell call "no man's land"?

A. Zone I
B. Zone II
C. Zone III
D. Zone IV
E. Zone V

Bunnell coined the term *no man's land* for the zone II portion of the flexor system because of the extreme difficulty in obtaining a good result with primary repair of tendons lacerated in this area. The classically termed *no man's land* is now termed *some man's land* (see Fig. 15-1).

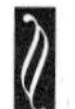

Answer: **B**

Strickland in Green, Hotchkiss, Pederson, p. 1851

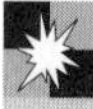

CLINICAL GEM:

Teno Fix is a new surgical repair technique for flexor tendon repairs that appears promising to allow for improved results with tendon repairs. The Teno Fix system is designed to allow patients to begin motion therapy faster after surgery, leading to an earlier return to normal motion and reducing the need for repeat surgeries caused by scarring. Visit www.ortheon.com for more information.

18. True or False: The vincula are folds of mesotendon carrying blood supply to the flexor tendons.

One way flexor tendons receive their blood supply is from the vincula, which are folds of the mesotendon. The vincular system exits on the dorsal surface of the tendons and is supplied by transverse communicating branches of the common digital artery. If the vincula are uninjured after tendon damage, clinical results are better than in cases in which the vincula are injured.

Answer: **True**

Strickland in Green, Hotchkiss, Pederson, p. 1851
Hunter, Schneider, Mackin, pp. 278-285
Hunter, Mackin, Callahan, p. 413
Pettengill, van Strien in Mackin, Callahan, Skirven, et al, pp. 433-434
Refer to Fig. 15-6

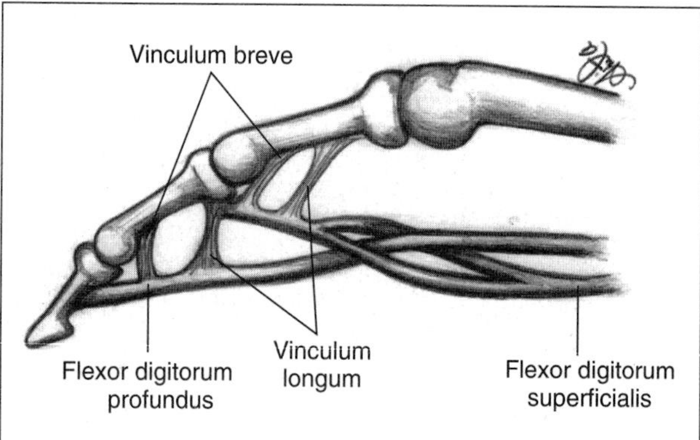

Fig. 15-6

19. A resident medical doctor calls from the operating room to set up the first postoperative therapy visit for a 21-year-old sheet metal worker who cut his hand at work. The lacerations of his FDP and FDS were repaired emergently. Knowing the optimal time frame for initiation of early mobilization to repaired flexor tendons, when will you schedule the patient's first therapy session?

A. Today (same day as the repair) because immediate initiation of ROM is crucial
B. At postoperative day 2 to 4 to allow edema to subside before starting the protocol
C. 1 week after the repair to allow time for the patient's pain to diminish
D. 3 weeks after the repair because you do not want to start ROM until the stitches are removed

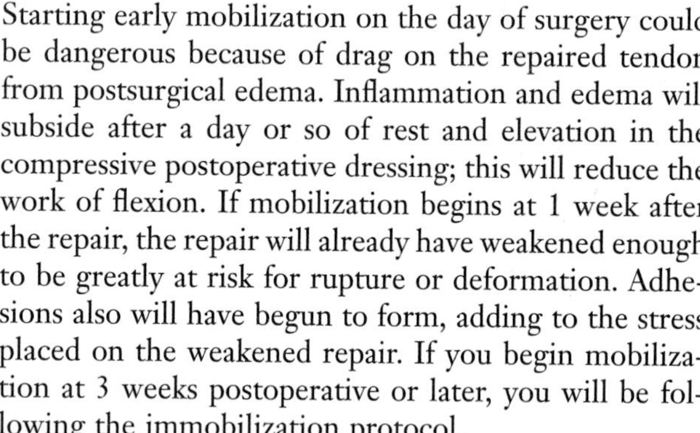

Starting early mobilization on the day of surgery could be dangerous because of drag on the repaired tendon from postsurgical edema. Inflammation and edema will subside after a day or so of rest and elevation in the compressive postoperative dressing; this will reduce the work of flexion. If mobilization begins at 1 week after the repair, the repair will already have weakened enough to be greatly at risk for rupture or deformation. Adhesions also will have begun to form, adding to the stress placed on the weakened repair. If you begin mobilization at 3 weeks postoperative or later, you will be following the immobilization protocol.

Answer: **B**

Culp, Taras in Mackin, Callahan, Skirven, et al, p. 416
Evans, Thompson, p. 277

20. Which statement is *false* regarding diagnostic signs of intact flexor tendons?

A. Squeezing the forearm musculature will demonstrate flexion of the digits
B. Tenodesis of the flexor tendons is performed when the wrist is placed in flexion, loss of digital flexion will be demonstrated if the flexor tendons are severed
C. An intact FDS to the index finger is demonstrated through pulp-to-pulp pinch with the thumb and index finger.
D. Cascade of flexion increases as one proceeds from the index finger to the small finger.
E. All of the above statements are true.

Assessing tenodesis of flexor tendons with the wrist in extension, not flexion, will demonstrate loss of finger flexion if flexor tendons are severed. All of the other statements are true. Isolated testing of the FDS to the index finger often is not applicable because of the independent muscle belly of the FDP. The FDS to the index finger can be demonstrated through pulp-to-pulp pinch with the thumb and index finger. Additionally, demonstration of PIP joint flexion of the index finger with the DIP joint fully extended or hyperextended also documents superficialis function to the index finger. In the normal hand, a cascade of flexion of the digits is noted, increasing as one proceeds from the index to the small fingers. Squeezing the forearm musculature to demonstrate flexion of the digits may also be helpful.

Answer: **B**
Culp, Taras in Mackin, Callahan, Skirven, et al, pp. 418-419

21. Flexor tendon injuries in which of the following zones would be most likely to have an associated median or ulnar nerve injury?

A. Zone II
B. Zone III
C. Zone IV
D. Zone V
E. Zones IV and V

Zone IV consists of that segment of flexor tendons covered by the transverse carpal ligament within the carpal tunnel. Concomitant injuries to the median and ulnar nerves may be associated with flexor tendon injuries in this zone. Zone V extends from the flexor musculotendinous junction in the forearm to the proximal border of the transverse carpal ligament. Associated neurovascular injuries are likely to occur at this level and may compromise results.

Answer: **E**
Culp, Taras in Mackin, Callahan, Skirven, et al, p. 418

22. True or False: The retinacular portion of the flexor tendon sheath (characterized by fibrous bands called *pulleys*) is of greater importance to flexor tendon function than the synovial portion (which provides a low-friction gliding system) because of the mechanical stability it provides to the tendon.

The digital flexor sheath is a synovial-lined fibroosseous tunnel. This system functions to hold the flexor tendons in close opposition to the phalanges, ensuring efficient mechanical function in producing digital flexion. It comprises retinacular and synovial tissue components. The pulleys create a firm opposing surface for the avascular volar side of the tendon during flexion and appear to provide a pumping mechanism for diffusion of nutrients to the tendon. The retinacular portion is characterized by annular and cruciate pulleys that provide mechanical stability to the system. The synovial portion of the sheath provides not only a low-friction gliding system but also provides nutrition to the tendon. Both portions of the sheath are interrelated and equally important in flexor tendon function.

Answer: **False**
Culp, Taras in Mackin, Callahan, Skirven, et al, p. 416
Pettengill, van Strien in Mackin, Callahan, Skirven, et al, p. 438
Refer to Fig. 1-12

23. True or False: A core suture alone can withstand early active motion without gap formation or rupture.

Active motion puts forces on the repair site that are greater than a core suture can withstand alone. With the addition of a running epitenon suture (Fig. 15-7, *D*), the tensile strength of the repair is increased, and early active motion can be performed more safely. It is important to note that these data are generated from cadaver tendons and do not account for the decreased pullout strength of the tendon ends (which occurs 4 to 10 days after surgery), the effect of cyclic stress, gap formation, or the effect of tendon sheath dissection. Some authors indicate that a core suture with epitendinous repair is not able to tolerate full fisting and recommend modified fisting instead. Continued research is needed in this area to provide our patients with safe early active motion programs.

Answer: **False**
Hunter, Schneider, Mackin, p. 322
Refer to Fig. 15-7

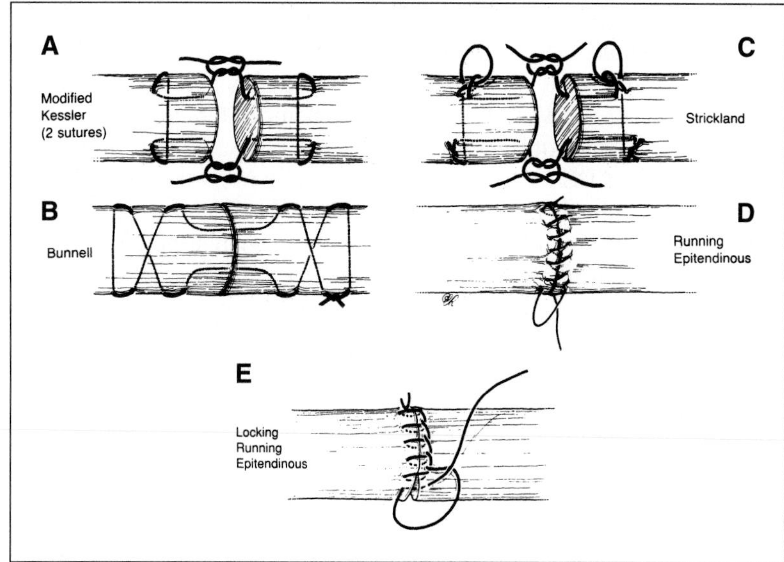

Fig. 15-7 ■ **A,** The modified Kessler; **B,** Bunnell; and **C,** Strickland techniques of core suture placement. Augmentation with a **D,** running, or **E,** locking running, epitendinous suture. (From Green DP, Hotchkiss R, Pederson WC: *Green's Operative hand surgery*, ed 4, New York, 1999, Churchill Livingstone.)

24. All but which of the following are true about suture techniques?

A. The strength of a tendon repair is roughly proportionate to the number of suture strands crossing the repair.
B. A six-strand repair is technically difficult for the physician.
C. A peripheral epitendinous suture reduces the tendency toward gap formation.
D. All of the above are true about suture techniques.

All of the above comments are applicable to suture techniques. The number of strands crossing the repair site is roughly proportional to the strength of the tendon repair; thus a two-strand repair is weaker than a four- or six-strand repair. Four- and six-strand repairs increase strength but add technical difficulty for the surgeon and increase the volume of suture material in the repair site. With horizontal mattress or running locked peripheral epitendinous sutures with four- and six-strand repairs, therapists enjoy the relative safety of both passive and light active digital motion during the entire healing process in an unswollen digit. A peripheral epitendinous suture repair assists in increasing repair strength and reduces the tendency toward gap formation at the repair site. The therapist must consult the surgeon regarding the type of repair used on the patient.

Answer: **D**

Hunter, Schneider, Mackin, p. 354
Strickland in Green, Hotchkiss, Pederson, p. 1860

25. Where is Camper's chiasm located?

A. Where the central slip inserts
B. Where the two FDS slips reunite
C. Where the FDP splits
D. Where the terminal tendon inserts

Camper's chiasm is where the two FDS slips reunite. This intersection of fibers is similar to the intersection of the neurofibers of the chiasm opticum of the second cranial nerve. The chiasma of Camper (also called the *chiasma tendinum of Camper* or *Camper's chiasm*) forms a plate beneath the flexor profundus and can be lifted off the periosteum and the capsule of the PIP joint.

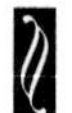

Answer: **B**

Hunter, Mackin, Callahan, p. 417
Pettengill, van Strien in Mackin, Callahan, Skirven, et al, p. 433
Hunter, Schneider, Mackin, pp. 245, 250
Spinner, p. 63
Refer to Fig. 15-8

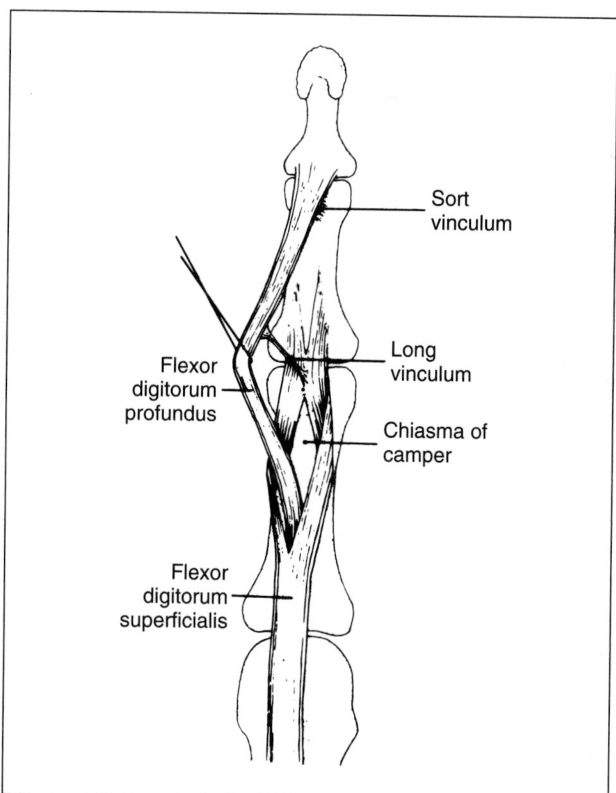

Fig. 15-8 ■ From Schneider LH: *Flexor tendon injuries,* Boston, 1985, Little Brown.

26. When does a tendon have the least tensile strength after it is surgically repaired?

A. 3 to 5 days
B. The first day
C. 10 to 14 days
D. 16 to 21 days

A tendon has the least tensile strength 3 to 5 days after surgical repair secondary to softening of the tendon ends. Its tensile strength is greater on the first day after repair. From days 5 to 21, tensile strength increases slowly as the collagen matures and cross-linking continues. Studies indicate that a decrease in tensile strength may not occur with early motion programs that allow for immediate controlled mobilization as early as 1 to 2 days after repair.

Answer: **A**
Strickland, 1989, pp. 30-41
Hunter, Mackin, Callahan, p. 438

27. The FDS in the small finger is absent in which percentage of the population?

A. 5%
B. 21%
C. 42%
D. 60%

The FDS of the small finger is variable and is absent in 21% of the population. It is important to note, however, that when the FDS and FDP are lacerated, it is necessary to repair both tendons. Advantages of repairing and maintaining both tendons include maintenance of the vincular blood supply, retention of a smooth gliding surface for the FDP, and the reduced possibility of hyperextension deformities at the PIP joint.

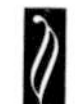

Answer: **B**
Hunter, Mackin, Callahan, pp. 420-421
Culp, Taras in Mackin, Callahan, Skirven, et al, p. 415

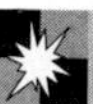

CLINICAL GEM:
Some authors report the FDS has a slip to the FDP and does not allow for independent FDS glide, and mimics the absence of the FDS tendon.

28. Which muscle is able to extend the IP joint of the thumb despite a rupture of the extensor pollicis longus?

A. The extensor pollicis brevis
B. The abductor pollicis longus
C. The abductor pollicis brevis
D. All of the above

Despite an extensor pollicis longus rupture, the IP joint can be extended by the intrinsic muscles through their contribution to the dorsal apparatus. The abductor pollicis brevis contributes to IP joint extension. The most disabling impairment after a rupture of the extensor pollicis longus is extension loss at the MCP joint. Retroposition, which is the ability to lift the thumb off the table into the extended position, also is lost.

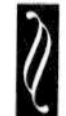

Answer: **C**
Hunter, Mackin, Callahan, p. 551
Rosenthal in Mackin, Callahan, Skirven, et al, pp. 528-529

29. A pullout suture using a button is a helpful procedure in which scenario?

A. When the distal FDP stump is extremely short after laceration
B. When both tendons are cut in zone II
C. When both slips of the FDS are cut and epitendinous repair is inappropriate
D. None of the above

When a patient sustains a laceration of the FDP and the distal stump is short or nonexistent, the tendon must be repaired to the distal phalanx. The suture is pulled through both the radial and ulnar aspects of the bone, exiting through the nail plate, and tied over the nail with a button (Fig. 15-9). The pullout suture and button are removed 4 to 6 weeks after repair. Rehabilitation with the button is the same as rehabilitation without the button for zone I tendon repairs.

Answer: **A**
Hunter, Mackin, Callahan, pp. 423-424
Culp, Taras in Mackin, Callahan, Skirven, et al, pp. 421-422
Mackin, Callahan, Skirven, et al, p. 443.

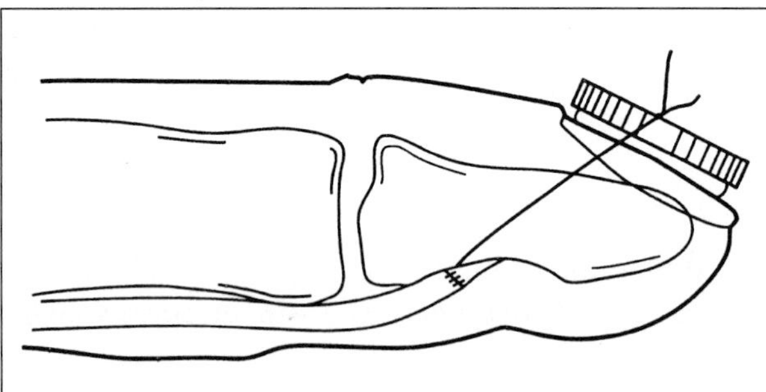

Fig. 15-9 ■ From Mackin EJ, Callahan AD, Skirven TM: *Rehabilitation of the hand and upper extremity*, ed 5, St Louis, 2002, Mosby.

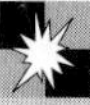

CLINICAL GEM:
Although a Kleinert program can be used with the application of the hook onto the button, it often is easier to use a Duran protocol for this repair. Evans has developed a specific protocol for repairs to zone I.

Mackin, Callahan, Skirven, et al, p. 443.

30. A 21-year-old lawn worker complains of an inability to flex his ring finger after his pull-start lawn mower backfired. Radiographs confirm an intraarticular fracture of the distal phalanx with rupture of the profundus insertion. The fragment involves less than 10% of the articular surface of the distal phalanx. Appropriate treatment would include which of the following?

A. Cast immobilization of the hand in a functional position
B. Dynamic flexion-assist splinting for 3 weeks to see whether the tendon heals in the appropriate position
C. Repair of the flexor tendon after excision of the fragment and Bunnell pullout-wire technique
D. All of the above

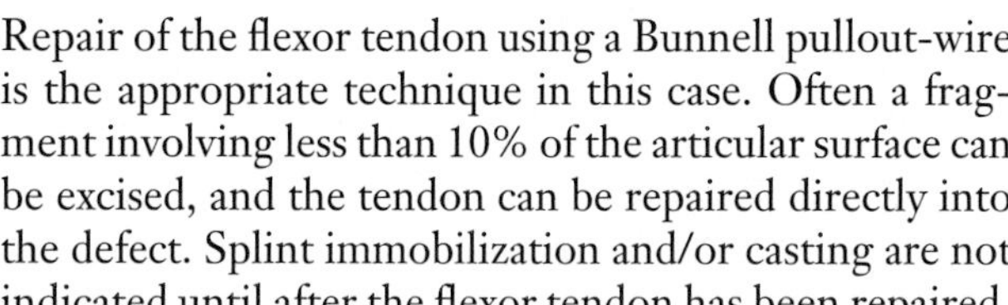

Repair of the flexor tendon using a Bunnell pullout-wire is the appropriate technique in this case. Often a fragment involving less than 10% of the articular surface can be excised, and the tendon can be repaired directly into the defect. Splint immobilization and/or casting are not indicated until after the flexor tendon has been repaired.

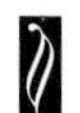

Answer: **C**
Schneider, pp. 277-285

31. Which protocol emphasizes controlled passive motion to treat flexor tendon injuries?

A. Kleinert
B. Duran
C. The Washington regime
D. McLean

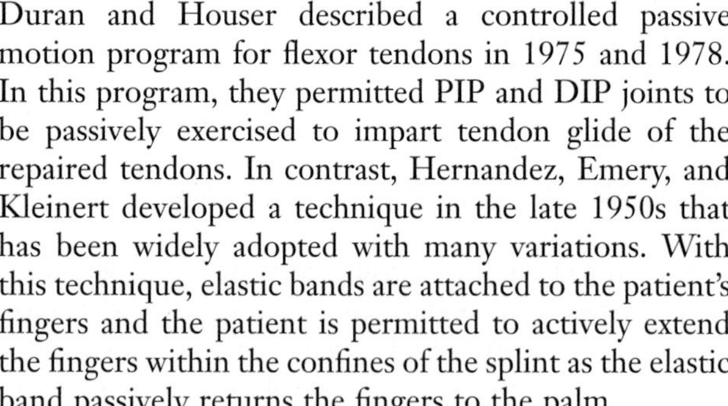

Duran and Houser described a controlled passive motion program for flexor tendons in 1975 and 1978. In this program, they permitted PIP and DIP joints to be passively exercised to impart tendon glide of the repaired tendons. In contrast, Hernandez, Emery, and Kleinert developed a technique in the late 1950s that has been widely adopted with many variations. With this technique, elastic bands are attached to the patient's fingers and the patient is permitted to actively extend the fingers within the confines of the splint as the elastic band passively returns the fingers to the palm.

Answer: **B**
Strickland, 1989, p. 71

32. True or False: Patients who "cheat" on their passive mobilization programs usually rupture their tendons.

Hand therapists often observe their patients "cheating" on their passive mobilization programs by actively flexing either during the passive exercises or inadvertently flexing between their exercise sessions. Contrary to our fears, many of these patients do exceptionally well. This reinforces the idea that light active flexor muscle contraction is beneficial.

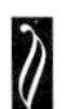

Answer: **False**

Hunter, Schneider, Mackin, p. 336
Evans in Mackin, Callahan, Skirven, et al, pp. 559-561

33. Your patient is a 30-year-old woman who had FDP repair in zone I of the middle finger. You note decreased tendon glide 7 weeks after surgery. You decide to teach home exercises to increase tendon glide. Which exercise provides the maximum profundus tendon excursion?

A. Straight fist
B. Full fist
C. Hook fist
D. All of the above provide equal profundus excursion.

The full-fist position provides maximum profundus tendon excursion. The straight-fist position provides maximum superficialis tendon excursion. The hook-fist position provides maximum differential gliding between the FDP and FDS tendons. Maximum tendon and joint motion can be obtained with tendon gliding exercises.

Answer: **B**

Wehbe, p. 164
Hunter, Mackin, Callahan, p. 443
Pettengill, van Strien in Mackin, Callahan, Skirven, et al, pp. 440-441
Refer to Fig. 15-2

34. Which of the following statements is false regarding the flexor pollicis longus (FPL) muscle?

A. It travels alone in its flexor sheath.
B. It has one vincula.
C. It has no associated lumbricals that originate on it.
D. It inserts on the base of the distal phalanx.
E. All of the above are true statements.

The anatomic differences between the FPL and the digital tendons and sheath have been described. The FPL spans only two digital joints and travels alone in its flexor sheath. These factors may explain improved results in FPL repair. The FPL has only one vincula and no associated lumbrical muscles.

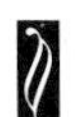

Answer: **E**

Culp, Taras in Mackin, Callahan, Skirven, et al, p. 424

35. True or False: Lacerations of the FPL in zones I and II are less likely to retract proximally into the palm compared with lacerations of the FDP to digits 2 to 5 in zones I and II.

The FDP of digits 2 to 5 has vascular supply from the vinculum brevis profundus and the vinculum longus profundus. The lumbrical muscles also originate on the FDP tendons at the palmar level. The checkrein effect of the vinculae and the lumbrical muscles typically prevents the tendon stump of the FDP from retracting into the palm. The FPL only has one vincula and no associated lumbrical muscles; therefore lacerations in zones I and II of the FPL are more likely to retract more proximally to the palm or wrist level.

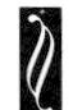

Answer: **False**

Culp, Taras in Mackin, Callahan, Skirven, et al, p. 424
Strickland in Green, Hotchkiss, Pederson, p. 1853
Boyer, Strickland, Engles, pp. 1685-1686

36. A 48-year-old female is referred to you in your acute care facility. She sustained a zone V flexor tendon injury from a laceration in a suicide attempt. She is being monitored in the psychiatric unit of your facility and is 3 days after flexor tendon repair. Which protocol would be most appropriate in this situation?

A. Modified Duran protocol with protective dorsal block splint
B. Kleinart protocol with traction to dynamically hold fingers in flexion
C. Immobilization cast for 3 to 4 weeks
D. Early active mobilization protocol

Early mobilization protocols are appropriate for alert, motivated patients who understand the exercise program and precautions. For patients younger than 10 years of age, those with cognitive deficits, and those who for any other reason are clearly unable or unwilling to participate in a complex rehabilitation program, immobilization is the treatment of choice. These patients will benefit from protection of the repair until adequate healing and adhesion formation has taken place.

Answer: **C**

Pettengill, van Strien in Mackin, Callahan, Skirven, et al, pp. 436, 439

37. Which of the following statements is false regarding the vincular system?

A. The vincula must be repaired if lacerated because they are the sole nutritional pathway for tendons.
B. The intact vincula can prevent tendons from retracting proximally.
C. The vincula are folds of mesotendon that carry blood supply to the tendons.
D. The vincula enter the tendons from the dorsal surface; therefore the optimal surgical technique is to place sutures on the volar surface of the tendon to preserve blood supply.
E. All are correct.

Investigators have shown that under certain conditions synovial fluid can provide the essential nutrition for tendon viability and the elements necessary for healing after tendon injury, even if detached from all blood supply. These studies demonstrated the role of synovial diffusion as an important pathway for tendon nutrition. A delicate balance between the two nutritional pathways (blood supply and synovial diffusion) is found within the tendon sheath. Therefore, repair of the vincula is not always necessary. The tendon can heal in the absence of the vincular system; however, its loss affects the nutritional balance, compromises tendon healing, and causes adhesion formation. When intact, vincula can prevent tendons from retracting proximally into the palm. Animal studies have shown a greater strength of repair with more dorsal placement of the core suture within the tendon stumps; however, its effect on the vascularity of the intrasynovial flexor tendon in humans is unknown.

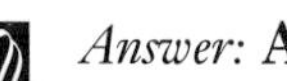

Answer: **A**

Culp, Taras in Mackin, Callahan, Skirven, et al, pp. 417, 421
Pettengill, van Strien in Mackin, Callahan, Skirven, et al, pp. 433–438
Boyer, Strickland, Engles, p. 1686
Strickland in Green, Hotchkiss, Pederson, p. 1853
Hunter, Schneider, Mackin, pp. 278-285
Refer to Fig. 15-6

38. In traditional management of an extensor tendon zone III acute closed injury (no surgery performed) the patient is treated with which of the following protocols?

A. Immobilization of the PIP joint at 0 degrees for 3 weeks
B. Immobilization of the PIP joint at 0 degrees for 6 weeks
C. Immobilization of the PIP joint slightly flexed to 10 degrees for 3 weeks
D. Immobilization of the PIP joint slightly flexed to 10 degrees for 6 weeks

Most authors recommend that traditional management of a zone III acute closed injury be managed with uninterrupted immobilization of the PIP joint at 0 degrees for 6 weeks. Injuries that require surgical repair are mobilized earlier—sometimes as early as 3 to 4 weeks—with protective splinting between exercise sessions. It is crucial for the splint to be positioned with the PIP joint at absolute 0 degrees to avoid gapping of the tendon in an elongated position.

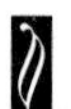

Answer: **B**

Hunter, Mackin, Callahan, pp. 576-579
Evans in Mackin, Callahan, Skirven, et al, p. 552

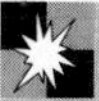

CLINICAL GEM:
The long finger is the most commonly injured extensor tendon, and zone V1—directly over the metacarpals—is the most commonly injured zone.

39. True or False: One method of treating a central slip extensor tendon surgical repair (zone III) is to begin early PIP joint motion within 1 week.

Thomes and Thomes advocate an early motion protocol using a hand-based dynamic extension splint with a lumbrical stop for central slip tendon repairs. The splint positions the MCP joint at 20 degrees of flexion with the PIP joint at neutral to slight hyperextension. Evans advocates short arc motion using template splints for PIP and DIP joint exercise sessions and resting the PIP and DIP joints at absolute 0 degrees between exercising.

In general, both protocols allow for 30 degrees of PIP joint flexion during the first 2 weeks, with a progression of 10 degrees for each following week, providing that no extensor lag develops. Some authors advocate no ROM restrictions at the PIP joint as early as week 4; others advocate some degree of caution until week 6.

Answer: **True**

Thomes, Thomes, p. 195
Hunter, Mackin, Callahan, p. 383
Evans in Mackin, Callahan, Skirven, et al, pp. 559-560

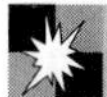

CLINICAL GEM:
If choosing the dynamic splint protocol, you may consider fabricating an additional finger gutter splint that fits under the sling to ensure proper positioning and avoid gapping.

40. What is the recommended wrist position for initiation of PIP joint active motion in Evan's immediate active short arc motion (SAM) protocol?

A. 40 to 50 degrees of flexion
B. 20 to 30 degrees of flexion
C. 40 to 50 degrees of extension
D. 20 to 30 degrees of extension
E. Wrist position does not matter

The movements of wrist flexion and finger extension are synergistic; finger extension is effectively increased as the wrist flexes. The position of wrist flexion reduces the passive tension of the digital extrinsic flexors; therefore the force required of the extensor communis to extend the digital joints is reduced. The action of the interossei muscles with the wrist flexed may further reduce the work requirement of the digital extensor mechanism in active extension of the IP joints. Based on these anatomical considerations, the SAM protocol is 30 degrees of wrist flexion during PIP joint exercise. This position reduces flexor resistance, facilitates interossei function to extend the PIP joint, and thus reduces the work requirement of the extensor digitorum communis (EDC) with active extension of the PIP joint.

Answer: **B**
Evans in Mackin, Callahan, Skirven, et al, p. 559-560
Refer to Fig. 15-10

41. True or False: Immediate active SAM protocol is the most traditionally and widely accepted method of treating postoperative repairs of the central slip.

Both SAM and immobilization protocols are used with success in zone III extensor tendon repairs. The use of immediate active motion is not a new or traditional technique. A number of variables need to be taken into account when considering the application of early mobilization. Physician preference, strength of the repair, quality of the tendon, and compliance issues with the patient are crucial to assess, in addition to experience of the therapist when choosing between the two treatment protocols. Several studies have shown that complicated and uncomplicated open central slip repairs can be treated postoperatively with 3 weeks of immobilization followed by 3 weeks of controlled flexion with good results. The immobilization protocol is easier to use, less expensive, and may be preferable for a patient population with compliance issues.

Answer: **False**
Pratt, Burr, Grobbleaar, p. 533
Evans, Thompson, p. 266

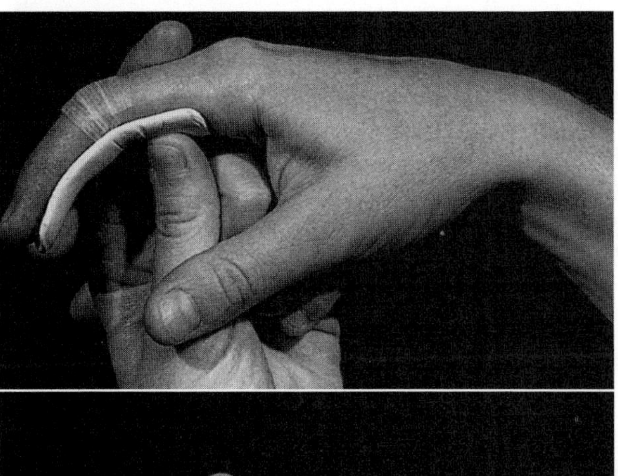

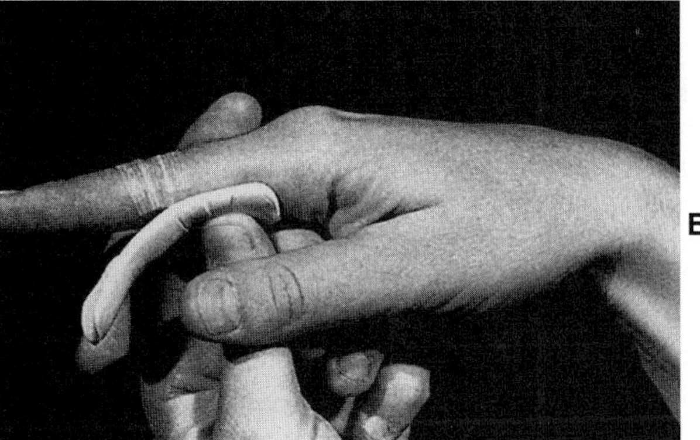

Fig. 15-10 ■ **A** and **B**, Template splint 1 allows 30 degrees at the PIP joint and 20 to 25 degrees at the DIP joint, thus preventing the patient from stretching the repair site by allowing only the precalculated excursion of the central slip. The wrist is positioned in 30 degrees of flexion; the digit is supported at the proximal phalanx by the contralateral hand; and the PIP joint is actively flexed and extended in a controlled ROM. (From Evans RB: Early active short arc motion for the repaired central slip, *J Hand Surg* [Am] 19(6):992, 1994.)

42. True or False: DIP joint flexion exercises can be advocated within the first week after a central slip extensor tendon surgical repair.

DIP joint flexion exercises, with the PIP joint at absolute zero, are advocated within the first week unless the lateral bands are involved. If the lateral bands are involved, DIP joint flexion is delayed until approximately the fourth week after surgery.

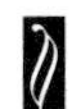

Answer: **True**
Maddy, Meyerdierks, p. 207
Hunter, Mackin, Callahan, p. 578
Evans in Mackin, Callahan, Skirven, et al, p. 555

CLINICAL GEM:
If the lateral bands were repaired, flexion of the DIP joint should be limited to 30 degrees of unrestrained motion for 3 to 4 weeks after surgery.

43. You are treating a patient with an extensor tendon repair to the ring finger in zone VI, just distal to the extensor retinaculum. Which of the following would be an appropriate splint?

A. Forearm-based splint, with wrist in extension, including the ring finger only
B. Hand-based splint extending the ring finger only
C. Forearm-based splint, with wrist in extension, including the middle, ring, and little fingers
D. Forearm-based splint, with wrist in slight flexion, including the middle, ring, and little fingers

A zone VI repair just distal to the extensor retinaculum requires a forearm-based splint with the wrist in 30 to 40 degrees of extension and the middle, ring, and little fingers extended. Many static and dynamic splinting protocols vary the degrees of wrist and digit extension. It is important to consider the juncturae tendinum, which are interconnections between the extensor communis on the dorsum of the hand. If the repair is proximal to the juncturae tendinum (Fig. 15-11), as in this situation, it is necessary to splint the affected and adjacent digits in extension to eliminate stress on the repair site. If the repair is distal to the juncturae tendinum, only the affected digit must be splinted, and the adjacent fingers can be splinted with the MCP joints at 30 degrees of flexion and the IP joints free. This position reduces stress at the repair site as it permits advancement of the proximal end of the severed tendon.

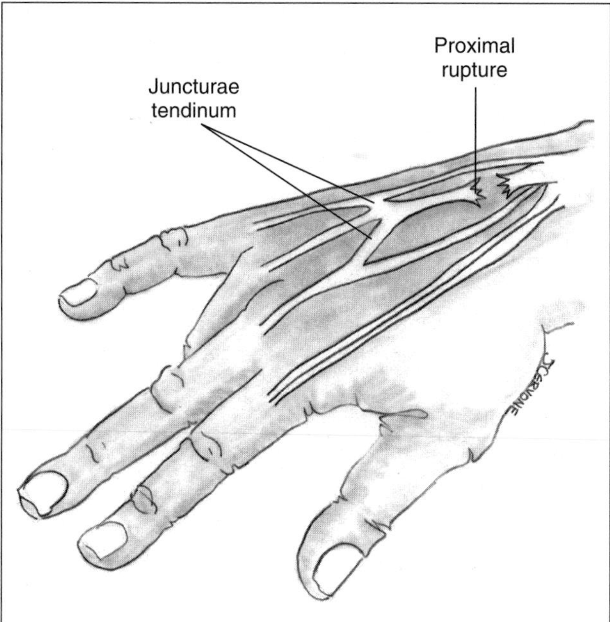

Fig. 15-11

Answer: **C**
Thomas, Moutet, Guinard, p. 310
Hunter, Mackin, Callahan, p. 588
Evans in Mackin, Callahan, Skirven, et al, pp. 563-564

44. A patient you have been treating status post flexor tendon repair is preparing for another surgery. This patient has an extensive amount of scar tissue, and an obvious loss of the pulley system as indicated by bowstringing. Which surgical procedure is most likely indicated for this patient?

A. Tenolysis
B. Reconstruction of the pulleys
C. Placement of a silicone tendon implant with reconstruction of the pulleys
D. Surgery is not a good option for this patient.

Placement of a silicone tendon implant would be a preparatory stage to allow for the formation of a favorable bed for tendon grafting. This procedure, which is a two-stage reconstruction, is indicated when the patient's original trauma was from a crushing injury and is characterized by an underlying fracture or overlying skin damage, when a patient displays excessive scarring of the tendon bed, when previous surgery has failed, when complications from a healed infection occur, and when there is significant loss of the pulley system.

In 1965, Hunter first published his personal experience with the tendon implant. In stage one, the silicone implant is placed in the hand and the pulley system is reconstructed. The implant is left in place for 3 months to allow a new bed to form. In stage two, the implant is removed, and a long tendon graft is placed in the newly formed sheath. This procedure is demanding and requires the postoperative care of a skilled hand therapist.

Answer: **C**
Hunter, Schneider, Mackin, pp. 518-521

45. True or False: The use of immediate active motion is a new technique that is widely accepted in clinical practice.

The use of immediate active motion is not a new or widely accepted technique. It is, however, a subject of renewed interest. Stronger suture techniques that are designed for active motion have now been developed. Early active motion with current popular suture techniques has not been recommended because most clinicians believe that these repairs do not provide enough tensile strength (with adequate safety margins) to tolerate the forces of full active motion.

Answer: **False**

Evans, Thompson, p. 266

46. A 6-year-old patient is referred to you for splinting 3 days after surgery for flexor tendon repair. Which of the following protocols would be most appropriate in this situation?

A. Immobilization splinting for 3 to 4 weeks
B. Kleinert protocol with traction to the fingers
C. Duran protocol with protected dorsal blocking splint
D. Early active motion protocol

As mentioned previously, immobilization protocols are the treatment of choice for patients younger than 10 years of age, patients with cognitive deficits, or patients who for any other reason are clearly unable or unwilling to participate in a rehabilitation program. Often the patient is casted for 3 to 4 weeks postoperatively. He or she may, however, be referred for an early dorsal blocking-type splint with complete immobilization. When the splint is applied, it should be a dorsal forearm-based splint with the wrist in 10 to 30 degrees of flexion, MCP joints at 40 to 60 degrees, and IP joints in full extension. At 3 to 4 weeks, the splint is modified to bring the wrist to a neutral position and the patient exercises in the splint hourly. At 4 to 6 weeks, the dorsal blocking splint is discontinued, and gentle blocking exercises and isolated gliding exercises are initiated.

Answer: **A**

Hunter, Mackin, Callahan, pp. 442-443
Pettengill, van Strien in Mackin, Callahan, Skirven, et al, pp. 439-442

47. The finger and wrist positions recommended by Evans while performing the early active motion "place and hold" component for repaired flexor tendons in zone I or II are which of the following?

A. Wrist in slight flexion, MCP joints at 70 degrees of flexion, PIP joints at 60 degrees of flexion, and DIP joints at 30 degrees of flexion
B. Wrist at 20 degrees of extension, with MCP joints at 83 degrees of flexion, PIP joints at 75 degrees of flexion, and DIP joints at 40 degrees of flexion
C. Wrist flexed 20 degrees with MCP joints at 80 degrees of flexion, PIP joints at 75 degrees of flexion, and DIP joints at 40 degrees of flexion
D. Wrist at 10 degrees of extension, with MCP joints at 43 degrees of flexion, PIP joints at 40 degrees of flexion, and DIP joints at 80 degrees of flexion

The position Evans recommends for the early active "place and hold" technique for zone I and II flexor tendon repairs using the MAMTT or SAM is wrist at 20 degrees of extension, MCP joints at 83 degrees of flexion, PIP joints at 75 degrees of flexion, and DIP joints at 40 degrees of flexion (Fig. 15-12, *A*). The therapist places the fingers and the wrist in the SAM position, and the patient is asked to gently maintain the placed position with minimal tension. The therapist can measure the tension with a force gauge (Fig. 15-12, *B*). A force of 15 to 20 g allows the force application tension to be reliable and repeatable, minimizing the risk of rupture using a standard two-strand with epitendinal suture (modified Kessler) technique. This protocol must be initiated within 24 to 48 hours postoperatively because presumably it is safer to move a tendon at this time than at day 5 or 10, when adhesions have formed.

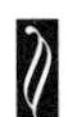

Answer: **B**

Evans, Thompson, pp. 275-277
Hunter, Schneider, Mackin, pp. 337, 362-391
Pettengill, van Strien in Mackin, Callahan, Skirven, et al, pp. 451-453

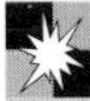

CLINICAL GEM:
The therapist must take a patient's edema into consideration. Edema can increase the force at the repair site with active motion. Therefore the therapist should carefully evaluate a patient's edema before initiating the SAM program. If edema is present, a modified position that requires less flexion at the MCP, PIP, and DIP joints is indicated.

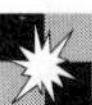

CLINICAL GEM:
Remember to always communicate with the hand surgeon about tendon repair techniques. It is essential to know how many strands cross the repair site and if an epitenon suture was used.

A

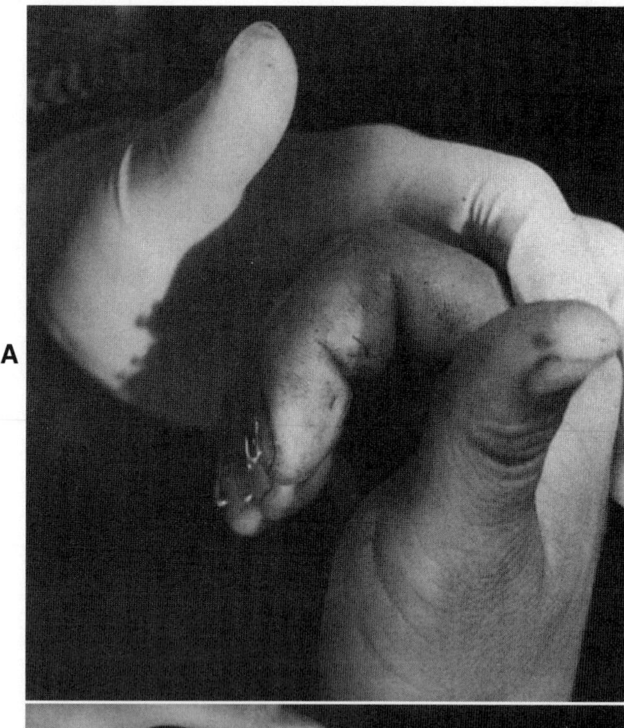

B

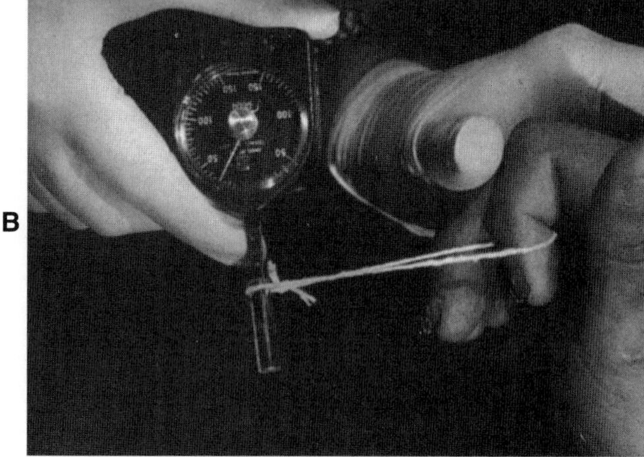

Fig. 15-12 ■ **A,** According to the MAMTT protocol, the active hold positions the digits in moderate flexion (MCP joint 83 degrees, PIP joint 75 degrees, DIP joint 40 degrees). **B,** Tension is limited to 50 g of force, which is measured with the Haldex gauge. (From Evans RB, Thompson DE: The application of force to the healing tendon, *J Hand Ther* 6:276, 1993.)

48. A patient is referred to you for treatment of extensor tendon subluxation of the ring finger. During the evaluation, you notice that the patient is able to hold the involved finger in the fully extended position only when it is placed there. When starting from the fisted position, the patient is unable to achieve full extension of the involved digit. The extensor lag with active extension is approximately 35 degrees. Which structure might be involved?

A. Extensor digitorum communis
B. Transverse retinacular ligament
C. Sagittal band
D. Central tendon

This patient is unable to extend the MCP joint actively; however, the patient is able to sustain active MCP extension, which indicates that the extensor tendon is intact. The structure that is damaged in this case is most likely the sagittal band because the patient is able to hold the digit in the fully extended position once the tendon is relocated over the MCP joint. Rupture is most often of the radial sagittal band and is common in the long finger where the extrinsic extensor tendon may dislodge from its weak attachment to the underlying sagittal fibers. The result is an ulnar displacement of the extensor tendon. Conservative, nonoperative treatment includes splinting of the wrist with the MCP joints in neutral for 4 weeks; often this is successful for an acute injury. However, surgery is indicated with complete rupture of the sagittal band and for chronic, recurrent cases (see Fig. 2-14 and Question 19 in Chapter 2).

Answer: **C**
Hunter, Mackin, Callahan, p. 531
Rosenthal in Mackin, Callahan, Skirven, et al, p. 507

49. True or False: Loss of independent index finger extension is highly probable if the extensor indicis proprius tendon is used for tendon transfer to the thumb.

Independent index finger extension was noted by Moore and colleagues in 20 of 27 patients after extensor indicis transfer. They suggested that the reason for the presence of independent action after the transfer was that the EDC in all cases had four distinct muscle bellies with separate and distinct innervation from the posterior interosseous nerve and that the juncture tendinum between the index and long fingers was filamentous and poorly developed in comparison with the more ulnar digits, which had well-developed and thick juncturae that limited independent extension.

Answer: **False**
Doyle in Green, Hotchkiss, Pederson, p. 1951

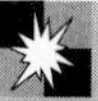

CLINICAL GEM:
The EDC tendon to the little finger is absent in approximately 50% of people. It is often replaced by a juncture tendinum from the ring finger.

50. After surgical repair, an early active mobilization protocol is not generally accepted practice for which of the following extensor tendon zones?

A. Zone I
B. Zone III
C. Zone IV
D. Zone VII
E. None of the above

Dynamic splinting and early active motion for extensor tendon injuries have been demonstrated to be useful for the postoperative management of both complex and simple extensor tendon injuries in zones V to VIII. This usefulness has been extended to zones III to IV. At this time, zone I and II injuries are best treated by static means.

Dynamic splinting is most likely to yield a good result in a cooperative patient under the supervision of an experienced hand therapist. The postoperative rehabilitation technique must be selected with care to match the needs of the patient and include the factors of age, general health and healing potential, and motivation of the patient in the decision-making process. Therapist expertise, surgical technique, timing of the repair, and initiation of therapy intervention are important considerations.

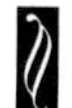

Answer: **A**

Doyle in Green, Hotchkiss, Pederson, p. 1961
Pettengill, van Strien in Mackin, Callahan, Skirven, et al, pp. 436-438
Evans in Mackin, Callahan, Skirven, et al, pp. 562, 575

51. True or False: A complex extensor tendon injury that includes concomitant crush or soft tissue is better treated with an immobilization protocol to reduce complications in healing associated with increased fibroblastic response.

Total immobilization should not be considered with extensor tendon injury associated with crush injury where the paratenon is extensively involved, with injury to the periosteum or adjacent soft tissues, or in hands with osteoarthritic or rheumatoid joints. The more complex injury can be expected to have more complications associated with increased fibroblastic response, and immobilization of the complex injury will add to those complications.

Answer: **False**

Evans in Mackin, Callahan, Skirven, et al, pp. 552, 562-563

52. You are treating a patient referred for evaluation and treatment after a football injury that resulted from grabbing his opponent's shirt. While evaluating the patient, you notice he is unable to bend the DIP joint of his ring finger. The appropriate treatment plan for this patient is which of the following?

A. Electrical stimulation to facilitate tendon glide of the scarred FDP tendon
B. Ultrasound of the tendon to improve flexor glide
C. A strengthening regime
D. Referral to a hand surgeon for Jersey finger repair
E. None of the above

A Jersey finger occurs in high-velocity injuries such as those that involve grabbing an opponent's shirt in rugby or football. The distal phalanx of the finger is passively hyperextended while the other fingers remain flexed. Therapy treatment for this patient would not be indicated because the flexor tendon is not intact. Surgical intervention should be considered.

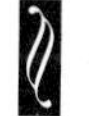

Answer: **D**

Tubiana, Thomine, Mackin, p. 217

53. A 35-year-old office worker sustained a laceration over the palmar aspect of her ring finger at the middle phalanx. She initially was treated with sutures in the emergency room and was told that no underlying structural damage to the hand had occurred and that she should follow up with her primary care doctor for suture removal. Four weeks after the injury, the patient was referred to hand therapy because of decreased strength. She complained to the hand therapist that her grip is weak and that it was hard for her to fully extend her MCP joint. The therapist noted that the patient was unable to flex her DIP joint. The patient was then referred to a hand surgeon. Which procedure would the hand surgeon most likely plan?

A. Long finger FDS transfer to ring finger FDP with lumbrical release
B. FDP tendon repair using modified Kessler technique
C. DIP fusion
D. FDP tendon repair using modified Kessler technique with lumbrical release
E. FDP tendon repair with DIP joint fusion

FDP tendons lacerated proximal to the insertion of or through the long vincula can retract all the way into the wrist. In this case, the patient likely experienced weakness and difficulty with MCP joint extension because of lumbrical tightness secondary to proximal FDP migration. Two and a half weeks after such an injury, the muscle is fibrosed and attempts to repair the severed tendon ends would likely result in quadrigia. In this situation, the lumbrical-plus deformity can be corrected with a lumbrical release and the FDP can be easily reconstructed with a transfer of the FDS from an adjacent finger. DIP fusion can be considered in cases of missed FDP laceration when prolonged rehabilitation should be avoided (e.g., for manual laborers or elderly patients).

Answer: **A**
Green, pp. 1853-1868

54. You are treating a patient with an extensor pollicis longus tendon repair in zone V. How much flexion is desired at the IP joint to produce a 5-mm passive glide of the extensor pollicis longus?

A. 20 degrees
B. 40 degrees
C. 60 degrees
D. 80 degrees

During treatment of an extensor pollicis longus repair in zone IV or V with a dynamic splinting protocol, the wrist is splinted in extension with the carpometacarpal joint in neutral, the MCP joint at 0, and the IP joint at 0 with dynamic extension (Fig. 15-13, *A*). The distal joint is actively flexed to 60 degrees to produce a 5-mm passive glide at the extensor pollicis longus tendon (Fig. 15-13, *B*). The traction then returns the distal phalanx to the resting position at 0.

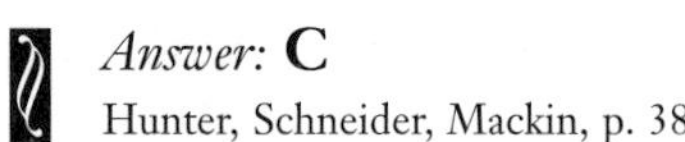

Answer: **C**
Hunter, Schneider, Mackin, p. 388

55. In which flexor zone should the wrist be splinted in neutral?

A. Zone I
B. Zone II
C. Zone III
D. Zone IV
E. Zone V

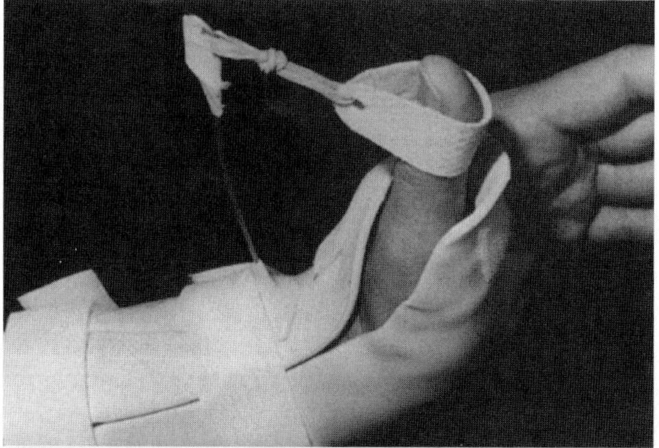

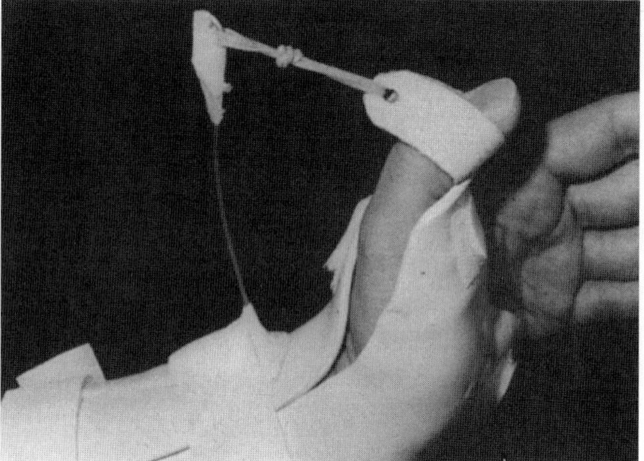

Fig. 15-13 ■ **A** and **B** from Evans RB, Burkhalter WE: A study of the dynamic anatomy of extensor tendons and implications for treatment, *J Hand Surg* (Am) 11(5):777, 1986.

After surgical repair of a flexor tendon in zone IV, the wrist should be splinted at a near neutral position with the MCP joints at 70 degrees of flexion. If the wrist is splinted in flexion, bowstringing can occur. If the wrist is splinted in extension, rupture may occur (see Fig. 15-1).

Answer: **D**
Hunter, Mackin, Callahan, p. 424
Culp, Taras in Mackin, Callahan, Skirven, et al, p. 424

56. True or False: It is important to always include all fingers in dynamic traction when treating flexor tendon injuries with a Kleinert-type protocol.

Several theories about including or not including all the fingers in dynamic traction exist. Some therapists propose keeping all of the fingers in traction with FDS repairs because passive flexion is easier to obtain and because inadvertent flexion of adjacent fingers is avoided. Other therapists hope that by leaving the adjacent, uninvolved fingers free the patient is more likely to have uninvolved finger flexion, allowing him or her to "cheat" in a helpful fashion. A choice of one protocol over another depends on the surgeon's preference as well as the therapist's comfort level with treating the diagnosis.

Answer: **False**

Hunter, Mackin, Callahan, p. 455
Pettengill, van Strien in Mackin, Callahan, Skirven, et al, p. 446

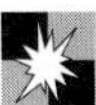

CLINICAL GEM:
The FDS tendons usually arise from individual muscle bellies and act independently, whereas the FDP tendons usually have a common muscle origin and produce simultaneous flexion of multiple digits. This may affect treatment of flexor tendon repairs in that all digits should be included in the dorsal block splint when an FDP tendon is repaired. If an isolated FDS is repaired, it may be safe to eliminate certain fingers from the dorsal block splint.

57. A patient is referred to you 3 days after extensor tendon repair in zone VI. Orders are to evaluate, treat, and splint. Which of the following protocols is best suited for this patient?

A. Treatment by immobilization with the wrist at 40 to 45 degrees of extension, with 0 to 20 degrees of MCP joint flexion and 0 degrees of IP joint flexion
B. Dynamic splint with wrist at approximately 40 to 45 degrees of extension, with the MCP and IP joints resting at 0 degrees in the slings
C. Same splint as in answer B with the application of immediate, MAMTT, as described by Evans
D. All of the above are appropriate protocols.

All of the above are possible protocols for treatment of this zone. The protocol used in your facility will depend on the physician's order, therapist's experience, suture techniques, and various other factors. Each protocol has pros and cons. The therapist must understand each protocol thoroughly before it is applied and understand which protocol may be most beneficial for each patient.

Answer: **D**

Hunter, Mackin, Callahan, pp. 590-596
Evans in Mackin, Callahan, Skirven, et al, pp. 562-570

58. You are treating a football player who 4 weeks ago sustained a closed zone III extensor tendon injury that resulted in a boutonnière deformity. He has been casted with his PIP joint in extension for the past 3 weeks, and he has been performing DIP joint active and passive flexion exercises hourly throughout the day. Which statement is true regarding progression of the immobilization protocol at zone III?

A. Schedule this patient for an appointment in 1 week to begin active movement of the PIP joint.
B. When active motion is initiated, encourage the patient to push PIP joint ROM through as much flexion as he can tolerate.
C. When active motion is initiated, extension splinting is completely discontinued.
D. When active motion is initiated, exercise should emphasize PIP joint extension with no more than 30 degrees of flexion.

Closed zone III extensor tendon injuries (central slip disruptions) are traditionally treated with uninterrupted immobilization of the PIP joint at 0 degrees of extension for 6 weeks. Therefore, beginning active motion of the PIP joint should be delayed, for the above patient, for 3 additional weeks. It is crucial that full PIP joint extension is achieved and maintained in the splint or cast; if not, the tendon may heal in the elongated position, resulting in potential extension lag at that joint. PIP joint flexion exercises should be initiated with caution. ROM should emphasize active PIP joint extension with flexion of the PIP joint to no more than 30 degrees. If no extension lag develops, motion can progress to 40 to 50 degrees in the second week. Forceful flexion exercises are not appropriate and development of an extension lag should be addressed with increased extension splinting and decreased increments of flexion.

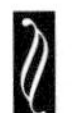

Answer: **D**

Evans in Mackin, Callahan, Skirven, et al, p. 552

59. You are seeing a 32-year-old office manager who cut the dorsum of her left hand while opening a box with a knife. She underwent zone V extensor tendon repair 3 days ago, and orders are to begin treatment following an early passive motion protocol. How will you proceed with treatment?

A. Fabricate a dorsal forearm-based dynamic extension splint with the wrist in 40 degrees of extension and the MCP joints in dynamic traction at 0 degrees of extension; instruct the patient to actively flex the digits at the MCP joints only and then to relax the digits, allowing the extensor outrigger to return the digits to 0 degrees.
B. Fabricate a volar forearm-based static splint with the wrist in 40 degrees of extension and the MCP joints in 0 to 20 degrees of flexion; instruct the patient to actively flex and extend the IP joints through full ROM while wearing the splint.
C. Fabricate a dorsal forearm-based dynamic extension splint with the wrist in 40 degrees of extension and the MCP joints in dynamic traction at 0 degrees of extension; instruct the patient in an "active hold" of the digital extensors with the hand passively placed by the therapist in 20 degrees of wrist flexion and all digital joints at 0 degrees of extension.
D. Fabricate a volar forearm-based static splint with the wrist in 30 degrees of extension and the MCP joints in 45 degrees of flexion; instruct the patient to actively flex and extend the MCP and IP joints synchronously; limit MCP joint flexion to 45 degrees (imposed by the splint) and MCP joint extension to 0 degrees.

All of the above are valid descriptions of various protocols used for zone V extensor tendon injuries. Answer A is a description of an early passive motion protocol, which allows active flexion of the MCP joints but *passive* digital extension. Answer B is a description of an immobilization protocol. Answer C is a description of an immediate active tension protocol. Answer D is a description of a controlled active mobilization protocol. The actual protocol used in your facility will depend on the tensile strength of the repair technique, physician preference, therapist experience, and your assessment of the patient's compliance level.

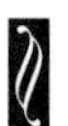
Answer: **A**
Evans in Mackin, Callahan, Skirven, et al, pp. 543, 562-570
Khandwala, Webb, Harris, p. 141

60. When is the earliest that a tenolysis should be considered after flexor tendon repair?

A. 6 weeks
B. 12 weeks
C. 24 weeks
D. 36 weeks

The proper timing for tenolysis after tendon repair is controversial. Studies on chicken tendons conclude that waiting a minimum of 12 weeks is optimum for the procedure. Other authors recommend waiting as long as 6 to 9 months after tendon repair. Most important to consider are the prerequisites for tenolysis. All fractures should be healed; wounds should have reached tissue equilibrium with soft and pliable skin; joint contractures must be overcome; near normal passive ROM must be achieved; and satisfactory sensation must be present. Another important factor is that a tenolysis must be performed on an extremely compliant patient who understands what is involved in the surgery and what is expected of him or her in rehabilitation.

Answer: **B**
Hunter, Schneider, Mackin, pp. 443-444
Evans in Mackin, Callahan, Skirven, et al, p. 457
Schneider in Green, Hotchkiss, Pederson, p. 1922

CLINICAL GEM:
It is important to consult with the surgeon regarding tendon integrity after tenolysis before initiating therapy. If the tendon is frayed, a frayed tendon protocol must be initiated.

61. True or False: The extensor indicis proprius and extensor digiti minimi tendons usually run on the ulnar side of the extensor digitorum communis tendon.

The extensor digitorum communis and the two independent extensor tendons pass underneath the extensor retinaculum on the back of the wrist. Both the extensor indicis and the extensor digiti minimi have independent muscles that allow independent function of the second and fifth digits, respectively. Both tendons run on the ulnar side of the extensor digitorum communis tendon.

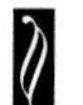
Answer: **True**
Hunter, Schneider, Mackin, p. 547

62. You are treating a patient after flexor tendon repair in zone II. At 3 weeks, active ROM is assessed. The patient is able to actively complete a fist. How should the program progress?

A. Continue splinting
B. Discontinue splinting and begin an active ROM program
C. Begin blocking exercises to further increase tendon glide
D. Initiate strengthening program because the patient has full ROM

A patient who demonstrates full active motion as early as week 3 has little to no adhesions limiting tendon glide and is at an increased risk for rupture. The patient should be further protected with splinting. Active ROM can be performed in the clinic under the supervision of a skilled hand therapist.

In contrast, if the patient exhibits little to no tendon glide at 3 weeks after surgery, a more aggressive program should be initiated. The heavily scarred patient may be able to start active or resistive exercises earlier under the close supervision of a skilled hand therapist. Protocols are helpful for an inexperienced therapist, but with time a therapist must make such judgments without relying on protocols to optimize treatment.

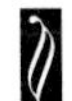

Answer: **A**

Hunter, Mackin, Callahan, p. 455
Schneider, Feldscher in Mackin, Callahan, Skirven, et al, p. 457

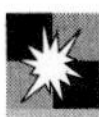

CLINICAL GEM:
In general, the more adherent a tendon, the safer it is to apply resistance to movement. This greater resistance applied to the flexors will elicit a strong muscle contraction, thus facilitating elongation of adhesions and improving flexor tendon glide. Caution must be taken, however, because excessive resistance may rupture the tendon.

63. Which early active program uses a tenodesis splint?

A. Strickland/Cannon
B. Silverskiold and May
C. Evans and Thompson
D. All of the above

All of the above programs use early active motion. The Strickland/Cannon program used at the Indiana hand center uses the tenodesis splint to allow the patient to exercise in a protected range.

Answer: **A**

Pettengill, van Strien in Mackin, Callahan, Skirven, et al, pp. 450-452
Refer to Fig. 15-14

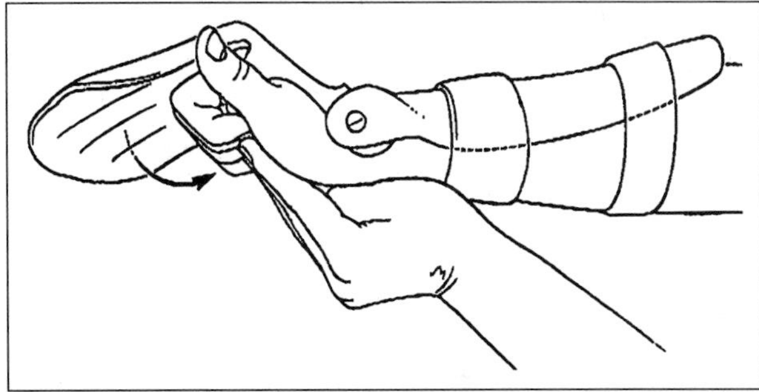

Fig. 15-14 ■ From Cannon NM: Post flexor tendon repair motion protocol, *Indiana Hand Center Newslett* 1:13-18, 1993.

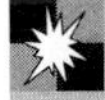

CLINICAL GEM:
Visit www.liveconferences.com to learn how to make a dorsal blocking hinge splint.

Chapter 16

Biomechanics and Tendon Transfers

1. When selecting a donor tendon for transfer, the hand surgeon is concerned with which of the following?

A. Strength
B. Amplitude of excursion
C. Direction of pull
D. Expendability
E. All of the above

The selection of donor tendons is based on several principles of tendon transfer. First, the tendon chosen for transfer must be strong enough to perform its new function in an altered position. The work capacity of different forearm muscles has been defined in the literature, and "classic" tendon transfers are based on these data. For a tendon transfer to provide full range of motion (ROM), the amplitude of tendon excursion must be adequate. Roughly, wrist extensors and flexors move about 33 mm; finger extensors and the extensor pollicis longus (EPL) move about 50 mm; and finger flexors move about 70 mm. Ideally, the most efficient tendon transfer is one that passes from a direct line from its own origin to the insertion of the tendon being substituted. Finally, sacrifice of the donor tendon should not result in functional deficit. Other muscles should exist that perform the same basic function as the donated muscle.

Answer: **E**
Curtis, pp. 231-242
Hunter, Schneider, Mackin, pp. 419-424

2. Match each of Newton's laws with the appropriate description.

Law

1. First law
2. Second law
3. Third law

Description

A. A body at rest tends to remain at rest; a body in motion will remain in such motion at a constant velocity unless acted on by an external force.
B. To every action there is always an equal reaction, and the forces of action and reaction between interacting bodies are of equal magnitude, opposite in direction, and have the same line of action.
C. A body with a force acting on it will accelerate in the direction of that force, and the magnitude of the acceleration will be proportional to the magnitude of the net force.

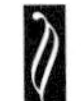
Answers: **1, A; 2, C; 3, B**
Ozkaya, Nordin, pp. 6-7

3. Match each of the following terms with the appropriate description.

Terms

1. Force
2. Moment
3. Velocity
4. Acceleration

Description

A. Action of one body against another
B. Time rate of increase of velocity
C. Time rate of change in position
D. Rotational, bending, or twisting action of one body on another

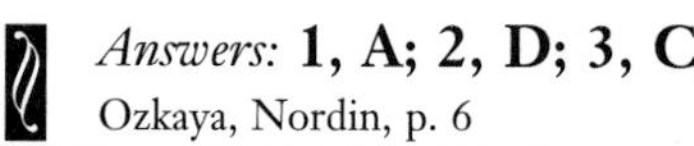

Answers: **1, A; 2, D; 3, C; 4, B**
Ozkaya, Nordin, p. 6

4. In a patient with an irreparable radial nerve palsy, which of the following functions has been lost and needs to be restored by tendon transfer?

A. Wrist extension
B. Finger (metacarpophalangeal [MCP] joint) extension
C. Thumb extension
D. All of the above

The primary extensors of the wrist are the extensor carpi radialis longus (ECRL), the extensor carpi radialis brevis (ECRB), and the extensor carpi ulnaris (ECU) muscles. The primary extender of the finger MCP joints is the extensor digitorum communis (EDC) muscle. The extensor indicis proprius (EIP) provides independent MCP extension to the index finger, and the extensor digiti minimi (EDM) provides MCP extension to the little finger. The EPL is the sole extensor of the thumb interphalangeal (IP) joint. Both the extensor pollicis brevis (EPB) and the EPL help to extend the MCP joint of the thumb. The ECRL and the ECRB are innervated by the radial nerve, whereas the remaining wrist and digital extensors are innervated by the posterior interosseous nerve (PIN), a branch of the radial nerve. Because all the muscles mentioned above are innervated by the radial nerve or a branch of the radial nerve, an irreparable injury to the radial nerve results in loss of all the muscles mentioned.

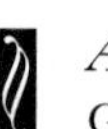

Answer: **D**
Green in Green, Hotchkiss, Pederson, p. 1481
Skirven, Callahan in Mackin, Callahan, Skirven, et al, pp. 601-603
Refer to Fig. 16-1

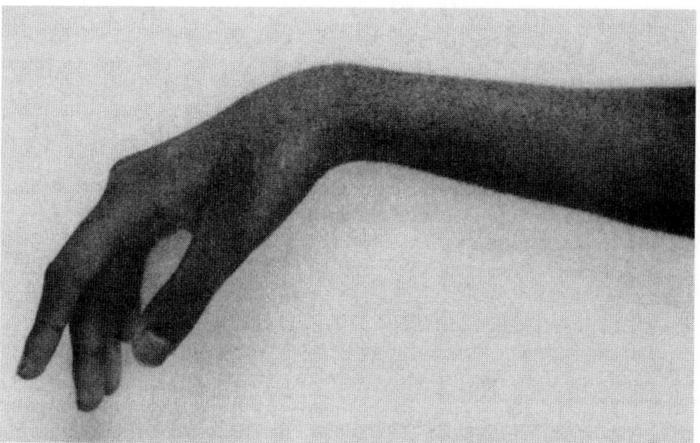

Fig. 16-1 ■ Wrist-drop deformity resulting from radial nerve injury. (From Stanley BG, Tribuzi SM: *Concepts in hand rehabilitation*, Philadelphia, 1992, FA Davis.)

5. The "standard" or most commonly used set of tendon transfers for radial nerve palsy includes which of the following?

A. Pronator teres (PT) to ECRB, flexor carpi ulnaris (FCU) to EDC, palmaris longus (PL) to EPL
B. PT to ECRL, flexor carpi radialis (FCR) to EDC, FCU to EPL
C. PT to EPL, PL to EDC, FCU to ECRB
D. PT to ECRL, FCR to EDC, PL to EPL

Multiple authors have described various methods for tendon transfer for radial nerve palsy, but it is important to understand what is most commonly seen in practice. Choice A is the correct answer. Some authors would suggest using the FCR instead of the FCU to the EDC. In choice B, both the FCU and FCR are used. This set of transfers is not a good choice because the PL is not strong enough to function effectively as the sole wrist flexor. C is not a good choice because the PL has a much lower work capacity than the EDC and is not strong enough to perform the duties of the EDC. Finally, in choice D, because the ECRB (which inserts at the base of the third metacarpal) is a more central tendon than the ECRL (which inserts at the base of the second metacarpal), transfer to the ECRB would provide better wrist extension, whereas transfer to the ECRL would result in radial deviation as well as wrist extension.

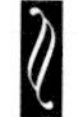

Answer: **A**
Green in Green, Hotchkiss, Pederson, pp. 1481-1496
Skirven, Callahan in Mackin, Callahan, Skirven, et al, p. 619

6. Which of the following transfers is part of the superficialis transfer ("Boyes transfer") for radial nerve palsy?

A. PT to ECRB
B. Flexor digitorum superficialis (FDS) III to EDC
C. FDS IV to EPL
D. FCR to abductor pollicis longus (APL)/EPB
E. All of the above

All of the above are part of the superficialis transfer for radial nerve palsy. With the standard transfers, the FCR or FCU is transferred to the EDC. However, because the wrist flexors have less amplitude of excursion (33 mm) in comparison with the finger extensors (50 mm), active extension of the fingers can only be achieved when the wrist is in volar flexion, relying on the tenodesis effect of the wrist. Thus wrist and finger extension cannot be achieved simultaneously. The FDS tendon has greater excursion (70 mm), which overcomes this limitation. In addition, use of the FDS allows the FCR to be used for thumb abduction. The FDS can be used because finger flexion is still provided by the flexor digitorum profundus (FDP).

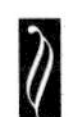

Answer: **E**

Boyes, pp. 958-969
Green in Green, Hotchkiss, Pederson, p. 1491
Refer to Fig. 16-2

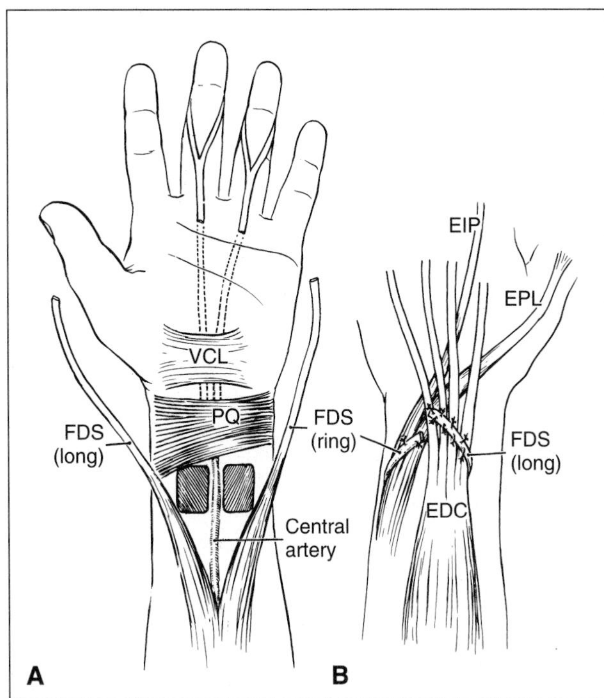

Fig. 16-2 ■ Transfer of the long and ring FDS tendons through the interosseous membrane for finger and thumb extension. The holes in the interosseous membrane must be large but must not damage the central artery on the volar side of the forearm. The long finger superficialis provides extension of the four fingers, whereas the ring finger superficialis provides extension of the thumb and index finger. (From Omer GE, Jr: *Am Acad Orthop Surg Instructional Course Lectures* 18 (J):93, 1962–1969.)

7. In addition to thumb opposition, what other functions are lost (and must be replaced) in a high median nerve palsy?

A. Thumb IP flexion
B. Thumb IP extension
C. Index and long distal interphalangeal (DIP) flexion
D. Index and long proximal interphalangeal (PIP) flexion
E. A, C, and D

The median nerve innervates the following musculature in the upper extremity: pronator teres, FCR, flexor pollicis longus (FPL), FDP (index and long fingers), FDS, pronator quadratus, abductor pollicis brevis (APB), flexor pollicis brevis (FPB), index and long finger lumbricals, and opponens pollicis (OP). In a high median nerve palsy, thumb opposition, thumb flexion, and flexion of the index and long fingers are all lost (flexion of the ring and little fingers is preserved because the FDP to these fingers are innervated by the ulnar nerve).

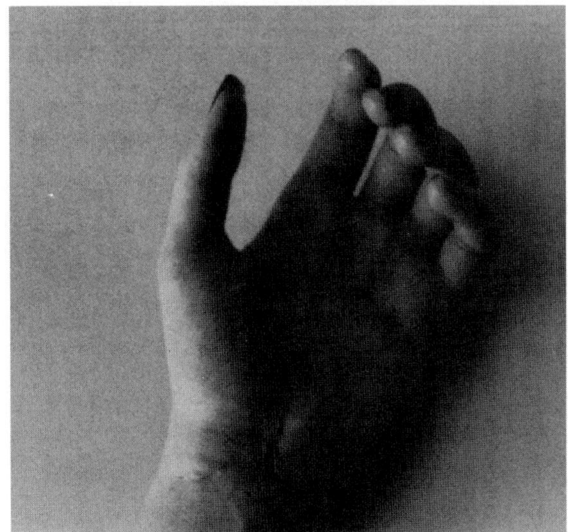

Fig. 16-3 ■ Median-nerve palsy with flattened thenar eminence. (From Stanley BG, Tribuzi SM: *Concepts in hand rehabilitation*, Philadelphia, 1992, FA Davis.)

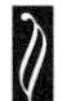
Answer: **E**
Davis, Barton in Green, Hotchkiss, Pederson, p. 1497
Skirven, Callahan in Mackin, Callahan, Skirven, et al, pp. 604-605
Refer to Fig. 16-3

8. All but which of the following can be used in the treatment of high median nerve palsy?

A. FDS ring to APB for thumb opposition
B. Extensor digiti minimi (EDM) to APB for thumb opposition
C. Brachioradialis (BR) to FPL for thumb IP flexion
D. FDP index and long to FDP of ring and little (side to side)

Although choice A is excellent for low median nerve palsy, this choice is poor in high median nerve palsy because the FDS is innervated by the median nerve and thus would not function in a high median nerve palsy. Therefore thumb opposition would have to be recreated with another tendon transfer such as choices B, C, and D. All of these transfers are used commonly for high median nerve palsy. The EDQ is innervated by the ulnar nerve; the BR by the radial nerve; and the FDP ring and little fingers by the ulnar nerve.

Answer: **A**
Green in Green, Hotchkiss, Pederson, p. 1519
Skirven, Callahan in Mackin, Callahan, Skirven, et al, pp. 604-605

9. A patient sustains a closed humeral shaft fracture with minimal displacement, angulation, and shortening. On initial physical examination, the patient is noted to have a complete radial nerve palsy. He is referred to occupational therapy. Initial management should be which of the following?

A. Splinting to immobilize the humerus fracture and elbow until open reduction and internal fixation (ORIF) of the fracture with exploration of the radial nerve can be performed
B. Splinting of the humerus fracture, including prolonged immobilization of the elbow, wrist, and MCP joints
C. Surgery for ORIF of the fracture and tendon transfers
D. Splinting to immobilize the humerus fracture with therapy to maintain ROM of the wrist, thumb, and fingers

A minimally displaced or angulated fracture of the humerus can be treated with a fracture brace (Sarmiento) (see Fig. 5, p. 349). Some physicians may include the elbow in the immobilization splint. The most important aspect of nonoperative management in a patient with radial nerve palsy is maintenance of full ROM in all joints of the wrist and hand, including the thumb-index web space. Splints are often provided that help maintain the wrist, thumb, and fingers in extension through the day. These splints are then removed to allow daily therapy to maintain ROM.

92% of radial nerve palsies resulting from closed humerus fractures will resolve. If no nerve function returns, nerve repair, nerve graft, or tendon transfers are considered. However, for these procedures to be effective, the joints in the hand and wrist must be kept supple.

Answer: **D**
Green in Green, Hotchkiss, Pederson, pp. 1482-1483
Pollack, Drake, Bovill, pp. 2392-2443

10. Match the biomechanical term to its correct description.

Biomechanical Term

1. Stress
2. Shear stress
3. Mechanical advantage
4. Axis

Description

A. Occurs when one force acting on a lever has doubled the moment arm of the opposing force
B. Force per unit area
C. Occurs in tissue that is subjected to two opposing forces that are not exactly in line
D. Two bones moving around each other at a joint and one line that does not move in relation to either bone

Answers: **1, B; 2, C; 3, A; 4, D**
Brand, Hollister, pp. 3-6

11. In relation to a muscle contraction, the resting length is which of the following?

A. Distance between the maximal stretch and the maximal contracture of a fiber
B. Maximal stretch of a muscle fiber
C. Optimal position for a muscle to generate a strong contraction
D. A and B
E. A and C

The resting length is the length that a sarcomere, or a muscle fiber, assumes when a limb is in its resting and balanced condition. Resting length is approximately equal to the distance between the maximal stretch and the maximal contracture of a fiber. The optimal strength of active contraction is obtained when the muscle is in the middle of its normal excursion (neutral). At the two extremes of maximal stretch and maximal contraction, the ability of a muscle to form an active contraction is close to 0. In contrast, when a muscle is at resting length, it has the maximal power to perform a strong contraction of a fiber.

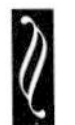

Answer: **E**
Brand, Hollister, p. 14
Tubiana, Thomine, Mackin, pp. 44-46

12. Match each term to the correct description.

Term

1. Force
2. Friction
3. Static friction
4. Coulomb friction
5. Radian

Description

A. Frictional force resulting between two surfaces that move relative to one another
B. Defined as that which will cause acceleration
C. A unit of angular measurement
D. A friction force produced when two surfaces do not move relative to one another
E. Resisting force parallel to and resulting from direct contact between two surfaces

Answers: **1, B; 2, E; 3, D; 4, A; 5, C**
Brand, Hollister, pp. 5-6
Giurintano, p. 84

13. Which of the following signs *will not* be present on low ulnar nerve palsy?

A. Pollock's sign (loss of extrinsic power of the ulnar innervated portion of the FDP, with an inability to flex the DIP joints of the ring and little fingers)
B. Claw hand (hyperextension of proximal phalanges, and flexion of the IP joints of the ring and little fingers)
C. Jeanne's sign (hyperextension of the thumb MCP joint with key pinch or gross grip)
D. Froment's sign (obligate flexion of the thumb IP joint to 80 to 90 degrees to pinch object between thumb and index finger)

Choice A is the correct answer. The only tendons that flex the DIP joints of the ring and little fingers are the ulnar portion of the FDP, which is innervated by the ulnar nerve. However, the innervation is in the proximal forearm and is not compromised in low ulnar nerve palsy. In claw hand, the intrinsic function of the ring and little fingers (dorsal and volar interossei, and third and fourth lumbricals) is lost. In a normal hand, these muscles allow MCP flexion and IP joint extension. Conversely, when compromised, the MCP joints will extend, and the IP joints will flex, thus causing a claw-like position of the hand if extrinsic function is normal (Fig. 16-4). With normal lateral pinch, the adductor pollicis helps the thumb adduct, flex at the MCP joint, and extend at the IP joint. In low ulnar nerve palsy, the adductor pollicis is compromised. Instead, the person will adjust and generate pinch strength by hyperextending the MCP joint 10 to 15 degrees. In low ulnar nerve palsy, the first dorsal interosseus muscle, which abducts the index finger, and the adductor pollicis do not function. Thus, when attempting to grasp an object between the thumb and index finger, the person will flex

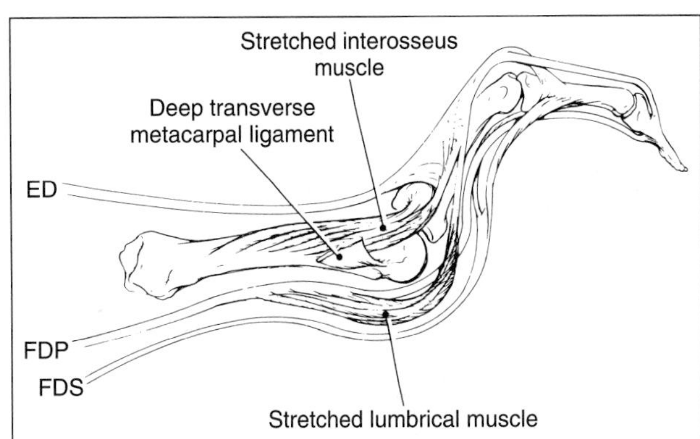

Fig. 16-4 ■ In ulnar palsy, the loss of intrinsic muscle control in the ring and little fingers allows the MCP joints to hyperextend. The denervated muscles are stretched in this claw position. *ED,* Extensor digitorum communis; *FDP,* flexor digitorum profundus; *FDS,* flexor digitorum superficialis. (From Mackin EJ, Callahan AD, Skirven TM, et al: *Rehabilitation of the hand and upper extremity,* ed 5, vol 2, St Louis, 2002, Mosby.)

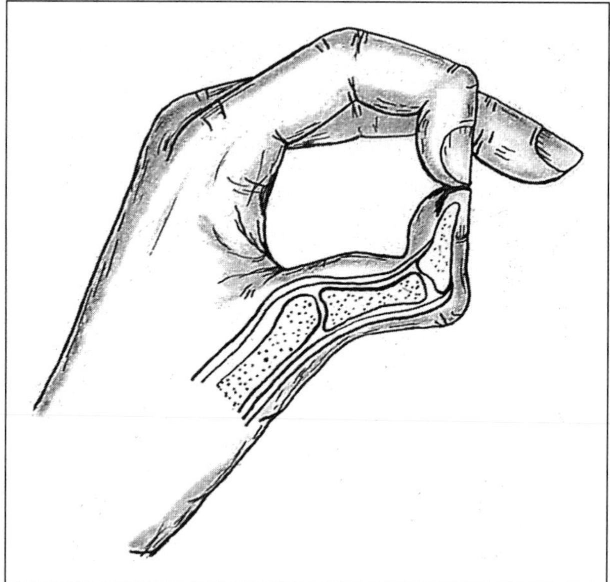

Fig. 16-5 ■ Froment's sign. (From Hunter JM, Schneider LH, Mackin EJ: *Tendon and nerve surgery in the hand: a third decade*, St Louis, 1997, Mosby.)

the IP joint of the thumb to use the FPL to pinch the object (Fig. 16-5).

Answer: **A**

Brown, pp. 323-342
Earle, Vlastou, pp. 560-565
Omer in Green, Hotchkiss, Pederson, p. 1526
Skirven, Callahan in Mackin, Callahan, Skirven, et al, pp. 608, 623-626
Hunter, Schneider, Mackin, p. 422

14. Occasionally, a low median nerve palsy will occur with a low ulnar nerve palsy. Essentially, this situation involves a total loss of intrinsic function. In this situation, muscles innervated by the radial nerve must be used. Match the donor tendon innervated by the radial nerve with the compromised tendon or function.

Donor Tendon

1. ECRB
2. APL
3. EIP
4. BR

Compromised Tendon or Function

A. Clawed fingers (MCP flexion)
B. Index abduction (first dorsal interosseus [DI])
C. Thumb adduction (adductor pollicis [AP])
D. Thumb opposition (APB)

The best donor tendon is the ECRB via tendon graft around the third metacarpal to the abductor tubercle for thumb adduction. The APL is attached to the first dorsal interosseous, and the EIP to the APB. A brachioradialis plus tendon graft to the lateral bands of clawed fingers may be performed.

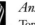

Answers: **1, C; 2, B; 3, D; 4, A**

Topper, p. 342

15. Match the terms with the appropriate description.

Term

1. Mechanics
2. Statics
3. Dynamics
4. Biomechanics

Description

A. Branch of physics concerned with motion and deformation of bodies that are acted on by mechanical disturbances called *forces*
B. Study of forces on rigid bodies in motion
C. Study of forces on rigid bodies at rest or moving at a constant velocity
D. The application of engineering mechanics with the fields of biology and physiology

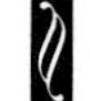

Answers: **1, A; 2, C; 3, B; 4, D**

Ozkaya, Nordin, pp. 3-4

16. Match the terms with the appropriate description.

Terms

1. Elastic body
2. Plastic body
3. Viscosity
4. Viscoelastic

Description

A. All deformations are recoverable after removal of external forces
B. Body maintains permanent deformity after removal of external forces
C. Quantitative measure of resistance to flow
D. Material that has both fluid and solid properties

To understand the difference between elastic and plastic behavior, consider the example of a spring. If a small force is applied and released, the spring will go back to its original shape. In this situation, the spring exhibits elastic behavior. However, if a large enough force is applied, the spring may become permanently deformed. When the heavy object is removed, it will recover somewhat, but the spring may be a little longer than it originally was. In this situation, the spring demonstrates plastic behavior.

To define viscosity and viscoelastics, we must first define a fluid. When a force is applied, a solid object will deform to a certain extent but the continuous application of the force will not necessarily continue to deform the object. In contrast, a fluid object will continue to deform in the face of a continuously applied force (flow). Viscosity is a fluid property that measures the resistance to this deformation or flow. In nature, most materials exhibit both fluid and solid properties. These materials are called *viscoelastic.*

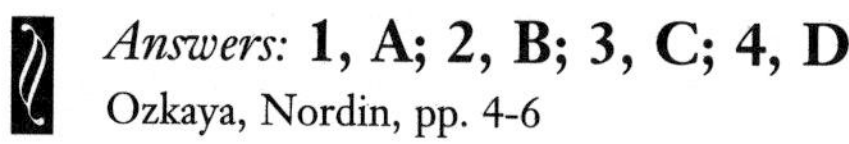

Answers: **1, A; 2, B; 3, C; 4, D**
Ozkaya, Nordin, pp. 4-6

17. Which of the following statements is true of a sarcomere?

A. It is the basic contractile unit.
B. It shortens during contraction.
C. It comprises interacting myosin and actin.
D. All of the above

A sarcomere is the basic contractile unit of muscle tissue in muscle fiber. It is composed of two overlapping filaments: the thick myosin filament and the thin actin filament. There is an overlap and interdigitation of actin and myosin molecules with a subsequent shortening of the sarcomere during active contraction.

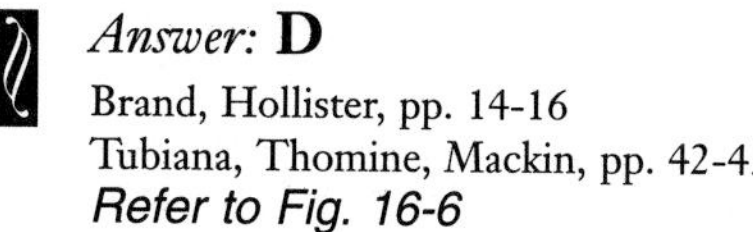

Answer: **D**
Brand, Hollister, pp. 14-16
Tubiana, Thomine, Mackin, pp. 42-45
Refer to Fig. 16-6

18. Match each term to its definition.

Term

1. Creep
2. Work
3. Drag
4. Hysteresis
5. Stress relaxation

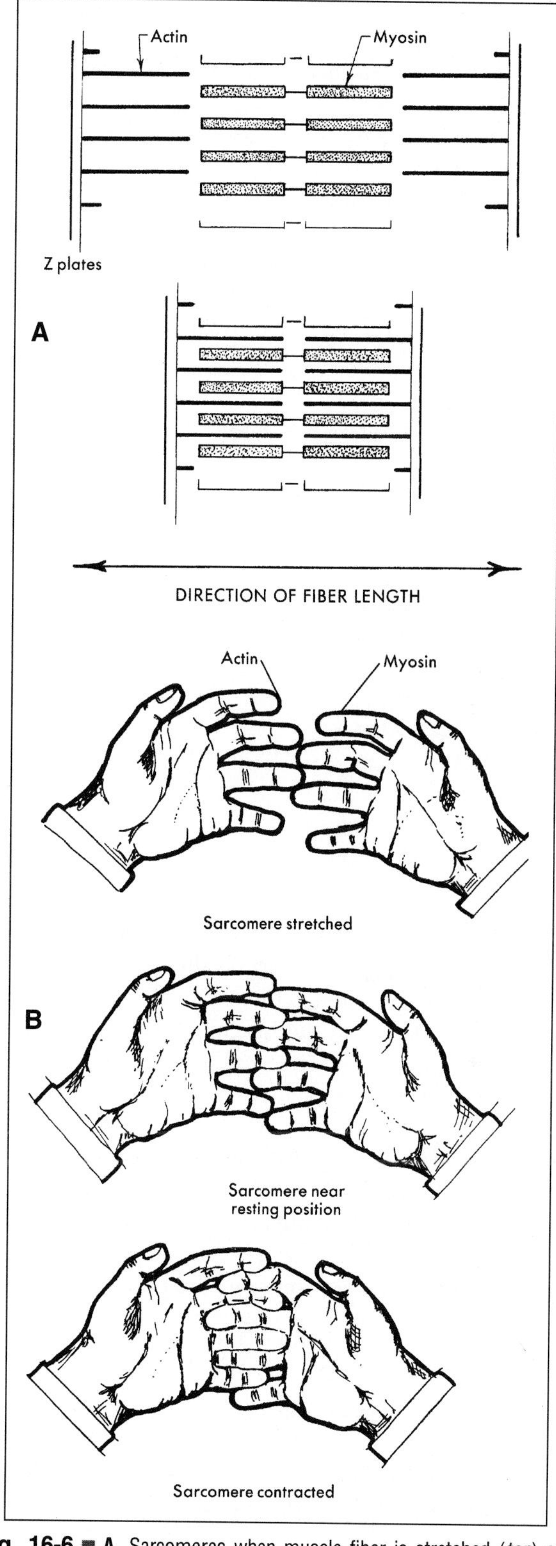

Fig. 16-6 ■ **A,** Sarcomeres when muscle fiber is stretched (*top*) and when it is contracted (*bottom*). **B,** Contraction of a sarcomere is similar to a pair of hands with interdigitating fingers (the fingers of one hand are actin and those of the other are myosin). (From Brand PW, Hollister A: *Clinical mechanics of the hand,* ed 2, St Louis, 1993, Mosby.)

Definition

A. Shear stresses resulting from the action of a fluid on a surface
B. Energy required to move a force through a distance
C. A decrease in stress after a material is initially strained and then held at a constant for a long time
D. A stretched, elastic material springing back to its original shape when stress is removed
E. Tissue permanently remaining in a lengthened state after being stretched and held under moderate tension for a long time

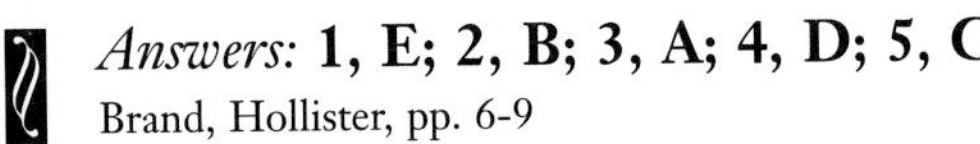

Answers: **1, E; 2, B; 3, A; 4, D; 5, C**
Brand, Hollister, pp. 6-9

19. The most common lever found in the human body is which of the following?

A. First-class lever
B. Second-class lever
C. Third-class lever
D. Force arm

A *lever* is defined as a rigid bar revolving around a fixed point or fulcrum. The force arm is the distance between the fulcrum and the applied force and the resistance arm is the distance between the fulcrum and the resistance. A first-class lever is characterized by a fulcrum between the force and the resistance, as in a teeter-totter, scissors, or, anatomically, the triceps. A second-class lever is the resistance between the fulcrum and the force, as in a wheelbarrow or a nutcracker. In a third-class lever, the force is applied between the fulcrum and the resistance (e.g., the biceps). The third-class lever is the most common lever found in the human body.

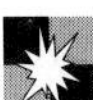

CLINICAL GEM:
The body uses the third-class lever system, and most splints are the second-class lever system, which gives splint makers an advantage. Therapists tend to have difficulty with this concept because we consider the design being the same as the action. Paul Van-Lede (Orfit) explains it simply in the following:

> Because all splints need to be attached to a proximal segment and act on a distal segment (with the pivot in the middle), they always have a first-class lever design. However, when one considers the action (efficiency) of the force on the distal segment, there is only the possibility of a second- or third-class level, depending on the distance of the attachment to the pivot (proximal or distal to the gravity point). Also, the muscles have either a second- or third-class lever action.

For additional clarification, refer to van Lede, van Veldhoven: *Therapeutic Hand Splints, A Rational Approach*, vol 1, *Mechanical and Biomechanical Considerations*, Antwerp, Belgium, 1998, Provan Buba.

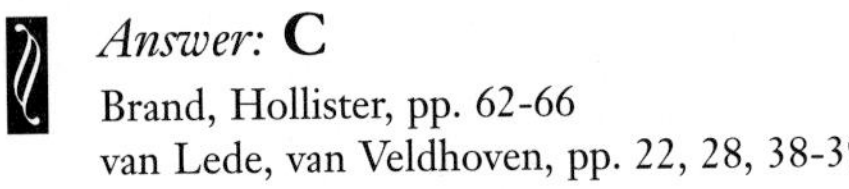

Answer: **C**
Brand, Hollister, pp. 62-66
van Lede, van Veldhoven, pp. 22, 28, 38-39

20. Which of the following types of stress typically occurs in a tendon or ligament?

A. Shear stress
B. Compression stress
C. Tension stress
D. Strain

Tension stress occurs when applied forces are colinear and act in opposite directions. Tendons use tension stress to produce joint movement and ligaments use tension stress to provide joint stability.

Sprains, strains, ruptures, and avulsions may occur if opposing forces exceed the ability of the materials to resist them. A strain is the deformation of an object or tissue.

Compression stress is present when a force presses perpendicular to a surface or when forces act toward each other. *Compression* and *pressure* are defined as force per unit area (i.e., pounds per square inch, or psi).

Shear stress is caused by forces that are parallel to a surface but are not exactly in line or colinear. Shear stress can occur within tissues beneath the skin or between skin and external forces (e.g., splints).

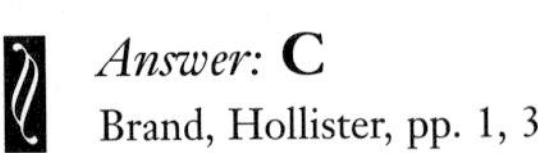

Answer: **C**
Brand, Hollister, pp. 1, 3

21. The clinical significance of applying heat to tissues before stretching exercises is related to which biomechanical principle?

A. Viscosity
B. Elasticity
C. Plastic change
D. Creep

All of the above can affect the outcome of stretching or lengthening exercises. Creep occurs when a tissue gradually changes its structure and remains in a lengthened state after being stretched and held under tension for a long time. Rising temperature may increase the amount of creep. Maximizing creep is the goal of stretching tissues.

Viscosity is the property of a material that causes it to resist movement. Viscosity does not prevent motion; it retards it. For example, a thick fluid offers greater resistance than a thin fluid and is thus more viscous.

Elasticity is the property that enables a material or tissue to return to its exact original shape after the removal of all stress; it allows a tissue to be deformed and then return to its resting state. Elastic tissues hinder the motion of a joint or tendon by maintaining the tissues' initial state. Collagen is elastic and can resist stretch.

Plastic change occurs when a tissue is stretched beyond its elastic limit and may be permanently deformed. Tendon attenuations, ruptures, avulsions, and stress fractures are examples of plastic change; these tissues never return to their original shape.

Answer: **D**
Brand, Hollister, pp. 5-7, 94-105

22. Which of the following variables is not measurably related to muscle tension capability?

A. Physiological cross-sectional area
B. Actin/myosin fibril ratio
C. Muscle fiber length
D. Mass

There are three measurable variables for each muscle: 1) mass, which is directly proportional to volume; 2) muscle fiber length, which is proportional to the potential for excursion; and 3) the physiological cross-sectional area, which is muscle volume divided by its mean fiber length and is proportional to total maximum tension.

The actin/myosin fibrils entwine within muscle sarcomeres as the fingers of one hand might interdigitate and overlap with the fingers of the other hand. When the sarcomere unit is activated by a motor nerve impulse, the actin and myosin exercise a strong attraction to one another, pulling together into deeper interdigitations. These fibrils are the basis of all muscle contractions but are not measurable with regard to strength of contraction.

Answer: **B**
Brand, Hollister, pp. 13-16, 26-28

23. True or False: Muscle tissues are best described by the term *elasticity* rather than *viscoelasticity*.

Elasticity allows soft tissues to be deformed and then immediately return to their resting shape. Viscoelasticity is a combination of both viscous and elastic properties and is characterized by hysteresis, which allows a material to spring back to its original shape more slowly when tension is removed. All muscles have a certain tone, even in the absence of apparent nerve stimulation. This tone is a combination of the elasticity of a muscle and the connective tissue that surrounds it. The term *viscoelasticity* is better suited to describe muscle tissue than *elasticity* because muscle behaves differently when it is subjected to fast movement than when it is subjected to slow movement.

Answer: **False**
Brand, Hollister, pp. 6-7, 21, 94-98, 115

24. A radian is approximately how many degrees?

A. 30
B. 57
C. 73
D. 91

Tendon excursion can be calculated geometrically through radians. A radian is an angle that is created when the radius lies along the circumference of the circle and is joined by a line at each end in the center of the circle. This angle is always equal to 57.29 degrees, or 1 radian.

It is important to understand the concept of radians when calculating extensor tendon excursions. For example, when the MCP joint is moved 1 radian (57.29 degrees), the MCP joint motion of 57.29 degrees will yield a 10-mm extensor tendon excursion. Therefore, as Duran and Gelberman suggested, to obtain the 5 mm of excursion to minimize extrinsic adhesions, a joint must be moved through 0.5 radian, or 28.64 degrees of rotation (flexion). It is important to know that joints have various tendon excursions, depending on their size. A small joint with a smaller moment arm produces less tendon excursion.

Answer: **B**
Hunter, Mackin, Callahan, p. 569
Brand, Hollister, pp. 67-68
Refer to Fig. 16-7

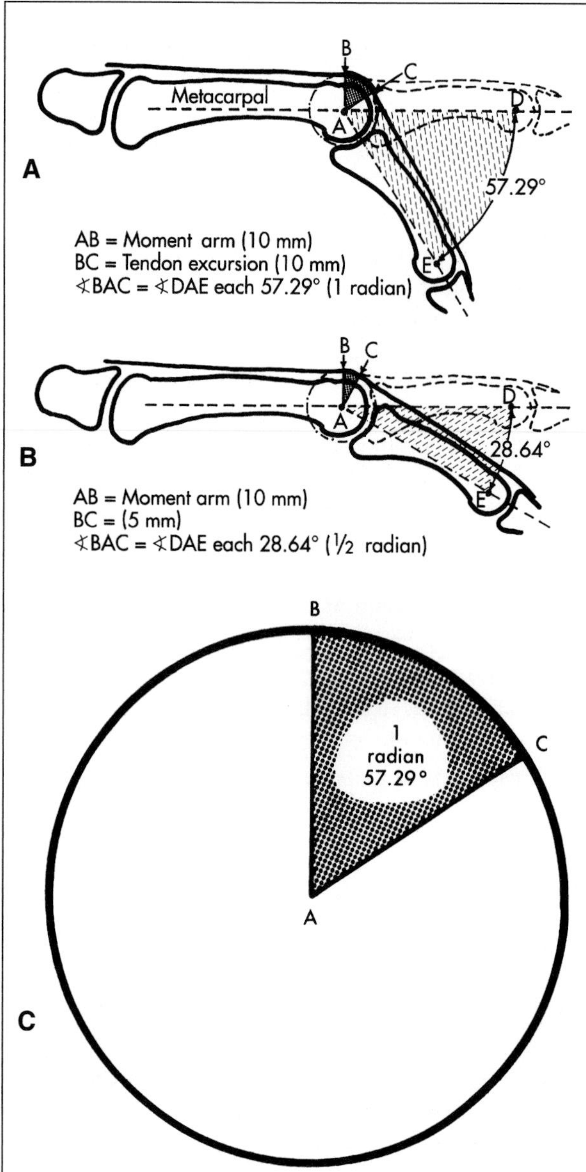

Fig. 16-7 ■ A, If the head of the metacarpal is considered in terms of a circle, the moment arm of the extensor tendon is equal to the radius of that circle. If MCP joint motion equals 57.29 degrees, or 1 radian, tendon excursion is equal to the moment arm, or AB = BC. If the moment arm equals 10 mm, angular change of 57.29 degrees affects 10 mm of extensor tendon excursion. **B,** Angular change of 0.5 radian or 28.3 degrees affects the 5 mm of extensor tendon excursion recommended for the early passive motion program. **C,** A radian is the angle that is created when the radius that lies along the circumference of a circle is joined by a line at each end in the center or axis of the circle. Angle *BAC* equals 1 radian, or 57.29 degrees. (**A** From Evans RB, Burkhalter WE: A study of the dynamic anatomy of extensor tendons and implications for treatment, *J Hand Surg* [Am] 11:776, 1986; **B** and **C** from Hunter JM, Mackin EJ, Callahan AD: *Rehabilitation of the hand: surgery and therapy*, ed 4, St Louis, 1995, Mosby.)

25. In a low ulnar nerve palsy, all but which of the following functions must be replaced with tendon transfers?

A. MCP joint flexion
B. Thumb adduction
C. Index abduction
D. DIP flexion of the ring finger

DIP flexion of the ring and little fingers is provided by the FDP, which is not compromised in low ulnar nerve palsy. Flexion at the MCP joint of the fingers is initiated by the intrinsic muscles, which are mostly innervated by the ulnar nerve (except for the lumbricals to the index and long fingers). Various tendon transfers have been described that transfer tendons into the lateral bands at the MCP joints, which allow MCP flexion and IP extension. The FDS, ECRL, EDQ, EIP, and FCR tendons have all been used in this fashion. Another option is to perform a MCP joint capsulodesis to hold the MCP joints in slight flexion and allow the extrinsics to provide the rest of the flexion.

The ECRB, ECRL, and BR have all been transferred to the AP to provide thumb adduction. Index abduction is provided by the EIP or APB to the first DI muscle.

Answer: **D**
Topper, p. 342

26. In a low median nerve palsy, the patient loses thumb opposition. Thumb opposition is a complex movement that involves which of the following?

A. Trapeziometacarpal supination, extension, adduction
B. Trapeziometacarpal pronation, extension, abduction
C. Trapeziometacarpal pronation, flexion, abduction
D. Trapeziometacarpal supination, flexion, adduction

Thumb opposition is the ability to place the pulp of the thumb opposite that of the middle finger such that the nail of the thumb is parallel to the volar surface of the finger. It is a complex movement of trapeziometacarpal joint *abduction*, *flexion*, and *pronation*. This motion is extremely important for function because it allows the patient to maintain a strong pincer grasp. In contrast, thumb retroposition involves trapeziometacarpal joint abduction, extension, and supination.

Answer: **C**
Cooney, Linscheid, An, pp. 777-786
Davis, Barton in Green, Hotchkiss, Pederson, p. 1497

27. In a high ulnar nerve palsy, what is the most common tendon transfer to provide flexion of the DIP joints of the ring and little fingers?

A. FDS to FDP
B. EIP to FDP
C. PL to FDP
D. FDP index and long to FDP of ring and little

The primary difference in high versus low ulnar nerve palsy is the loss of the ability to flex the DIP joints of the ring and little fingers. The FDP tendons share a common muscle belly. By simple tenodesis of the ring and little finger tendons to the tendons of the long and index finger, DIP flexion can be restored (Fig. 16-8). In addition, some wrist flexion and ulnar deviation is lost with high ulnar nerve palsy because the FCU is compromised. This loss of function is usually not significant and can be compensated for without a tendon transfer.

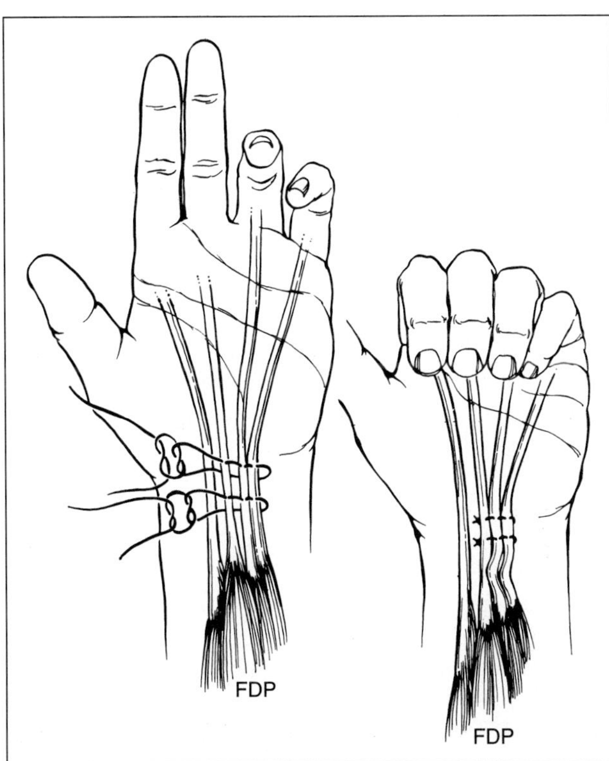

Fig. 16-8 ■ Tenodesis of the ulnar-innervated profundus tendons of the ring and little fingers to the active median-innervated FDP of the long finger to increase power for gross grip. A double line of sutures is important to prevent "whipsawing" of the tendons during power grip. (From Green DP, Hotchkiss RN, Pederson WC: *Green's Operative hand surgery*, ed 4, New York, 1999, Churchill Livingstone.)

Answer: **D**
Topper, p. 342
Omer in Green, Hotchkiss, Pederson, p. 1538

28. Match the terms with the appropriate description.

Terms

1. Force
2. Moment
3. Velocity
4. Acceleration

Description

A. Action of one body against another
B. Time rate of increase of velocity
C. Time rate of change in position
D. Rotational, bending, or twisting action of one body on another

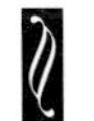

Answers: **1, A; 2, D; 3, C; 4, B**
Ozkaya, Nordin, p. 6

29. After a standard tendon transfer for a radial nerve palsy, when should an AROM program be initiated?

A. Immediately
B. 2 weeks
C. 4 weeks
D. 3 months

In the operating room, a long-arm splint is applied that immobilizes the forearm in 15 to 30 degrees of pronation, the wrist in approximately 45 degrees of extension, the MCP joints in 10 to 15 degrees of flexion, and the thumb in maximum extension and abduction. The splint and sutures are removed at 10 to 14 days. A long-arm cast is reapplied in the position noted above. At 4 weeks, the cast is removed and a removable short-arm splint to hold the wrist, fingers, and thumb in extension is made. At this point, a well-supervised hand therapy program is initiated. Between therapy sessions, the removable splints are worn. Patients typically achieve good control of function by 3 to 6 months.

Answer: **C**

Green in Green, Hotchkiss, Pederson, p. 1489

30. A 55-year-old female, who was recently treated for a nondisplaced distal radius fracture in a cast, presents with an acute onset of wrist pain and inability to extend the IP joint of the thumb. The patient has no other functional deficit. What is the most appropriate treatment?

A. Therapy to keep thumb MCP and IP joints supple while awaiting return of function of neuropraxia
B. Tendon transfer of the EIP to the EPL
C. Modalities, resting, splinting and gentle ROM to facilitate resolution of tenosynovitis
D. B or C

This patient had a spontaneous rupture of the EPL tendon after a nondisplaced distal radius fracture. It is hypothesized that nondisplaced fractures of the distal radius cause localized swelling and hematoma in the third dorsal compartment of the wrist (which contains the EPL), leading to ischemia and weakening of the tendon. Intraoperatively, a direct repair of the tendon can be attempted if the repair will not be under undue tension. Usually, because of the degenerative nature of this condition, such a repair will not be possible and the EIP is transferred to the EPL. Choices A and C are incorrect because this patient does not have a neurologic injury or a tenosynovitis.

Answer: **B**

Bonatz, Kramer, Masear, pp. 118-122
Gelb, pp. 411-422

31. True or False: A muscle will always drop a grade (on a manual muscle test scale of 0 to 5) after tendon transfer.

A widely quoted rule in the past was that when a muscle-tendon unit was transferred, its strength would drop one level; however, this generalization is accepted no longer. Diminished effectiveness of muscles after transfer is more likely to be a function of scar adhesion, drag (force resulting from action of a fluid on a surface), and/or imperfect reeducation than of actual loss of muscle tension capability. However, if a muscle has been weakened by disease or paralysis, it is unwise to expect a better performance after transfer.

Answer: **False**

Brand, Hollister, p. 30

32. The strongest muscle that crosses the wrist is which of the following?

A. ECRB
B. FCU
C. ECRL
D. FDP

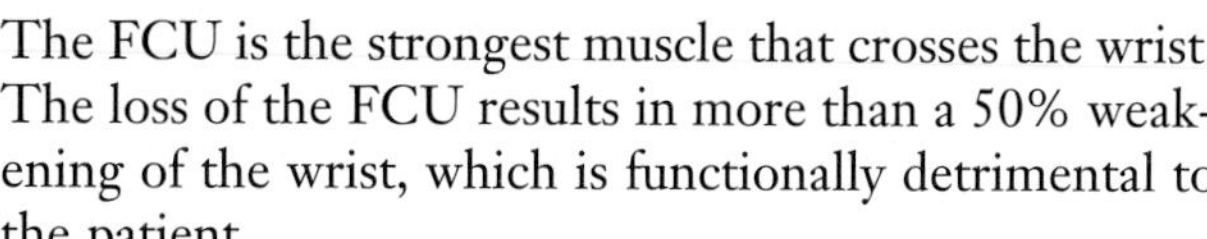

The FCU is the strongest muscle that crosses the wrist. The loss of the FCU results in more than a 50% weakening of the wrist, which is functionally detrimental to the patient.

The ECRB is the strongest and most efficient wrist extensor; the ECRL has the greatest capacity for sustained work. The FDP flexes the DIP joint and may assist as a weak wrist flexor.

Answer: **B**

Brand, Hollister, pp. 189, 267, 276, 311-315
Hunter, Mackin, Callahan, p. 523
Rosenthal in Mackin, Callahan, Skirven, et al, p. 501

33. True or False: You have a patient who underwent a proximal row carpectomy in which the scaphoid, lunate, triquetrum, and tip of the radial styloid were excised. After surgery and rehabilitation, this patient is expected to achieve normal strength.

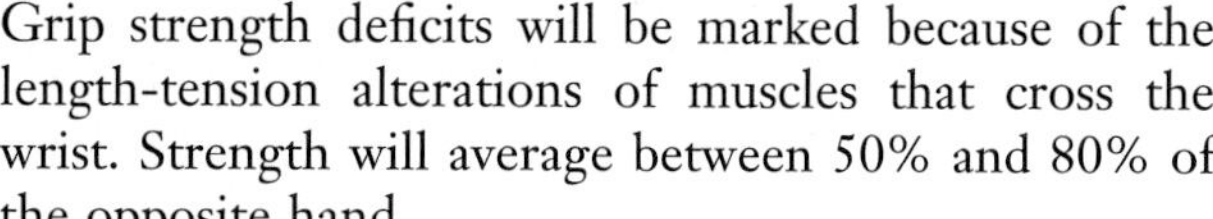

Grip strength deficits will be marked because of the length-tension alterations of muscles that cross the wrist. Strength will average between 50% and 80% of the opposite hand.

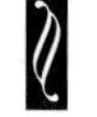

Answer: **False**

Wright, Michlovitz, pp. 149-151

34. True or False: The Blix curve depicts two curves of muscle tension: one by active contraction and the other by passive recoil.

When a muscle is stretched, it stores potential energy in a way similar to the elastic band. When it is released, the muscle contracts. Passive recoil is an elastic passive contracture that is not controlled by the nervous system but is an important component of total muscle tension.

The Blix curve (Fig. 16-9) depicts two different tension curves—one of active contracture (contractile tension) and the other of elastic (passive) stretch and passive recoil in the same fiber.

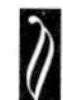

Answer: **True**

Brand, Hollister, pp. 17-18
Tubiana, Thomine, Mackin, pp. 42-44

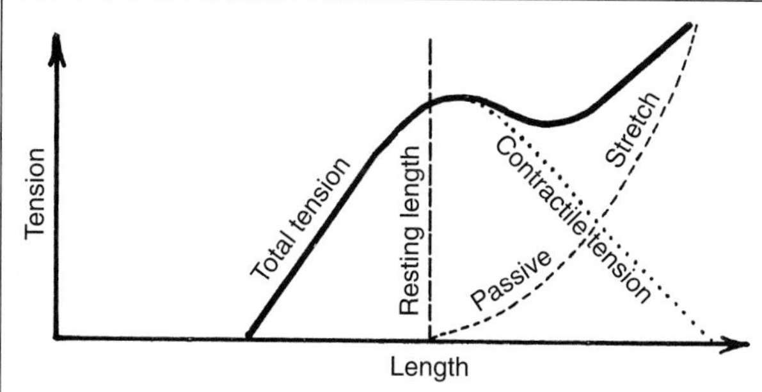

Fig. 16-9 ■ From Brand PW, Hollister A: *Clinical mechanics of the hand,* ed 2, St Louis, 1993, Mosby.

35. True or False: The motor muscles of the wrist have a tendinous excursion of approximately 3.5 cm.

Tendon excursion depends on muscular contractions. Other factors that influence tendon excursion are adherence of muscles to the aponeurosis, the freedom of a tendon gliding with its paratenon, the changes in direction around a pulley, and the crossing of one or more articulations. Tendon excursion for the wrist is approximately 3.5 cm. The common extensors of the fingers along with the long flexor of the thumb have an excursion of approximately 4 to 5 cm. The tendons of the long flexors of the fingers have the greatest excursion of all of the muscles in the hand—approximately 7 cm.

Answer: **True**

Tubiana, Thomine, Mackin, p. 53

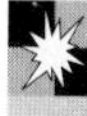

CLINICAL GEM:

The following is a quick reference to tendon excursion:

Excursion	Anatomical part
3 cm	Wrist
5 cm	Common finger extensors
7 cm	Long finger flexors

36. Which of the following tendons can be transferred to the APB to restore thumb opposition in a low median nerve palsy?

A. FDS
B. PL
C. EIP
D. Abductor digiti quinti (ADQ)
E. All of the above

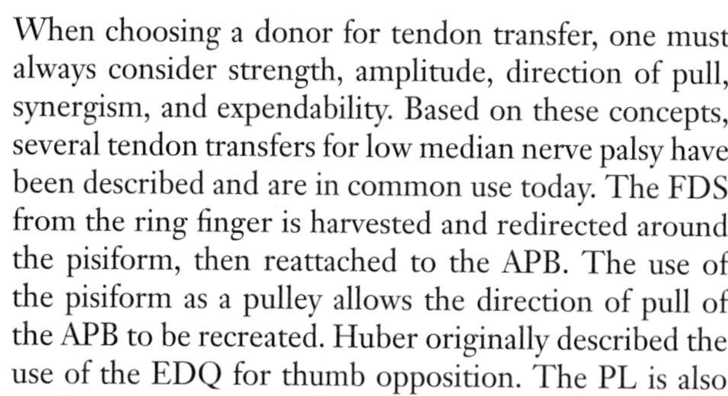

When choosing a donor for tendon transfer, one must always consider strength, amplitude, direction of pull, synergism, and expendability. Based on these concepts, several tendon transfers for low median nerve palsy have been described and are in common use today. The FDS from the ring finger is harvested and redirected around the pisiform, then reattached to the APB. The use of the pisiform as a pulley allows the direction of pull of the APB to be recreated. Huber originally described the use of the EDQ for thumb opposition. The PL is also used to connect to the APB. This was originally described by Bunnell in 1924 and Camitz in 1929. The EIP and ECU have also been used for treatment of low median nerve palsy (Fig. 16-10).

Answer: **E**

Davis, Barton in Green, Hotchkiss, Pederson, pp. 1498, 1500-1501

37. Match each of Newton's laws with the appropriate description.

Terms

1. Stress
2. Strain
3. Young's modulus
4. Yield strength
5. Ultimate strength

Description

A. Stress/strain
B. Change in length/total length
C. Force per unit area
D. Level of stress, if exceeded, will cause a material to have permanent deformation when the external force is removed
E. Level of stress, if exceeded, will cause a material to break

When a force is applied to an object, that force is distributed over an area. The magnitude of the force over

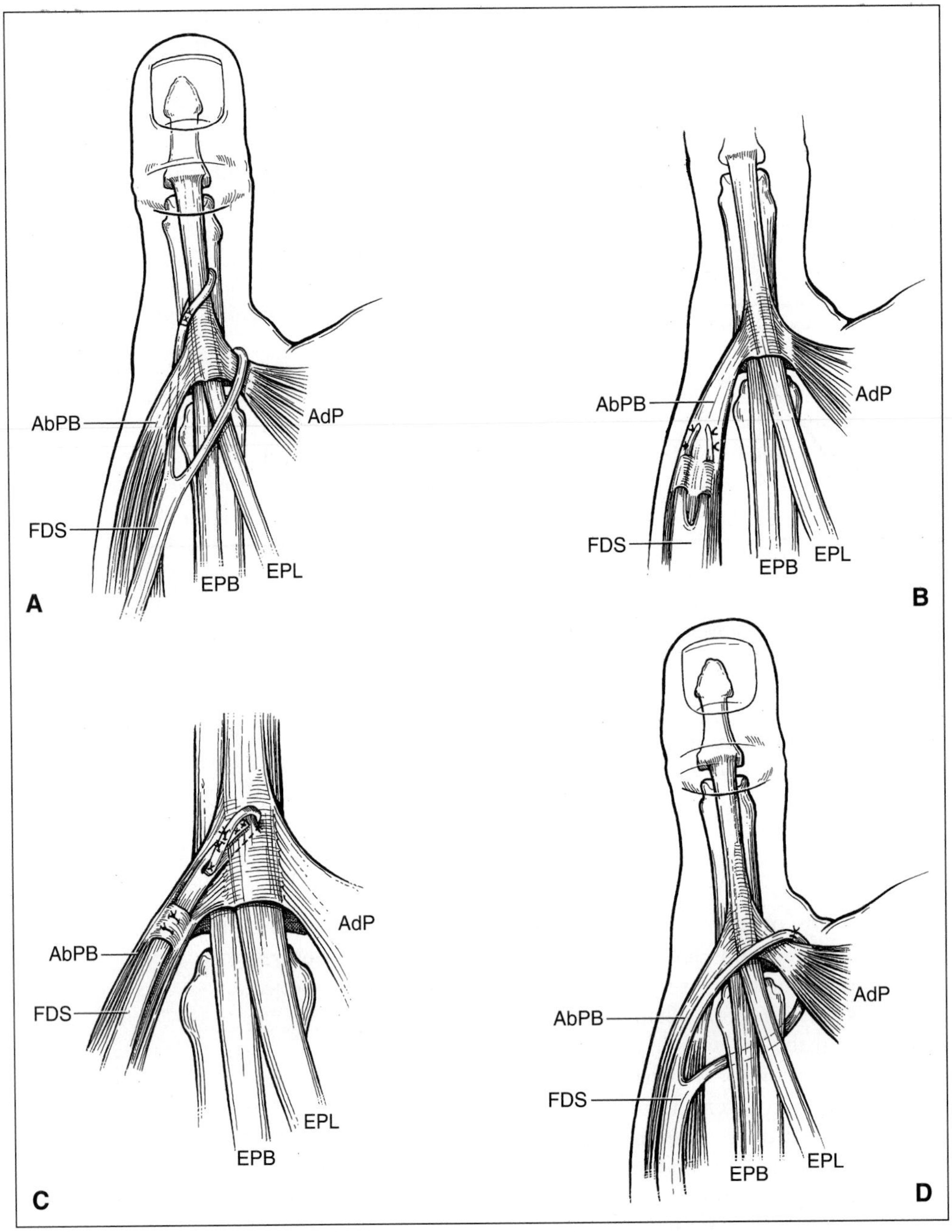

Fig. 16-10 ■ Techniques of distal attachment as described by Brand, Littler, Riordan, and Royle-Thompson. (From Green DP, Hotchkiss RN, Pederson WC: *Green's Operative hand surgery,* ed 4, New York, 1999, Churchill Livingstone.)

the surface area is the stress that the force exerts on that object. *Strain* is defined as a change in length of an object divided by the object's original length when a force is applied. The more rigid or stiff an object, the less strain that object will experience for a given stress. When the stress of a force is plotted against strain as a result of that force on a graph, the slope of that relationship is the Young's modulus (stress/strain). The higher the Young's modulus, the stiffer the object (the less strain will be generated by a given stress). In the elastic portion of a curve, when a stress is removed, the object will return to its original length. However, when the yield strength is surpassed, that object is permanently deformed and will have a longer resting length when the force is removed. If the stress applied is greater than the ultimate strength, the object will not only stretch—it will break.

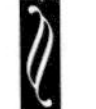

Answers: **1, C; 2, B; 3, A; 4, D; 5, E**
Ozkaya, Nordin, pp. 265-266

38. The Steindler flexorplasty is performed for which of the following conditions?

A. High median nerve palsy
B. Low median nerve palsy
C. Radial nerve palsy
D. Brachial plexus palsy

In brachial plexus injuries, several functions of the upper extremity are lost. Often this includes flexion of the elbow. Most authors agree that elbow flexion is the single most important motion to restore in order to provide a maximally functional extremity. In 1918, Steindler described a procedure to help restore elbow flexion in patients suffering from brachial plexus palsies. The Steindler flexorplasty transposes the flexor-pronator origin proximally on the humerus. This transposition gives the flexor-pronator mass a greater moment arm, allowing the patient to flex the elbow against gravity. However, strength is still severely limited, with approximately 5 pounds as the maximum weight that the patient can move after this transposition.

Answer: **D**
Marshall, Williams, Birch, pp. 577-582
Steindler, pp. 117-119

39. The prime muscle of thumb opposition is which of the following?

A. APB
B. FPB
C. OP
D. AP

The APB originates from the scaphoid and trapezoid bones and inserts on the radial aspect of the base of the proximal phalanx of the thumb. It is generally recognized as the primary muscle of thumb opposition. The tendon transfers most commonly used today to provide thumb opposition in median nerve palsy are designed to recreate the action of this muscle.

Answer: **A**
Cooney, Linscheid, An, pp. 777-786

40. Which of the following transfers augments finger flexion in a person with high median nerve palsy?

A. ECRL to FDP
B. PT to FDP
C. BR to FDP
D. EIP to FDP

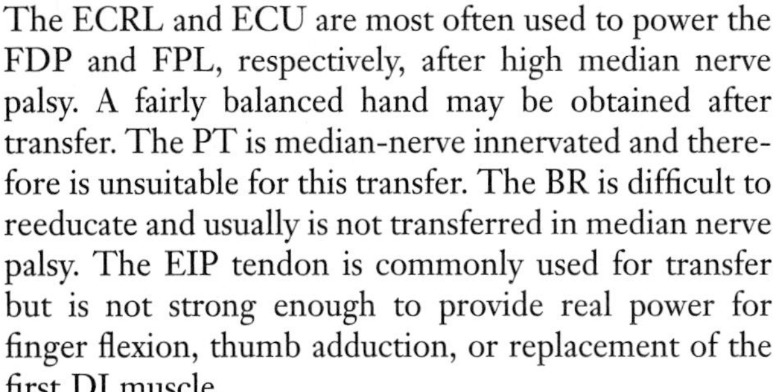

The ECRL and ECU are most often used to power the FDP and FPL, respectively, after high median nerve palsy. A fairly balanced hand may be obtained after transfer. The PT is median-nerve innervated and therefore is unsuitable for this transfer. The BR is difficult to reeducate and usually is not transferred in median nerve palsy. The EIP tendon is commonly used for transfer but is not strong enough to provide real power for finger flexion, thumb adduction, or replacement of the first DI muscle.

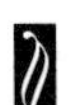
Answer: **A**
Brand, Hollister, pp. 214-215, 322-323

41. Match each opposition transfer with the surgeon(s) for which it is named.

Surgeon

1. Royle-Thompson
2. Huber
3. Bunnell
4. Phalen/Miller
5. Camitz

Opposition Transfer

A. ECU to the thumb through the pisiform/FCU pulley
B. Ring finger FDS to the thumb through the pisiform/FCU pulley
C. PL to the thumb
D. Ring finger FDS to the thumb MCP joint
E. Abductor digiti minimi to the thumb MCP joint

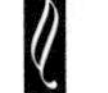
Answers: **1, D; 2, E; 3, B; 4, A; 5, C**
Davis, Barton in Green, Hotchkiss, Pederson, pp. 1498-1525

42. Which tendon transfer would best replace the FPL after a high median nerve injury?

A. ECRL
B. ECRB
C. FCR
D. BR

A hand with a high median nerve palsy lacks the FPL, FDS, FDP to the index and middle fingers, PL, FCR, and the pronators. Major functional losses include opposition, flexion of the IP joint of the thumb, and flexion of the DIP joints of the index and middle fingers. An excellent transfer to regain thumb IP joint flexion is the BR to the FPL. The ECRL to the FDP of the index and middle fingers also is a useful transfer with this nerve palsy. Opposition transfers are presented in the previous question.

Answer: **D**

Hunter, Schneider, Mackin, p. 215
Skirven, Callahan in Mackin, Callahan, Skirven, et al, p. 619

43. A patient suffers a supracondylar humerus fracture. The patient developed a compartment syndrome of the forearm flexor compartment. On emergent fasciotomy, it is apparent to the surgical team that extensive ischemic necrosis has developed in the flexor compartment mass. Subsequent debridement, infarct excision, and contracture release leave no functioning flexor mechanism. To best restore finger flexion to this patient, which of the following procedures will be necessary? Hint: There is more than one answer.

A. Transfer of the ECRL to FDP tendons
B. Direct repair of the median nerve
C. Free neurotized muscle transfer with the gracilis muscle
D. Nerve grafting of the median nerve

In this situation, the muscles of the flexor-pronator mass have been lost. To restore function, the best option is either to transfer functioning extensor tendons or transfer a healthy functioning free neurotized muscle into place. The most common causes of muscle death in the forearm are direct injury and ischemic necrosis secondary to compartment syndrome.

For free muscle transfers to work, certain conditions must exist: full passive motion of the digits and wrist, stable wrist joint, intrinsic muscle function, viable tendons to connect, and undamaged local motor nerves. The most commonly used muscle transfer to the upper extremity is the gracilis. The donor nerve is the anterior division of the obturator nerve, and the donor artery is a branch of the medial femoral circumflex artery. The muscle and neurovascular bundle is harvested and then placed in the forearm. The muscle is connected to the local tendons, the artery is connected to a local artery, and the anterior division of the obturator nerve is connected to a viable motor nerve in the upper extremity.

Postoperatively, the wrist and fingers are splinted in flexion to put less tension on the repair. Postoperative 3 weeks, passive extension is begun by the therapist. As reinnervation develops, active flexion is performed. Finally, when ROM approaches normal, resistive exercises are begun.

Answer: **A, C**

Manklelow, Anastakis in Green, Hotchkiss, Pederson, pp. 1209-1212

44. A patient presents to your clinic with classic "wrist drop." Which nerve is injured?

A. Median nerve
B. Ulnar nerve
C. Musculocutaneous nerve
D. Radial nerve

In a patient with a radial nerve paralysis, the forearm is pronated in the classic "wrist drop" position (Fig. 16-11). The patient's grip strength is substantially reduced because the inactive wrist extensors create an unstable wrist and minimize the finger flexors' power. The patient also displays an inability to extend the fingers of the MCP joints, which prevents the grasp and release of large objects.

Answer: **D**

Hunter, Mackin, Callahan, p. 753
Golditz in Mackin, Callahan, Skirven, et al, p. 632
Reynolds in Mackin, Callahan, Skirven, et al, p. 821

45. True or False: In a high radial nerve palsy, wrist extension always should be restored by transferring the PT tendon into both the ECRL and ECRB tendon insertions.

The ECRL has a smaller moment arm for wrist extension than the ECRB, unless radial deviation also occurs. It is better to put the PT into only the ECRB (Fig. 16-12) or the patient will be forced into radial deviation every time he or she tries to extend the wrist. If one muscle has multiple insertions, all of the muscles will always move together. In high median and ulnar palsy, for example, the ECRL may be used to power all of the finger flexors. If one finger flexes, all will flex. If one is prevented from flexion by stiffness, none of the fingers will be able to flex.

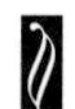

Answer: **False**

Brand, Hollister, pp. 75, 183
Green in Green, Hotchkiss, Pederson, p. 1488

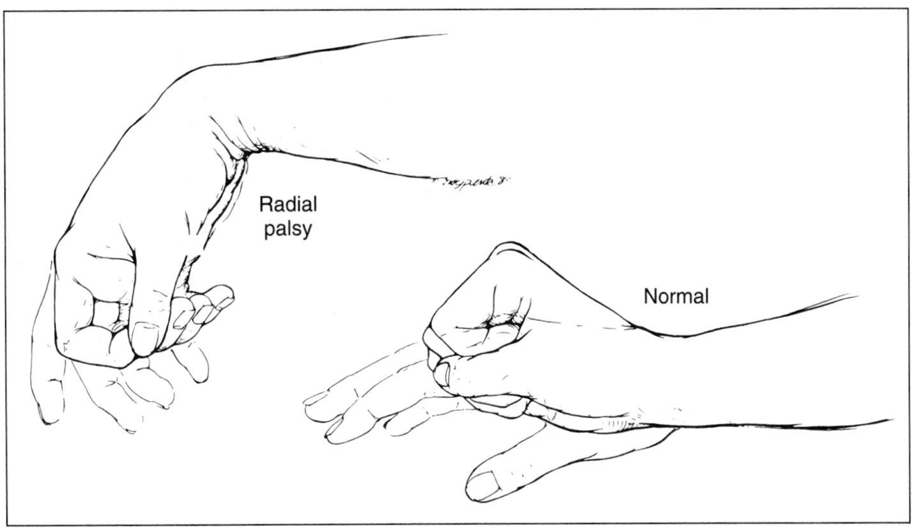

Fig. 16-11 ■ From Colditz J: *J Hand Ther* 1:19, 1987.

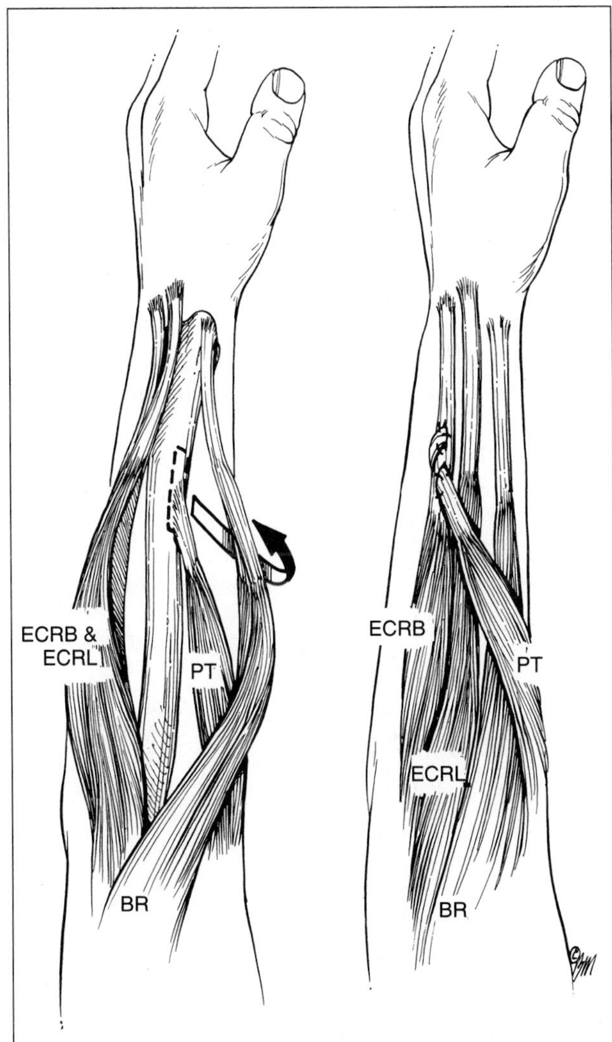

Fig. 16-12 ■ PT to ECRB transfer. It is important to take a strip of periosteum in continuity with the PT insertion to ensure adequate length for the transfer. (Copyright Elizabeth Roselius. From Green DP, Hotchkiss RN, Pederson WC: *Green's Operative hand surgery*, ed 4, New York, 1999, Churchill Livingstone.)

46. You are treating a patient with a radial nerve palsy and you note that he is able to supinate. You recall your anatomy and remember that the supinator is innervated by the radial nerve. Why is this patient still able to supinate?

A. The PT can act as a supinator
B. The FCR can act as a supinator
C. The biceps brachii can act as a supinator
D. The PL can act as a supinator

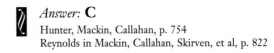

The patient is still able to supinate despite the radial nerve palsy because of the action of the biceps brachii. This muscle is innervated by the musculocutaneous nerve; therefore supination is not completely lost even with the loss of the supinator muscle. To eliminate the biceps and assess the supinator function, the therapist should extend the elbow completely before evaluating the supinator's function.

Answer: **C**
Hunter, Mackin, Callahan, p. 754
Reynolds in Mackin, Callahan, Skirven, et al, p. 822

47. A patient with cerebral palsy (CP) has severe bilateral wrist and finger flexion contractures and thumb-in-palm deformity. Occupational therapy, night splints, and botulinum toxin injections have all failed to improve the patient's low level of hand function. Local hygiene has become difficult because of the contractures. At this point, which of the following procedures should the surgeon perform?

A. FDS to FDP transfer (superficialis to profundus [STP] transfer)
B. FPL lengthening
C. Release/lengthening of the AP, first dorsal interosseous, FPB, FPL
D. Transfer of the BR, PL, FDS to improve thumb abduction and extension
E. A and B

In addition to flexion deformity of the wrists and fingers and thumb-in-palm deformity, patients with severe CP will also often have pronated forearms, flexed elbows, and internally rotated and adducted shoulders.

In severe contractures, when the fingers cannot be passively extended even with the wrist fully flexed, the STP transfer should be considered. The superficialis tendons are transected distally and the profundus tendons are divided proximally and then sutured to one another, thus providing a single lengthened digital flexor for each finger. However, in patients with functional hands, the STP transfer should not be performed because it will significantly decrease grip strength.

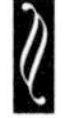
Answer: **E**
Topper, p. 341

48. A patient is referred to the hand therapist after a recent tendon transfer. Which of the following needs to be considered in the postoperative treatment protocol?

A. Edema reduction measures
B. Gentle passive ROM
C. Active-assisted ROM
D. Activities to restore function and coordination
E. All of the above

For most tendon transfers, small, gentle, passive ROM exercises are begun 3 to 4 days to 1 week postoperatively. This prevents adhesion formation and loss of ROM. This also allows the development of a new mesotenon of appropriate length at a time when the fibrovascular tissue is still immature. Over the first 2 weeks, sessions should be four times a day with gradual increase in the magnitude of the motion.

At 3 to 4 postoperative weeks, after adequate passive ROM is attained, neuromuscular reeducation is initiated. The therapist asks the patient to perform the motion the transferred muscle originally performed. The therapist blocks this motion, while the new motion is appreciated by the patient. Eventually, the new motion for this muscle is ingrained in the patient. As soon as these motions are mastered, functional training is begun. Active-assisted training is slowly incorporated with increased resistance. At 6 to 8 weeks, prolonged stretching (10 to 20 minutes four times per day) is also incorporated.

Answer: **E**
Kottke, Stillwell, Lehmann, pp. 833-834

49. What muscle is most commonly used to restore extension of the wrist after radial nerve palsy?

A. FCR
B. FCU
C. PT
D. PL

One "standard" set of tendon transfers for radial nerve palsy is the PT to the ECRB (refer to Fig. 16-12), the FCU to the EDC (Fig. 16-13) two through five, and the PL to the extensor pollicis longus EPL (see part *A* of the following Clinical Gem). However, the best combination of transfers has not been agreed upon.

Some authors feel that the sublimis tendon is a more ideal tendon for finger extensors, by using the third FDS tendon to the EDC, the fourth FDS to power the EPL and EIP, and the FCR to power the EPB and APL is an alternative method of transfer. The PT is still used to power the ECRL and ECRB (Clinical Gem, part *B*).

Another set of authors uses the following combinations: the PT to the ECRB; the FCR to the EDC; and the PL to the EPL (Clinical Gem, part *C*).

These three sets of tendon transfers currently are considered the most feasible alternatives.

Answer: **C**
Green, p. 1488

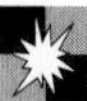
CLINICAL GEM:
The following is quick reference to radial nerve tendon transfers:

(A) PT to ECRB
FCU to EDC
PL to EPL
(B) PT to ECRB, ECRL
Middle FDS to EDC
Ring FDS to EPL and EIP
FCR to EPB and APL
(C) PT to ECRB
FCR to EDC
PL to EPL

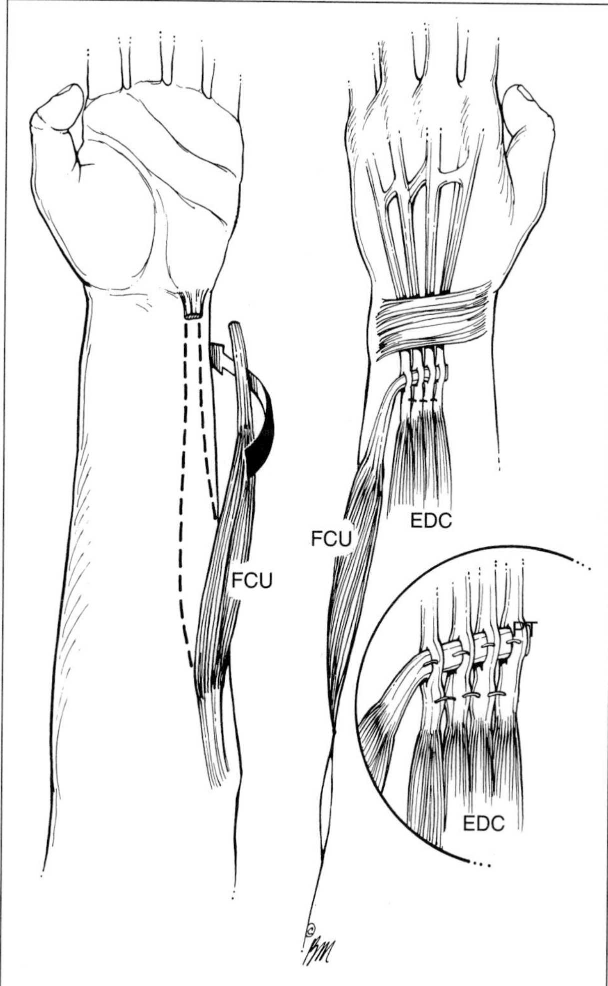

Fig. 16-13 ■ FCU to EDC transfer. The FCU must be freed up extensively to create a direct line of pull from its origin to the new insertion into the EDC tendons just proximal to the dorsal retinaculum. End-to-side juncture is shown here. Moberg and Nachemson have suggested that 4 to 5 cm of the paralyzed EDC tendons be resected proximal to the juncture, thus allowing an end-to-end suture and a more direct line of pull. (Copyright Elizabeth Roselius. From Green DP, Hotchkiss RN, Pederson WC: *Green's Operative hand surgery*, ed 4, New York, 1999, Churchill Livingstone.)

50. After a radial nerve tendon transfer, in which position should the arm be immobilized?

A. Elbow flexed to 90 degrees; forearm pronated; wrist extended 30 to 45 degrees; MCP joints neutral; and IP joints free

B. Elbow flexed to 30 degrees; forearm supinated; wrist extended 30 to 45 degrees; MCP joints neutral; and IP joints free

C. Elbow flexed to 70 degrees; forearm supinated; wrist extended 50 to 60 degrees; MCP joints neutral; and IP joints free

D. Elbow flexed to 90 degrees; forearm pronated; wrist at neutral; MCP joints neutral; and IP joints free

After tendon transfers of the wrist and digital extensors, the extensors of the arm are usually immobilized in a cast for 4 weeks. The typical position of immobilization is with the elbow flexed to 90 degrees, the forearm pronated naturally, the wrist extended 30 to 45 degrees, the MCP joints extended to neutral, and the IP joints free. If transfers were completed for the thumb, the thumb also is immobilized, with the IP and MCP joints completely extended, and the thumb abducted and extended at the carpometacarpal joint.

The purpose of a long-arm cast is to prevent supination of the forearm and protect the PT transfer. This position takes tension off of the tendon transfers, thus allowing healing to occur without overstretching or rupturing transfers. Four weeks after surgery, reeducation exercises are initiated. A custom-made, removable splint is fabricated at this time to protect transfers between exercise sessions. The splint is used for an additional 3 to 4 weeks.

Four weeks after surgery, the focus should be on MCP joint flexion to avoid debilitating extension contractures. In the second week of rehabilitation (5 weeks postoperatively), the focus should be on the tendon transfers themselves. Reeducation is challenged most when finger flexors are transferred to finger extensors. Exceptional patient concentration and cooperation are needed to achieve extension of the digits when sublimis transfers are used. Seven weeks after surgery, dynamic or static progressive splinting can be initiated if there is a need to increase flexion of the MCP joint. At 8 weeks after surgery, protective splinting is discontinued and resistive exercises are initiated.

Answer: **A**

Hunter, Mackin, Callahan, p. 758
Reynolds in Mackin, Callahan, Skirven, et al, p. 827

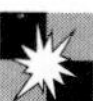

CLINICAL GEM:
Because of the limited tendon excursion, the ability to simultaneously extend the fingers and wrist is *not* possible after a radial nerve palsy tendon transfer (FCU to EDC). Hence the patient uses the tenodesis effect by active volar flexion of the wrist to enhance the excursion to achieve active extension of fingers (Fig. 16-14).

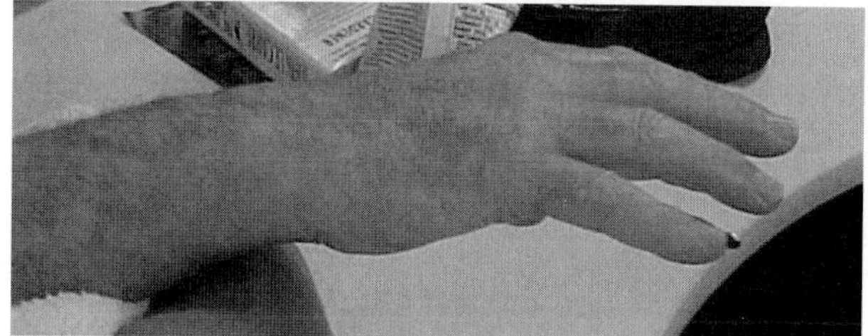

Fig. 16-14 ■ Courtesy Dr. Marvin Susskind.

51. You are evaluating a patient with a nerve palsy. During your evaluation, the patient reveals a positive Froment's sign. Which nerve is injured?

A. Median
B. Radial
C. Ulnar
D. Musculocutaneous

A positive Froment's sign occurs in a patient with an ulnar nerve palsy. A Froment's test is performed by putting a piece of paper between the thumb and the radial side of the index finger, using the lateral pinch. While the paper is being grasped, the thumb IP joint hyperflexes to hold or stabilize the paper because of the imbalance from lost intrinsic muscles. Usually lost are half of the FPB, the first DI, and the AP muscles.

Answer: **C**

Hunter, Mackin, Callahan, p. 733
Bell-Krotoski in Mackin, Callahan, Skirven, et al, p. 804
Refer to Figs. 16-5 and 16-15

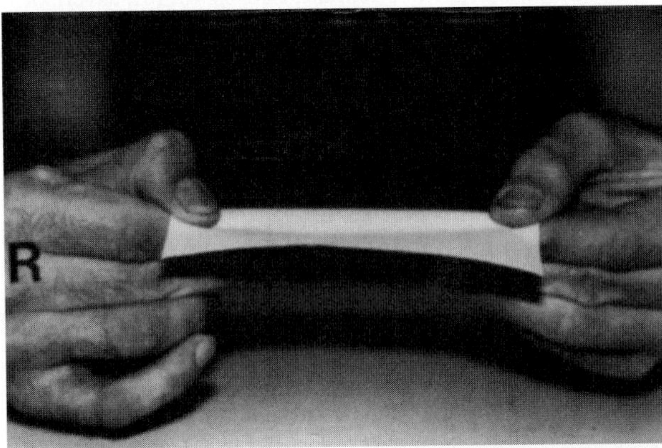

Fig. 16-15 ■ Right hand demonstrates a positive Froment's sign. (From Mackin EJ, Callahan AD, Skirven TM, et al: *Rehabilitation of the hand and upper extremity*, ed 5, vol 2, St Louis, 2002, Mosby.)

52. You are treating a patient 6 months after a complete ulnar nerve laceration 3 inches proximal to the wrist. The patient does not exhibit clawing. Why doesn't the patient exhibit clawing?

A. Patient stretches regularly
B. Patient has a Riche Cannieu anastomosis
C. Patient has made an internal splint using stronger tendons to overcome the clawing
D. None of the above

A Riche Cannieu anastomosis is a connection between the motor branch of the ulnar nerve and the recurrent branch of the median nerve in the hand. This anomalous neural pattern permits a hand to present without deformity, even with a complete ulnar nerve palsy. There is no clawing in the digits if the median nerve innervates all of the lumbricals and interossei through the Riche Cannieu anastomosis.

Answer: **B**

Green, p. 1450

53. After repair of a nerve, what is the estimated rate of nerve regeneration?

A. 1 mm/day
B. 1 mm/week
C. 1 mm/month
D. 1 cm/day

Seddon published data that show repaired nerves will regenerate at a rate of approximately 1 mm/day. Based on these data, more proximal nerve injuries will take a longer time to recover because they have a further distance to travel. This number is also important because it allows the surgeon and therapist to estimate the amount of time nerve recovery will require. If the nerve has not recovered in its predicted time frame, it is likely that the repair has failed and tendon transfer surgery is indicated. Nerve regeneration often can be followed clinically by a Tinel's sign, a tingling sensation elicited in the regenerating nerve end by tapping on the skin.

Answer: **A**

Green in Green, Hotchkiss, Pederson, p. 1485
Spinner, p. 28

54. Successful treatments for the intrinsic minus hand include which of the following?

A. Dorsal MCP joint blocking splints
B. FDS to A1 pulley attachment
C. FDS to lateral bands attachment
D. All of the above

The intrinsic minus hand deformity is called *claw hand* because the extensor tendons overact in an attempt to extend the fingers. The ulnar paralyzed intrinsic muscles are unable to stabilize the MCP joints on the flexor side (refer to Fig. 16-4, Question 13). Anything that limits extension of the MCP joints—including splinting, capsulodesis, or even a scar on the palm—can assist the long extensors in extending the PIP joints. Unless they are controlled, almost all cases of low ulnar palsy develop into a progressive deformity because the unopposed extensor pull stretches the volar plate, skin, and other soft tissues over time. There often is a delay in correcting the clawing because the deformity is not apparent at first. If the FDS is attached to the A1 pulley, it serves as a tenodesis to hold the MCP joints just short of full extension. Likewise, the FDS may be attached to the lateral bands so that it becomes a PIP joint extensor and MCP joint flexor.

Answer: **D**
Brand, Hollister, pp. 189, 203-204
Colditz in Mackin, Callahan, Skirven, et al, pp. 624-627

55. Which of the following procedures uses a "lasso" technique to correct clawing in ulnar nerve palsy?

A. Huber
B. Camitz
C. Royle-Thompson
D. Zancolli

The Zancolli technique uses the FDS in a "lasso" procedure through a transverse incision at the level of the distal palmar crease. The proximal pulley (A1) of the flexor sheaths is exposed, and the FDS tendons are used in sections and divided into two slips for each finger. Each tendon slip is volarly retained to the deep transverse metacarpal ligament and looped through the A1 pulley and sutured to itself. The MCP joint is pulled down into approximately 45 degrees of flexion. This transfer should be carried out to all four fingers because weakness is not limited to the clawing fingers.

All of the other transfers listed as choices are used for median nerve palsy to restore opposition.

Answer: **D**
Omer in Green, Hotchkiss, Pederson, pp. 1530-1531

56. Which function is lost after low ulnar nerve palsy?

A. Lateral or key pinch
B. Proficient grip
C. Tip pinch
D. All of the above

With a low ulnar nerve palsy, a patient displays a loss of flexion of the proximal phalanges from paralysis of the interossei and other intrinsic muscles. Clawing results from the extrinsic muscles hyperextending the proximal phalanges and from the pull of the proximally innervated FDP, which contributes to poor grasp. A flat metacarpal arch, which also contributes to poor grasp, may be noted with ulnar nerve palsy because of the paralysis of the opponens digiti quinti and the decreased range of the little finger MCP joint. Loss of lateral or key pinch of the thumb is caused by paralysis of the AP muscle. The patient also loses distal stability and rotation for tip pinch between the thumb and index finger. This loss is caused by paralysis of the first dorsal and second palmar interossei as well as the AP muscle.

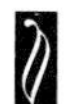
Answer: **D**
Green, pp. 1526-1541
Colditz in Mackin, Callahan, Skirven, et al, pp. 624-626

57. Which of the following is not innervated by the PIN?

A. ECRL
B. EDC
C. Extensor digiti minimi (EDM)
D. APL

The radial nerve proper innervates the BR, ECRL, ECRB, and anconeus. It then branches into a purely sensory superficial branch of the radial nerve and the PIN. The PIN innervates the EDC, EDM, ECU, supinator, APL, EPB, EPL, and EIP. Some authors believe the ECRB can also be innervated by the PIN. Knowledge of radial nerve anatomy is essential to determine the location of the injury as well as the appropriate treatment.

Answer: **A**
Green in Green, Hotchkiss, Pederson, p. 1481

58. The median innervates all but which of the following intrinsic muscles of the hand?

A. APB
B. OP
C. First and second interossei
D. First and second lumbricals

The ulnar nerve innervates most of the intrinsic muscles of the hand. However, the median nerve also contributes to the innervation of intrinsic muscle of the hand. In particular, the median nerve innervates the APB, OP, and first and second lumbricals. The FPB has a dual innervation by the median as well as the ulnar nerve in most individuals. Anatomic studies suggest some variation of thenar musculature innervation. One study states the median nerve supplies all three muscles in 63% of hands and only the APB and OP in 30% of hands. Others claim the superficial head of the FPB has a dual innervation in 30%, whereas the deep head of the FPB has a dual innervation in 79% and a sole ulnar nerve innervation in 19% of hands. It is important to understand the variability in innervation, as this explains why thumb abduction and opposition can be maintained after median nerve injury in some individuals.

Answer: **C**

Davis, Barton in Green, Hotchkiss, Pederson, p. 1497
Olave, Prates, Del Sol, pp. 441-446

59. Which of the following structures is not innervated by the ulnar nerve?

A. FCU
B. AP
C. Third lumbrical
D. Second lumbrical

Although anomalous nerve patterns are described, it is important to know all the muscles the ulnar nerve innervates. Such knowledge allows the surgeon and therapist to understand what deficit the patient has and what needs to be replaced with surgery and subsequent therapy.

The ulnar nerve begins in the shoulder as a terminal branch of the medial cord of the brachial plexus. At the arm, it passes from the anterior compartment to the posterior compartment by passing through the intermuscular septum. It then passes behind the medial epicondyle of the elbow and enters the flexor carpi ulnaris in the proximal forearm. The FCU is first muscle the ulnar nerve innervates. In the forearm, the ulnar half of the FDP is also innervated by the ulnar nerve. In the hand, all the intrinsic muscles of the hand are innervated by the ulnar nerve with a few exceptions (APB, OP, first and second lumbrical, FPB [partial innervation with ulnar nerve]). These ulnar nerve intrinsic muscles include the palmaris brevis, adductor digiti minimi (ADM), flexor digiti minimi (FDM), opponens digiti minimi (ODM), third and fourth lumbricals, interossei, and AP.

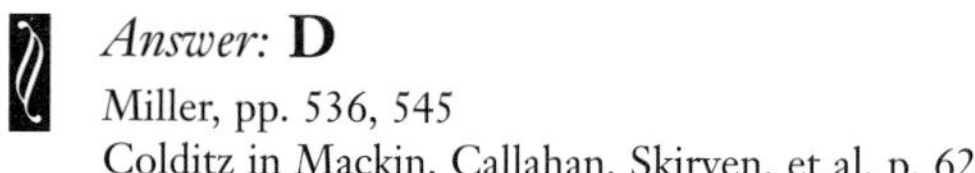

Answer: **D**

Miller, pp. 536, 545
Colditz in Mackin, Callahan, Skirven, et al, p. 626

60. To treat a patient with an ulnar nerve peripheral neuropathy, which splint should be applied?

A. Passive MCP joint flexion splint to the ring and small fingers
B. Passive MCP joint flexion splint to the index and middle fingers
C. Passive MCP joint extension splint to the index and small fingers
D. Passive MCP joint extension to the ring and small fingers

After ulnar nerve injury, the splint should focus on restoring the longitudinal arch by providing a means of passive MCP joint flexion to the ring and small fingers (Fig. 16-16). After MCP joint flexion is established, the intact extrinsic finger extensors are actively able to extend the IP joints of the fourth and fifth fingers, thus reducing the risk of IP joint flexion contractures. If the patient already has IP joint contractures, serial casting is an effective means of improving passive ROM. Prevention is the best means of intervention when treating a patient with ulnar nerve paralysis or any nerve palsy (see Fig. 1, p. 349).

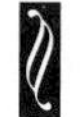

Answer: **A**

Hunter, Schneider, Mackin, p. 97
Mackin, Callahan, Skirven, et al, p. 626

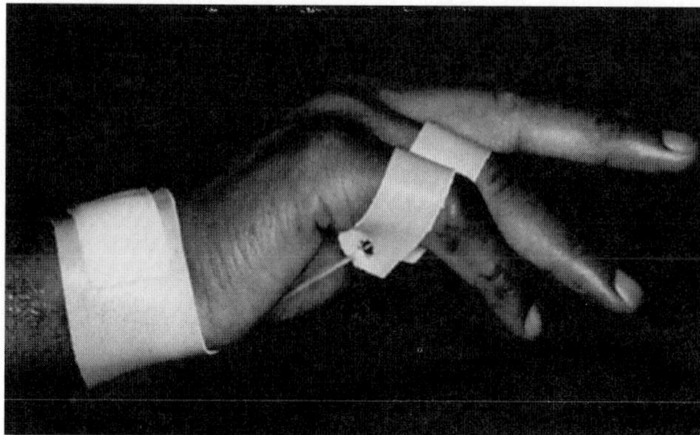

Fig. 16-16 ■ An ulnar palsy splint may be made of leather wrist and finger cuffs with a static line to block MCP hyperextension. (From Mackin EJ, Callahan AD, Skirven TM, et al: *Rehabilitation of the hand and upper extremity*, ed 5, vol 2, St Louis, 2002, Mosby.)

61. In median nerve palsy, what soft tissue contractures of the thumb should be anticipated?

A. Adduction
B. Supination
C. Abduction
D. B and C
E. A and B

Patients with median nerve palsy develop adduction and supination contractures of the thumb. Contractures can be prevented with passive thumb abduction and opposition exercises and by abduction splints. Established soft tissue contractures need to be corrected before opponensplasty by therapy, splinting, or surgical release.

Answer: **E**

Davis, Barton in Green, Hotchkiss, Pederson, p. 1498

62. What type of splint would you use for a patient to assist with prehension tasks after a radial nerve palsy occurs in his dominant hand?

A. Dorsal spring coil wrist extension splint
B. Low-profile dynamic splint with thumb, MCP joint, and wrist extension assist components
C. Volar-based wrist support orthotic
D. Dynamic MCP joint extension assist splint

A variety of splints have been designed for radial nerve palsy. In some instances, a simple cock-up wrist splint will do (volar-based wrist support). Other splints available include those with outriggers to provide dynamic finger (Fig. 16-17) and thumb extension to enhance hand function while awaiting nerve recovery or tendon transfer surgery. The best answer is B because it includes thumb, finger, and wrist extension (see Fig. 16-17). However, keep in mind the patient's functional needs. Usually, if the nondominant hand is involved, a simple wrist support splint is sufficient. If the patient's dominant hand is involved, a dynamic assist splint is a good option in addition to a wrist support splint. However, most patients find the dynamic splints bulky for continuous wear.

Answer: **B**

McKee, Morgan pp. 112-114
Skirven, Callahan in Mackin, Callahan, Skirven, et al, pp. 610-615

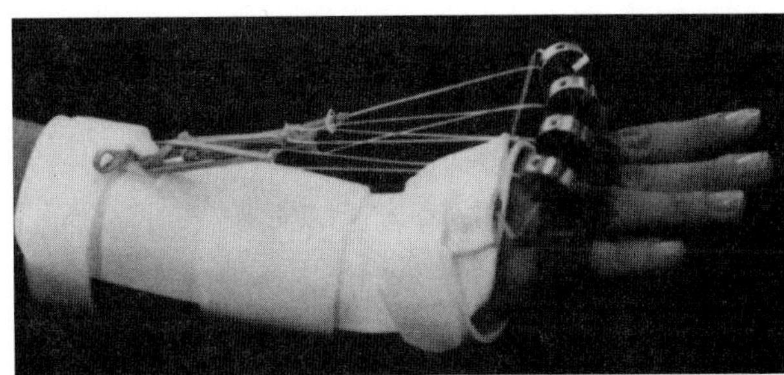

Fig. 16-17 ■ From Stanley BG, Tribuzi SM: *Concepts in hand rehabilitation,* Philadelphia, 1992, FA Davis.

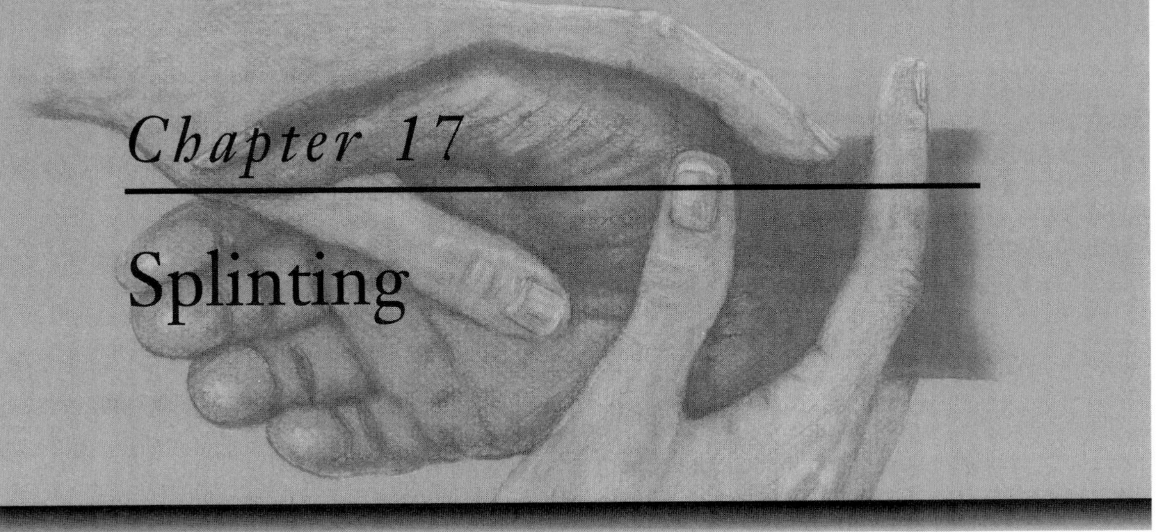

Chapter 17

Splinting

1. In a coaptation circuit splint or device that is intended to flex fingers, joint mobilization occurs in which of the following ways?

A. From proximal to distal
B. From distal to proximal
C. From stiffest to softest joint
D. Randomly

A coaptation circuit splint or device works like a flexion glove (Fig. 17-1, *A*), which allows all involved joints to be mobilized together, but because the segments are of different sizes, the largest (the metacarpophalangeal [MCP]) is mobilized first. After the MCP joint has achieved maximum flexion, it should be removed from the circuit to allow the distal joints to flex further (Fig. 17-1, *B*).

Answer: **A**
Van Lede, van Veldhoven, pp. 22-33
Fess in Mackin, Callahan, Skirven, et al, pp. 1821-1823

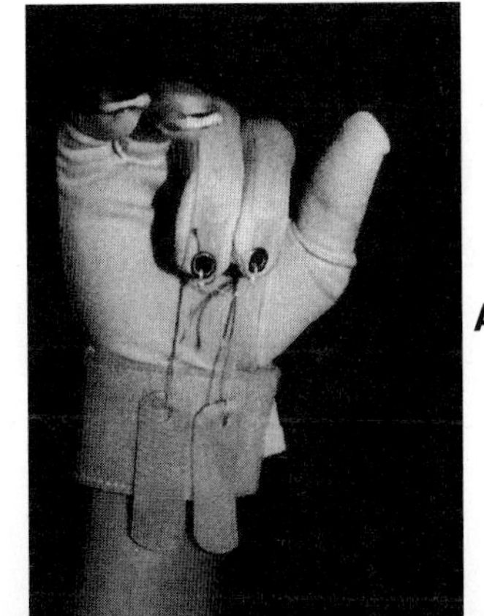

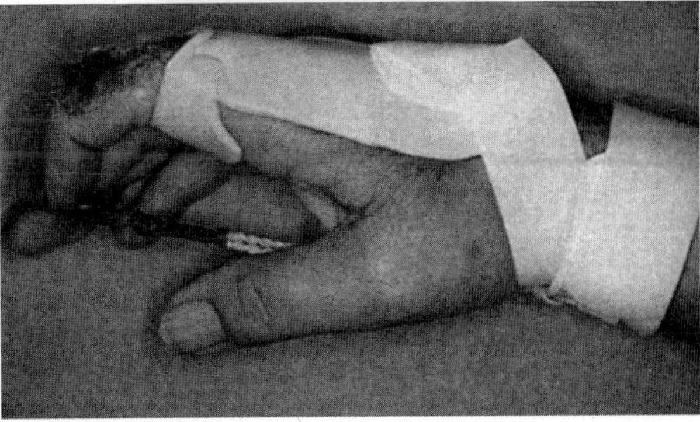

Fig. 17-1 ■ **A,** A flexion glove is a form of a coaptation circuit splint that is designed to flex the digits from the MCP joint to the distal interphalangeal (DIP) joint (proximal to distal). **B,** The normal MCP joint is immobilized in this IP flexion mobilization splint, type 1, thus allowing the flexion force to be directed to the IP joints. (**A** From Jacobs MA, Austin NM: *Splinting the hand and upper extremity: principles and process*, Baltimore, 2003, Lippincott Williams & Wilkins; **B** from Fess EE, Philips CA: *Hand splinting: principles and methods*, ed 2, St Louis, 1987, Mosby.)

2. True or False: To extend a flexed stiff finger joint, a dorsal splint is not appropriate because of the high pressure on the joint.

To extend a flexed finger joint, some pressure on the dorsal aspect of the joint is inevitable. If the pressure per square centimeter is intolerable, it suffices to increase the surface area. Proper anatomical molding of the splint material with padding (prepadding before molding) assists in decreasing pressure.

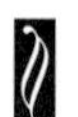

Answer: **False**

Van Lede, van Veldhoven, pp. 62, 68, 143-145
Wilton, Dival, p. 53

3. Patients appreciate circumferential splints because they are which of the following?

A. Lightweight (thin)
B. Comfortable
C. Stable
D. All of the above

Circumferential splints (Fig. 17-2) immobilize joints in all planes of motion, and because of the cylindrical shape they are stable in all planes. They are made out of thin, flexible material and are lightweight and comfortable.

Answer: **D**

Van Lede, van Veldhoven, p. 66
Wilton, Dival, p. 63
McKee, Morgan, p. 53

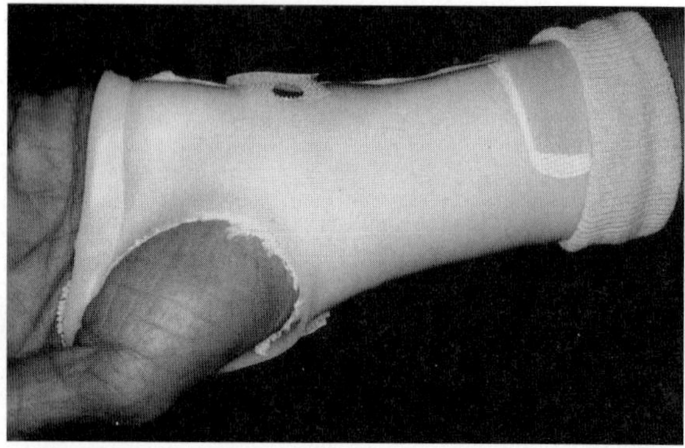

Fig. 17-2 ■ Courtesy Judy C. Colditz, OTR/L, CHT, FAOTA, HandLab, a Division of RHRC, Inc.

4. True or False: Material that is not drapeable enough will cause folds/creases in areas such as the elbow.

When thermoplastics are heated, the polymers come loose and allow shifting into a third dimension, which is necessary to conform to the anatomical shape of the body. A splint material that is not drapeable enough will end up with folds/creases in areas such as the elbow. Materials that are *not* drapeable should not be used to make cylindrical splints because pressure points can easily develop.

Answer: **True**

Van Lede, van Veldhoven, p. 83
McKee, Morgan, pp. 72-73
Refer to Fig. 17-3

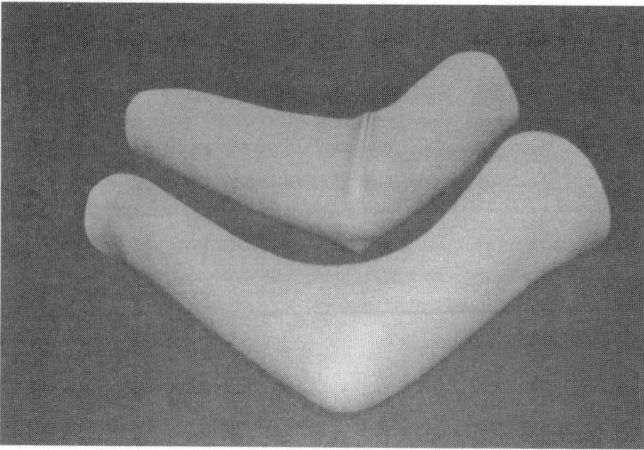

Fig. 17-3 ■ From van Lede P, van Veldhoven G: *Therapeutic hand splints: a rational approach*, Antwerp, 1998, Provan.

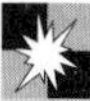

CLINICAL GEM:
Paradoxically, materials that are nonmoldable or have less drape are easy to handle and are often preferred by beginners or inexperienced splint makers.

5. True or False: Dynamic splinting approaches require more time to gain motion than static progressive approaches to produce an increase in range of motion (ROM).

Clinical experience reported by Shultz-Johnson has shown that dynamic approaches to splinting require more time to gain motion than static progressive approaches do. Static progressive approaches to passive ROM limitations offer the fastest results without additional tissue trauma. The therapist can also design splints that combine approaches.

Answer: **True**

Jacobs, Austin, p. 295

6. Which of the following is *not* a contraindication to mobilization splinting?

A. Acute inflammation
B. Infection
C. Myositis ossificans
D. All are contraindications.

Common contraindications to mobilization splinting include all of the above as well as joint instability, avascular necrosis, unstable fractures, demineralisation, heterotopic ossification, exostosis formation, and a loose body in the joint.

Answer: **D**
Fess in Mackin, Callahan, Skirven, et al, pp. 1827-1829

7. Which of the following is a disadvantage of using plaster of Paris in splinting?

A. It is nonconforming.
B. Pressure points are more likely to develop.
C. Chance of skin maceration is increased.
D. It is not water-resistant.

All of the above statements are false except statement D. Plaster of Paris is conforming; this minimizes the chance that the patient will develop pressure points. It also allows for adequate circulation of air, which minimizes skin maceration. The major disadvantage of plaster of Paris is that it is not water-resistant. When it becomes wet it softens and loses its strength and integrity.

Answer: **D**
Tribuzi in Mackin, Callahan, Skirven, et al, p. 1829

8. Match each arch of the hand with the correct definition.

Arch

1. Longitudinal arch
2. Distal transverse arch
3. Proximal transverse arch

Definition

A. Consists of the distal row of carpal bones. It is rigid and acts as a stable pivot point for the wrist and long finger flexor muscles.
B. Deepens with flexion of the fingers, is mobile, and passes through the metacarpal heads
C. Allows distal interphalangeal (DIP) joints, proximal interphalangeal (PIP) joints, and MCP joints to flex

Answers: **1, C; 2, B; 3, A**
Coppard, Lohman, pp. 50-51
Refer to Fig. 17-4

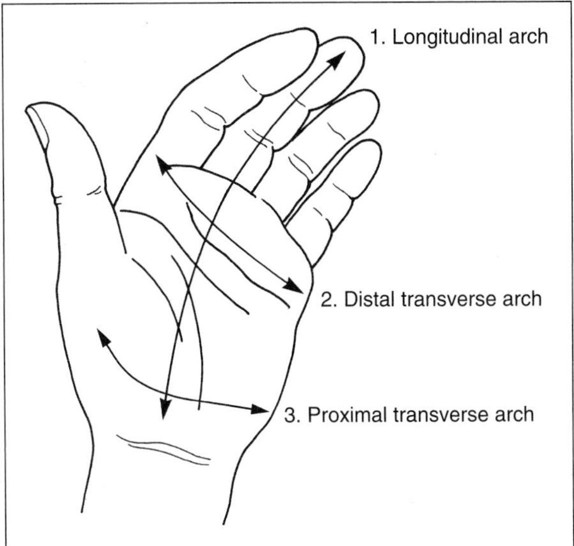

Fig. 17-4 ■ From Coppard BM, Lohman H: *Introduction to splinting: a clinical-reasoning and problem-solving approach,* ed 2, St Louis, 2001, Mosby.

9. True or False: The proximal palmar crease is an important landmark for splinting a patient in a wrist support splint.

The skin on the volar aspect of the hand is thick, tough, and inflexible. These characteristics (especially the inflexibility) account for palmar creases. The distal palmar crease is an important landmark for splinting because it marks the distal edge for splint application when applying a wrist support splint. When the splint is positioned proximal to this crease, it allows for full MCP joint flexion. Below the distal palmar crease is the proximal palmar crease, which is not a significant landmark for splinting in a wrist support.

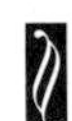

Answer: **False**
Coppard, Lohman, p. 51
Malick, p. 16
Refer to Fig. 17-5

10. True or False: Open-cell padding is nonabsorbent.

The two basic types of padding are open- and closed-cell foam. Closed-cell foam is nonabsorbent and is easily washed and towel-dried. A therapist can apply closed-cell foam padding to thermoplastic material before molding. This is important to know when planning splint fabrication because padding may cause the splint

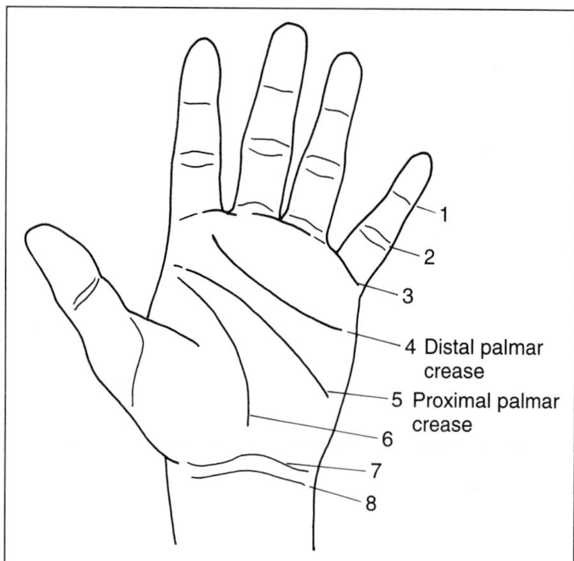

Fig. 17-5 ■ Creases of the hand. *1,* Distal digital crease; *2,* middle digital crease; *3,* proximal digital crease; *4,* distal palmar crease; *5,* proximal palmar crease; *6,* thenar crease; *7,* distal wrist crease; *8,* proximal wrist crease. (From Coppard BM, Lohman H: *Introduction to splinting: a clinical-reasoning and problem-solving approach*, ed 2, St Louis, 2001, Mosby.)

to be tighter, thus compromising the fit. For example, if 1/16-inch padding is added after fabrication, the splint will be 1/16 of an inch too tight. Open-cell padding absorbs moisture; therefore it is more difficult to keep clean and can be a breeding ground for bacteria. Open-cell padding usually is softer and more conforming than closed-cell padding.

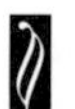

Answer: **False**
Coppard, Lohman, p. 238

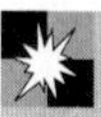

CLINICAL GEM:
Samons Preston Rolyan has splint material with pre-embedded padding for convenience and comfort.

11. When treating joint contractures with static progressive splinting, what mechanical phenomenon occurs?

A. Creep
B. Stress relaxation
C. Viscoelasticity
D. Shear fracture

Stress relaxation is the continued decrease in stress needed to maintain a given deformation. Stress relaxation occurs over time when tissues are stretched and held at *constant length*, such as in static progressive splinting.

Creep results from stretching tissue under a *constant load* and is the continued deformation of a material under constant stress. Creep occurs with dynamic splinting.

Viscoelasticity is a combination of both viscous and elastic properties and is characterized by hysteresis. Hysteresis occurs when an elastic material immediately springs back to its original shape after stretch or compression. A viscoelastic material returns to its original shape more slowly.

Answer: **B**
Brand, Hollister, pp. 6, 7, 21, 98, 101-105

CLINICAL GEM:
Studies have indicated that when stress relaxation is employed, a viscoelastic material becomes softer or more pliable sooner than when creep or dynamic splinting is employed.

12. The application of the splint in Fig. 17-6 uses what theory of tissue elongation?

A. Creep
B. Stress relaxation
C. TERT
D. None of the above

The Joint Active Systems splints (including the one in Fig. 17-6) use stress relaxation as it is the most efficient way to produce a permanent elongation of soft tissue. The accepted protocol requires wearing the splint three times a day for 30-minute sessions with incremental "tissue stress" or stretch increases.

Creep-based modality systems (dynamic splints) require a longer wearing time to create tissue change. Creep occurs after 8 to 12 hours of wear time.

Total end range time (TERT) is a concept popularized by Flowers and LaStayo that theorizes to promote tissue growth via the length of time a joint is held at its end range.

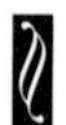

Answer: **B**
McKee, Morgan, pp. 4, 10, 27
Jacobs, Austin, pp. 50, 68, 449

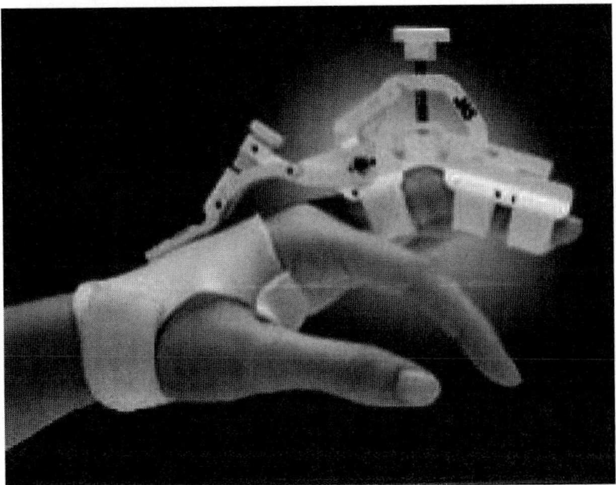

Fig. 17-6 ■ Static progressive (SPS) device. (Courtesy Joint Active Systems, Inc., Effingham, IL.)

13. True or False: Splinting materials with elastic properties have memory, thus allowing repeated remolding of the splint regardless of the time lapse evolved. The inconvenience of memory is that the splinting material tends to oppose the molding and makes contouring harder.

Memory is a combination of elasticity and activation and is not time-bound. Materials overstretch or tear when they lack cross-links or when cross-links have limited elasticity. Splints that are highly elastic are more difficult to mold and best used when there is a need for frequent remodeling. On the contrary, splints that have low elasticity overstretch easily and cannot be remolded frequently and repeatedly.

Answer: **True**
Van Lede, van Veldhoven, pp. 84-85
Jacobs, Austin, p. 80

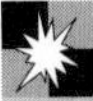

CLINICAL GEM:
High-elasticity splints tolerate fingerprints, whereas low-elasticity splints fingerprint easily. Coated elastic material can provide a temporary bond to help mold against gravity; once dried, it can easily be popped apart.

14. The most essential part of a dynamic splint is which of the following?

A. The gauge and length of the kinetic energy (spring/elastic)
B. The perfect contour of the base
C. The exact placement of the fixation straps
D. The height and length of the outrigger
E. The strength of the outrigger

Dynamic splints are used to substitute biodynamic deficiency (i.e., positioning the digits in extension for a radial nerve palsy) or to increase ROM. Both the power (gauge) and excursion possibilities (length) of the substitution item (rubber band/spring) are the essentials parts of a dynamic splint.

Answer: **A**
Van Lede, pp. 192-201
Refer to Fig. 17-7

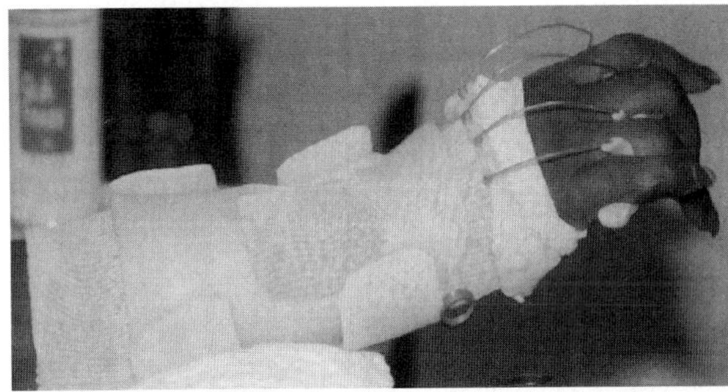

Fig. 17-7

15. True or False: Finger cuffs should always be made of soft material with a smooth surface.

Soft cuffs attached to single slings tend to tilt during movement, digging the edge into the flesh (Fig. 17-8, *A*). They also exert lateral pressure on the finger, which could impede blood flow. With rigid cuffs (Fig. 17-8, *B*), lateral pressure is avoided, and with a cuff attachment at the middle of the finger (see Fig. 17-8, *B*) tilting is prevented. If the cuff cannot slide, it can tilt, affecting the plane of support (Fig. 17-8, *C*).

Answer: **False**
Van Lede, van Veldhoven, pp. 121-122
Brand, Hollister, pp. 140-144

16. A patient with acute burns of the whole upper half of the body is brought to the hospital for treatment in a sterile room. Hand splints are

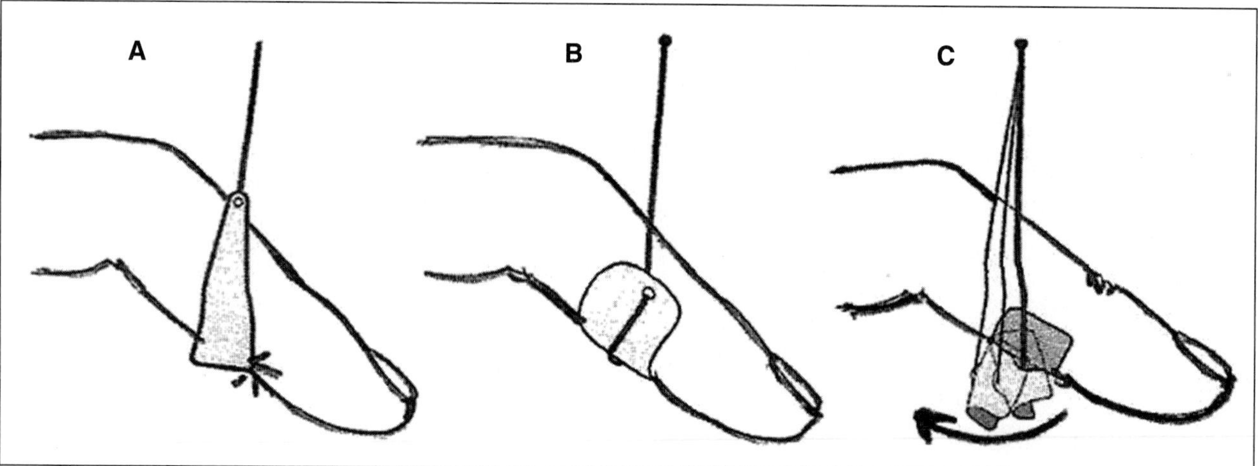

Fig. 17-8 ■ From van Lede P, van Veldhoven G: *Therapeutic hand splints: a rational approach*, Antwerp, 1998, Provan.

advocated to promote proper hand positioning. However, no splinting material is available, so it is decided to use a prefabricated design from the shelf rather than delay. True or False: This is a good decision.

Because of the stereotypical positioning of most burns and the voluminous dressing being changed every day, it makes sense to use a well-adapted prefabricated splint rather than delay the treatment and face dramatic contractures while waiting for splint material to arrive.

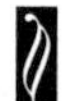
Answer: **True**
Van Lede, van Veldhoven, pp. 85, 91, 143
Jacobs, Austin, pp. 450-452

17. The length of a splint's forearm trough when fabricating a wrist extension splint should be approximately which of the following?

A. One fourth the length of the forearm
B. One half the length of the forearm
C. Two thirds the length of the forearm
D. Full length of the forearm

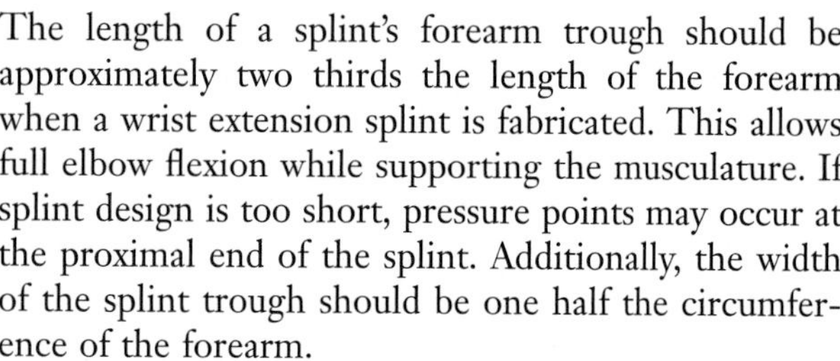

The length of a splint's forearm trough should be approximately two thirds the length of the forearm when a wrist extension splint is fabricated. This allows full elbow flexion while supporting the musculature. If splint design is too short, pressure points may occur at the proximal end of the splint. Additionally, the width of the splint trough should be one half the circumference of the forearm.

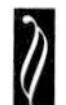
Answer: **C**
Coppard, Lohman, p. 60

CLINICAL GEM:
Because the dorsal musculature is firmer than the volar musculature, a shorter lever arm for a dorsal splint is allowed. Therefore dorsal splints do not have to be two thirds the length of the forearm.

18. All but which of the following are goals of static splinting?

A. Immobilization
B. Preventing deformity
C. Preventing soft-tissue contractures
D. All of the above are goals of static splinting.

The goals of static splinting include immobilizing joints to allow them to rest, thus preventing deformity progression by maintaining an improved position when the splint is applied and preventing soft-tissue contracture by positioning in a protective fashion. Static splints are used for patients with diagnoses such as rheumatoid arthritis, carpal tunnel syndrome, fractures, and soft-tissue repairs, to name a few. They are the most frequent splints therapists fabricate. If it is not contraindicated, static splints should be removed intermittently to perform ROM exercises to decrease stiff joints and associated complications.

Answer: **D**
Coppard, Lohman, pp. 4-9
Jacobs, Austin, p. 5

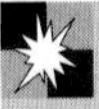

CLINICAL GEM:
When securing Velcro, carefully heat the sticky side of the Velcro and/or the splinting material for better adhesion.

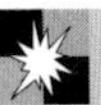

CLINICAL GEM:
Chlorine removes ink marks from splints.

19. You are treating a patient with a diagnosis of carpal tunnel syndrome. A wrist support splint is fabricated and applied. The patient returns to the clinic 2 days later with tenderness over the radial styloid. He removes the splint and the area is red. The redness persists for 30 minutes after splint removal and then subsides. What should be done in this situation?

A. Because the redness resolved in 30 minutes, it is acceptable. The splint should not be adjusted.
B. The splint should be padded around the radial styloid.
C. The splint should be flared out around the radial styloid.
D. The splint should be discontinued because it obviously is not working.

If redness persists around a bony prominence for 20 minutes or longer after splint removal, an adjustment is necessary to decrease pain and pressure on the soft tissue and to increase patient compliance. Padding a splint around the radial styloid without increasing the available space may actually increase pressure. Therefore in this case, the best option is to flare the splint out around the radial styloid.

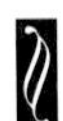

Answer: **C**
Coppard, Lohman, pp. 95-97

CLINICAL GEM:
The following is a quick reference to common pressure areas one must consider when fabricating splints:

- Dorsum of the MCP joints
- Head of the ulna
- Base of the thenar eminence
- Radial styloid
- Proximal end of a splint

20. True or False: Application of a small constant force has been shown to be beneficial when mobilizing joints.

Application of low amounts of constant force has been shown to be beneficial versus high, strong, damaging forces, causing ischemia and pain. Techniques that use strong damaging force can set up a vicious cycle of inflammation, increased scarring, and contractures proving detrimental to recovery.

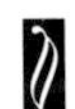

Answer: **True**
Fess, Philips, p. 59
Fess, Gettle, Philips, et al, pp. 96-99

21. True or False: Dynamic splints are best used when a patient has moderate to severe tissue contractures.

Dynamic or elastic splints are most effective in the early stages of joint stiffness. After a patient has moderate to severe tissue contractures, static progressive or serial static splinting will have better results.

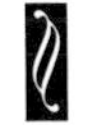

Answer: **False**
Fess, Gettle, Philips, et al, p. 109

22. You are treating a patient with a PIP joint flexion contracture of 50 degrees. You decide to fabricate a static progressive PIP joint extension splint with a low-profile outrigger. Two weeks later you remeasure the PIP joint and note a 10-degree increase in range. What should you do next?

A. Discard the splint because it already has helped sufficiently.
B. Leave the splint alone; it is working fine.
C. Modify the outrigger.
D. None of the above

Because the patient has shown a 10-degree increase in his ROM, the splint is no longer pulling at a 90-degree angle, and some element of joint compression or distraction may be occurring. The splint should be regularly modified to retain a perpendicular angle (90 degrees) of pull. It is important to know that when the outrigger is at a 90-degree angle of pull, the translational force is 0, thus resulting in an absence of joint compression or distraction. Splinting should be continued as long as the patient's ROM is improving.

Answer: **C**

Fess, Philips, p. 136

Refer to Fig. 17-9

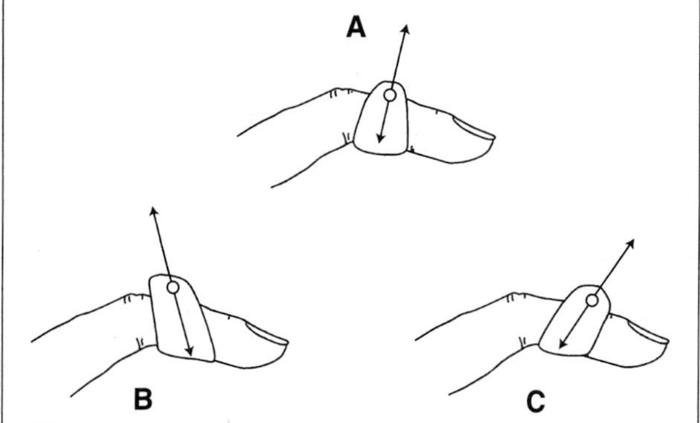

Fig. 17-9 ■ **A,** Angle of approach is 90 degrees to the middle phalanx, thus ensuring that force is not dissipated when the PIP joint is pulled into extension. **B,** An angle of approach less than 90 degrees to the axis of the middle phalanx compresses the joint. **C,** An angle of approach greater than 90 degrees to the axis of the middle phalanx distracts the joint. (From Pedretti LW, Early MB: *Occupational therapy: practice skills for physical dysfunction*, ed 5, St Louis, 2001, Mosby.)

23. You are treating a patient who has been provided with a thumb spica splint after a ligament reconstruction tendon interposition is performed. The patient complains of pain over the base of the thumb. True or False: The best way to relieve pressure over this area is to cut a hole in the splint over the area of pain.

A common mistake made by therapists is attempting to relieve pressure from a splint by cutting material away and leaving a hole. Cutting holes in splints to relieve pressure can result in greater forces around the circumferential border of the cut-out area. This creates a potential for soft tissue injury (Fig. 17-10). A better way to approach this problem is to *bubble out* the area over the bony prominence or problem area and pad the newly bubbled-out area if needed. When the splint in Fig. 17-10 was applied, it could have been assumed that the MCP area was going to be problematic due to edema from pin removal. The therapist can prevent this problem by adding a pad or piece of putty to the patient's potential problem area, thus *bubbling out* this area during splint fabrication. After the splint is fabricated, the pad or piece of putty should be removed from the potential problem area and discarded.

CLINICAL GEM:

The following is a quick reference to decreasing a pressure area:

- Mark the patient's skin over the pressure area with lipstick
- Reapply the splint
- Remove the splint
- Look for smudged lipstick on the splint
- Bubble out the smudged area with a heat gun
- Reapply the splint
- Reevaluate the pressure area

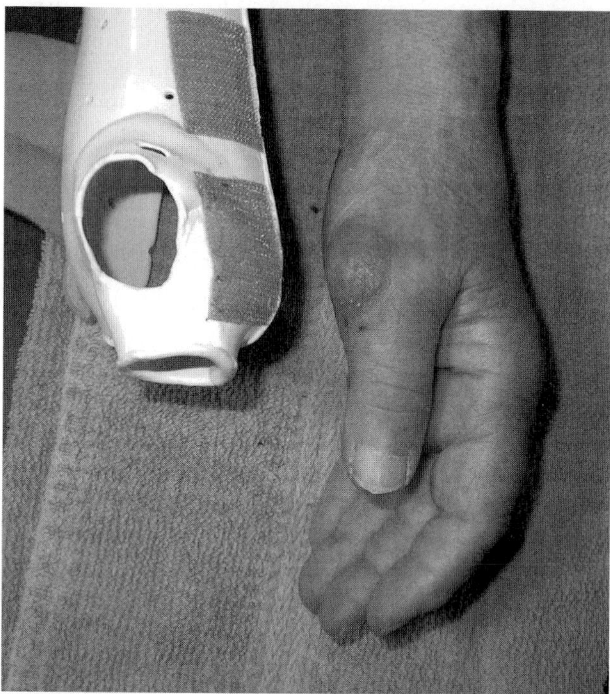

Fig. 17-10

Answer: **False**

Fess, Philips, p. 247

24. Which of the following is considered the safe position for fingers that have not undergone surgical repair but require immobilization after trauma?

A. MCP joints at 30 degrees of flexion and interphalangeal (IP) joints at 0 to 20 degrees of flexion

B. MCP joints at 80 degrees of flexion and IP joints at 30 to 40 degrees of flexion

C. MCP joints at 70 to 90 degrees of flexion and IP joints at 0 to 10 degrees of flexion

D. None of the above is a safe position.

Immobilization after trauma of fingers that have not undergone surgical repair should involve protection in the safe position splint. The safe position is with the MCP joints flexed at 70 to 90 degrees of flexion and the IP joints at 0 to 10 degrees of flexion. This position considerably decreases the potential for ligamentous contractures with subsequent limitation of articular motion.

Answer: **C**
Fess, Philips, p. 273

25. True or False: All metacarpal neck fractures should be splinted with this splint (Fig. 17-11, *A*).

A custom-molded fracture brace (Fig. 17-11, *A*) that widely distributes pressure typically is recommended for isolated midshaft fractures, *not* metacarpal neck fractures. This splint holds the four metacarpals as a unit, allowing full digital motion. The brace stabilizes the fracture with direct pressure over the bone; the pressure is distributed widely rather than concentrated. Fractures of the metacarpal neck are splinted (Fig. 17-11, *B*) with the MCP joint in flexion to provide a stabilizing force to the distal fracture fragment. Flexing the MCP joint to 90 degrees will provide fracture stability and assist with maintaining collateral ligament length. Additionally, this position puts the intrinsics in an effective position to pull the IPs into full extension, which is a common problem after immobilization. Full IP joint flexion and extension is encouraged.

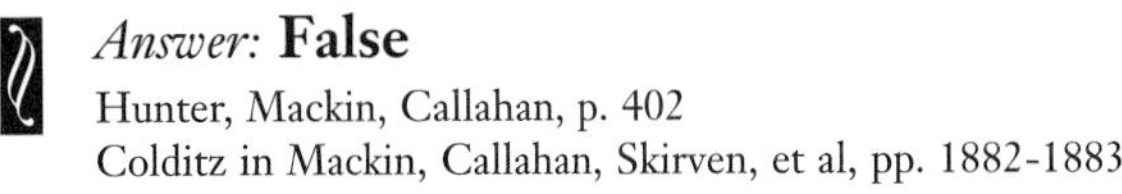

Answer: **False**
Hunter, Mackin, Callahan, p. 402
Colditz in Mackin, Callahan, Skirven, et al, pp. 1882-1883

26. A patient with a mild Dupuytren's contracture of the MCP in the fourth finger of the right hand is referred for conservative treatment. You decide to splint him with which of the following?

A. A palmar supportive splint
B. A dorsal corrective splint
C. A functional dynamic extension splint
D. A circumferential compression splint
E. No splint is effective for this diagnosis.

All attempts to influence the progression of Dupuytren's contracture via splinting have failed so far. Dupuytren's contracture does not respond to low-load prolonged stress. Therefore no splint is indicated for the conservative management of this disorder.

Answer: **E**
Coppard, Lohman, p. 195
Jacobs, Austin, p. 297

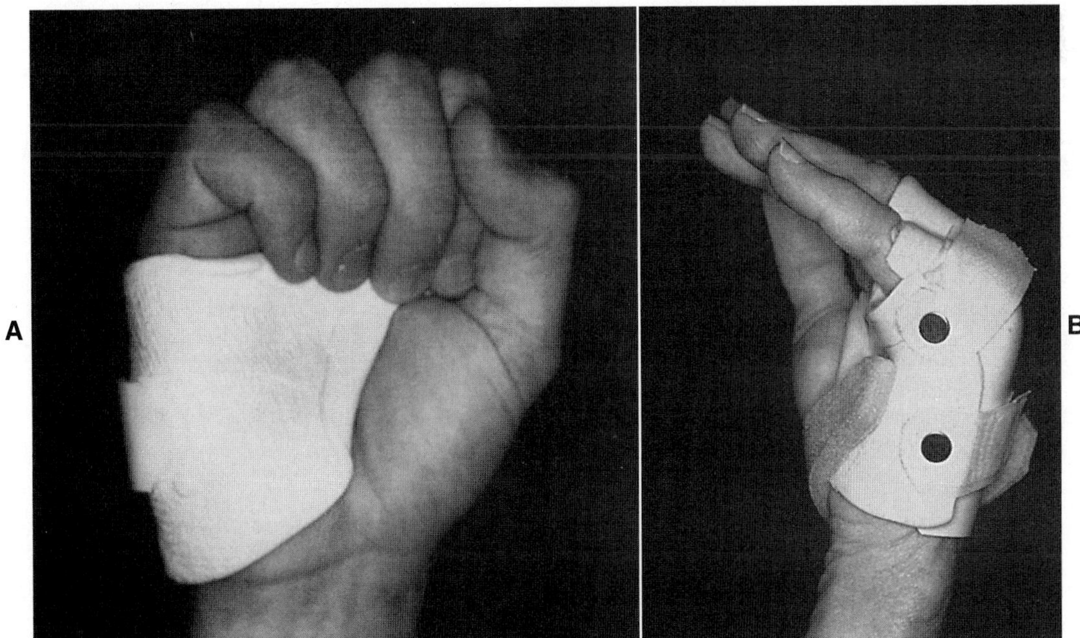

Fig. 17-11 ■ Custom-molded fracture brace. (**A** From Mackin EJ, Callahan AD, Skirven TM, et al: *Rehabilitation of the hand and upper extremity,* ed 5, St Louis, 2002, Mosby; **B** from Mackin EJ, Callahan AD, Skirven TM, et al: *Rehabilitation of the hand and upper extremity,* ed 5, St Louis, 2002, Mosby.)

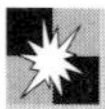

CLINICAL GEM:
Using collagenase for conservative treatment of Dupuytren's contracture proposes to retard the disease and decrease contractures.

27. A patient suffering from a humeral fracture and an accompanying radial nerve palsy is brought to therapy for splinting. What do you advise?

A. A static wrist and MCP extension splint
B. A dynamic wrist and MCP extension splint with elastic kinetic force
C. A tenodesis wrist splint
D. Any of the above splints could be applied.

Radial nerve palsy affects the dynamics of wrist and MCP extension ability and can often benefit from a substitutional device. Deciding which device would perform best depends on the patient's personality, motivation, and physical needs. The therapist will make the suggestion after careful evaluation of the patient and his or her needs. Any of these splints could be applied.

Answer: **D**
Van Lede, van Veldhoven, p. 195
Jacobs, Austin, pp. 69, 395-396

28. Which of the following is a correct argument favoring traction application to all fingers when a single tendon is repaired?

A. Improvement of physical gliding of the tendon
B. Decreased stress on the suture of the tendon
C. Enhanced biological response on the suture site
D. Facilitation of the functional prehension pattern

All fingers are often placed in traction to decrease stress on the sutured tendon. Flexing and extending of all the fingers together drags the paratenon, which otherwise could constrain the gliding of a single tendon and put stress on the suture. However, many therapists advocate traction to only the involved finger after tendon repair.

Answer: **B**
Van Lede, van Veldhoven, pp. 162, 171-172

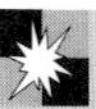

CLINICAL GEM:
Interestingly, when only one finger is in traction, the patient can sometimes "cheat" a little and get a bit of active glide; these patients often end up with excellent results.

29. You are treating a patient with a grade II dorsal dislocation of the PIP joint of the long finger. This patient has been referred to you for a splint. What type of finger splint should be applied?

A. Dorsal splint with the PIP joint in 25 degrees of flexion
B. Dorsal splint with the PIP joint in 60 degrees of flexion
C. Volar splint with the PIP joint at 0 degrees
D. Volar splint with the PIP joint at 5 to 10 degrees of flexion

Application of the dorsal finger splint with 25 degrees of PIP joint flexion should be sufficient to sustain reduction of a grade II subluxation. Radiographs should be obtained after application of the splint to confirm reduction. The application of this dorsal splint allows the patient to begin flexion exercises and avoid stiffness (see Fig. 11-10).

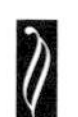

Answer: **A**
Hunter, Mackin, Callahan, pp. 378, 383
Campbell, Wilson in Mackin, Callahan, Skirven, et al, p. 405

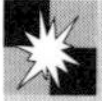

CLINICAL GEM:
A quick reference guide to dorsal dislocation grade, description, and splint follows:

Dorsal dislocation grade	Description	Splint
I	Proximal phalanx head damages central attachments distally. Critical corner integrity is maintained (the critical corner is where the volar plate, proper collateral ligament, and accessory collateral ligament merge). Refer to Fig. 2-24.	Dorsal finger splint with 25 degrees of flexion for 3 to 10 days; follow up with buddy taping
II	Disrupts the critical corner	Same splint as for grade I; worn for 2 to 4 weeks
III	Instability occurs volarly and laterally.	Dorsal splint with greater flexion for 6 to 8 weeks Surgical intervention may beindicated.

30. You are treating a patient with an acute MCP joint grade II collateral ligament injury. How should this patient's MCP joint be splinted?

A. Neutrally
B. With 20 degrees of flexion
C. With 50 degrees of flexion
D. With 90 degrees of flexion

MCP joint collateral ligament injuries occur less frequently than injury to the PIP joint. However, when injury occurs, the MCP joint should be immobilized in 50 degrees of flexion to maintain soft tissue length for 3 weeks. Some authors recommend including adjacent MCP joints. An additional 3 to 6 weeks of buddy taping minimizes stress on the injured ligament.

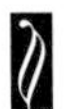
Answer: **C**
Hunter, Mackin, Callahan, p. 387

31. You are treating a patient with chronic MCP joint extension contractures. Which splinting technique would be most helpful for this patient?

A. Dynamic MCP joint flexion splinting
B. Serial cast with the MCP joints in flexion
C. Static progressive flexion splinting of the MCP joints
D. Splinting would not be helpful for this patient. This patient should be referred for surgery.

Static progressive splinting is especially beneficial for chronic stiffness such as occurs in MCP joint extension contractures because dynamic splinting is *not* as effective with chronically stiff joints. If there is no progress after several months of static progressive splinting, surgical intervention may be considered.

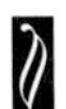
Answer: **C**
Hunter, Mackin, Callahan, p. 1131
Innis in Mackin, Callahan, Skirven, et al, pp. 1053-1054

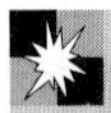
CLINICAL GEM:
According to Karen Shultz-Johnson, a MerIT component is a helpful device for static progressive splinting. You may use the total end range time concept developed by P. LaStayo and K. Flowers or the stress relaxation technique with this device. This device is available through U.E. Tech (see Appendix 3).

CLINICAL GEM:
In contrast to the theory of low-load prolonged stress, Bonutti et al report that static progressive splinting can be applied for a short duration with a low-load force to restore ROM through stress relaxation using Joint Active System splints.

32. The patient in the previous question was treated with static progressive splinting for 4 months and had less than 50 degrees of active ROM at his MCP joints. A capsulectomy was performed. When can splinting be reinitiated to maintain the gains made in surgery?

A. Within 72 hours after surgery
B. 3 to 5 days after surgery
C. 14 days after surgery, when sutures are removed
D. Splinting would not be indicated because the surgeon corrected the restrictions.

This patient was a good candidate for a capsulectomy because he had less than 65 degrees of flexion at the MCP joints. Therapy and splinting should be initiated within 72 hours after surgery. Mobilization splinting should be applied intermittently, after surgery, to pull the proximal phalanx into flexion. Dynamic splints can be used during the day as an adjunct to the patient's active exercise program, as well as to protect weakened structures. Some therapists advocate mobilization splints for night use, placing the MCP joints at near end range of obtainable flexion. The safe position splint is another option for use at night. All splints must be monitored and adjusted frequently. The therapist must pay careful attention to extension lags; if they develop, flexion splinting must be alternated with extension splinting.

Answer: **A**
Hunter, Mackin, Callahan, pp. 1132-1134
Wright, Rettig in Mackin, Callahan, Skirven, et al, p. 2084

33. A patient is referred to you with a diagnosis of tennis elbow. His physician has recommended a wrist support splint. In which position would you apply this splint?

A. Volar wrist splint with the wrist positioned at 5 degrees of dorsiflexion
B. Volar wrist splint with the wrist positioned at 45 degrees of dorsiflexion
C. Volar wrist splint with the wrist at neutral
D. Volar wrist splint with the wrist at 20 degrees of flexion

The purpose of a wrist splint for treatment of lateral epicondylitis is to place the wrist extensor muscles in a position of rest. A volar wrist splint is applied with the wrist in 45 degrees of dorsiflexion. For a very acute lateral epicondylitis or when a patient experiences pain with elbow flexion or extension, a posterior elbow splint with 90 degrees of elbow flexion and moderate wrist extension can be worn continuously for 2 to 3 weeks to reduce inflammation and pain.

Answer: **B**
Hunter, Mackin, Callahan, p. 1817

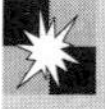
CLINICAL GEM:
Although 45 degrees of wrist extension is advocated, this position may be uncomfortable and may put the median nerve of the wrist at risk for compression. Monitor and re-assess frequently.

34. A patient with rheumatoid arthritis is referred to you for a resting hand splint for night wear. Which splint position is recommended for this patient?

A. Wrist at 10 to 30 degrees of extension with the thumb palmarly abducted; metacarpal joints at 15 to 25 degrees of flexion; and the digits in slight flexion
B. Wrist at 30 to 50 degrees of extension with the thumb radially abducted; metacarpal joints at 30 to 40 degrees of flexion; and the digits in slight flexion
C. Wrist at 40 to 50 degrees of extension with the thumb palmarly abducted and metacarpal joints at neutral; and the digits in slight flexion
D. Wrist at slight flexion with the thumb radially abducted; metacarpal joints at 10 to 20 degrees of flexion; and the digits in slight flexion

In an inflammatory condition such as rheumatoid arthritis, a resting hand splint is recommended. The resting hand splint places the wrist at 10 to 30 degrees of extension, with the thumb in palmar abduction, metacarpal joints at 15 to 25 degrees of flexion, and the digits in slight flexion. For patients with severe deformity or exacerbation from rheumatoid arthritis, the resting splint can be modified to position the wrist at neutral or slight extension with slight ulnar deviation. The thumb should be positioned midway between radial and palmar abduction for increased comfort. The recommended thumb position for splinting the rheumatoid hand (at any time) varies among authors.

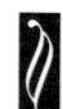
Answer: **A**
Hunter, Mackin, Callahan, p. 1349
Biese in Mackin, Callahan, Skirven, et al, pp. 1574-1575
Coppard, Lohman, pp. 190-193

35. True or False: It is important for all patients with radial nerve palsy to receive dynamic splinting regimes.

The most important rationale for splinting a high radial nerve injury is to support the wrist in extension, enhance hand function, and prevent overstretching of the extensors. For many patients, the use of a simple wrist extension splint (not pictured) is sufficient to allow satisfactory hand function because the lumbricals and interossei are able to extend the IP joints. Oftentimes this splint will extend further to include the MCPs for more support in dynamic splinting. Extension outriggers for the digits and thumb should be used in situations in which full digital extension is required for successful completion of specific tasks (Fig. 17-12). However, these splints often are considered bulky and excessive and may be discontinued by the patient. Choose patients wisely before fabricating this splint.

Answer: **False**
Fess, Philips, p. 346

36. True or False: An effective way to finish the edges on your splint is to use moleskin.

This is a common method of edge finishing, but it is inappropriate. The moleskin may look nice and feel soft at first, but it will quickly become dirty, smelly, and rough. Moleskin does not wash or dry easily and retains moisture. To produce a smooth edge use 1/16-inch self-adhesive Plastazote, Aquaplast Ultra Thin Edging

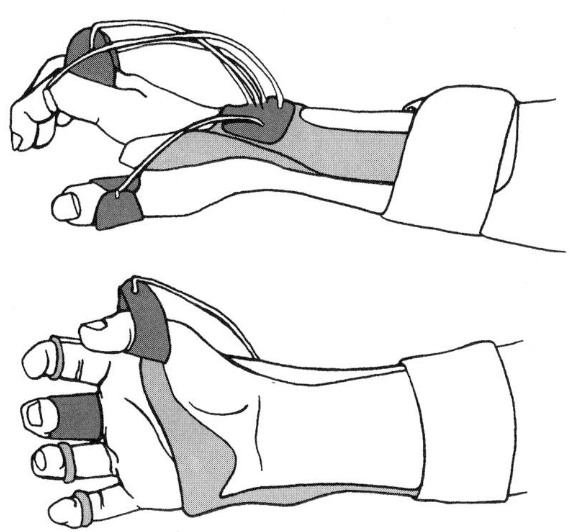

Fig. 17-12 ■ From McKee P, Morgan L: *Orthotics in rehabilitation: splinting the hand and body*, Philadelphia, 1998, FA Davis.

Material, or microfoam tape, which is a closed-cell tape that conforms to contours. These materials produce a smooth, nonirritating, washable edge.

Answer: **False**
McKee, Morgan, p. 129
Refer to Fig. 17-13

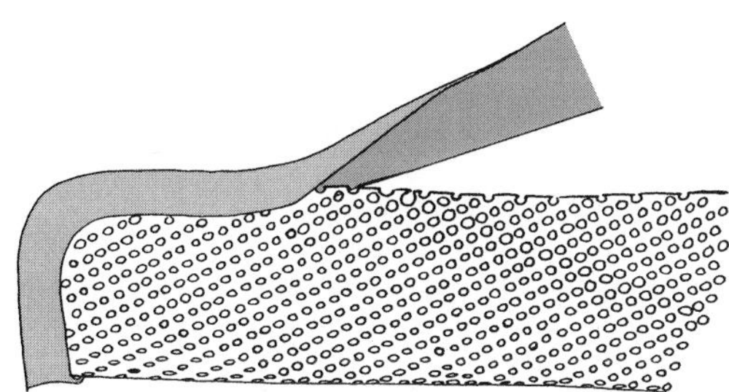

Fig. 17-13 ■ Edge covering. Covering the rough edge of a maxi-perforated thermoplastic with a smooth, washable, nonirritating covering. (From McKee P, Morgan L: *Orthotics in rehabilitation: splinting the hand and body*, Philadelphia, 1998, FA Davis.)

37. You are treating a patient with a 6-month-old fixed PIP joint flexion contracture. Which of the following is the best technique for increasing the ROM of this joint?

A. Dynamic PIP joint extension splint, hand-based
B. Dynamic PIP joint extension splint, forearm-based
C. Serial cast
D. No splint. This is a fixed contracture and requires surgical intervention.

Casting is one of the most helpful techniques for treating older injuries when remodeling has already taken place. In the case of a fixed contracture, serial casts often are the only form of treatment other than surgical release that provides satisfactory correction. Serial casting often is used preoperatively to improve the chances of successful surgery by reversing the contracture to maximal soft-tissue length. The cast should be changed every other day or a minimum of two times a week to allow exercise and to monitor skin status.

Answer: **C**
Fess, Philips, pp. 453-457
Refer to Fig. 17-14

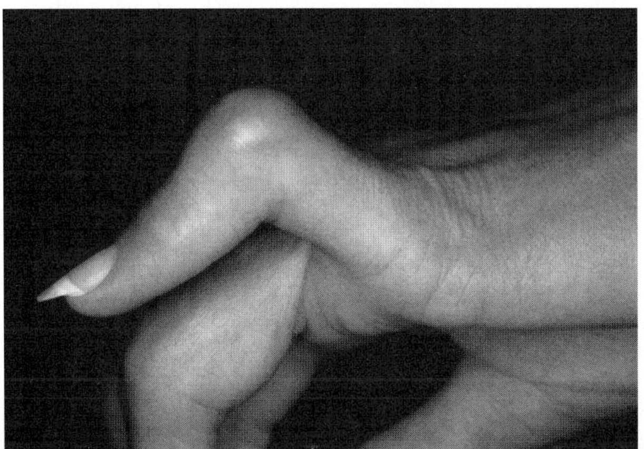

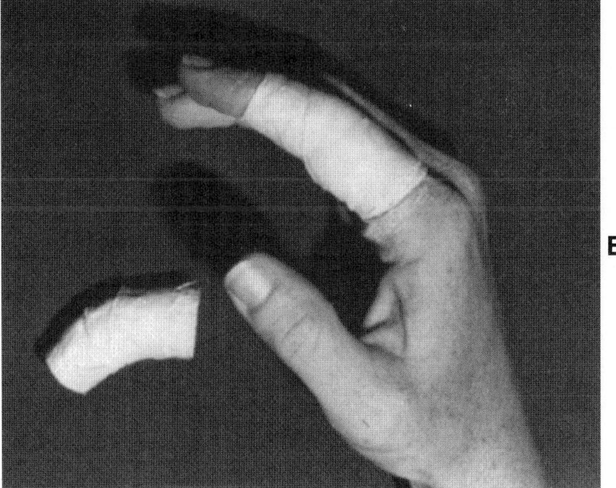

Fig. 17-14 ■ **A**, PIP joint contracture. **B**, Progressive casting of the index IP joint into extension. (From Mackin EJ, Callahan AD, Skirven TM, et al: *Rehabilitation of the hand and upper extremity*, ed 5, St Louis, 2002, Mosby.)

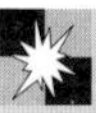

CLINICAL GEM:
Preconditioning before cast application is achieved with passive exercise, joint mobilization, or other modalities that help bring the tissue to its end range for several minutes. After preconditioning, cast application should be immediate because the tissues will quickly return to their pre-stretch length.

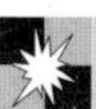

CLINICAL GEM:
For serial casting, either plaster of Paris or a low-temperature, thermoplastic material such as Plastofit by Orfit may be used.

38. Golfer's elbow (medial epicondylitis) is treated with which type of wrist splint?

A. Volar wrist splint with the wrist at 30 degrees of extension
B. Volar wrist splint with the wrist at neutral
C. Volar wrist splint with the wrist flexed at 20 to 30 degrees
D. No splint will help this condition.

Golfer's elbow is a tendinitis that affects the muscles that originate from the medial epicondyle. During the acute phase, the goal is to reduce inflammation and promote the healing of microscopic tears. A volar wrist splint with the wrist at neutral is applied and worn for 10 to 14 days continuously. After the acute phase, the splint is used for protection or on an as-needed basis for pain.

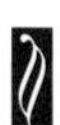

Answer: **B**

Hunter, Mackin, Callahan, pp. 1811-1812
Wright, Rettig in Mackin, Callahan, Skirven, et al, pp. 2078-2079

39. A machinist with "thick, working hands" and well-developed intrinsic muscles was diagnosed with carpal tunnel syndrome. He has been treated for 3 weeks with wrist-control splinting, antiinflammatory medications, oral vitamins, and instructions to avoid provocative wrist positions and repetitive motions. Despite conservative management, his symptoms of low median nerve compression persist. Provocative testing of the cervical spine and proximal upper extremity is negative. The patient fears surgery and resists any suggestion of it. Which of the following would be your next treatment technique for achieving symptom relief?

A. Adding ice massage to treatment and reassessing the patient in 2 weeks
B. Initiating therapy three times a week to improve strength for return to work
C. Incorporating extension of the MCP joints into the wrist extension splint
D. Providing patient education to convince him that surgery is required

Although ice massage is an effective modality for relief of pain and inflammation, this patient has already been taking antiinflammatory medications and has altered provocative activities. Therapy for muscle conditioning is not advisable because repetitive finger flexion exercises and sustained grip can increase median nerve compression by increasing pressure in the carpal canal. Although surgery may ultimately be required, conservative treatment for persistent symptoms should include splinting the MCP joints in extension to pull the lumbricals—which take their origin from the flexor digitorum profundi—up out of the carpal tunnel. Studies have shown that the lumbricals lie distal to the carpal tunnel and do not affect intratunnel pressures until finger flexion occurs. Wrist-control splinting alone may not be sufficient to reduce carpal tunnel pressures and digital flexion also may need to be restricted.

Answer: **C**

Evans, pp. 17-18

40. You are treating a patient who was referred to you with a humeral shaft fracture. The doctor orders a splint for this patient. Which type of splint would you fabricate?

A. Airplane splint
B. Sarmiento fracture brace
C. Abduction wedge brace
D. Splinting is not indicated for this patient.

The humerus is an ideal candidate for functional fracture bracing. A cylinder applied externally to a fractured long bone restrains soft-tissue expansion, thus directing force equally in all directions during muscle contraction (see Fig. 5 in Question 44). Sarmiento describes this as a "pseudohydraulic environment." The internal force mechanically stabilizes the fracture. The Sarmiento fracture brace is fastened circumferentially. Active pendulum exercises can be initiated 1 week after humeral shaft fracture—with or without brace application.

Answer: **B**
Hunter, Mackin, Callahan, pp. 396-398
Colditz in Mackin, Callahan, Skirven, et al, p. 1876
Refer to Fig. 17-15

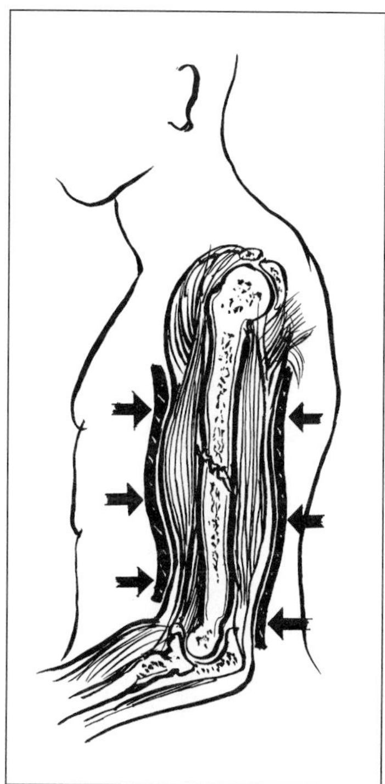

Fig. 17-15 ■ Schematic drawing of a humeral fracture brace (Sarmiento fracture brace) shows how the compressed soft tissue stabilizes a humeral fracture. (Redrawn from Sarmiento A, Latta L: *Closed functional treatment of fractures,* New York, 1981, Springer-Verlag.)

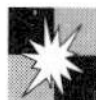

CLINICAL GEM:
Pendulum or passive exercises are permitted during the first few weeks after humeral shaft fracture. Early active exercise should be avoided until the fracture stabilizes because active exercise can contribute to fracture angulation.

41. A patient with a grade I skier's thumb injury is treated with a splint for 3 weeks. What type of splint is recommended?

A. Hand-based thumb immobilization (short opponens), MCP at neutral to slight flexion, and the carpometacarpal (CMC) joint palmarly abducted 25 to 30 degrees
B. Hand-based thumb immobilization (short opponens), MCP at 30 degrees of flexion, and the CMC joint palmarly abducted 60 to 70 degrees
C. Hand-based thumb immobilization with the MCP free and the CMC joint palmarly abducted to 25 to 30 degrees
D. A splint is not needed for a grade I injury.

Ulnar collateral ligament injuries at the thumb MCP joint can be classified as grade I, II, or III. Acute grade I injuries (e.g., gamekeeper's or skier's thumb) are common and are treated with a hand-based thumb immobilization splint (short opponens). The MCP is held at neutral to slight flexion and the CMC joint is palmarly abducted 25 to 30 degrees for 3 weeks (Fig. 17-16). The IP joint is left free to allow for early motion of this joint. Gentle ROM exercises to the MCP joint are initiated 3 weeks after injury. In a grade II injury, the ligament is partially torn and requires longer immobilization than is needed for a grade I injury, approximately 4 to 5 weeks. A grade III injury is characterized by a complete ligament rupture that requires surgical intervention and is often casted and then splinted after cast removal.

Answer: **A**
Coppard, Lohman, pp. 226-227

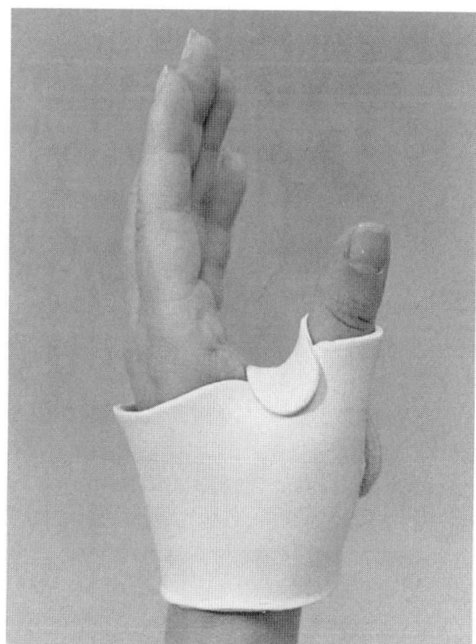

Fig. 17-16 ■ From Coppard BM, Lohman H: *Introduction to splinting: a clinical-reasoning and problem-solving approach,* ed 2, St Louis, 2001, Mosby.

17 SPLINTING

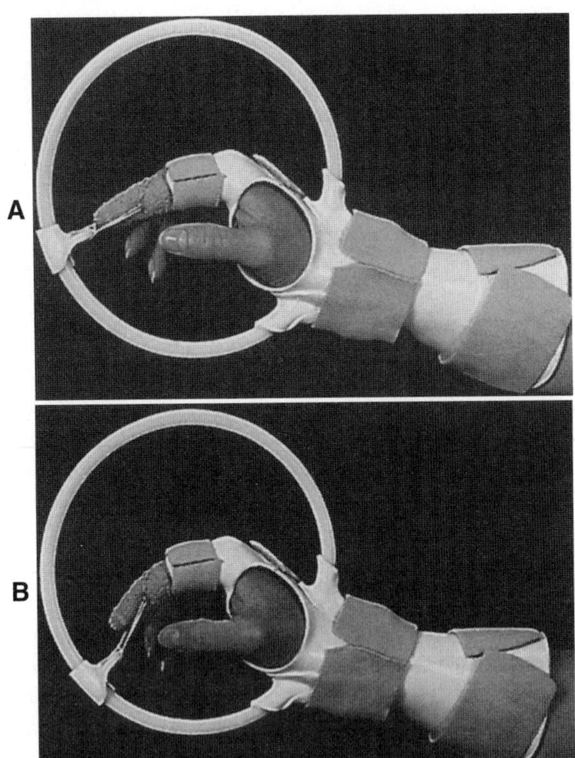

Fig. 17-17 ■ From Jacobs MA, Austin NM: *Splinting the hand and upper extremity: principles and process,* Baltimore, 2003, Lippincott Williams & Wilkins.

42. Fig. 17-17 is used to treat what diagnosis?

A. Metacarpal shaft fractures
B. PIP joint intraarticular fractures
C. P3 fractures
D. None of the above

This is a dynamic traction splint, also known as a *Schenck splint.* This splint provides gentle, controlled distal distraction to assist in reduction of an intraarticular fracture of the PIP joint. The arc of motion is set with the surgeon, and tension is carefully set by the therapist. This splint can also be used to treat intra-articular MCP, thumb MCP, and IP joint injuries, pilon fracture of the PIP joint, fracture dislocation of the PIP joint, condylar fractures, and oblique or spiral phalangeal shaft fractures.

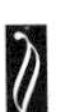
Answer: **B**
Jacobs, Austin, p. 192

43. A patient is referred to you with the diagnosis of mild basal joint arthritis. She reports pain at the base of the thumb with functional task performance. Which type of splint should you fabricate?

A. Short opponens
B. Ulnar gutter
C. Wrist support splint
D. No splint

The basal joint, or first CMC joint, commonly is affected by osteoarthritis. A short opponens splint (Fig. 17-18) can be applied to reduce dorsoradial subluxation at the first CMC joint. Patients with arthritis in this joint often are greatly relieved by using this small splint during functional activities. The molding must be precise at the base of the first metacarpal to ensure adequate stabilization of the CMC joint during active use of the thumb.

Answer: **A**
Hunter, Mackin, Callahan, pp. 1164-1165
Colditz in Mackin, Callahan, Skirven, et al, p. 1881
Weiss, LaStayo, Mills, pp. 218-219

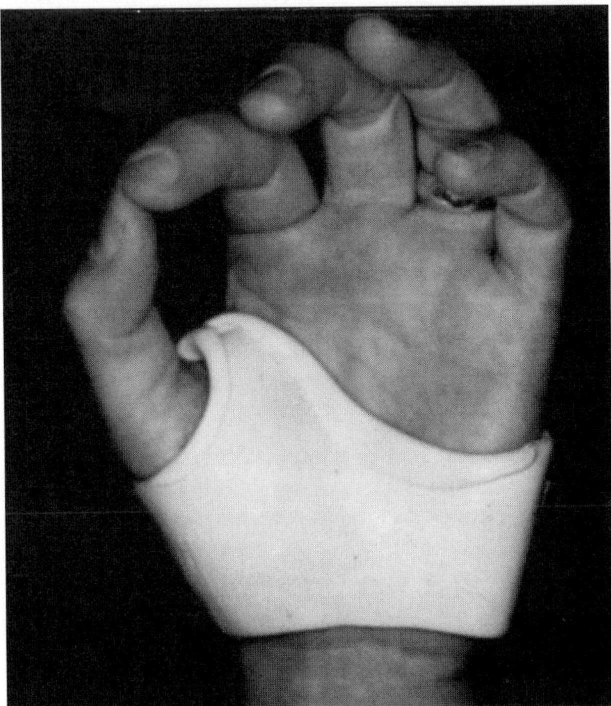

Fig. 17-18 ■ From Mackin EJ, Callahan AD, Skirven TM, et al: *Rehabilitation of the hand and upper extremity,* ed 5, St Louis, 2002, Mosby.

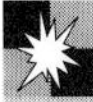

CLINICAL GEM:
Recent research has indicated that patients will choose a neoprene CMC joint splint over the short opponens for comfort when they have symptoms at the first CMC joint. The neoprene splint is efficient at reducing dorsoradial subluxation at the first CMC joint.

44. Name the following splints.

Splint

1.

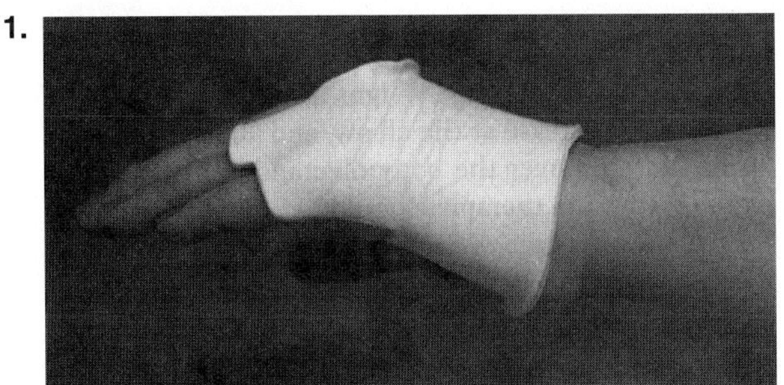

From Coppard BM, Lohman H: *Introduction to splinting: a clinical-reasoning and problem-solving approach*, ed 2, St Louis, 2001, Mosby.

2.

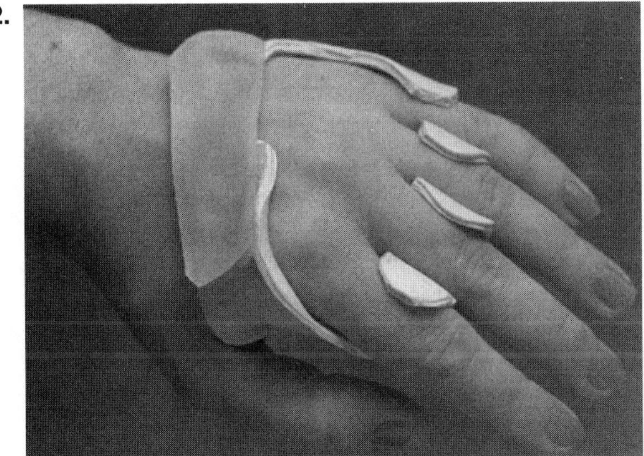

From Coppard BM, Lohman H: *Introduction to splinting: a clinical-reasoning and problem-solving approach*, ed 2, St Louis, 2001, Mosby.

3.

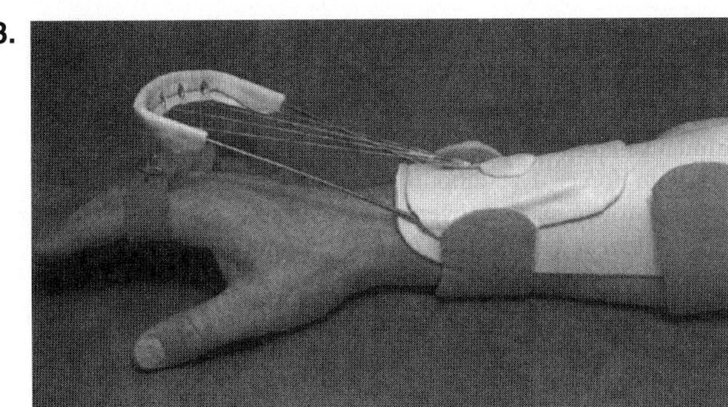

From Coppard BM, Lohman H: *Introduction to splinting: a clinical-reasoning and problem-solving approach*, ed 2, St Louis, 2001, Mosby.

4.

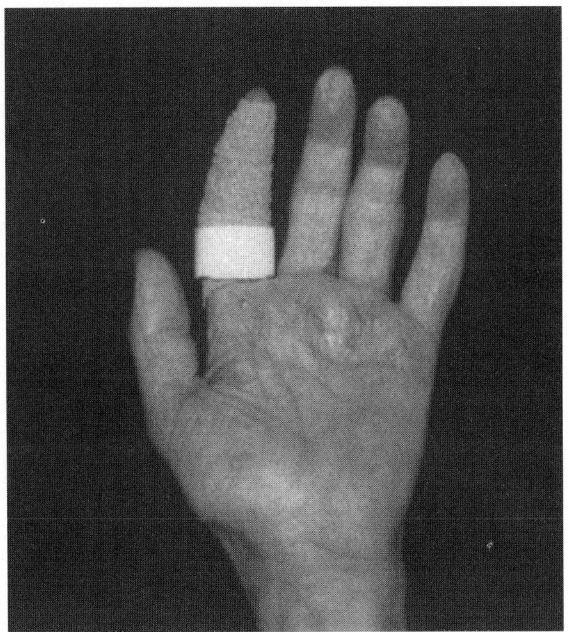

From Hunter JM, Mackin EJ, Callahan AD: *Rehabilitation of the hand: surgery and therapy*, ed 4, St Louis, 1995, Mosby.

5.

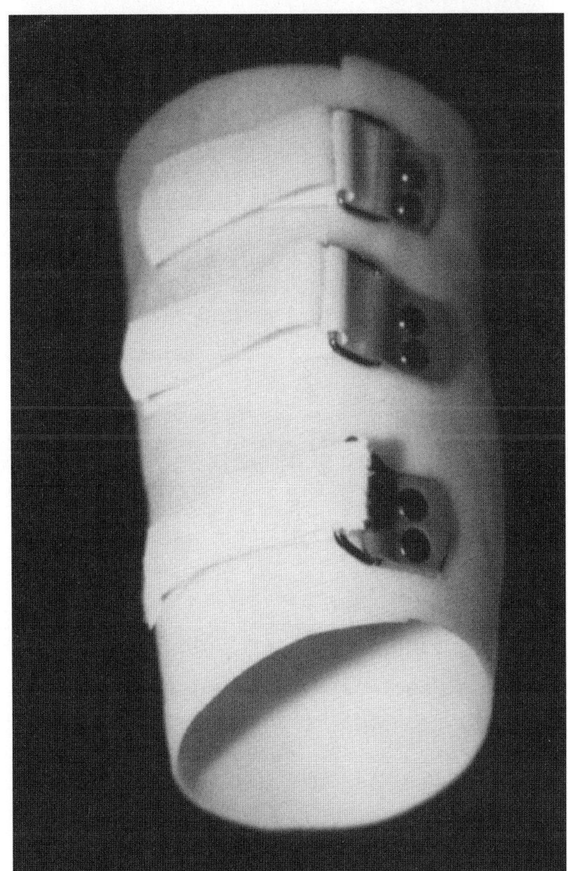

From Mackin EJ, Callahan AD, Skirven TM, et al: *Rehabilitation of the hand and upper extremity*, ed 5, St Louis, 2002, Mosby.

6.

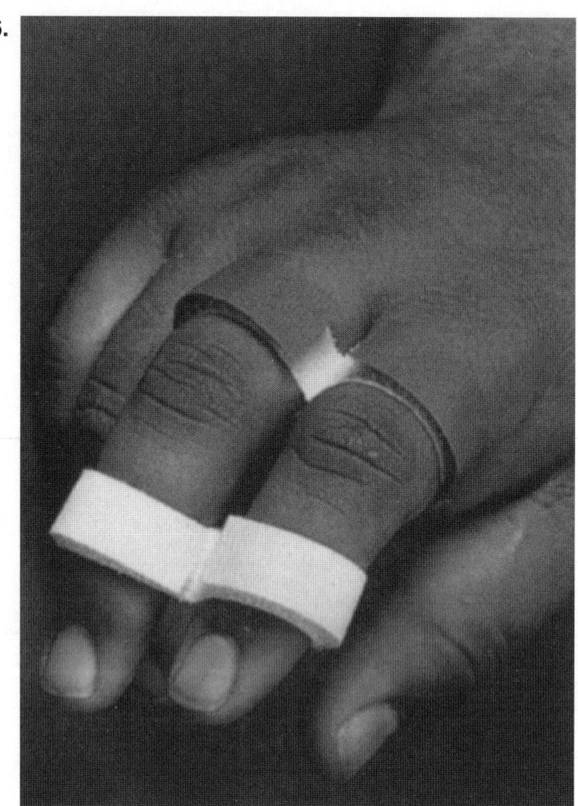

From Mackin EJ, Callahan AD, Skirven TM, et al: *Rehabilitation of the hand and upper extremity*, ed 5, St Louis, 2002, Mosby.

Name

A. Pulley ring splint
B. Ulnar nerve injury splint
C. Budding strapping
D. Sarmiento fracture bracing
E. Ulnar deviation splint
F. Radial nerve palsy

Answers: **1, B; 2, E; 3, F; 4, A; 5, D; 6, C**
Hunter, Mackin, Callahan, pp. 318, 399, 470
Campbell, Wilson in Mackin, Callahan, Skirven, et al, p. 399
Colditz in Mackin, Callahan, Skirven, et al, pp. 1879-1880
Coppard, Lohman, pp. 6-7, 278, 307

45. CMMS stands for which of the following?

A. Casting minimal motion splints
B. Casting motion to mobilize stiffness
C. Casting mainly to manage stiffness
D. Casting to maintain motion from splinting

CMMS stands for casting motion to mobilize stiffness. This a technique that uses plaster of Paris to selectively immobilize joints in an ideal position so that they move in a desired direction and range. This technique mobilizes stiff joints, reduces edema, and directs a new pattern of motion to revive the cortical representation of productive motion. According to Colditz, this technique is very effective with a chronically stiff hand.

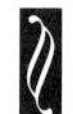

Answer: **B**
Colditz in Mackin, Callahan, Skirven, et al, p. 1039

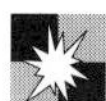

CLINICAL GEM:
To learn how to apply the CMMS technique, visit www.handlab.com for courses by Judy Colditz.

Chapter 18

Cumulative Trauma

1. True or False: The *only* indicator of a positive upper limb tension test (ULTT) is ability to reproduce the patient's symptoms.

Reproduction of the patient's symptoms is only one indicator of a positive ULTT. A positive result may also be identified by a difference in range of motion (ROM), resistance encountered, and/or symptom response during movement in the upper extremity (UE) in comparing involved and uninvolved sides.

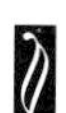

Answer: **False**

Butler, pp. 162-163

Walsh in Mackin, Callahan, Skirven, et al, p. 770

2. Which technique would you choose for treatment of adverse neural tension in the UE?

A. Nerve gliding
B. Nerve tensioning
C. Nerve elongation
D. A and C
E. All of the above

All of the above techniques can be used to treat neural tension. Nerve gliding is placing tension on the nerve at one point while releasing it at the other. This leaves the resting tension and strain on the nerve unchanged. Gliding can occur within the nerve itself or between the nerve and its interfacing tissue. Treatment is kept tension free in a pain-free ROM and is recommended for patients in the irritated "acute" phase.

Nerve tensioning or elongation is pulling on both ends of the nerve to unfold the nerve. This technique has effects on neurophysiology because of alterations in vascular and axoplasmic flow and is recommended during the nonirritated phase or when pain is absent at rest. As irritability decreases, the therapist can work through the tissue barriers to restore movement and increase function.

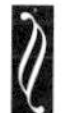

Answer: **E**

Mackin, Callahan, Skirven, et al, pp. 764-774

Refer to Fig. 18-1

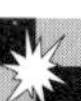

CLINICAL GEM:
Precautions and Contraindications

Precautions

- Irritable conditions
- Spinal cord signs
- Severe unremitting night pain that lacks a diagnosis
- Recent paresthesia/anesthesia/complex regional pain syndrome type I or II
- Mechanical spine pain with peripheralization

Contraindications

- Recently repaired peripheral nerve
- Malignancy
- Active inflammatory conditions
- Neurologic: acute inflammatory/demyelinating diseases

From Mackin EJ, Callahan AD, Skirven TM, et al: *Rehabilitation of the hand and upper extremity*, ed 5, St Louis, 2002, Mosby.

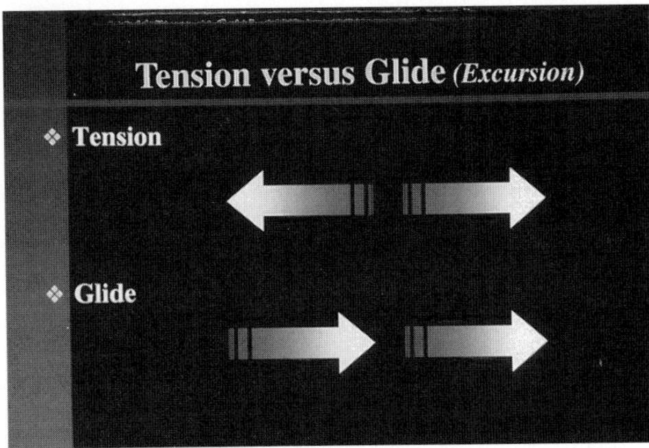

Fig. 18-1 ■ From Mackin EJ, Callahan AD, Skirven TM, et al: *Rehabilitation of the hand and upper extremity*, ed 5, St Louis, 2002, Mosby.

3. True or False: Adverse tension testing can always identify the location of neural dysfunction.

Adverse tension testing, along with additional objective examination, can help the examiner use clinical reasoning to prove or disapprove the source or location of adverse tension signs and symptoms (i.e., intraneural, extraneural; Table 18-1). It cannot *always* identify the location of neural dysfunction. It can be difficult to pinpoint the location of dysfunction when distribution of symptoms is widespread or with the possibility of multiple sites along the nervous system and the contributions of nonneural structures.

Answer: **False**
Butler, pp. 165-166

CLINICAL GEM:
Patients presenting with a history of prolonged upper extremity pain or guarding postures will most likely present with adverse neural tension along the UE and proximal musculature dysfunction that limits ROM and may contribute to distal pain.

4. A 36-year-old man is referred to you with the diagnosis of lateral epicondylitis. After conservative treatment that included iontophoresis, trigger point treatment of the supinator, the wrist and finger extensors, and stretching and progressive strengthening exercises, the patient no longer reports palpable tenderness at the lateral epicondyle. He only reports noting pain/discomfort in the lateral epicondyle region after working out, especially after performing pushups. Which muscle can be a source of continued referred pain to the lateral epicondyle?

A. Pectoralis major
B. Brachioradialis (BR)
C. Pectoralis minor
D. Tricep

Table 18-1

Some Signs and Symptoms That May Indicate Intraneural and Extraneural Sites of Adverse Neural Tension: a Hypothesis

	Extraneural	Intraneural	
		Conducting tissues	**Connective tissues**
Description and distribution	Catches, twinges around vulnerable areas	Burning, tingling, electric feelings in innervation field	Lines of pain, along trunks, nondermatomal
Constancy	Intermittent → constant short symptom duration	More constant, longer symptom duration	Intermittent → constant
Recognition	Familiar	Unfamiliar, bizarre, nervy	More familiar
Aggravating/easing factors	↑ With movement of interface	↑ With tension of nervous system	↑ With tension ↑↓ With movement
Physical signs	Comparable signs in interfacing structures	Neurological signs and symptoms	Palpation → local pain
Tension test symptom response	↑ or ↓ With movement	↑ With tension	↑ With movement ↑ With tension
Examples	Tight scalenei → irritation of the nervous system	Neuroma and immature axons in scarred endoneurium	Irritated epineurium

From Butler DS: *Mobilisation of the nervous system*, New York, 1991, Churchill Livingstone.

An active trigger point in the triceps (lateral head) will refer pain to the lateral epicondyle. Although the BR also refers pain to the lateral epicondyle, in this case the triceps was most likely activated by the overenthusiastic performance of pushups, because the tricep's function is to extend the forearm at the elbow.

Answer: **D**

Travell, Simons, pp. 462-463
Kostopoulous, Rizpoulos, p. 130

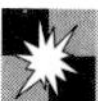

CLINICAL GEM:
Patients will complain of referred pain (pain that is proximal or distal to the origin of pain), and sometimes of localized pain, burning, and tenderness on the involved muscle. Each involved muscle has a characteristic referred pain pattern in distal or proximal locations. It is helpful to know these patterns because they will help direct you to the appropriate muscle to treat. The taut band on the muscle will be tender. Also, the trigger point itself will demonstrate nodularity and exquisite pain. With increased pressure or the progressive pressure technique on the trigger point nodule, a referred pain pattern will present itself.

Kostopoulos, Rizopoulos, p. 25

5. A 40-year-old man is referred to you with the diagnosis of lateral epicondylitis. He reports the onset of pain after carrying his luggage on a business trip. Which muscle is most likely the source of the referred pain to the lateral epicondyle in this case?

A. BR
B. Supinator
C. Extensor carpi radialis brevis (ECRB)
D. Extensor carpi radialis longus (ECRL)

An active trigger point in the supinator will refer pain to the lateral epicondyle. In this case, the supinator was most likely activated when the patient was walking while carrying his luggage; the supinator stabilizes the straight elbow while extended, as would occur while carrying swinging luggage.

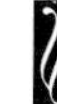

Answer: **B**

Travell, Simons, p. 514

6. Another name for the arcuate ligament is ____.

A. Transverse retinacular ligament
B. Arcade of Frohse
C. Osborne's band (ligament)
D. Ligament of Struthers

The roof of the cubital tunnel is the arcuate ligament or Osborne's band (ligament). It also can be called the *humeral ulnar aponeurotic arcade* or the *triangular ligament.* The floor of the tunnel is formed from the medial collateral ligament and the walls are formed by the medial epicondyle and the olecranon.

Answer: **C**

Idler, p. 379
Refer to Fig. 18-2

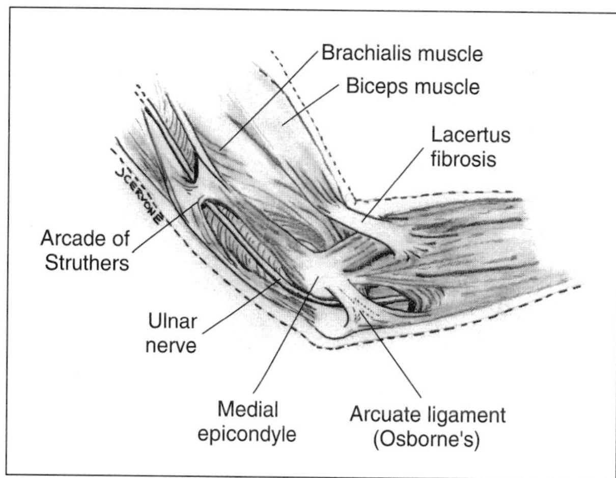

Fig. 18-2

7. Trigger finger is associated with which of the following?

A. Middle-aged women
B. Rheumatoid arthritis
C. Using tools with hard or sharp edges
D. All of the above

Trigger finger is associated with all of the above. It is caused from stenosis (thickening) at or around the A1 pulley (see Fig. 1-12). If the patient has sufficient swelling in this region, the tendon can become locked in flexion and can cause a snap (often painful) as it pulls under the A1 pulley. The most commonly affected digit is the thumb. A thickened pulley and an hourglass enlargement of the tendon are consistent findings with trigger finger. Conservative treatment includes steroid injection and a splinting regime (Fig. 18-3). Operative treatment is performed if conservative management has failed.

Answer: **D**

Putz-Anderson, p. 16
Hunter, Mackin, Callahan, pp. 1007-1009
Lee, Nasser-Sharif, Zelouf in Mackin, Callahan, Skirven, et al, pp. 938-942

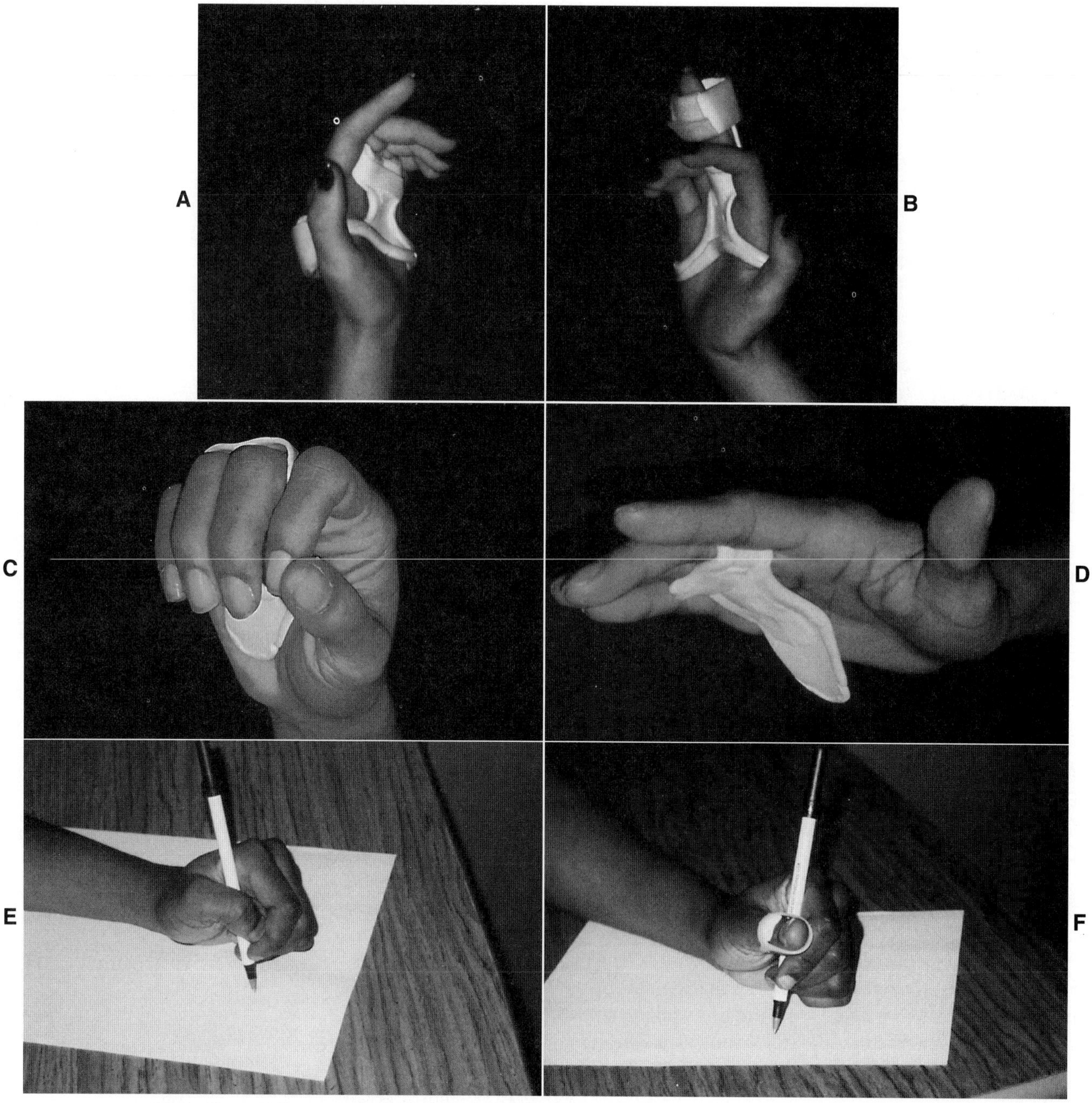

Fig. 18-3 ■ Splinting options for trigger digits. **A,** Hand-based MCP extension splint. **B,** For PIP contracture, dorsal component for static progressive extension. **C** and **D,** Paddle design blocks extreme flexion but allows more freedom in extension and allows easier donning and doffing. **E,** Excessive thumb IP flexion during writing by a man with trigger thumb. **F,** Three-point extension splint for thumb IP joint prevents excessive flexion.

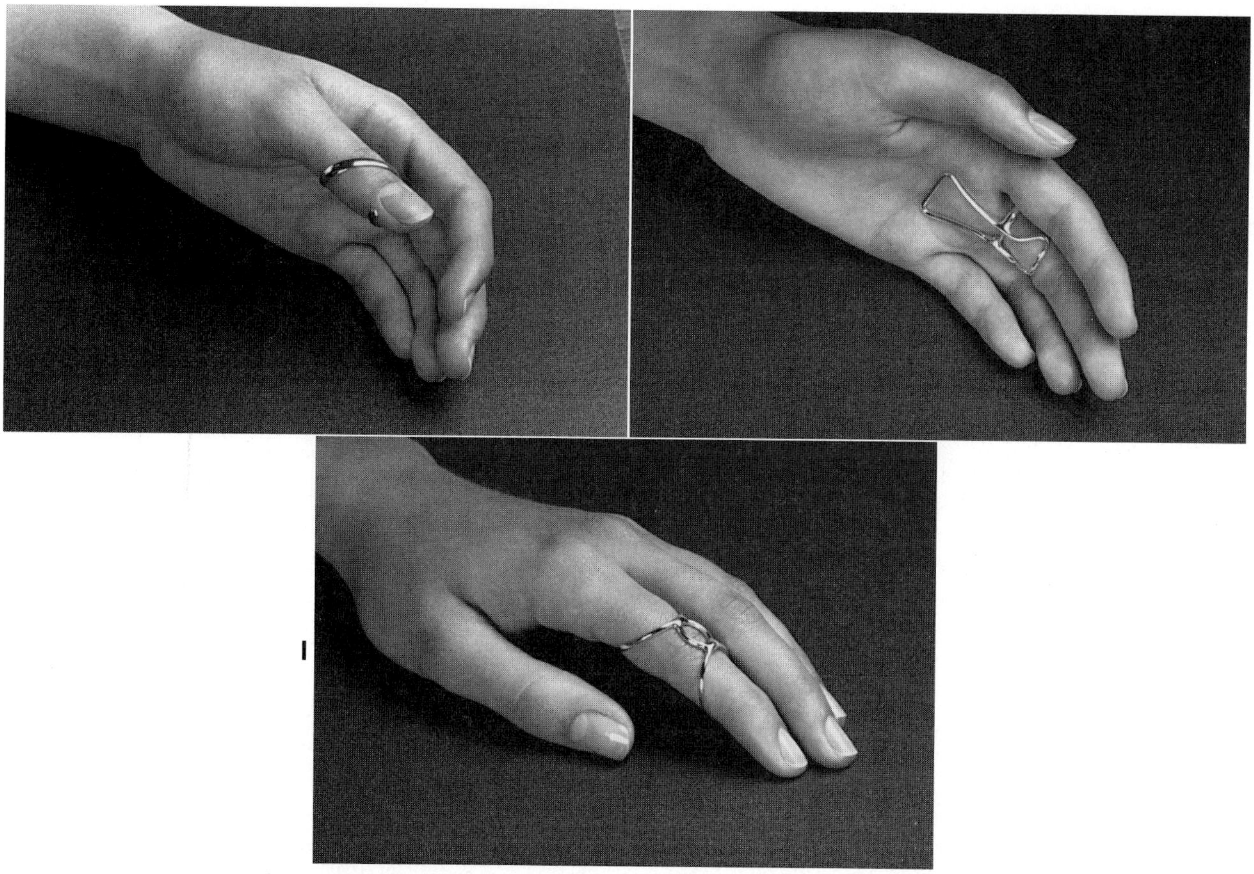

Fig. 18-3 ■ cont'd G through **I,** Silver ring splints for chronic triggering. (**C** and **D** Based on design by Linder-Tons and Ingell, 1998; From Mackin EJ, Callahan AD, Skirven TM, et al: *Rehabilitation of the hand and upper extremity,* ed 5, St Louis, 2002, Mosby; **F** courtesy 3-Point Products, Inc., 1610 Pincay Court, Annapolis, MD 21401, [410] 349-2649, e-mail the3ptprod@aol.com; courtesy Silver Ring Splint Company, P.O. Box 2856, Charlottesville, VA 22902-2856, e-mail cindy@silverringsplint.com, fax 804-971-8828.)

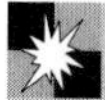
CLINICAL GEM:
Stenosing tenosynovitis is also termed *stenosing tendovaginitis. Tendovaginitis* (tendon sheath + inflammation) is considered to be a more accurate term then tenosynovitis to describe the inflamed and thickened retinacular sheath that characterizes these conditions. However, tenosynovitis is generally and broadly defined and has been used to describe the many vague aching conditions of the upper extremity.

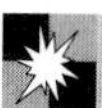
CLINICAL GEM:
The most common tendovaginitides are de Quervain's disease and trigger digits.

CLINICAL GEM:
The following is a quick reference to trigger-finger rehabilitation:

- Splint the MCP joint in extension, with PIP and DIP joints free, for 3 to 6 weeks
- Perform passive ROM to MCP joint to avoid stiffness
- Use modalities to reduce pain and inflammation
- Use Coban to reduce edema

8. de Quervain's disease is a tenosynovitis (*tendovaginitis*) of which tendons?

A. Abductor pollicis longus and extensor pollicis brevis
B. Abductor pollicis longus and palmaris brevis
C. Palmaris brevis and extensor pollicis brevis
D. Extensor pollicis longus and abductor pollicis longus
E. Extensor pollicis longus and abductor pollicis brevis

In the 1893 edition of *Gray's Anatomy*, "washerwoman's sprain" was first described. In 1895, Fritz de Quervain further described this condition as a stenosing tenosynovitis. The tendons of the abductor pollicis longus and the extensor pollicis brevis (Fig. 18-4, *A*) are housed in the first of six compartments residing beneath the extensor retinaculum. Pain usually is the predominant symptom, with tenderness and swelling noted proximal to the radial styloid. de Quervain's disease typically is caused from overuse of the hand and wrist, especially when the patient has combined pinch with wrist motion and forearm rotation. Metabolic abnormalities such as diabetes, hypothyroidism, and rheumatoid arthritis may be associated with this disease. Pregnancy also may be associated with de Quervain's disease. A positive Finkelstein's test usually is noted with de Quervain's disease (Fig. 18-4, *B*).

Answer: **A**

Hunter, Mackin, Callahan, pp. 1012-1014
Lee, Nasser-Sharif, Zelouf in Mackin, Callahan, Skirven, et al, pp. 944-947

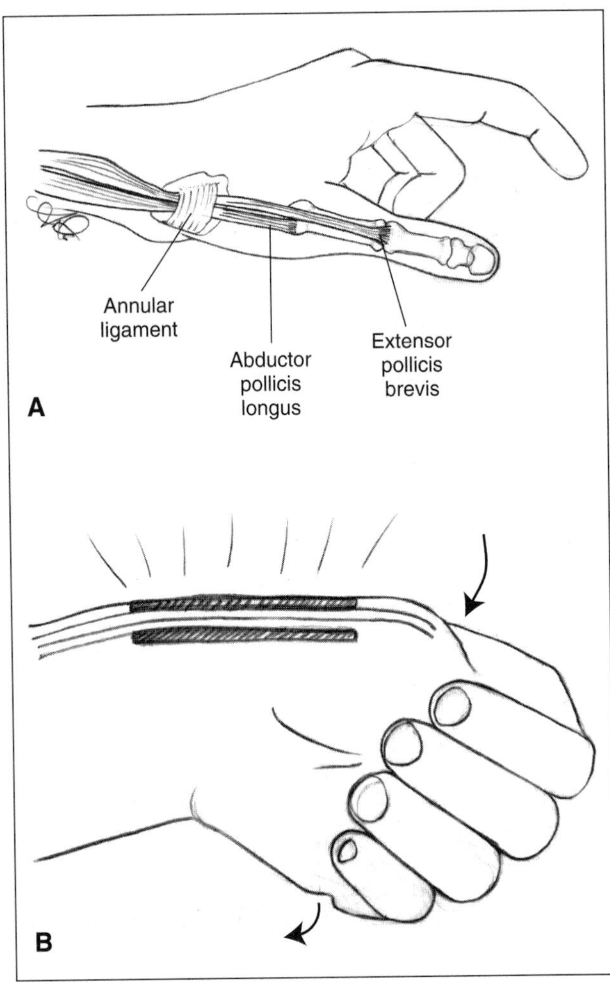

Fig. 18-4

9. Which of the following should be avoided or modified to reduce the risk of developing cumulative trauma disorders (CTDs)?

A. Tool vibration
B. Extreme or awkward joint postures
C. Repetitive finger action
D. All of the above

All of the above contribute to CTDs and should be decreased when possible. Avoiding or modifying high-contact forces and static loading also reduces the chance of acquiring CTDs. In addition force, temperature extremes, mechanical compression, and duration/recovery time are basic risk factors.

Answer: **D**

Putz-Anderson, p. 10
Berg Rice, pp. 162-163

CLINICAL GEM:
Did you know that pain elicited with resisted thumb extension at the MCP joint is referred to as a positive "hitchhiker's test"? This test indicates inflammation of the extensor pollicis brevis tendon in the first dorsal compartment.

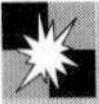

CLINICAL GEM:
The following is a quick reference to performing a Finkelstein test:

- Place patient's thumb across his palm
- Wrap patient's fingers around his thumb
- Passively move the patient's wrist into ulnar deviation
- Excruciating pain around the radial styloid indicates a positive test.

10. Gantzer's muscle is an accessory muscle of which of the following?

A. Extensor pollicis longus
B. Abductor pollicis longus
C. Flexor pollicis longus
D. Extensor pollicis brevis
E. Flexor digitorum superficialis

Gantzer's muscle is an accessory slip off the origin of the flexor pollicis longus muscle. It can be a site of compression in anterior interosseous nerve (AIN) pathology.

Answer: **C**
Spinner, p. 339
Refer to Fig. 18-5

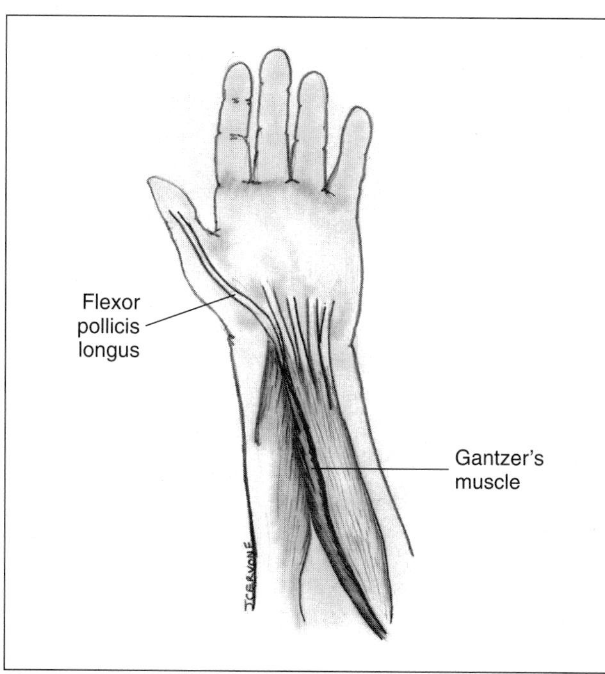

Fig. 18-5

11. What causes nocturnal pain with carpal tunnel syndrome (CTS)?

A. Sleeping position
B. Vascular stasis
C. Thenar atrophy
D. A and B
E. All of the above

Patients with CTS often complain of nocturnal pain that awakens them. They relieve this symptom by shaking their hands. Sleeping posture can cause nocturnal pain because of the flexed position of the wrist that often is assumed during the night. Vascular stasis, which can occur in the canal at night from inactivity, contributes to compression of the median nerve by increasing canal pressure as the blood vessels become full, thus causing pain.

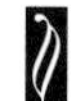

Answer: **D**
Hunter, Mackin, Callahan, pp. 909-910
Hayes, Carney, Wolf, et al, in Mackin, Callahan, Skirven, et al, pp. 645-646

12. Which type of splint should be used on a patient referred to you with de Quervain's disease?

A. Wrist support splint
B. Thumb spica splint with the interphalangeal (IP) joint free
C. Thumb spica splint, including the IP joint
D. Elbow extension splint
E. Short opponens splint

A patient with de Quervain's disease is splinted in a thumb spica with the IP joint free. Immobilizing the IP joint is unnecessary because the extensor pollicis longus tendon is not an offender in this disorder. Steroid injections commonly are used in conjunction with splinting to reduce inflammation. As the pain subsides, the patient can move from the rigid splint (Fig. 18-6, *A*) to a flexible splint and/or kinesiotape (Fig. 18-6, *B*) to allow for maximal flexibility. Wrist position for splinting ranges from neutral, with the thumb in radial abduction, to the wrist at 20 degrees of extension with the thumb in extension.

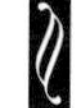

Answer: **B**
Hunter, Mackin, Callahan, p. 1013
Lee, Nasser-Sharif, Zelouf in Mackin, Callahan, Skirven, et al, pp. 945-946

13. Intersection syndrome involves which dorsal wrist compartments?

A. First and second
B. First and third
C. Third and fifth
D. Fourth and fifth
E. Fifth and sixth

Intersection syndrome is a condition triggered by repetitive use of the wrist or a traumatic incident. This syndrome tends to be more common among weightlifters, people who row or canoe, and writers. Patients complain of pain and tenderness in the distal forearm with localized swelling about 4 cm proximal to the wrist. In severe cases pain may be accompanied with redness and crepitus. The cause of pain appears to be from the ECRL and ECRB tendons (second dorsal wrist compartment) crossing over the extensor pollicis brevis and

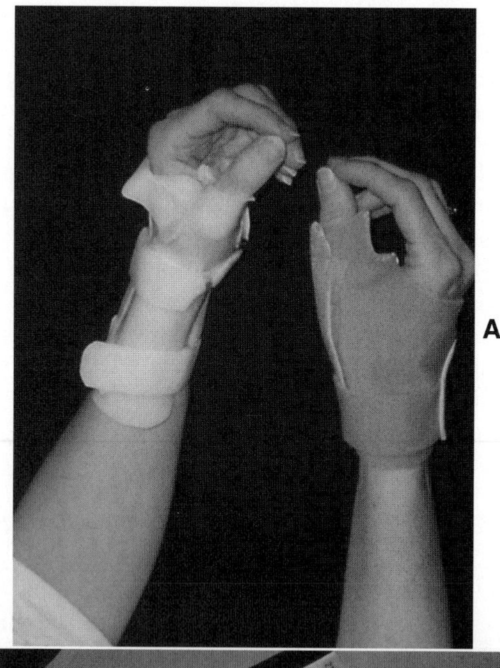

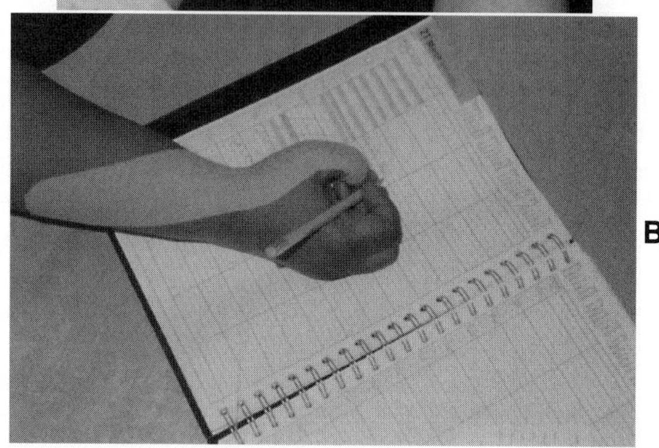

Fig. 18-6 ■ **A,** Courtesy 3-Point Products, Inc., 1610 Pincay Court, Annapolis, MD 21401, (410) 349-2649, e-mail the3ptprod@aol.com; **B,** from Mackin EJ, Callahan AD, Skirven TM, et al: *Rehabilitation of the hand and upper extremity*, ed 5, St Louis, 2002, Mosby.

abductor pollicis longus tendons (first dorsal wrist compartment) and/or with peritendnous bursal inflammation. Treatment includes thumb spica splinting with the wrist in approximately 15 degrees of extension, anti-inflammatory medications, steroid injections, ice, and avoidance of provocative activities.

Answer: **A**

Hunter, Mackin, Callahan, pp. 1012-1013
Lee, Nasser-Sharif, Zelouf in Mackin, Callahan, Skirven, et al, pp. 944-945
Refer to Fig. 18-7

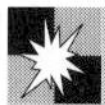

CLINICAL GEM:
Intersection syndrome can also be termed "squeaker's wrist."

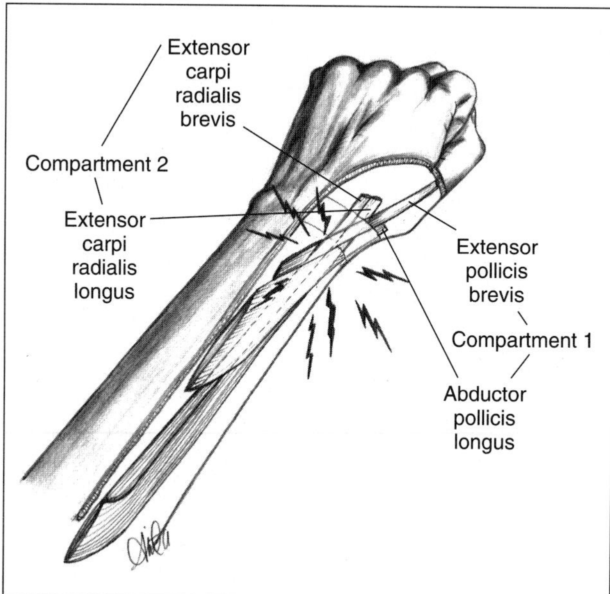

Fig. 18-7

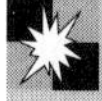

CLINICAL GEM:
Some researchers have discovered that the basic pathology in intersection syndrome is a tendosynovitis of the second dorsal compartment.

Green, Hotchkiss, Pederson, p. 2038

14. Injury of the posterior interosseous nerve (PIN) presents with all but which of the following?

A. Weak extensor digitorum muscle
B. Weakness of the triceps
C. Weakness of the extensor indicis muscle
D. Weakness of the wrist extensor muscles

The triceps is innervated by the radial nerve before it branches into the PIN. As the deep branch of the radial nerve exits from the supinator, it becomes the PIN. PIN syndrome elicits pain in the dorsal forearm, weakness of the metacarpophalangeal (MCP) joint extensors, and weak wrist extension because of loss of the extensor carpi ulnaris and of the ECRB in half of all cases. There is no sensory loss. The PIN is vulnerable for a variety of reasons, whether traumatic or nontraumatic. Some areas of entrapment include the following: 1) soft tissue tumors; 2) radial head fractures; 3) compression at the arcade of Frohse; 4) radiocapitellar joint; 5) vascular leash of Henry; 6) proximal edge of the ECRB; and 7) band of the proximal middle supinator. The most common areas of compression are arcade of Frohse and the supinator.

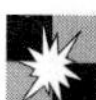

Answer: **B**

Prasartritha, Liupolvanish, Rojanakit, p. 107
Omar, Spinner, Van Beek, p. 521
Refer to Fig. 18-8

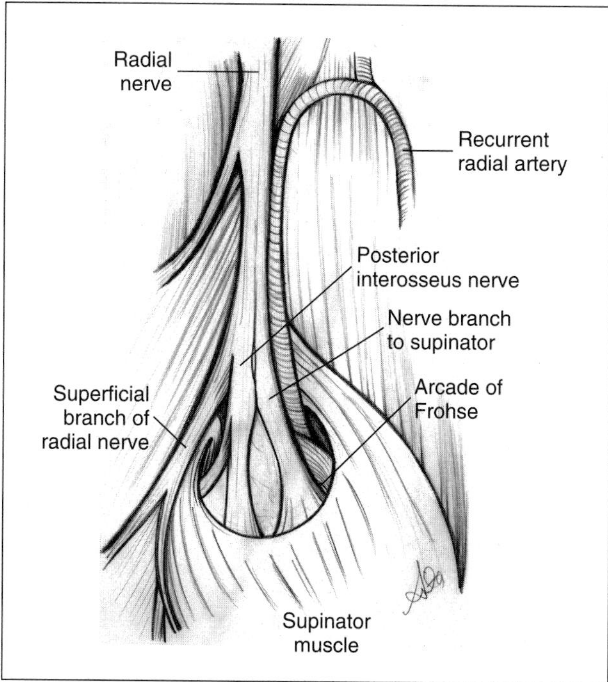

Fig. 18-8

CLINICAL GEM:
Rheumatoid arthritis is another disease that can cause compression of the PIN because of the common synovitis in the radiohumeral joint. Do not forget that with rheumatoid arthritis, tendon ruptures can look like a partial paralysis of the PIN.

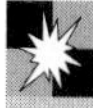

CLINICAL GEM:
The ECRB's tendinous origin places additional force on the supinator when the forearm is in pronation.

15. True or False: Golfer's elbow is another name for medial epicondylitis.

Medial epicondylitis involves the flexor muscles in the forearm and also is termed *golfer's elbow*. Patients report aching or burning at the flexor carpi ulnaris and flexor carpi radialis origins (the most commonly involved tendons). Conservative management is similar to that of lateral epicondylitis, except that the wrist is splinted at neutral and the air cast is applied to the flexors rather than the extensors.

Answer: **True**

Hunter, Mackin, Callahan, p. 1812
Woodsworth in Mackin, Callahan, Skirven, et al, p. 1268
Fedorczyk in Mackin, Callanan, Skirven, et al, p. 1279

16. Which of the following is *not* a factor in injury risk for patients to develop CTDs?

A. Heredity
B. Developmental
C. Lifestyle
D. All of the above are factors.

All of the above can influence a person's risk of developing CTDs. Heredity factors might include a predisposition to arthritis or a tendency towards hypermobility. Developmental or acquired factors could include poor posture, such as kyphosis or scoliosis, or a history of a previous injury. Lifestyle factors may include smoking, diet, and amount of exercise. Understanding personal factors related to injury is important because it helps develop a sense of individual responsibility. It shows patients that they have some control over events that will affect their outcome.

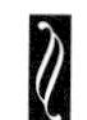

Answer: **D**

Wilson, p. 63

17. A patient is referred to you with the diagnosis of lateral epicondylitis. The patient sustained the injury when a swinging door slammed against his elbow at work. The patient reports a constant burning ache with intermittent sharp stabs. The air cast provided by the physician increased his symptoms. Which of the following tests should also be included in your evaluation?

A. Elbow flexion test
B. ULTT (radial nerve bias)
C. ULTT (median nerve bias)
D. Phalen test

Burning is a common complaint associated with nervous system involvement, as described by Butler. Because the radial nerve comes across the lateral elbow before bifurcating, the ULTT test (radial nerve bias) assists in identifying adverse neural tension as the source of comparable signs and symptoms in this region.

Answer: **B**

Butler, pp. 85, 155

Refer to Fig. 18-9

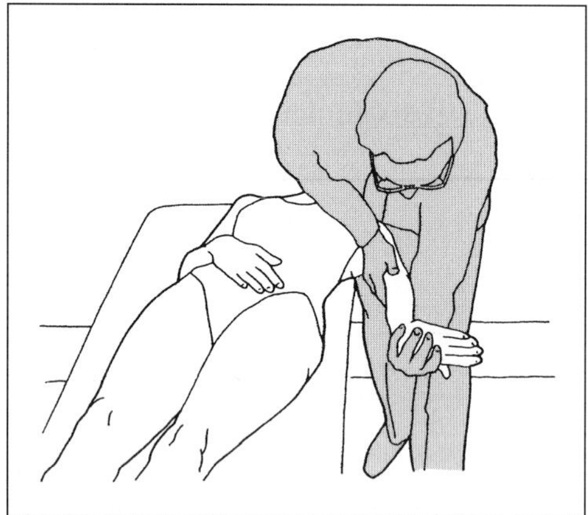

Fig. 18-9 ■ From Butler DS: *Mobilisation of the nervous system,* New York, 1991, Churchill Livingstone.

Clinical Gem:

Other tests to asses for tennis elbow are pressure algometer, ROM, grip strength, Cozen's test, Mills' test, simple handshake test, chair test, and the dumbbell test. See Mackin, Callahan, Skirven, et al, pp. 1274-1276, for details on each of these tests.

18. A primary-care physician refers you a 56-year-old woman with the diagnosis of wrist pain. She complains of constant radial wrist pain that increases when she abducts the thumb while working on her keyboard. She also has pain with writing notes. She has no symptoms of numbness or pain in the proximal arm. Further history reveals that she has performed this job for 8 years. After reviewing the patient's history, which one of the following problems may be the source of pain?

A. Basal joint osteoarthritis (BJOA) (carpometacarpal [CMC] joint)
B. Scapholunate instability
C. de Quervain tenosynovitis
D. Wartenberg's disease

Osteoarthritis of the first CMC joint can be caused by microtrauma incurred by repetitive stress and hypermobility. Repetitive thumb abduction may cause stress on the basal joint (first CMC joint), thus resulting in ligament attrition and articular changes. Dorsoradial subluxation of the basal joint occurs and is especially noted with pinch and prehension tasks. A residual adduction deformity will eventually occur.

Answer: **A**

Bozentka in Mackin, Callahan, Skirven, et al, pp. 1643-1648

Refer to Fig. 18-10

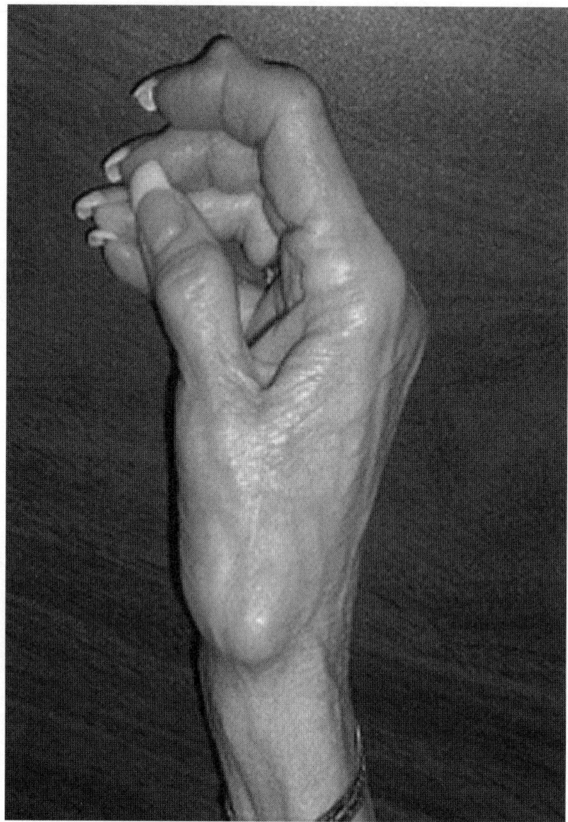

Fig. 18-10 ■ First CMC joint osteoarthritis—CMC joint dislocation and a positive "shoulder sign."

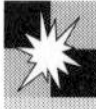

Clinical Gem:

Basal joint arthritis is commonly overlooked as the source of continued thenar region pain after carpal tunnel release and radial wrist pain after de Quervain's release.

19. Which tendon is most commonly involved in lateral epicondylitis?

A. ECRL
B. ECRB
C. Supinator
D. Extensor carpi ulnaris

The ECRB is the extensor tendon most commonly injured in lateral epicondylitis. The supinator and extensor carpi ulnaris also may be involved in lateral epicondylitis. The ECRL usually is not involved because its origin is proximal to the lateral epicondyle.

Answer: **B**

Stanley, Tribuzi, p. 430
Refer to Fig. 18-11

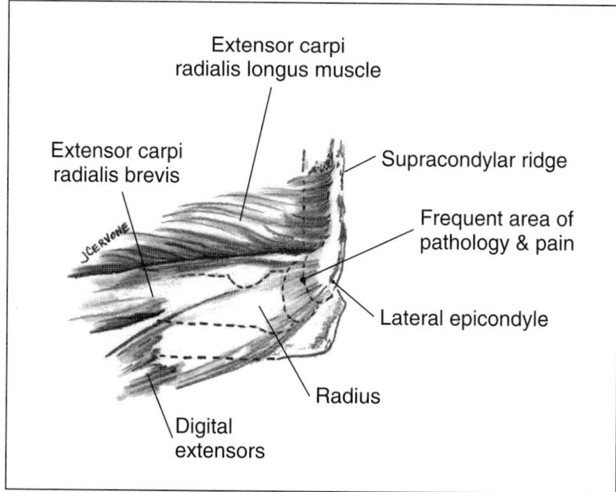

Fig. 18-11

20. A 46-year-old woman is referred to you with a diagnosis of acute lateral epicondylitis. If you decide to include a splint in your treatment plan, which splint is best?

A. Wrist immobilization splint with the wrist in 20 to 45 degrees of extension
B. Elbow flexion block splint
C. Wrist immobilization splint with the wrist neutral to 10 degrees of flexion
D. Forearm-based splint in supination

Most cases of lateral epicondylitis are treated conservatively. The goals of therapy are decreasing pain and inflammation and restoring functional use. This may be accomplished by applying a wrist immobilization splint (20 to 45 degrees of extension), which allows the common extensor muscles to rest. During the acute phase, ice, rest, and education are mandatory. Wrist immobilization may be used with severe/acute pain and is worn for a brief period (10 to 21 days). After the pain and inflammation have decreased, you may begin gentle stretching for both the extensor and flexor muscles of the forearm. At this point, a proximal pneumatic air splint may be worn in conjunction with the wrist immobilization splint. The air cast is proposed to counterforce the loading to the wrist extensors. After the patient's pain is managed and is not exacerbated easily, strengthening exercises can progress.

Interestingly, 85% of cases are successfully treated conservatively. However, 40% report certain tasks or motions elicit discomfort or pain.

Answer: **A**

Stanley, Tribuzi, p. 431
Mackin, Callahan, Skirven, et al, pp. 1277-1278

CLINICAL GEM:
Air casts used for lateral epicondylitis may cause compression of the PIN. The therapist must watch for symptoms of PIN irritation. The air cast should not be placed directly over the PIN.

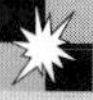

CLINICAL GEM:
To achieve optimal functional grip strength, O'Driscoll recommends the patient be splinted with the wrist at 35 degrees of extension. NOTE: This position is for grip strength, not optimal wrist position.

21. A 39-year-old woman presents with complaints of chronic ulnar wrist pain. With forearm rotation you notice a snapping on the ulnar side of the wrist. The patient reports increased pain with excessive wrist motion. What might this patient have?

A. Subluxation of the extensor carpi ulnaris
B. Rupture of the extensor digiti quinti
C. Tendinitis of the triangular fibrocartilage complex
D. Tendinitis of the intrinsic muscles

The extensor carpi ulnaris inserts on the fifth metacarpal base and constitutes the sixth dorsal compartment; it also has a separate compartment that is deep to the extensor retinaculum. Traumatic rupture of the extensor carpi ulnaris retinaculum causes subluxation of the extensor carpi ulnaris. Patients also can have a chronic subluxation that becomes symptomatic with excessive wrist ROM. During physical examination, the therapist can palpate the extensor carpi ulnaris coming out of the ulnar groove while inspecting forearm rotation.

Answer: **A**

Millender, Louis, Simmons, p. 137

Refer to Fig. 18-12

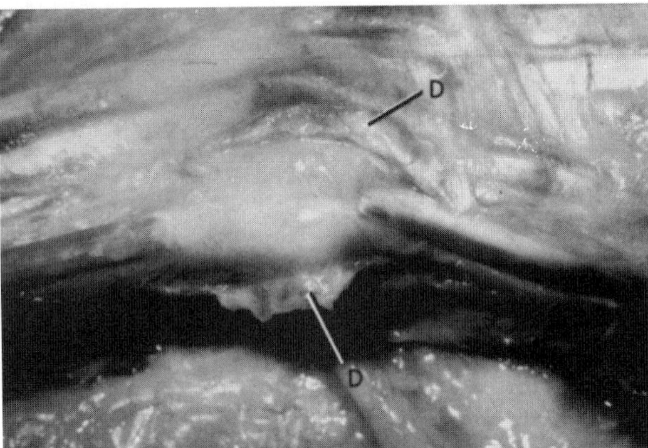

Fig. 18-12 ■ Sixth dorsal compartment. Supratendinous extensor retinaculum is seen reflected. Extensor carpi ulnaris tendon is fixed distal to the ulna by synovial-lined tunnel of fascia derived from the infratendinous retinaculum. Angulation of the tendon increases displacement forces during supination. Insertion of the tendon is on the fifth metacarpal to right. **D**, Extensor retinaculum. (From Mackin EJ, Callahan AD, Skirven TM, et al: *Rehabilitation of the hand and upper extremity,* ed 5, St Louis, 2002, Mosby.)

22. What would be your first recommendation for treatment of the patient in the previous question?

A. Splint or cast in pronation with slight dorsiflexion and radial deviation
B. Splint in slight flexion and ulnar deviation
C. Fluidotherapy for desensitization
D. Strengthening

Conservative treatment for extensor carpi ulnaris subluxation involves splinting or casting in pronation with dorsiflexion and radial deviation to determine whether the sheath will heal. Often subluxation continues and surgical reconstruction is needed.

Answer: **A**

Millender, Louis, Simmons, pp. 136-138
Thorson, Szabo, p. 425

CLINICAL GEM:
A circumferential wrist cuff with padding pressing on the extensor carpi ulnaris may help decrease subluxation and allow for greater function than a long-arm cast or splint.

23. In which position should a patient's wrist be splinted for conservative management of CTS?

A. Wrist extension (20 degrees)
B. Wrist neutral (0 degrees)
C. Wrist flexion (20 degrees)
D. Wrist flexion (40 degrees)

CTS traditionally was splinted with the wrist in a "cock-up" splint, with moderate amounts of wrist extension. It is recommended that the wrist be at neutral to reduce pressure in the carpal canal (Table 18-2). Other studies indicate the optimal position for wrist control splinting is neutral with the wrist postured at 2 degrees of flexion and 3 degrees of ulnar deviation (Fig. 18-13, *A*). This gives patients more relief of symptoms than the original protocol of wrist cock-up splinting (Fig. 18-13, *B*).

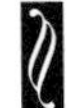

Answer: **B**

Ranney, p. 70
Gilberman, p. 747
Evans in Mackin, Callahan, Skirven, et al, p. 663

Table 18-2

Wrist Position Correlation with Carpal Canal Pressure

Wrist position	Carpal canal pressure
Neutral	18 mm Hg
20 degrees of extension	35 mm Hg
20 degrees of flexion	27 mm Hg
40 degrees of flexion	47 mm Hg

24. What muscle can occupy the space within the carpal tunnel when the fingers are flexed?

A. Lumbricals
B. Dorsal interossei
C. Palmar interossei
D. Adductor polices

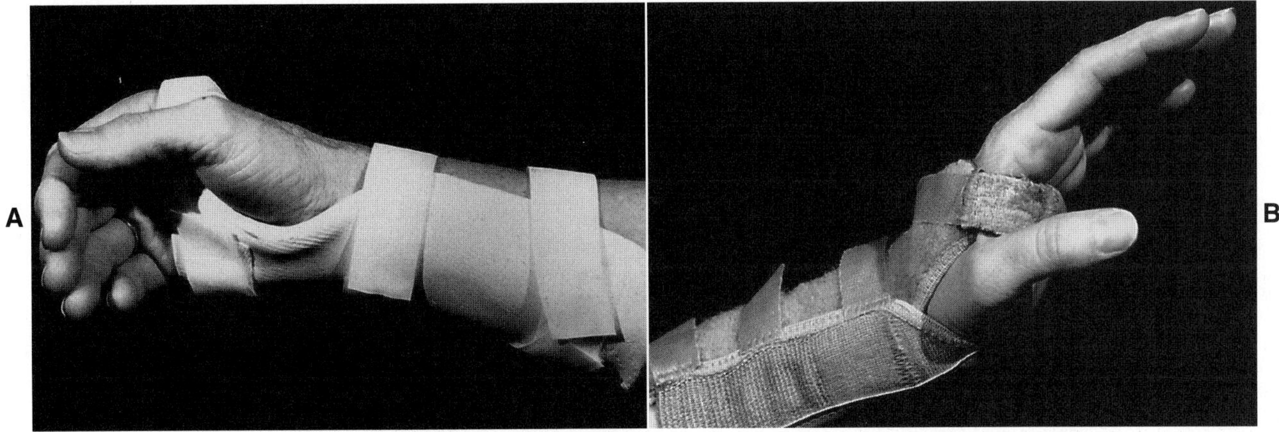

Fig. 18-13 ■ **A,** The proper position for wrist control splinting to minimize carpal tunnel pressures is neutral with the wrist postured at 2 degrees of flexion and 3 degrees of ulnar deviation. **B,** Improper splint position may elevate carpal tunnel pressure by 30 to 40 mm Hg. (From Mackin EJ, Callahan AD, Skirven TM, et al: *Rehabilitation of the hand and upper extremity*, ed 5, St Louis, 2002, Mosby.)

Scientific discussion has included the role of the lumbricals as space-occupying structures within the carpal tunnel when the fingers are flexed. This can lead to compression of the median nerve. Therefore, standard wrist immobilization splints may not be adequate for patients who sustain finger flexion during functional activities. This is especially common in manual laborers due to hypertrophy of the lumbricals. The method of splinting that would be helpful in these cases is to add the MCPs in the splint at 20 to 40 degrees of flexion (Fig. 18-14) to decrease the lumbrical pressure in the carpal canal.

Answer: **A**

Hayes, Carney, Wolf, et al, in Mackin, Callahan, Skirven, et al, p. 644

Evans in Mackin, Callahan, Skirven, et al, pp. 663-665

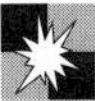

CLINICAL GEM:

A positive Berger test occurs when the patient has swelling at the volar wrist, thus indicating a flexor synovitis or a "compulsive gripper."

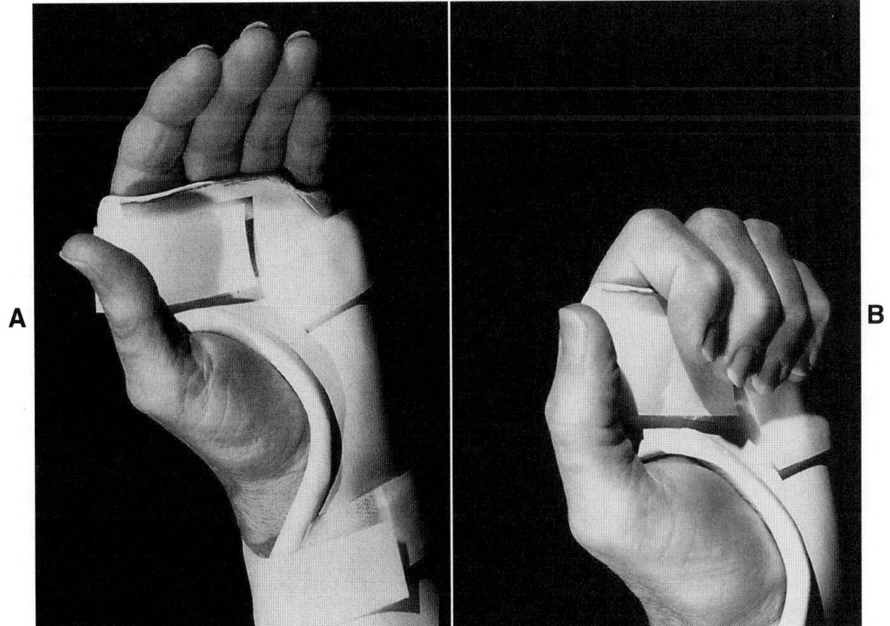

Fig. 18-14 ■ From Mackin EJ, Callahan AD, Skirven TM, et al: *Rehabilitation of the hand and upper extremity*, ed 5, St Louis, 2002, Mosby.

25. True or False: Putty is an excellent choice for conservative rehabilitation of CTS.

Research has shown that when the fingers are flexed more than 50%, the lumbricals can move into the carpal canal with flexor digitorum profundus contraction, which exacerbates compression of the median nerve. Therefore gripping exercises (e.g., putty) would amplify symptoms of CTS. Strengthening should not be a part of conservative management for acute and intermittent CTS. (See Question 24 for details.)

Answer: **False**

Evans, p. 17
Evans in Mackin, Callahan, Skirven, et al, p. 665

26. True or False: Microtrauma to soft tissue that causes common pain problems occurs only from high-velocity movements.

Daily activities that overstretch, overshorten, or overload muscles may cause microtrauma. Microtrauma can occur through repetitive or continuous low-velocity movements, and it can also occur through poor and asymmetrical postures. Microtrauma does not occur from sudden high-velocity movements.

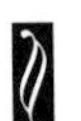

Answer: **False**

Kostopoulos, Rizopoulos, pp. 20, 25, 41

27. True or False: A *myofascial trigger point* is defined as "a hyperirritable spot on skeletal muscle that is associated with a hypersensitive palpable nodule in a taut band. The spot is painful on compression and can give rise to characteristic referred pain, referred tenderness, motor dysfunction and autonomic phenomena."

The description is the definition of a myofascial trigger point as defined by Travell and Simons. Trigger points can also be described as a local inflammatory response, muscular hardness, local ischemia, and connective tissue irritation.

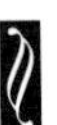

Answer: **True**

Travell, Simons, pp.
Kasch in Mackin, Callahan, Skirven, et al, p. 1013
Refer to Fig. 18-15

CLINICAL GEM:

The *progressive pressure technique* is performed by using the thumbs or four fingers of one or both hands and applying a steady pressure, moving inward toward the center. Applied pressure may start with a few ounces and go up to a couple of pounds. After tissue resistance is felt, stop and wait until the resistance dissipates. At this point, you may feel a slow release or "melting away" sensation of the tissue under the treating fingers. You should then proceed with further steady pressure, moving again inward toward the center. After new tissue resistance appears, you should stop and wait with steady force against the tissue, then repeat the cycle several times. At the end, either further relaxation of the tissue will be felt or no new gains will be achieved.

Kostopoulos, Rizopoulos, p. 52
Refer to Fig. 18-15

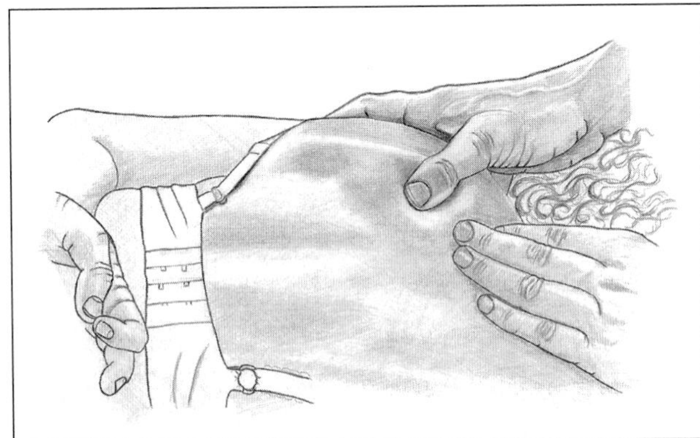

Fig. 18-15 ■ From Wilson A: *Effective management of musculoskeletal injury: a clinical ergonomics approach to prevention, treatment, and rehabilitation*, New York, 2002, Churchill Livingstone.

28. True or False: Myofascial trigger points can affect muscle flexibility.

Myofascial trigger points may decrease muscle flexibility, produce muscle weakness, and distort proprioception. In addition, muscle contraction slows down, thus decreasing, neuromuscular coordination and exposes muscle to the danger of reinjury and further injury.

Answer: **True**

Kostopoulos, Rizopoulos, pp. 19, 25

29. The radial nerve enters the forearm between the two heads of which muscle?

A. Flexor carpi ulnaris
B. Pronator teres
C. Supinator
D. BR

The radial nerve arises from the posterior cord of the brachial plexus and winds posterior to the humerus. The radial nerve subdivides at the elbow into the superficial sensory branch and a deep motor branch termed the *PIN*. The latter dives between the two heads of the supinator as it enters the forearm.

Answer: **C**
Hunter, Mackin, Callahan, pp. 70-73
Refer to Fig. 18-16

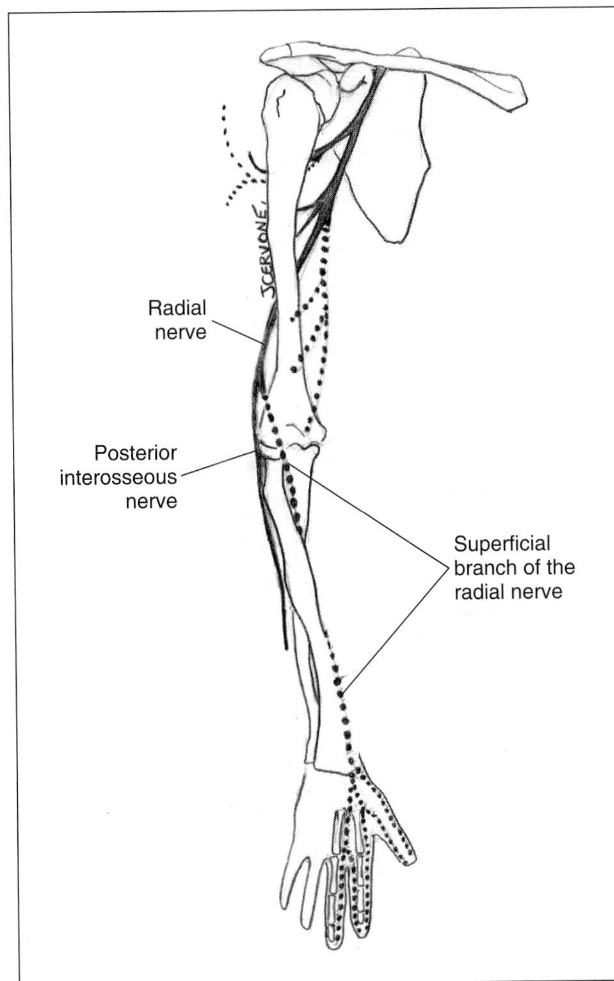

Fig. 18-16

30. Which nerve emerges between the BR and the ECRL tendons in the forearm and may become irritated after de Quervain's release?

A. PIN
B. Superficial branch of the radial nerve
C. Recurrent branch of the median nerve
D. Ulnar nerve

The superficial branch of the radial nerve (SBRN, see Fig. 18-16) emerges in the proximal forearm between the tendons of the BR and the ECRL. It is not uncommon for this nerve to become irritated or compressed with the release of the first dorsal compartment, a tight cast or splint, or repetitive forearm pronation with wrist ulnar deviation and flexion. Irritation of the SBRN may be misdiagnosed as de Quervain's tenosynovitis. Dellon and Mackin suggest testing with the patient's elbow in extension, forearm in hyperpronation, and wrist in ulnar flexion for 1 minute. A positive test for the SBRN results in numbness and tingling over the dorsoradial aspect of the hand. A positive Tinel's sign over the course of the nerve also may be present.

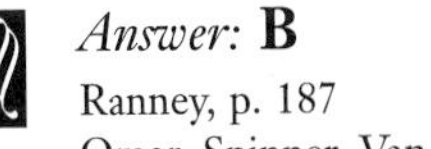

Answer: **B**
Ranney, p. 187
Omer, Spinner, Van Beek, p. 524

31. Wartenberg's syndrome is which of the following?

A. Compression of the ulnar nerve
B. Compression of the SBRN
C. Compression of the digital nerve to the thumb
D. Intrinsic weakness
E. Intrinsic muscle wasting

Wartenberg's syndrome also is known as *radial sensory nerve entrapment*. Patients complain of hypersensitivity, dorsal hand and radial wrist pain, and possibly dysesthesia of the dorsal thumb/index fingers on the dorsum of the hand. A positive Tinel's sign around the radial styloid often is present. Compression occurs at one of two sites: 1) 8 cm proximal to radial styloid at the fascial edge of the BR and ECRB; or 2) at the subcutaneous position of the radial styloid.

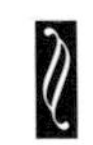

Answer: **B**
Ranney, p. 187
Omer, Spinner, Van Beek, pp. 524-525

CLINICAL GEM:
Cheiralgia paresthetica is another term for Wartenberg syndrome.

32. For treatment of a patient with acute Wartenberg's syndrome (disease), a recommended site of neural mobilization is which of the following?

A. Neck
B. Elbow
C. Wrist
D. All of the above
E. A and B

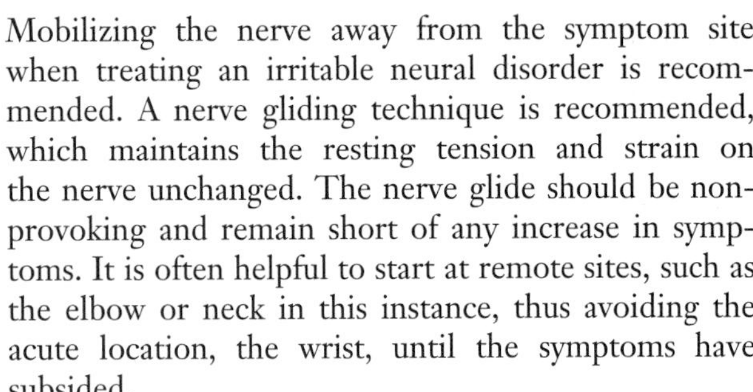

Mobilizing the nerve away from the symptom site when treating an irritable neural disorder is recommended. A nerve gliding technique is recommended, which maintains the resting tension and strain on the nerve unchanged. The nerve glide should be nonprovoking and remain short of any increase in symptoms. It is often helpful to start at remote sites, such as the elbow or neck in this instance, thus avoiding the acute location, the wrist, until the symptoms have subsided.

Answer: **E**
Evans in Mackin, Callahan, Skirven, et al, pp. 663-765

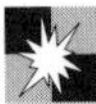

CLINICAL GEM:
Other helpful treatments for this diagnosis include thumb spica splinting, modalities, and modification of provocative activities.

33. True or False: Cumulative trauma injuries can benefit from a general exercise program (i.e., aerobic fitness).

Cumulative trauma injuries can benefit from appropriate exercises and a general exercise program. Beginning exercise with a person suffering chronic musculoskeletal symptoms should be performed carefully. Exercises should ease or reduce dysfunction. Exercise should be rhythmic, should involve active joint movements, should start away from injured tissues, and should allow for long periods of recovery before the next session. Poor circulation appears to be a factor in developing cumulative trauma; therefore restoration of circulation is crucial. Patients need to increase light aerobic activity and decrease consumption of caffeine, nicotine, and alcohol.

Answer: **True**
Wilson, p. 90
Skirven, Osterman in Mackin, Callahan, Skirven, et al, p. 1104

34. A 29-year-old woman is referred to you from her primary-care physician with a diagnosis of dorsal hand and wrist pain. She complains of decreased sensation in the dorsal thumb and index. Evaluation reveals point tenderness at the distal forearm on the radial side, an inconsistent positive Tinel's sign at the site of pain, mild edema along the distal radial forearm, and a 4.31 reading with the Semmes-Weinstein monofilament for the dorsal thumb. The patient's job requires repetitive forearm pronation with wrist flexion and ulnar deviation. Her primary-care physician issued a prefabricated wrist support splint, which increased her symptoms. What might you conclude?

A. The patient is experiencing de Quervain's tenosynovitis. Her primary-care physician should refer her to a hand surgeon for surgical consultation.
B. The patient is experiencing median nerve compression. Her primary-care physician should refer her to a hand surgeon.
C. The patient is experiencing Wartenberg's syndrome. The appropriate splint should be applied.
D. Current splint protocol should be continued. The patient needs time to adjust to the brace.

This patient has Wartenberg's syndrome (disease). Her splint increased her symptoms because the splint did not protect the thumb and may have increased the pressure on the nerve. This patient needs a radial thumb spica splint to protect from excessive thumb and wrist ROM.

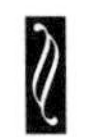

Answer: **C**
Ranney, p. 187
Skirven, Osterman in Mackin, Callahan, Skirven, et al, p. 1104

35. True or False: Radial tunnel syndrome (RTS) presents with symptoms of muscle paralysis in the wrist extensors.

RTS presents with pain in the posterior forearm (Fig. 18-17, *A*) without associated muscle paralysis. RTS is recognized with irritation of the PIN at the arcade of Frohse. The characteristics of RTS include pain at the lateral elbow without motor loss (paralysis) and localized tenderness with pressure on the arcade of Frohse.

Clinical tests include the resisted wrist extension test, the resisted supination test, and the resisted middle-finger extension test. These provocative tests also may be used to determine lateral epicondylitis and are positive if pain is reproduced during the examination. The key to differentiation between lateral epicondylitis and RTS is point tenderness. There is pain and tenderness with palpation over the supinator and the radial neck region with RTS; with lateral epicondylitis, the pain usually is over the ECRB origin, radial head, and lateral epicondyle.

Common sites of compression in RTS include the following: 1) the radial nerve against the capitellum by the ECRB (see Fig. 18-17); 2) arcade of Frohse (see Fig. 18-17, *A*); 3) leash of Henry (fan-shaped vessels); and 4) fibrous bands anterior to the radial head. Treatment for RTS is similar to treatment for lateral epicondylitis and includes decreasing wrist motion, splinting (wrist support), modification of activity, modalities, and a balance between activity and rest.

Answer: **False**

Ranney, p. 183
Hunter, Mackin, Callahan, p. 1816
Wright, Rettig in Mackin, Callahan, Skirven, et al, p. 2083
Omer, Spinner, Van Beek, pp. 521-523

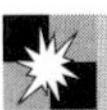

CLINICAL GEM:
RTS can coexist in 10% to 15% of lateral epicondylitis cases (Fig. 18-17, *B*), perhaps because of radiocapitellar bursitis and recurrent inflammation contracting the arcade of Frohse.

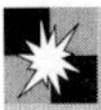

CLINICAL GEM:
Conservative treatment for RTS can include rest via splinting (elbow flexed at 90 degrees, forearm supinated and wrist extended at 20 to 30 degrees) (Fig. 18-18), avoidance of exacerbating activities, oral antiinflammatory medication, ultrasound, phonophoresis, electrical modalities (high-volt, ionto, and/or TENS), cryotherapy, and ROM exercises.

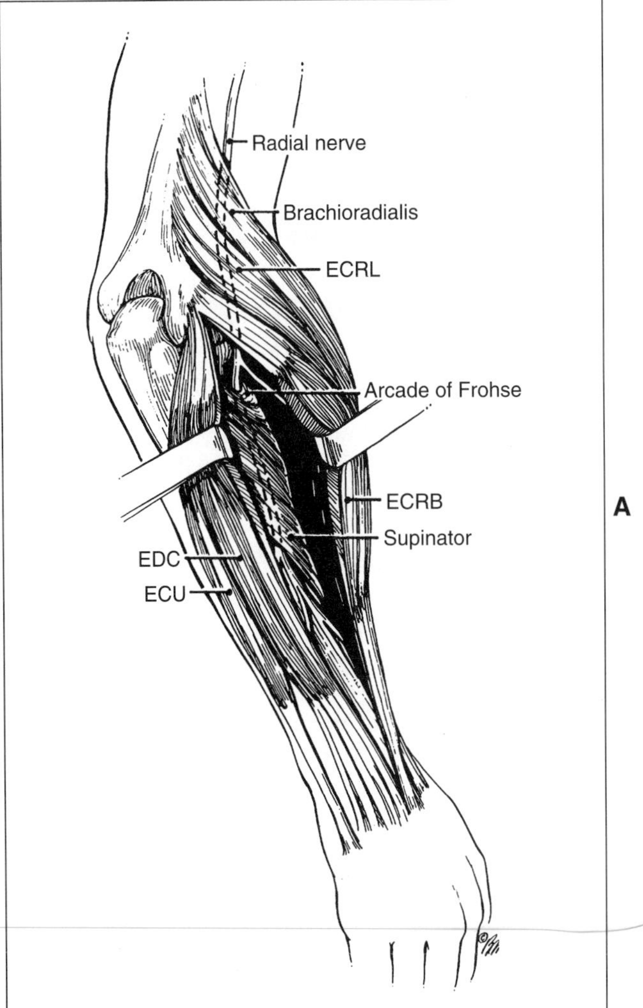

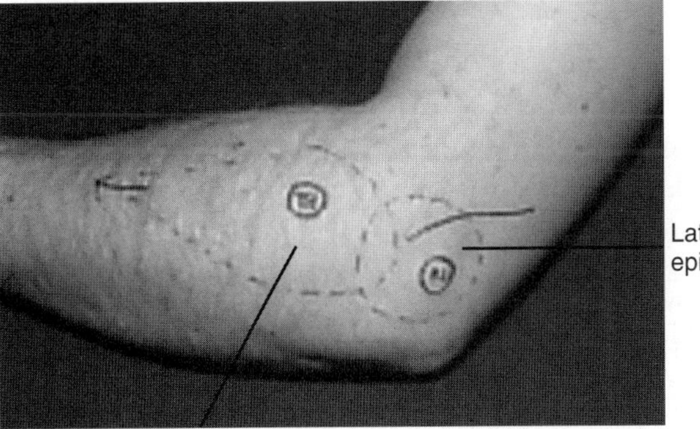

Fig. 18-17 ■ **B,** Areas of point tenderness to differentiate between lateral elbow tendonitis and RTS. (**A** Copyright Elizabeth Roselius, 1993; from Eversmann C: Entrapment and compression neuropathies. In Green DP, ed: *Operative hand surgery,* New York, 1993, Churchill Livingstone; **B** from Mackin EJ, Callahan AD, Skirven TM, et al: *Rehabilitation of the hand and upper extremity,* ed 5, St Louis, 2002, Mosby.)

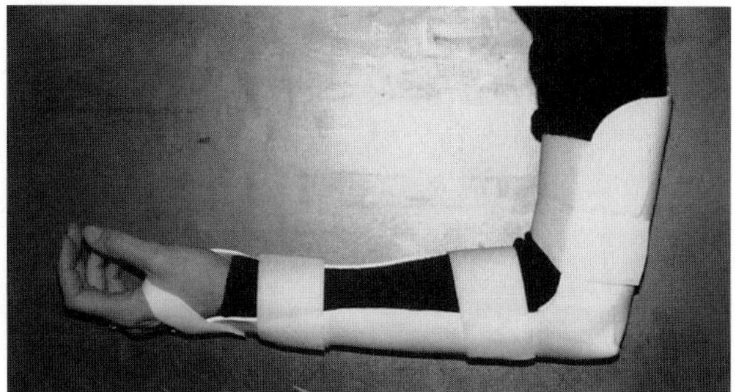

Fig. 18-18 ■ From Mackin EJ, Callahan AD, Skirven TM, et al: *Rehabilitation of the hand and upper extremity*, ed 5, St Louis, 2002, Mosby.

36. True or False: When testing for acute lateral epicondylitis, grip strength will be increased with the elbow extended.

Lateral epicondylitis, also known as *tennis elbow*, occurs from excessive loading to the extensor mass and/or a rapid grasp. One way to test lateral epicondylitis is to test grip strength with the elbow flexed and then with the elbow extended. If grip strength is significantly diminished with the elbow extended, the test for lateral epicondylitis is positive. This extended position puts increased tension on the extensor tendons. An increase in grip strength with the elbow extended has been found to correlate significantly with a satisfactory clinical outcome.

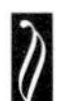

Answer: **False**

Hunter, Mackin, Callahan, p. 1816
Fedorczyk in Mackin, Callahan, Skirven, et al, p. 1274
Wright, Rettig in Mackin, Callahan, Skirven, et al, p. 2083

37. John H. is a patient referred to you with complaints of hand weakness and numbness in the ring and small fingers. Your sensory tests reveal diminished sensation of digits four and five, both volarly and dorsally. This patient might have nerve compression at which of the following points?

A. Guyon's canal
B. The cubital tunnel
C. The carpal tunnel
D. The arcade of Frohse

This patient has ulnar nerve symptoms; this knowledge narrows your choices to Guyon's canal or the cubital tunnel. You can rule out Guyon's canal because of the dorsal numbness. The dorsal cutaneous branch of the ulnar nerve comes off proximal to Guyon's canal. Dorsal sensory involvement of these digits indicates a problem proximal to the wrist, such as in the cubital tunnel (see Fig. 18-2). Patients typically present with motor weakness predominately in the hand intrinsics or sensory abnormalities of the ulnar nerve (as stated in the question). Causes of compression include the following: external pressure, synovitis, osteophytes, masses, fracture callus, perineural adhesions, hematomas, nerve instability, or adomalous muscles.

Answer: **B**

Reiner, Lohman, pp. 11-13
Omer, Spinner, Van Beek, p. 518

CLINICAL GEM:

The anconeus epitrochlearis is an uncommon cause of ulnar nerve compression at the elbow, which may be bilateral. It is a vestigial muscle originating from the medial border of the olecranon and inserting into the medial epicondyle. It crosses the ulnar nerve over the cubital tunnel and reinforces the aponeurosis of the two heads of the flexor carpi ulnaris and may cause compression of the ulnar nerve.

38. Handlebar palsy compresses which nerve?

A. AIN
B. Median nerve
C. Ulnar nerve
D. PIN

Clinical manifestation of handlebar palsy (a compression of the ulnar nerve at Guyon canal) can present with sensory deficits, intrinsic weakness, or both. The patient describes decreased pinch and grip and pain over the volar wrist and fifth digit. There is a classification system with three types of lesions. Type I involves both motor and sensory branches proximal to the wrist. Type II involves the motor branch at the hook of the hamate and at the distal part of the canal. Type III involves the superficial sensory branch. Compression occurs most commonly with types I and II. This palsy does not include the dorsal sensory branch because it branches off proximal to the wrist. Treatment includes rest, splinting, modifying the patient-bicycle fit, padding the handlebars, wearing gloves, and varying hand position while riding.

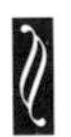

Answer: **C**

Hunter, Mackin, Callahan, pp. 1825-1826
Blackmore in Mackin, Callahan, Skirven, et al, pp. 680-684
Wright, Rettig in Mackin, Callahan, Skirven, et al, pp. 2092-2093
Omer, Spinner, Van Beek, pp. 516-517

39. A patient is diagnosed with cubital tunnel syndrome and receives orders for night splinting. The patient's elbow should be splinted in which position?

A. 0 degrees of flexion
B. 30 degrees of flexion
C. 50 degrees of flexion
D. 90 degrees of flexion

The cubital tunnel has the least amount of nerve tension with the elbow fully extended, but this position would be intolerable for most patients. Therefore the recommended position is between 30 to 45 degrees of flexion. It is helpful to include the wrist in the splint—not only for patient comfort but also to relax the flexor carpi ulnaris tendon. Other treatments that might be helpful include antiinflammatory drugs prescribed by the physician, modalities, and/or a nerve-gliding program. Patient education is important because the patient must fully understand the pathology in order to modify work, play, and rest.

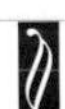

Answer: **B**

Hunter, Mackin, Callahan, p. 670
Refer to Fig. 18-19

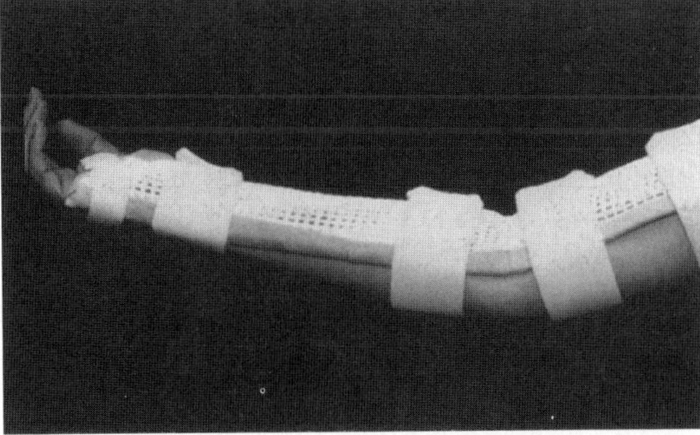

Fig. 18-19 ■ From Mackin EJ, Callahan AD, Skirven TM, et al: *Rehabilitation of the hand and upper extremity*, ed 5, St Louis, 2002, Mosby.

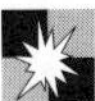

CLINICAL GEM:
An alternative to a splint is to roll up a towel, place on the volar arm, and secure with an elastic wrap with arm extension. Additionally, the pillow splint is a comfortable alternative to thermoplastic splinting.

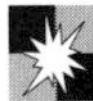

CLINICAL GEM:
Conservative treatment for cubital tunnel syndrome, including nighttime splinting and activity modification, should result in a decrease of symptoms within 3 weeks.

40. Active ROM therapy after cubital tunnel release with epicondylectomy should be started at which of the following? (Pick the best answer.)

A. Immediately (same day of surgery)
B. 14 days after surgery
C. 21 days after surgery
D. Therapy is not indicated for this procedure.

The literature does not have clear guidelines as to when therapy should be initiated after cubital tunnel release. According to Warwick and Seradge, if ROM is started at day 3, patients will have full ROM and minimal chance of flexion contracture. It is not unusual, however, to see a patient immobilized for 14 days before being sent to therapy. According to Sailer, therapy should be initiated at 7 to 10 days after surgery, with end-range stretching started at 4 weeks. According to Mackin, Callahan, Skirven, et al, ROM begins at 2 weeks. ROM should not begin on the same day as surgery (Answer A) and should not be delayed until day 21 (Answer C).

Answer: **B**

Warwick, Seradge, p. 245
Sailer, p. 239
Hunter, Mackin, Callahan, p. 671
Omer in Mackin, Callahan, Skirven, et al, pp. 676-677
Blackmore in Mackin, Callahan, Skirven, et al, pp. 683-689
Omer, Spinner, Van Beek, p. 519
Refer to Fig. 18-20

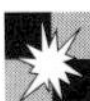

CLINICAL GEM:
Other procedures include a subcutaneous transposition and or submuscular transposition; the patient will usually have his elbow immobilized in 90 degrees of flexion with the forearm pronated for 3 weeks.

Omer in Mackin, Callahan, Skirven, et al, p. 677

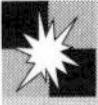

CLINICAL GEM:
For a quick reference chart on rehabilitation after cubital tunnel release, refer to the chart provided by Mackin, Callahan, Skirven, et al, in *Rehabilitation of the hand and upper extremity: surgery and therapy*, ed 5.

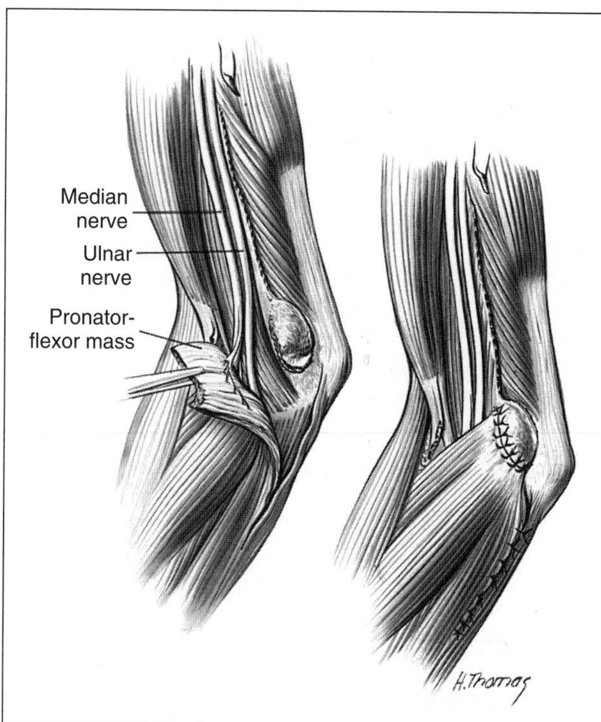

Fig. 18-20 ■ In any transposition of the ulnar nerve, a thorough decompression of the ulnar nerve must be performed. In a submuscular transposition, the ulnar nerve is translocated anterior and deep to the flexor-pronator muscles. The ulnar nerve is placed adjacent and parallel to the median nerve. The flexor-pronator muscles are loosely resutured to their origin. (From Spinner M: *Injuries to the major branches of peripheral nerves of the forearm*, ed 2, Philadelphia, 1978, WB Saunders.)

41. Trigger point therapy can include all but which of the following?

A. Progressive pressure technique
B. Dry needling
C. Injections using a local anesthetic
D. Acupuncture
E. Myofascial release

Acupuncture is not used for trigger point therapy. On the other hand, acupuncture points often correlate with trigger points (see the following Clinical Gem). Acupuncture is a traditional system of Chinese medicine that has been practiced for more than 2000 years. Classical acupuncture points are identified as precise points along specific meridians (except extrameridians and achi points) as defined by ancient Chinese documents. These points are used for the diagnosis and treatment of pathological conditions, including visceral and systemic dysfunction. Pain relief is achieved through the release of endorphins to balance the body's energy levels.

All of the other techniques above are used for trigger point therapy. In addition, postisometric relaxation, reciprocal inhibition, contract-relax techniques, muscle energy techniques, strain-counterstrain techniques, and massage are useful trigger point therapy techniques.

CLINICAL GEM:
There is a 71% correlation between trigger points and acupuncture points for the treatment of pain.

Melzak, Stillwell, Fox, pp. 3-23

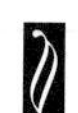
Answer: **D**
Kostopoulos, Rizopoulos, pp. 7-8

42. Effective trigger point therapy should be followed by which of the following?

A. Myofascial stretching exercises
B. Posttreatment modalities
C. Progressive resistive exercises
D. Proprioceptive retraining
E. All of the above

All of the above are appropriate treatments to follow trigger point therapy. Myofascial stretching exercises lengthen muscle fibers that are shortened by trigger point mechanisms. Stretching exercises help restore the musculotendonous unit to optimal resting length. The application of cold decreases sensitivity to areas of soreness. Strengthening exercises and proprioceptive retraining restore muscle strength and coordination. In addition, ongoing patient education and active participation in a home exercise program reinforce follow-through for a successful outcome.

Answer: **E**
Kostopoulos, Rizopoulos, p. 54

43. A 35-year-old medical office manager is referred to you for evaluation and treatment. Her diagnosis is CTD. She presents with complaints of pain to two distinct areas: the posterolateral neck and along her medial scapula and posterior shoulder. Further discussion of her daily work activities reveals that she spends most of her day scheduling patients on a handset phone. In addition, she tells you that she is a part-time student at a local community college and that she carries her heavy books and laptop computer in a shoulder bag. Which muscles are the likely sources of her reported pain? Pick two answers.

A. Scalenus
B. Rotator cuff
C. Upper trapezius
D. Levator scapulae

The upper trapezius refers pain to the posterolateral lateral aspect of the neck, behind the ear, to the temporal area (temporal headaches), and up to the zygoma. The levator scapulae refers pain to the angle of the neck, along the vertebral border of the scapula, and to the posterior shoulder. Active overstretching of these muscles occurs when stabilizing a phone handset between the neck and shoulder and when carrying a heavy bag supported with a belt-type over-the-shoulder strap.

Answers: **C and D**
Kostopoulos, Rizopoulos, pp. 90, 92

44. True or False: AIN syndrome is a motor syndrome.

The AIN is a branch of the median nerve that innervates the flexor pollicis longus, the flexor digitorum profundus to the index and long fingers, and the pronator quadratus. The AIN syndrome is characterized by an inability to make an "O," which requires thumb IP joint flexion and index finger distal interphalangeal (DIP) joint flexion (Fig. 18-21). Patients assume an abnormal pinch. In addition to paralysis, some patients report pain in the proximal forearm. No sensory loss is reported. Treatment includes rest and splinting. If unresolved within 90 days, surgery is indicated.

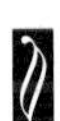
Answer: **True**
Hunter, Mackin, Callahan, pp. 632-633
Colditz in Mackin, Callahan, Skirven, et al, pp. 629-630

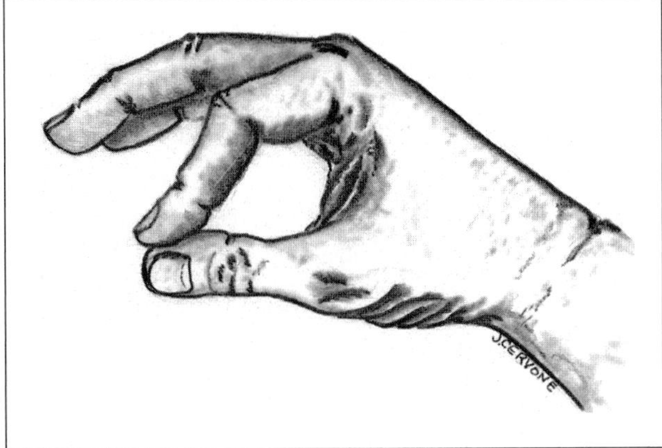

Fig. 18-21

CLINICAL GEM:
Fig. 18-22 depicts small splints to improve pinch.

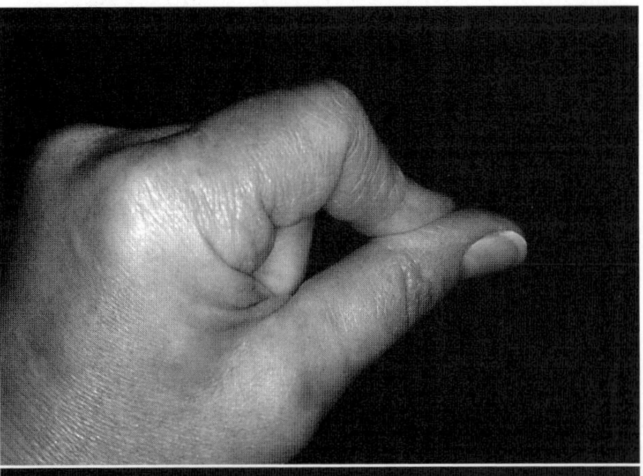

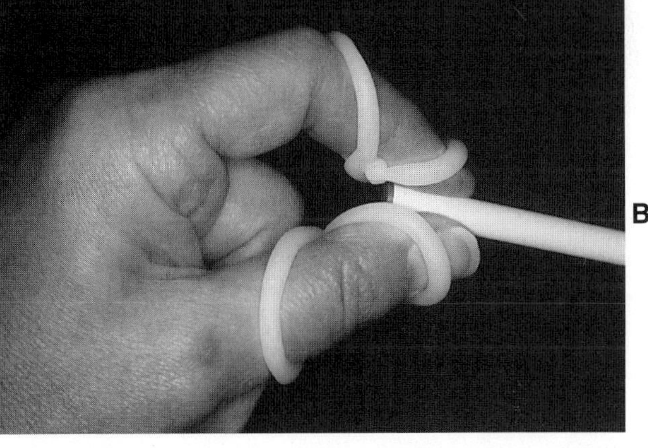

Fig. 18-22 ■ From Mackin EJ, Callahan AD, Skirven TM, et al: *Rehabilitation of the hand and upper extremity*, ed 5, St Louis, 2002, Mosby.

45. You plan to perform a job-site analysis on a patient with a CTD in the upper extremity. The patient's employer provides a job description. Which of the following will give you specific information to assist with performing an on-site analysis?

A. Occupational Safety and Health Administration guidelines
B. Local library
C. *Dictionary of Occupational Titles*
D. None of the above

The *Dictionary of Occupational Titles*, first published in 1939, is an excellent source for on-site analysis. It was developed to serve as a source for standardized occupational information. The information is divided into seven parts to present data regarding jobs in a systematic manner. These parts include the following: 1) occupational code number; 2) occupational title; 3) industry designation; 4) alternate titles; 5) the body of the definition; 6) undefined related titles; and 7) a definition trailer.

Answer: **C**
Dictionary of titles, ed 4

46. True or False: With respect to proper work surface heights and positioning, a general rule is to keep elbows close to the body and avoid full elbow extension.

Anthropometry (measurements of body size) is used as a basis for designing tools, equipment, and work and living places to reduce the incidence of CTDs. Positioning elbows close to the body is recommended. Work should be kept within arm's reach, and full elbow extension should be avoided. The general work surface should be 5 to 10 cm (2 to 4 inches) below the elbows. For precision work, higher surfaces decrease overstrain; for heavier work, lower surfaces are recommended.

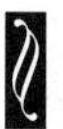

Answer: **True**
Falkenburg, Schultz, pp. 263-270
Refer to Fig. 18-23

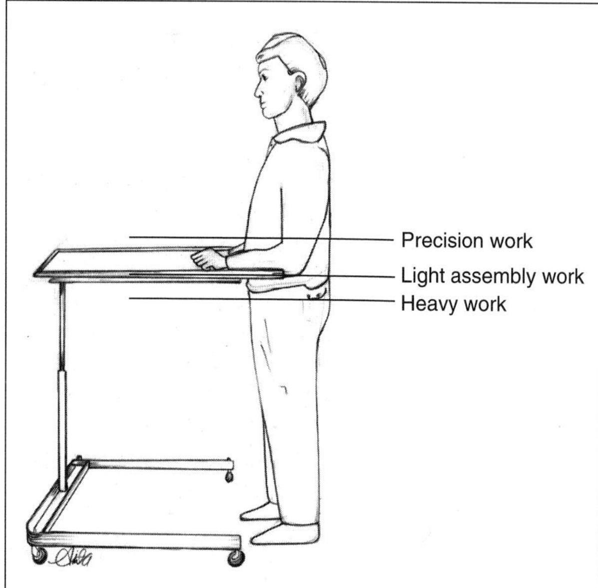

Fig. 18-23

47. True or False: Temperature is not a risk factor in the development of CTDs.

Temperature extremes increase vulnerability to developing CTDs. Cold affects dexterity and coordination, and heat increases fatigue. According to the National Institute of Safety and Health, favorable working temperatures are 68° F to 78° F with 20% to 60% humidity.

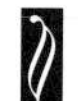

Answer: **False**
Falkenburg, Schultz, pp. 263-270

48. True or False: The handle of an ergonomic tool should be at least 9 cm in length.

A tool handle should distribute the force over the thenar and hypothenar eminences and digits two through five. If the handle is too short (Fig. 18-24), it may compress the median or ulnar nerve at the palm or the digital neurovascular structures. The tool length should accommodate the average hand width (9 to 12 cm, or 4 to 5 inches), thus allowing for evenly distributed forces to help reduce exposure to CTDs.

Answer: **True**
Johnson, pp. 299-310

49. Which tool might be used during a job-site analysis to measure the amount of force required to push and pull?

A. Dynamometer
B. Pedometer
C. Chatillon gauge
D. Ergonomic dynamometer

The Chatillon gauge is a valuable tool for performing a job-site analysis to measure the forces required to push or pull certain objects.

Answer: **C**
Hunter, Mackin, Callahan, pp. 1788-1789
Refer to Fig. 18-25

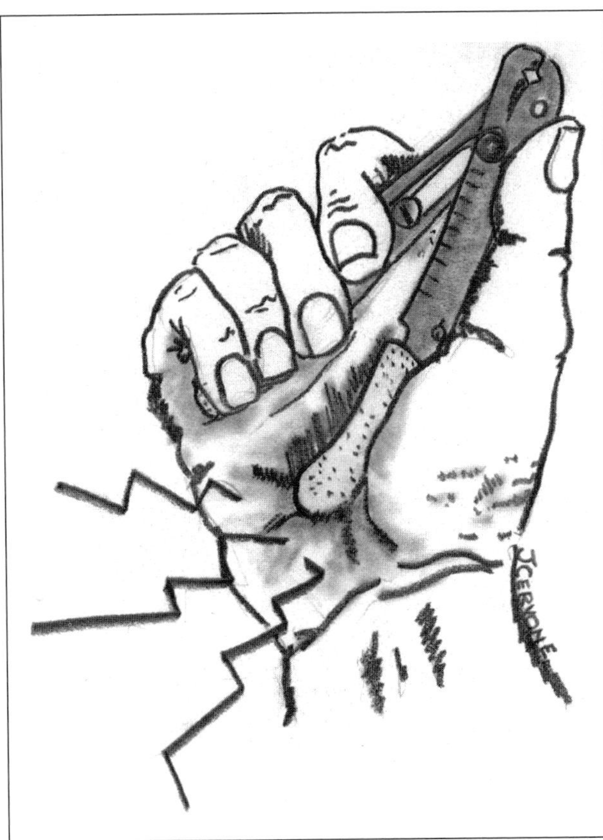

Fig. 18-24

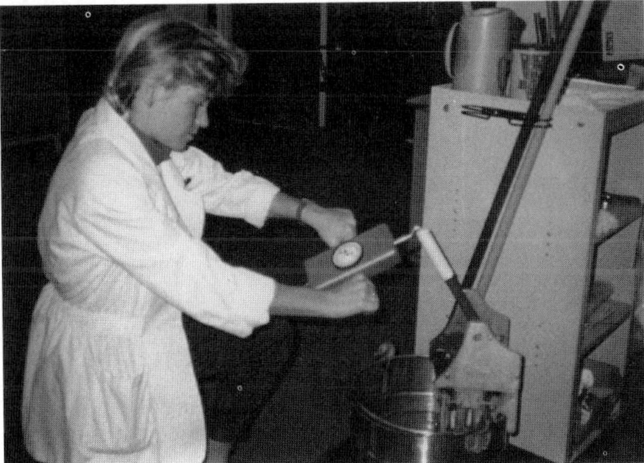

Fig. 18-25 ■ From Hunter JM, Mackin EJ, Callahan AD: *Rehabilitation of the hand: surgery and therapy,* ed 4, St Louis, 1995, Mosby.

50. All but which of the following are important for healthy computer use?

A. Maintaining the wrist in neutral position
B. Taking frequent breaks
C. Always using a wrist rest
D. Stretching frequently

All of the above are good rules to follow, except C. A common mistake people make is to rest the wrist while typing. This can cause direct pressure on the carpal canal and can put undue stress on the flexor tendons. Wrist rests are better termed *wrist guides*. One should only "rest" the wrist on the support when not typing.

Answer: **C**
Pascarelli, Quilter, pp. 178-181

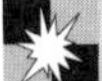

CLINICAL GEM:
An excellent device to issue for median nerve protection is the soft flex splint/support. This splint keeps pressure off the median nerve, aids in edema management, and allows full digital motion. This support can be ordered from durable medical equipment distributors such as AliMed and Northcoast, or directly through Softflex.

51. A 42-year-old woman is referred for therapy with a diagnosis of "wrist pain." After obtaining her history, you learn that she has recently started a new job that requires repetitive wrist flexion. During the evaluation, you note that the patient has volar ulnar wrist pain and tenderness over the ulnar carpus, specifically the pisiform, as well as pain along the ulnar forearm. Increased pain with resisted wrist flexion and passive wrist extension also is noted. You might conclude that she has which of the following?

A. Extensor carpi ulnaris tendinitis
B. Flexor carpi ulnaris tendinitis
C. Radial nerve entrapment
D. Lunate fracture

Flexor carpi ulnaris tendinitis, whether acute or chronic, presents with ulnar wrist pain. It is not uncommon to see this condition when individuals begin a new job that requires frequent wrist flexion or lifting heavy objects. The pain is over the flexor carpi ulnaris tendon, especially at the pisiform, where it inserts. Conservative treatment usually is successful, with no recurrence of symptoms. If a wrist splint is used, the wrist should be positioned at neutral to 25 degrees of flexion with slight ulnar deviation. Job modification also may be beneficial. The physician may prescribe nonsteroidal antiinflammatory drugs (NSAIDs) or give an injection to reduce inflammation. In some cases surgery is indicated.

Answer: **B**
Millender, Louis, Simmons, p. 131
Thorson, Szabo, p. 425

52. True or False: Pain over the thenar and hypothenar eminences after carpal tunnel release is referred to as *pillar pain.*

Pillar pain is a well-recognized complication after carpal tunnel release. Pillar pain must be distinguished from incisional or scar tenderness. However, a clear definition of pillar pain has yet to be established. It is variously described as the following:

- Pain in the thenar *and* hypothenar eminences
- Pain in the thenar *or* hypothenar eminences
- Discomfort in the area of the surgical incision
- Radial and ulnar tenderness

Pillar pain is thought to occur after release of the transverse carpal ligament (TCL), thus causing the muscles to fall apart and altering the muscle origins. It causes edema around the cut "raw" edges of the ligament. Pillar pain can occur with all surgical techniques (mini, open, endoscopic). Treatment includes soft tissue mobilization, vibration, modalities, desensitization, and/or splinting. The treatment goal is to control the magnitude and/or duration of the symptoms. Sometimes a steroid injection may be helpful.

Answer: **True**
Hunter, Schneider, Mackin, p. 150
Ludlow, Merla, Cox, pp. 277-281
Chase in Mackin, Callahan, Skirven, et al, p. 65
Hayes, Carney, Wolf, et al, in Mackin, Callahan, Skirven, et al, p. 656

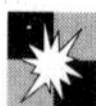
CLINICAL GEM:
It is not uncommon for pillar pain to persist for as long as 6 months. Reassure your patients that the pain will subside.

53. What area of sensibility may be abnormal with pronator syndrome but will not be with CTS?

A. Fingernail of index finger
B. Middle finger proximal phalanx
C. Thenar eminence
D. All of the above are affected in both syndromes.

The thenar eminence is affected in pronator syndrome but not in CTS. The thenar eminence is innervated by the palmar cutaneous branch, which arises around 5 to 7 cm proximal to the wrist; therefore in CTS the thenar eminence has already been innervated and thus will not be affected.

Answer: **C**
Szabo in Green, Hotchkiss, Pederson, p. 1418
Weinzweig, p. 110
Refer to Fig. 18-26

54. All but which of the following are potential compression sites for pronator syndrome?

A. Lacertus fibrosis
B. Ligament of Struthers
C. Pronator teres
D. Tendinous origin of the flexor digitorum superficialis
E. Arcade of Struthers

The median nerve is vulnerable to compression at several sites near the elbow. These sites include the following: 1) between the supracondylar process and the ligament of Struthers; 2) at the lacertus fibrosis, which crosses over the median nerve at the elbow; 3) within the pronator teres muscle; and 4) at the tendinous origin of the flexor digitorum superficialis. The majority of cases are from compression of the median nerve as it passes between the two heads of the pronator teres muscle.

Patients complain of pain in the volar proximal forearm and decreased sensation to the median—nerve innervated digits. Sensory disturbances are often present in the thenar eminence. Often patients report an occupational onset from repetitive use of the arm, especially resisted pronation. Treatment may include splinting, cessation of the provocative activity, and rest. Because minimal synovitis is present, steroid injections have not been proved to be effective. Surgical intervention often is not required. A differential diagnosis from CTS is made when there are negative Phalen's and Tinel's signs at the wrist but no complaints of nocturnal pain. Answer E, the arcade of Struthers, is involved with ulnar nerve entrapment.

Answer: **E**
Blair, pp. 754-763
Omer, Spinner, Van Beek, p. 514

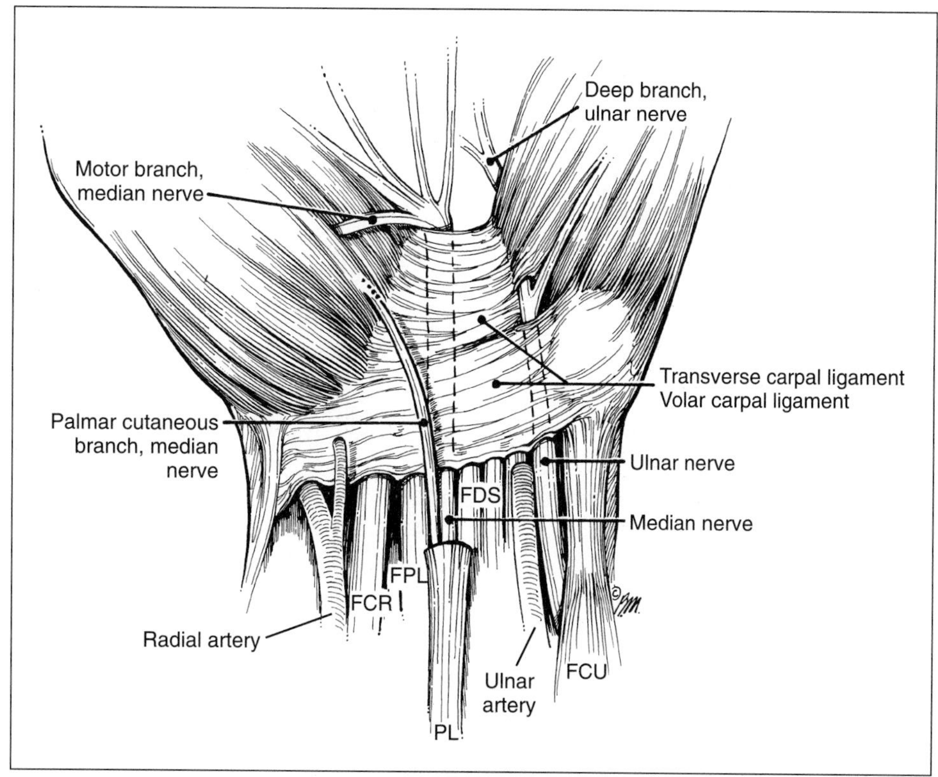

Fig. 18-26 ■ The palmar cutaneous branch of the median nerve lies radial to the median nerve and ulnar to the flexor carpi radialis tendon. It may pierce either the volar carpal or transverse carpal ligament or the antebrachial fascia before it becomes subcutaneous. (From Green DP, Hotchkiss, RN, Pederson WC: *Green's Operative hand surgery*, ed 4, New York, 1999, Churchill Livingstone.)

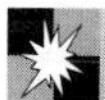
CLINICAL GEM:
To assess for pronator compression, see Fig. 18-27.

55. The cause of white finger is which of the following?

A. Vibration
B. C8 nerve compression
C. Peripheral neuritis
D. Diabetes

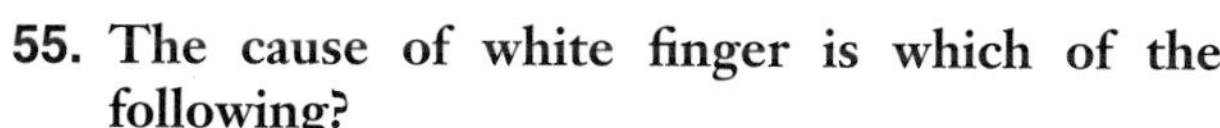

White finger is a vascular problem caused by industrial overuse of vibratory tools. With the use of vibratory tools, grip force often is doubled because of distortion of position sense. This disorder causes muscle fatigue, pain, numbness, and blanching of the affected fingers and may cause vascular insufficiencies.

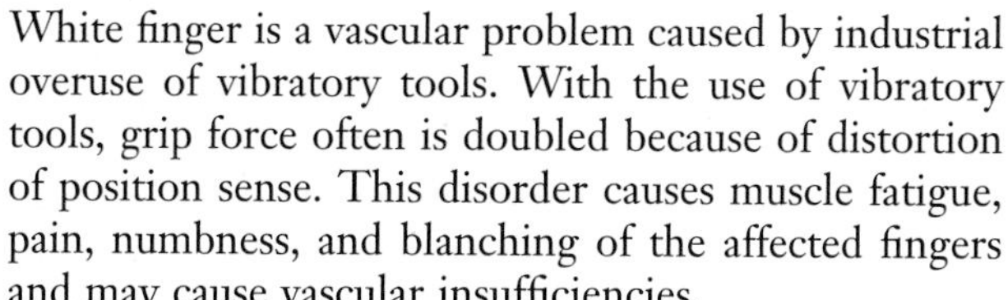

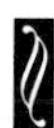
Answer: **A**
Ranney, pp. 187-188

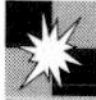
CLINICAL GEM:
Interestingly, 50% of people in occupations using vibration tools, such as jackhammers, report symptoms of Raynaud's phenomenon.

56. You are evaluating a patient who complains of distal volar forearm pain that is aggravated when DIP joint flexion of the index finger is blocked during active thumb flexion. What pathology exists with this patient? Hint: it occurs because of an anomaly between two tendons.

A. Drummer's palsy
B. Lindburg's syndrome
C. Intersection syndrome
D. None of the above

Lindburg's syndrome involves hypertrophic tenosynovium between the flexor pollicis longus and digital flexor tendons in the distal forearm or tenosynovitis of the flexor pollicis longus and index flexor digitorum

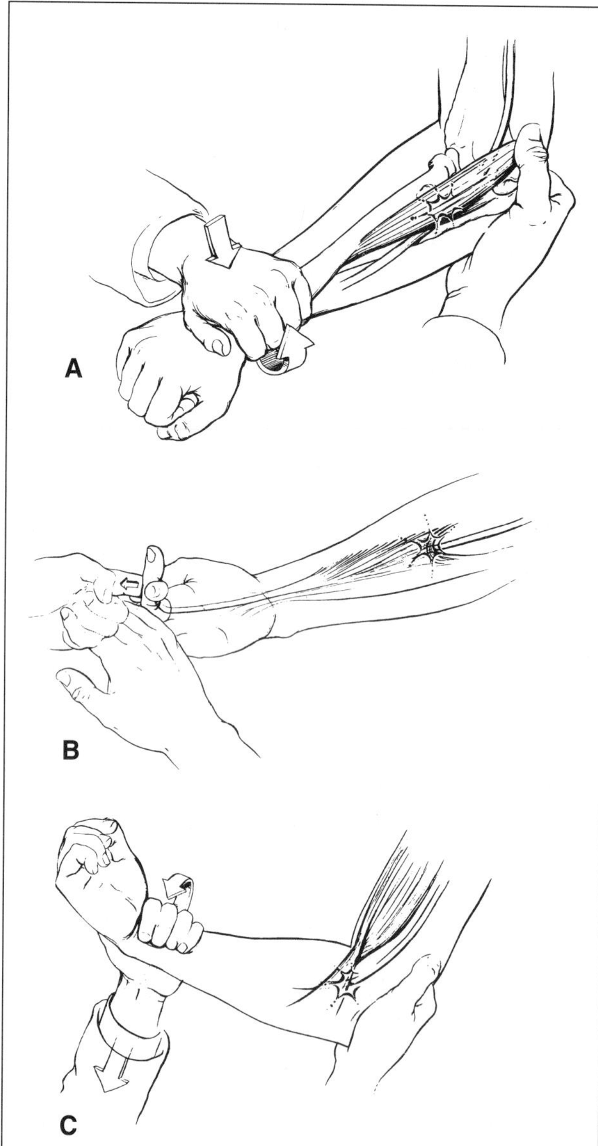

Fig. 18-27 ■ Tests for the site of compression in pronator syndrome. **A,** When the forearm pain is reproduced by resistance to pronation of the forearm and is aggravated by extending the elbow, the localization is at the pronator teres. **B,** When the pain occurs on resistance to flexion of the flexor digitorum superficialis of the long finger, the examiner's fingers keep the patient's remaining fingers in extension and resistance to flexion of the PIP joint of the long finger. This test localizes the compression to the flexor superficialis arch. **C,** When the forearm pain is reproduced by resistance to flexion of the elbow and supination of the forearm, the bicipital aponeurosis (lacertus fibrosus) is the offending fibrous structure. (From Spinner M: *Injuries to the major branches of peripheral nerves of the forearm*, ed 2, Philadelphia, 1978, WB Saunders.)

profundus with an associated anomaly between the two tendons (called *Linburg's anomaly*). The patient will have distal volar forearm pain that is intensified when DIP joint flexion of the index is blocked as the thumb is actively flexed into the palm.

Drummer's palsy is another name for extensor pollicis longus rupture after chronic tenosynovitis and tendinous attrition. Intersection syndrome is described earlier in this chapter.

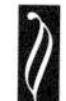
Answer: **B**
Jebson, p. 73

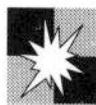
CLINICAL GEM:
Conservative treatment of Lindburg's syndrome involves rest, NSAIDs, and cortisone injections. Surgical treatment includes division of any tendinous inerconnections and tenosynovectomy.

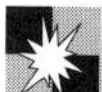
CLINICAL GEM:
CTS often coexists with Lindburg's syndrome.

57. True or False: Inflammatory edema and pooling stasis edema are considered the same thing.

These two types of edema are distinct and treated differently. Inflammatory edema is a result of a cellular response in a tissue producing increased fluid in conjunction with vasodilation, heat, and pain. Treatment includes elevation, avoiding exercising the inflamed muscle or tendon unit, avoiding muscle pumping, and rest to allow tissue healing.

When pooling (stasis) edema is present, you should produce a muscle contraction to assist with fluid drainage. The pooling-type edema (noninflammatory stasis edema) contains nonproteinaceous fluid, occupies space, and decreases joint motion. There is no vasodilation or pain with pooling edema.

Answer: **False**
Omer, Spinner, Van Beek, p. 101

58. A patient has CTS and you chose low-level laser therapy (LLLT). Which of the following is not a physiological effect of LLLT?

A. Improved blood circulation and vasodilation
B. Analgesic effect
C. Biostimulation, including improved metabolism and increase of cell metabolism
D. All of the above are physiological effects of LLLT.

LLLT is now Food and Drug Administration– (FDA-) cleared to treat CTS. LLLT is backed by over 12 years of clinical research. Low-level lasers supply energy to the body in the form of nonthermal photons of light. Light is transmitted through the skin's layers at all wavelengths in the visible range. The light waves in the near-infrared ranges penetrate the deepest of all light waves in the visible spectrum. LLLT light waves penetrate deeply, thus optimizing the immune responses of our blood. This has both antiinflammatory and immunosuppressive effects. It is a scientific fact that light transmitted to the blood in this way has benefits such as supplying oxygen and energy to cells. Additional physiological effects include antiinflammatory and antiedematous effects, wound healing, generation of new and healthy cells and tissue, increased blood supply, and relief of acute and chronic pain.

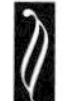

Answer: **D**

Department of Health and Human Services, FDA Re: K010175
Anderson, Good, Kerr
Whintraur, pp. 268-277

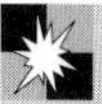

CLINICAL GEM:
LLLT is a new, internationally accepted term for biostimulation with low-energy lasers in order to achieve the desired therapeutic effect.

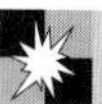

CLINICAL GEM:
LLLT is also called *cold laser*.

59. True or False: In relation to LLLT for treating CTS, the wavelength of 830 nm and power output of 90 mw laser has penetration of approximately 5 cm with a 3-cm lateral spread.

Since the FDA approved LLLT, many laser units have reached the market. One considers penetration and output for CTS with LLLT. The ML830 is one of the LLLTs that can provide nonthermal laser treatment and can penetrate 5 cm with a 3-cm lateral spread.

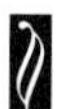

Answer: **True**

www.laserhealthproducts.com

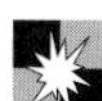

CLINICAL GEM:
Contact LaserHealth products to learn about microlight and LLLT at www.laserhealthproducts.com.

Chapter 19

Dupuytren's Disease and Tumors

1. Which of the following tasks are easier after correction of Dupuytren's disease?

A. Wearing gloves
B. Getting items out of your pocket
C. Shaking hands
D. All of the above are easier.

After successful release of Dupuytren's disease, all of the activities mentioned are easier to perform. These activities are often taken for granted and make a big difference in daily life skills for patients.

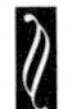
Answer: **D**
Lubahn, p. 134

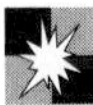
CLINICAL GEM:
Well-known people with Dupuytren's disease include former U.S. President Ronald Reagan and former British Prime Minister Margaret Thatcher.

2. Which is not a type of operation typically performed on patients with Dupuytren's disease?

A. Fasciotomy
B. Regional fasciectomy
C. Ray resection
D. All of the above are typically performed.

A ray resection is only performed as a salvage procedure for Dupuytren's disease and is not often performed. Amputations for Dupuytren's disease, when performed, are often at the level of the proximal phalanx rather than the whole ray.

A *fasciotomy* is performed under local anesthesia with immediate results. A fasciotomy is made by making an incision over the diseased cord and dividing every strand of diseased fascia under direct vision. This procedure is not as successful with proximal interphalangeal (PIP) joint releases. It is a minor operation and a good procedure to use with the elderly when recurrence is unlikely.

Regional fasciectomy is an operation in which the diseased fascia is removed and the rest of the fascia is left undisturbed. It is most often used when the disease is confined to the ring and small fingers.

An *extensive fasciectomy* is a more radical operation in which potentially diseased as well as obviously diseased tissue is removed. The surgical insult to the hand is greater in this procedure.

Finally, a dermofasciectomy is another procedure that can be used and is discussed in Question 12.

Answer: **C**
McFarlane, MacDermid in Mackin, Callahan, Skirven, et al, pp. 974-975

CLINICAL GEM:
One way to remember the terms is to know that *-ectomy* means removal of, or to cut out; *-otomy* means a surgical incision or to cut into.

3. True or False: It is important to be very aggressive the first few days after surgery when treating Dupuytren's disease to avoid stiffness and recurrence of flexion contracture.

Active exercises are initiated a few days postoperatively and should not be too aggressive. Overzealous exercise regimes can lead to a "flare reaction," which can result in reflex sympathetic dystrophy (RSD) or complex regional pain syndrome (CRPS). A "flare reaction" occurs in patients who have an increase in inflammatory response with more redness and swelling than expected. Roz Evans has challenged that therapists who treat with overaggressive therapy may contribute to a patient's poorer immediate results and to extension of the disease. Therefore respecting the tissues is very important for treatment of postoperative Dupuytren's disease.

Answer: **False**

McFarlane, MacDermid in Mackin, Callahan, Skirven, et al, pp. 974-975

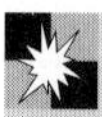

CLINICAL GEM:
Loss of flexion after surgery for Dupuytren's disease has been reported to occur in as many as 40% of patients.

4. What is the initial manifestation of Dupuytren's disease?

A. Nodule
B. Cord
C. Band
D. Pain

The initial presentation of Dupuytren's disease is a firm nodule in the palm near the distal palmar crease. Dupuytren's disease, which typically affects the palmar fascia, is a progressive disease often seen in men of northern European descent. It typically occurs during the fifth decade in men and during the sixth decade in women and is more common in men. Dupuytren's disease is causally associated with insulin-dependent diabetes mellitus, epilepsy, and chronic alcoholism. Both manual work and a single injury to the hand have also been causally implicated with Dupuytren's disease.

Answer: **A**

McFarlane, pp. 8-13
Rajon, p. 89
McFarlane, MacDermid in Mackin, Callahan, Skirven, et al, p. 971
Refer to Fig. 19-1

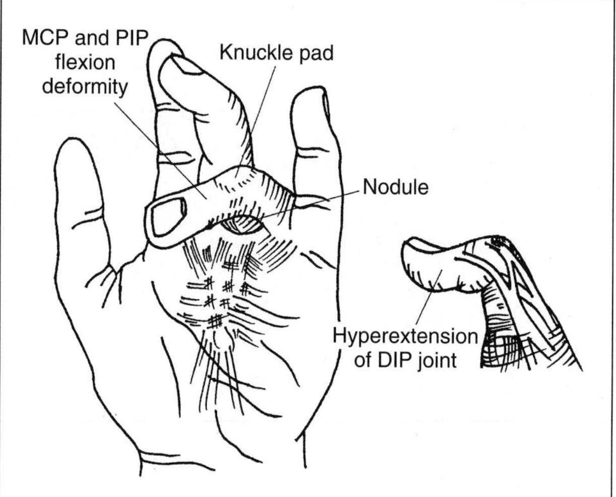

Fig. 19-1 ■ Features of the Dupuytren's hand can include palmar cords and nodules, interdigital web contracture, flexion deformity at the MCP and/or PIP joints, and hyperextension deformity of the DIP joint and knuckle pads. (Note the skip area, where the skin is not tethered by the disease. Fat between the skin and the disease in this skip area will often contain the neurovascular bundle). (From Boscheinen-Morrin J: *The hand: fundamentals of therapy*, ed 3, Boston, 2001, Butterworth-Heinemann.)

CLINICAL GEM:
Although Dupuytren's disease appears most commonly in fair skinned, blond-haired individuals, little evidence can substantiate the belief that Dupuytren's originated in Northern Europe; most evidence is anecdotal. The disease is widespread through Europe, and proof of origin would most likely be impossible.

5. What is the most common benign bone tumor of the hand?

A. Tophus
B. Lipoma
C. Carpometacarpal (CMC) boss
D. Enchondroma

An enchondroma (Fig. 19-2), which is a benign growth of cartilage that arises in the metaphysis of a bone, is the most common benign bone tumor of the hand. It may account for as many as 90% of bone tumors in the hand. A tophus is a gouty deposit. A lipoma is a tumor that is composed of benign fat cells or lipid cells and that is slow-growing and usually asymptomatic. A CMC boss is a rounded eminence on the surface of a bone, which is most often seen at the second and third CMC joints.

Answer: **D**

Hunter, Mackin, Callahan, p. 1017
Athanasian in Green, Hotchkiss, Pederson, p. 2233

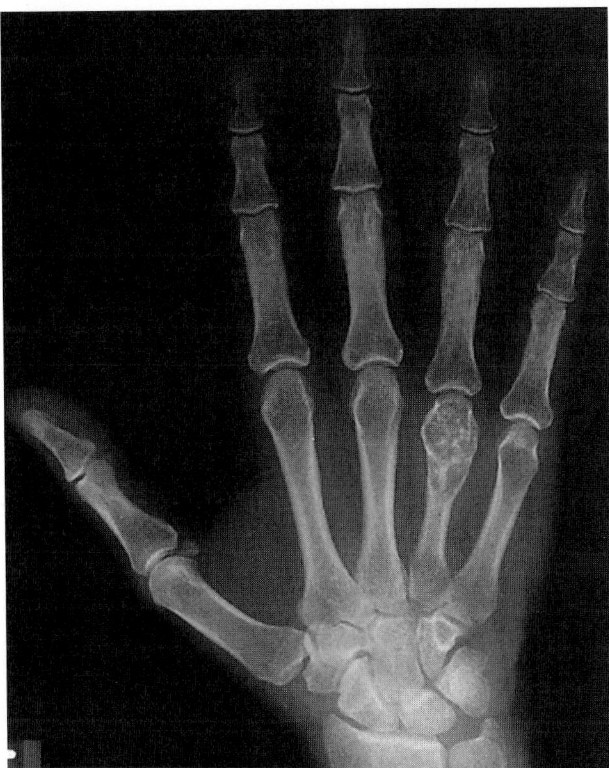

Fig. 19-2 ■ An enchondroma is demonstrated in this posteroanterior view. Note the decreased bone density of the fourth metacarpal head and shaft, which also are increased in size. Within the area of decreased bone density are stippled calcifications—a classic finding in this type of lesion. (From Mackin EJ, Callahan AD, Skirven TM: *Rehabilitation of the hand and upper extremity*, ed 5, St Louis, 2002, Mosby.)

6. Match each disorder to the appropriate definition.

Disorder

1. Fibroma
2. Bowen disease
3. Pyogenic granuloma
4. Lymphangiomas
5. Neurilemoma
6. Sarcoma

Definition

A. Tumors arising from lymph channels
B. Malignant tumor
C. Skin lesion, either benign or malignant
D. Vascular tumor protruding through the skin that bleeds easily
E. Nerve tumor
F. Benign tumor

Answers: **1, F; 2, C; 3, D; 4, A; 5, E; 6, B**

Hunter, Mackin, Callahan, pp. 1027-1031
Bush in Mackin, Callahan, Skirven, et al, pp. 961-962, 966

7. What is the initial degree of metacarpophalangeal (MCP) contracture that most patients begin to notice functional difficulty and consider the hand a nuisance?

A. 10 degrees
B. 30 degrees
C. 50 degrees
D. 70 degrees

A 30-degree contracture at the MCP joint is a significant amount of flexion and can interfere with shaking hands and putting the hand into one's pocket; it can become a nuisance overall. Operation is not urgent because MCP joint contractures can be corrected regardless of how long the patient has had the contracture.

PIP joint flexion contractures, on the other hand, are more difficult to correct because of the fascial bands involved with the contracture. The longer the joint is contracted at this level, the more difficult it is to fully correct. Nevertheless, surgery is not advised until the patient has a 30-degree or larger contracture. PIP joint contractures are often improved after surgery, but not completely corrected. When operations are performed with contractures of less than 30 degrees, the operation itself produces more scar tissue and often makes things worse rather then better.

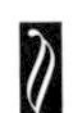

Answer: **B**

McFarlane, MacDermid in Mackin, Callahan, Skirven, et al, pp. 973-974
Green, p. 567
McGrouther in Green, Hotchkiss, Pederson, p. 570

8. After a Dupuytren's contracture is surgically released at the PIP joint, a splint is worn continuously for how long, excluding during daily hygiene and exercises?

A. 1 week
B. 3 weeks
C. 6 weeks
D. 12 weeks

A splint is indicated after surgical release of the PIP joint in all instances, regardless of the type of surgical correction. Splinting usually is initiated 2 or 3 days postoperatively.

During the first 3 weeks after PIP joint surgery, the splint is worn at all times, except during exercises and hygiene. To maintain extension gains, night splinting is continued for 2 or 3 additional months, and some authors recommend splinting for 6 months.

However, a splint is not always required after surgical correction of the MCP joint, especially if the MCP joint was fully corrected and the patient presents in the clinic with full correction. A skilled therapist must assess the situation and make a clinical judgment in collaboration with the referring physician.

Various authors propose a variety of splints—including dorsal- and volar-based splinting and splinting with the MCP joint flexed at 30 to 40 degrees—while extending the interphalangeal (IP) joints fully to avoid overstressing the tissues, especially the vascular tissues. As wound healing progresses, the MCP joints can be extended to neutral. Positioning the wrist in the splint to minimize tension on the flexor tendons also has been suggested.

Answer: **B**

McFarlane, pp. 8-13
Hunter, Mackin, Callahan, p. 990
McFarlane, MacDermid in Mackin, Callahan, Skirven, et al, pp. 982-984
Green, p. 589
Refer to Fig. 19-3

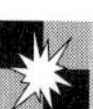

CLINICAL GEM:
Some people prefer dorsal-based splints because they minimize pressure on the surgical wound while maintaining full extension of the digit, whereas others prefer the palmar-based splint with the thought that increased pressure to the surgical site is useful for scar management.

9. What is the most common origin of the wrist ganglion?

A. Scapholunate (SL) ligament
B. Flexor tendons
C. Lunotriquetral ligament
D. Extensor tendons

The dorsal wrist ganglion accounts for a large percentage of hand and wrist ganglions. The most frequent site for this cyst is over the SL ligament. The dorsal cyst also may arise between extensor tendons or from other carpal joints but commonly has attachments to the SL ligament. Many problems arise from the excision of ganglions. Recurrence is common. Nerve problems, stiffness, and persistent pain are very common sequelae of primary excision. Ganglion cysts are the most common soft tissue tumor of the hand/wrist.

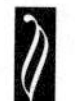

Answer: **A**

Green, p. 2159
Angelides in Green, Hotchkiss, Pederson, p. 2172
Bush in Mackin, Callahan, Skirven, et al, p. 957

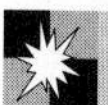

CLINICAL GEM:
A safe approach for treating ganglia is to aspirate, splint, procrastinate, and then reaspirate.

10. When should wrist range of motion (ROM) begin after a dorsal wrist ganglion is surgically removed?

A. Same day as surgery
B. In 5 days
C. In 14 days
D. In 21 days

Early motion for the wrist is important, especially for flexion, and is initiated at day 5, when the dressing is debulked. Sutures are removed approximately 14 days after surgery, and therapy continues until full ROM is attained.

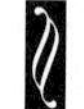

Answer: **B**

Green, pp. 2160, 2166
Angelides in Green, Hotchkiss, Pederson, p. 2174

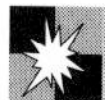

CLINICAL GEM:
The most common complication of ganglion surgery is early recurrence caused by inadequate and incomplete excision.

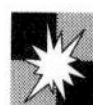

CLINICAL GEM:
A CMC boss is an osteoarthritic spur that develops at the base of the second and third metacarpal and often is mistaken for a dorsal wrist ganglion. After a carpal boss is removed, the wrist is immobilized for 3 to 6 weeks to allow for ligamentous healing and to avoid CMC stress.

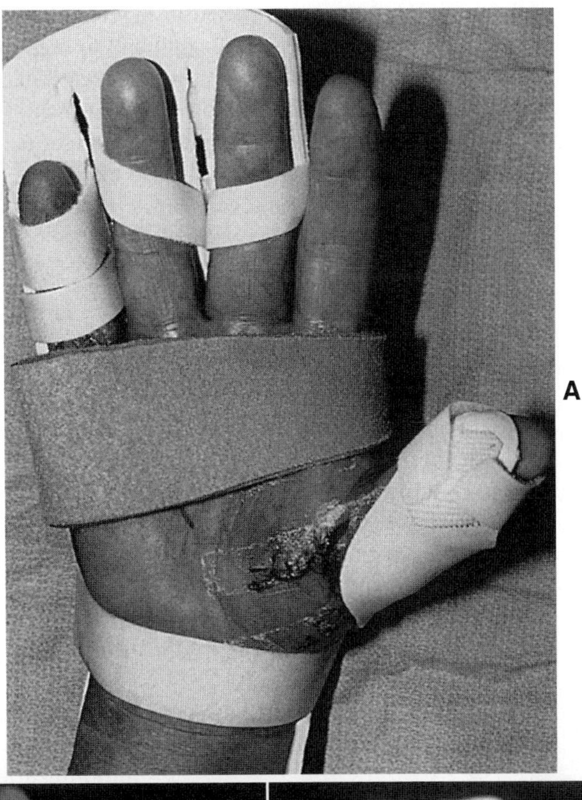

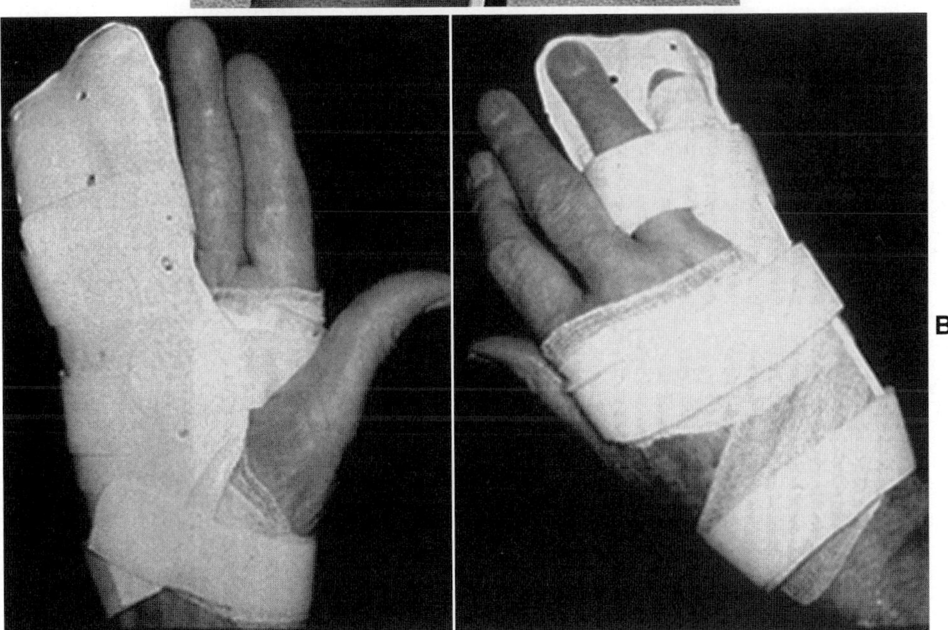

Fig. 19-3 ■ **A,** Dorsal splint. **B,** Volar hand-based splint. (From Mackin EJ, Callahan AD, Skirven TM: *Rehabilitation of the hand and upper extremity*, ed 5, St Louis, 2002, Mosby.)

11. Which two fingers does Dupuytren's disease typically affect?

A. Thumb and/or index fingers
B. Index and/or middle fingers
C. Index and/or ring fingers
D. Ring and/or little fingers

In approximately one half of patients with Dupuytren's disease, both hands are affected; the ring and/or little fingers are the digits most commonly involved. The tendon of the abductor digiti minimi often is involved.

Answer: **D**

Conrad, Enneking, pp. 12, 14
Taber's cyclopedic medical dictionary
Hunter, Mackin, Callahan, pp. 981-982
McFarlane, MacDermid in Mackin, Callahan, Skirven, et al, p. 971
Smith, p. 523
Refer to Fig. 19-4

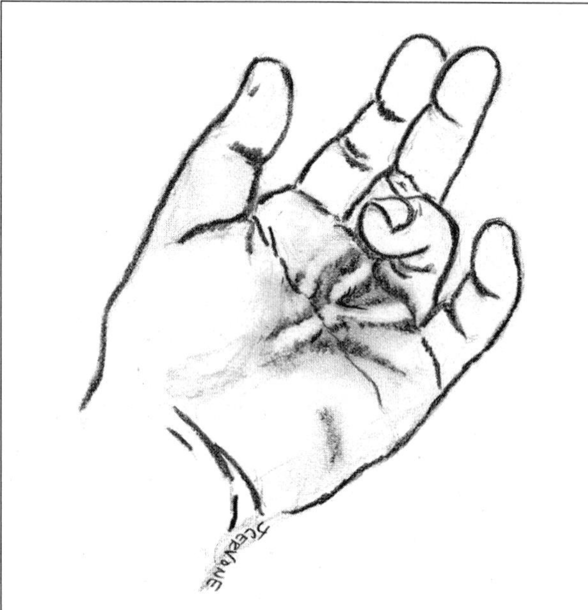

Fig. 19-4

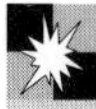

CLINICAL GEM:
Areas other than the palm that are affected by fibromatosis are the following: 1) dorsum of the penis (Peyronie's disease); 2) plantar fascia (Lederhosen disease); and 3) knuckle pad (Garrod's nodes). The presence of these suggests a more aggressive disease. In addition, a young age of onset, strong family history, radial-sided hand involvement, and rapid progression may also contribute to the severity of the disease.

CLINICAL GEM:
Dupuytren's disease is usually painless.

12. You are treating a patient who has had a dermofasciectomy. When can ROM exercises begin?

A. 7 to 10 days
B. 21 days
C. 4 weeks
D. 8 weeks

A dermofasciectomy is a surgical procedure that involves removal of the skin overlying the diseased tissue as well as the underlying fascia. A full-thickness skin graft (FTSG) is performed for coverage. This procedure is indicated in patients who have had a recurrent contracture, severe PIP joint contracture, and evidence of radial disease. A splint is applied postoperatively to ensure graft adherence, and ROM can being after 7 to 10 days of immobilization. Some physicians immobilize patients for 2 to 3 weeks. With a responsible patient, very gentle ROM can be performed a few times a day during the immobilization period to prevent extreme stiffness.

Strengthening typically begins 3 to 4 weeks postoperatively for release with primary closures, approximately 4 weeks after skin grafting (dermofasciectomy), and 4 to 6 weeks after an open-palm technique.

Answer: **A**

Lubahn, p. 134
McFarlane, MacDermid in Mackin, Callahan, Skirven, et al, pp. 978, 986
Smith, p. 535
Refer to Fig. 19-5

13. A 16-year-old patient presents with a painful soft tissue swelling in the arm after sustaining a blunt trauma while playing hockey. The patient has a mass that originates in the muscle. The diagnosis might be which of the following?

A. Schwannoma
B. Ganglion cyst
C. Fibroma
D. Myositis ossificans

When ossification occurs in a muscle, the term *myositis ossificans (MO)* is appropriate. This tumor is more preva-

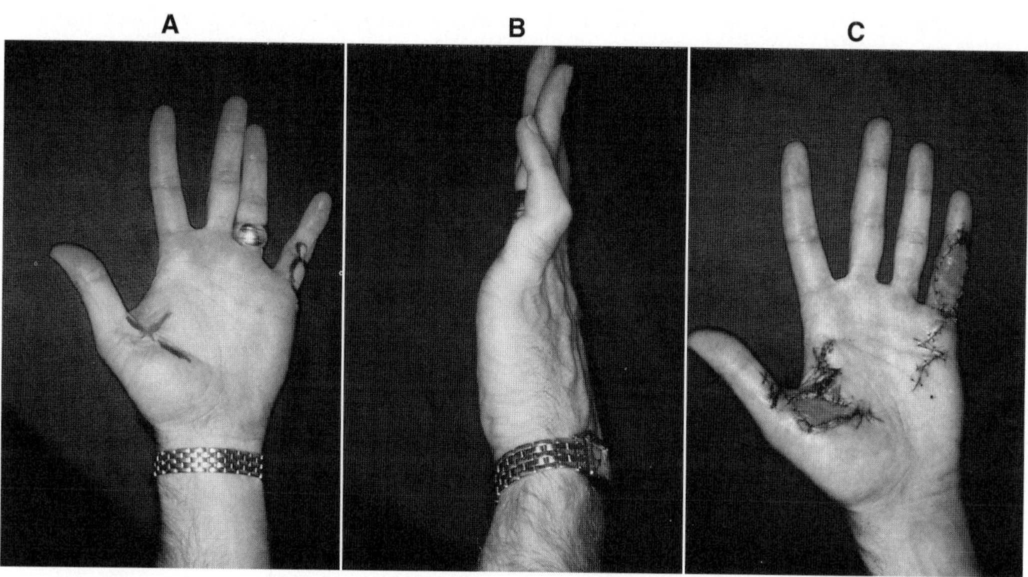

Fig. 19-5 ■ A patient with increased diathesis evidenced by radial disease **(A)** and marked PIP flexion contracture of the small finger **(B)** is a candidate for dermofasciectomy **(C)**. (From Mackin EJ, Callahan AD, Skirven TM: *Rehabilitation of the hand and upper extremity*, ed 5, St Louis, 2002, Mosby.)

lent in patients younger than 30 years who complain of increasing pain within 3 to 4 weeks after the incident. An erythematous mass develops over the injured area. Surgery is indicated when nerve compression is evident. Treatment involves rest and therapy. Differential diagnoses include malignant tumors. A correct diagnosis is imperative because treatment for a malignant tumor often is radical amputation.

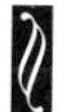

Answer: **D**

Giannakopoulos, Sotereanos, Tomaino, p. 195
Taber's cyclopedic medical dictionary

14. True or False: The most common site for Maffucci's syndrome is in the hand.

Maffucci's syndrome is a rare disease that was first described in 1881. Patients present with radiographic findings of multiple enchondromata (benign cartilaginous tumors), and the disease is often accompanied by multiple hemangiomas (vascular anomalies). Stiffness and deformity may occur with Maffucci's syndrome. Ollier disease was described in 1900 and is similar to Maffucci's syndrome without the vascular involvement. Both Maffucci's syndrome and Ollier disease are nonhereditary. The hands are the most common site of involvement for both diseases.

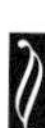

Answer: **True**

Floyd, Troom, p. 127
Hunter, Mackin, Callahan, p. 1433
Athanasian in Green, Hotchkiss, Pederson, p. 2235

15. What is the sole source of MCP joint contraction in Dupuytren's disease?

A. Nodule
B. Pretendinous bands
C. Natatory ligament
D. Cords

The most commonly contracted joint in Dupuytren's disease is the MCP joint. With contractures of 30 degrees or more, many patients report a hindrance with daily activities. MCP joint contracture is caused by the pretendinous bands (Fig. 19-6, *A*) of the palmar aponeurosis. The cords (spiral/lateral/central and/or retrovascular) (Fig. 19-6, *B*) cause PIP joint contractures. The cords develop from the normal components of the digital fascia. The natatory ligament (Fig. 19-6, *A*) can cause web space contractures. Web space contractures are common.

Answer: **B**

Hunter, Mackin, Callahan, p. 983
McFarlane, MacDermid in Mackin, Callahan, Skirven, et al, p. 974

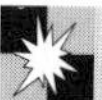

CLINICAL GEM:
Grayson's and Cleland's ligaments prevent rotary movement of the skin around the fingers, thus allowing grasp of objects, but Grayson's ligament is indicated in the pathology of PIP joint flexion contractures in Dupuytren's disease.

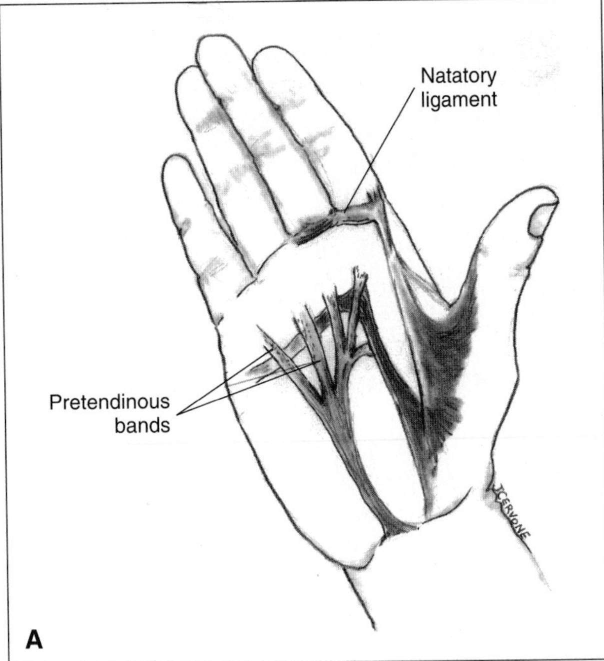

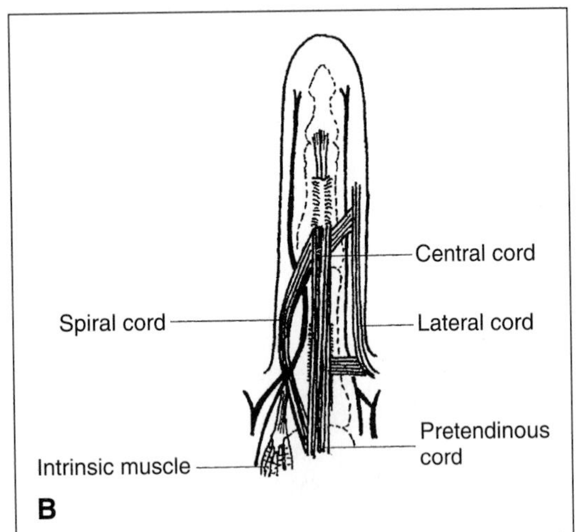

Fig. 19-6 ■ **B,** From Boscheinen-Morrin J: *The hand: fundamentals of therapy*, ed 3, Boston, 2001, Butterworth-Heinemann.

16. A penetrating injury that drives a fragment of epithelium into the subcutaneous tissue can result in which of the following?

A. Herpetic whitlow
B. Inclusion cyst
C. Enchondroma
D. Xanthoma

Inclusion cysts are traumatic in origin. These cysts may be present for years and result from a penetrating injury that drives a fragment of epithelium into the subcutaneous tissue. The cells grow over months to years to produce a painless swelling most often in the fingertip. When patients have a decline in function, these cysts are removed.

A xanthoma, also known as a *giant cell tumor*, is a solid tumor commonly found in the hand. It is a painless, slow-growing tumor that develops in a few months. An enchondroma is the most common primary bone tumor.

A herpetic whitlow is a viral infection that commonly is found in dental personnel and usually is treated nonoperatively.

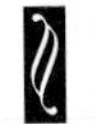

Answer: **B**
Green, pp. 1026, 2225-2227, 2235
Athanasian in Green, Hotchkiss, Pederson, p. 2223

17. What is the major advantage of using the McCash open-palm technique for treating Dupuytren's disease?

A. Decreased risk of hematoma
B. Does not require dressing changes
C. No scar management required
D. Acceleration of postoperative recovery

The open-palm technique (Fig. 19-7) for treating Dupuytren's disease is favored by many physicians because of the simplicity and flexibility it allows. The wound closes by secondary intention; it drains well; and skin sloughs are rarely seen. Thus hematomas do not occur. Additional benefits to the patient include decreased pain, decreased edema, and decreased stiffness. Closure usually occurs in 3 to 5 weeks.

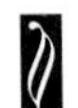

Answer: **A**
Hunter, Mackin, Callahan, p. 996
McFarlane, MacDermid in Mackin, Callahan, Skirven, et al, p. 986
Green, pp. 563-590
Smith, p. 531

18. True or False: Whirlpool with povidone-iodine is recommended for patients who have had McCash procedures.

Whirlpool treatment after a McCash procedure is performed at 98° F to 100° F to prevent increased edema. Povidone-iodine (Betadine) has been used in the past; however, it is not recommended because evidence suggests that it reduces epithelialization. A clear rinse is used when treating with whirlpool in a sterile whirlpool bath.

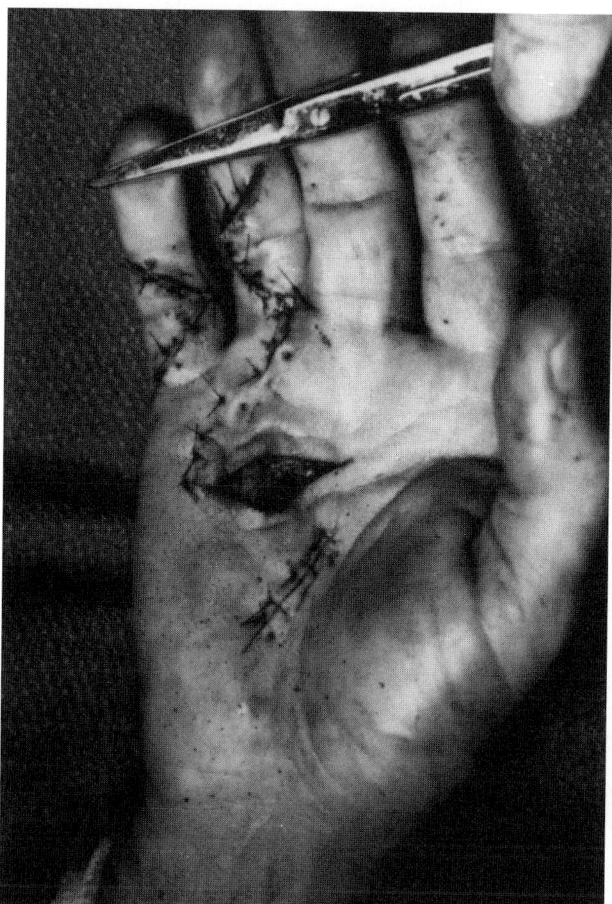

Fig. 19-7 ■ From Hunter JM, Mackin EJ, Callahan AD: *Rehabilitation of the hand: surgery and therapy,* ed 4, St Louis, 1995, Mosby.

Answer: **False**

McFarlane, MacDermid in Mackin, Callahan, Skirven, et al, p. 987

19. True or False: RSD/CRPS is a serious complication of Dupuytren's disease after surgical release.

RSD/CRPS is a serious complication of Dupuytren's disease and is best treated if detected early. If RSD/CRPS is diagnosed, your protocol should be modified to focus on resolving the acute RSD/CRPS before it becomes chronic; for example, splinting should be modified to reduce tension or discontinued because aggressive passive ROM is contraindicated. Other complications of Dupuytren's disease after surgical release include wound dehiscence, hematoma, infection, adhesions, PIP joint flexion contractures, poor flexion, and joint stiffness.

Answer: **True**

Prosser, Conolly, pp. 344-348
McFarlane, MacDermid in Mackin, Callahan, Skirven, et al, p. 981

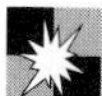

CLINICAL GEM:
RSD/CRPS occurs after about 5% of operations and is twice as likely in women.

20. True or False: Collagenase injections are a promising treatment for patients with Dupuytren's disease.

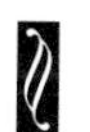

Studies of the effects of collagenase injections have been ongoing, and the results are extremely encouraging. More than 90% of MCP contractures and 66% of PIP contractures have shown excellent results. Recurrence has not been a problem. A study in the *Journal of Hand Surgery* in February of 2000 showed preliminary phase-two results of the injections that indicate its safety and effectiveness for treating Dupuytren's disease. The most common side effects observed to date are tenderness to pressure at the injection site, edema, and minimal hematoma.

Answer: **True**

Hurst, Badalamente, pp. 103-104
Refer to Fig. 19-8

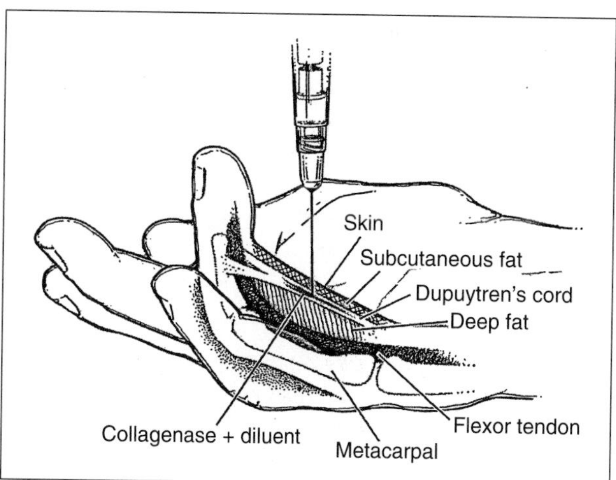

Fig. 19-8 ■ Central cord injection. Note that the collagenase and diluent must stay in the cord. If a small amount gets between the skin and cord, no harm is caused but the Dupuytren's cord may not rupture. No collagenase should go dorsal to the cord and into the deep fat. Injection of the flexor tendon must be avoided. With the needle in the cord, injection must be gentle and slow, and part of the volume put in three different contiguous positions to avoid forcing liquid through the Dupuytren's cord and into the deep fat over the flexor tendons. (From *Hand Clin* 15(1):104, 1999.)

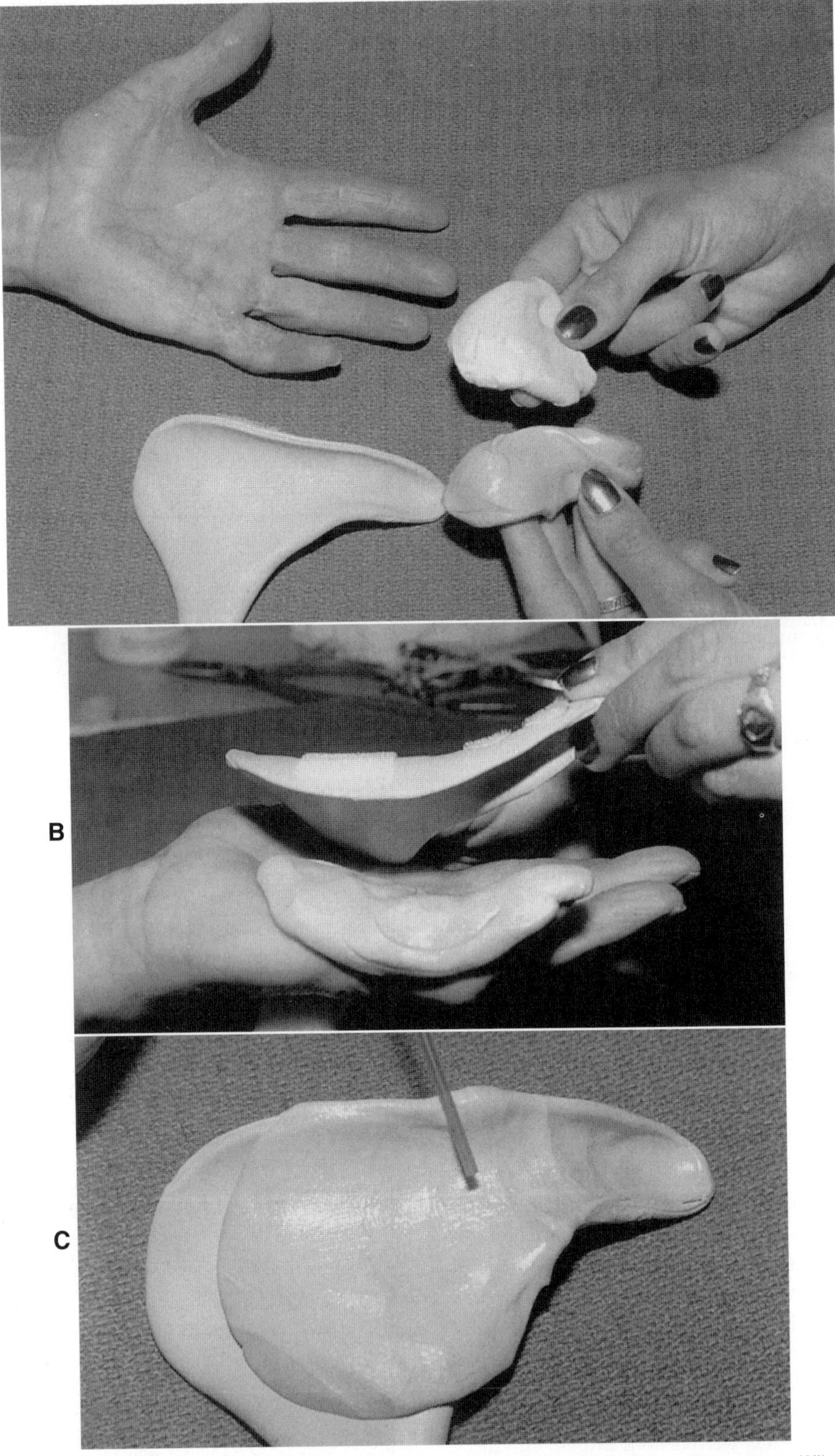

Fig. 19-9 ■ **A**, Equal parts of the 50/50 mix elastomer putty (Smith & Nephew Rolyan, Germantown, WI) are mixed to begin formation of the scar pressure insert. **B**, The soft putty is molded against the skin and the splint is placed against the putty. **C**, After the putty hardens, each line of the scar is visible. (From *Hand Clin* 15(1):172, 1999.)

21. True or False: Silicone gel sheets are helpful to manage scar after a Dupuytren's release.

The use of a silicone or putty elastomer insert applies pressure to the scar and can help manage nodular scar tissue. This scar tissue can interfere with ROM and functional grasp and must be managed. Elastomer putty or silicone inserts (Fig. 19-9) are often used between the hand and a splint. This treatment is often used for 3 to 6 months until the scar matures and softens.

Answer: **True**
Mullins, pp. 170-171

22. Mr. X, a 62-year-old male, presents to the clinic with a diagnosis of trigger finger. The physician injected the patient's finger with cortisone. Therapy treatment consists of splinting, ultrasound, and activity modification. Treatment fails to produce the expected progress. What might you suspect?

A. Dupuytren's disease
B. Peyronie's disease
C. Raynaud's disease
D. Lederhosen disease

Dupuytren's may be misdiagnosed as a stenosing tenosynovitis (trigger finger). The patient's symptom of triggering may be the primary presenting feature of Dupuytren's disease. Involvement of the deep fibers of the longitudinal fascia as they wrap around the A1 pulley may result in triggering, thus leading to the incorrect diagnosis of a trigger finger. Unfortunately, progressive development of Dupuytren's contracture may follow a surgical release of the A1 pulley, thus resulting in dismay between patient and physician. Therefore it is advisable that any case of trigger finger that fails to make expected progress should be examined for Dupuytren's disease.

Answer: **A**
Smith, p. 523

Chapter 20

Congenital Anomalies/ Amputations/Prosthetics

1. Fig. 20-1 depicts which of the following?

A. A hypoplastic index finger
B. Hypoplastic index finger and wrist
C. An amputated index finger
D. Failure of formation of carpals
E. None of the above

The x-ray in Fig. 20-1 is of a normal 15-month-old child. The index finger appears to be amputated or hypoplastic, but the child is merely bending his finger at the proximal interphalangeal (PIP) joint. This is not considered a good film because of the bent finger (this is a tricky x-ray). Fig. 20-2, *A*, is an acceptable radiograph of the same child, and Fig. 20-2, *B*, is the child. Note that an infant's hand is present only in cartilage because ossification centers appear at different ages. Refer to Table 20-1 for a reference to ossification centers.

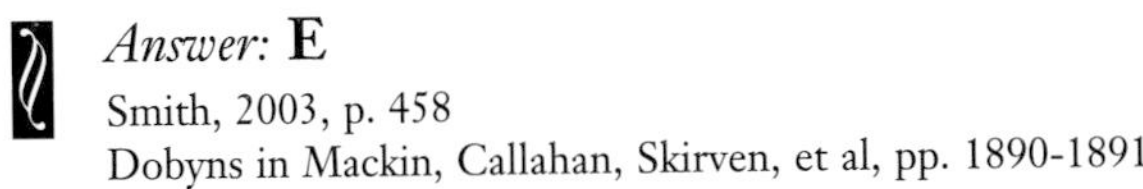

Answer: **E**
Smith, 2003, p. 458
Dobyns in Mackin, Callahan, Skirven, et al, pp. 1890-1891

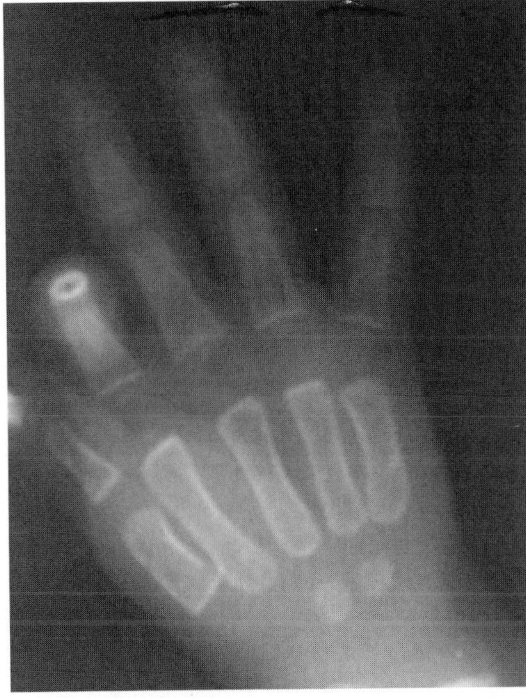

Fig. 20-1 ■ Hand x-ray, Jake Weiss.

2. Which of the following goals is included in a preprosthetic therapy program?

A. Addressing residual limb shrinkage and shaping
B. Maintaining normal joint range of motion (ROM)
C. Increasing muscle strength
D. Participating in myoelectric muscle site testing
E. All of the above

Atkins notes that the occupational therapist is the primary person who will manage the preprosthetic program. The program should begin when the sutures are removed and medical clearance is given from the treating physician. All of the above are goals to address in the preprosthetic program. Other goals to focus on include desensitizing the residual limb, proper hygiene of the limb, maximizing independence, orienting to prosthetic options, changing dominance training (if needed), and exploring the client's future goals.

Answer: **E**
Atkins, Alley, p. 2
Pillet, Mackin in Mackin, Callahan, Skirven, et al, pp. 1461-1472

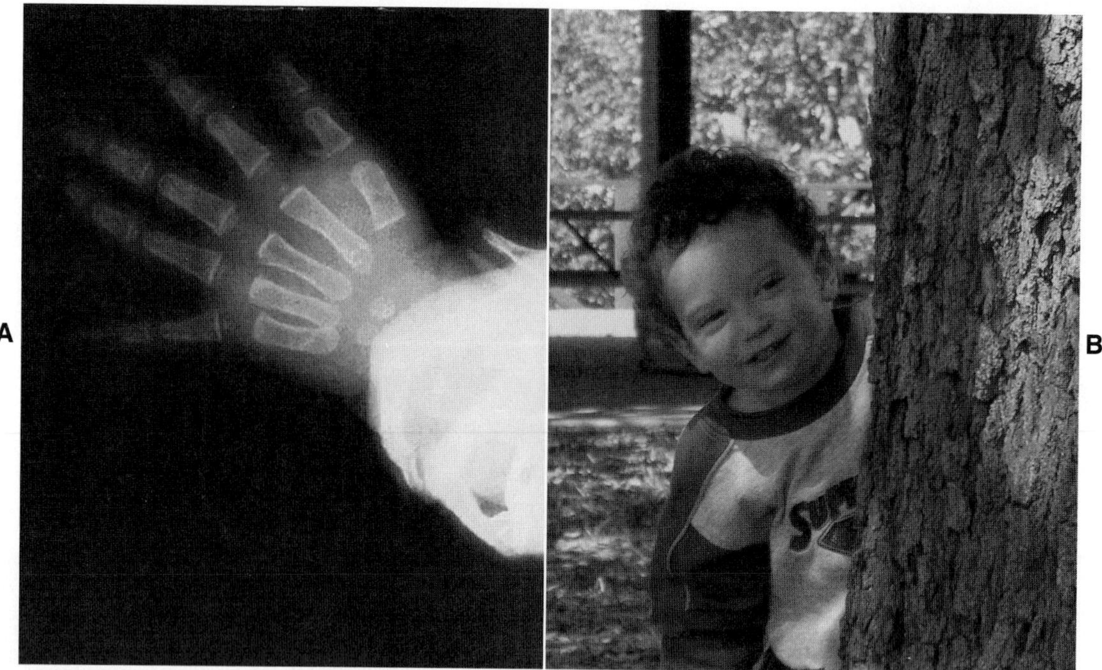

Fig. 20-2 ■ A and B, 15-month-old Jake Weiss. (Courtesy Jake Weiss.)

Table 20-1

Age of Appearance of Ossification Centers*

Ossification center	Age of onset
CARPUS	
Capitate and hamate	2 months
Triquetral	1.7 years
Lunate	2.6 years
Scaphoid, trapezium, trapezoid	4.1 years
METACARPUS AND PHALANGES (EPIPHYSEAL CENTERS)	
Metacarpophalangeal joints of the fingers (both centers)	All by 1.5 years
Metacarpal of thumb	1.6 years
Proximal phalanx of thumb	1.7 years
Middle phalanges	All by 2.0 years
Distal phalanges	All by 2.5 years

From Smith P: *Lister's The hand: diagnosis and indications*, ed 4, New York, 2002, Churchill Livingstone.

*Figures are for the 50th percentile in girls; centers appear later in boys by a multiplication factor of 1.55 ± 0.14 SD.

3. True or False: The therapist-prosthetist relationship is the key to a successful outcome for clients who are using an upper extremity prosthesis.

Atkins states that the therapist-prosthetist alliance may indeed be the best hope for successful outcomes in the future. As payers begin to look to outcome measures as the key to determine whether a particular device will be authorized, the need for successful results will be crucial. Payers will look at ways of achieving success based on methodology rather than componentry.

Answer: **True**
Atkins, Alley, p. 6
Pillet, Mackin in Mackin, Callahan, Skirven, et al, pp. 1461-1472

4. True or False: Improper positioning is the main reason that a person with an amputation finds difficulty in using a prosthesis.

Improper positioning is the main reason that a person with an amputation finds difficulty using his or her prosthesis. A person with a prosthesis should be instructed to orient the components of the prosthesis in space to a position that resembles that of a normal limb engaged in the same task. Practicing activities of daily living that are useful and purposeful such as cutting food, using scissors, dressing, opening a jar or bottle, washing dishes, hammering a nail, and driving a car should be pursued so that the individual automatically uses the prosthesis in daily routines.

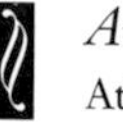

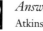

Answer: **True**
Atkins, p. 285

5. True or False: The prosthesis in a unilateral amputee plays a nondominant, functional role.

The sound limb performs fine motor prehension activities, whereas the prosthetic terminal device (TD) is most useful for gross prehension activities. It is unreasonable to expect the prosthesis to assume any more than 30% of the total function of the task in bilateral upper-extremity activities. The therapist must be realistic with the client in viewing the prosthesis as a "helper."

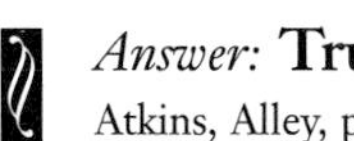

Answer: **True**

Atkins, Alley, p. 2

6. Match each congenital deformity with the proper classification (pick two deformities for each classification).

Classification

1. Failure of formation (arrest of development)
2. Failure of differentiation (separation)
3. Duplication
4. Overgrowth
5. Undergrowth
6. Congenital constriction band syndrome
7. Generalized skeletal abnormalities

Congenital Deformity

- **A.** Thumb-clutched hand
- **B.** Polydactyly
- **C.** Madelung's deformity
- **D.** Transverse deficiencies
- **E.** Maffucci's syndrome
- **F.** Kirner's deformity
- **G.** Macrodactyly
- **H.** Triphalangism
- **I.** Brachydactyly
- **J.** Phocomelia
- **K.** Hypoplasia
- **L.** Gigantism
- **M.** Compression neuropathy
- **N.** Acrosyndactyly

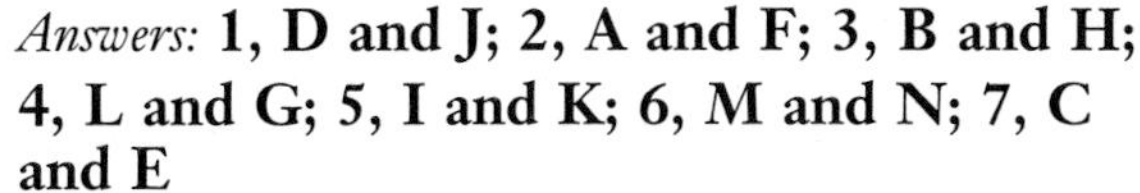

Answers: **1, D and J; 2, A and F; 3, B and H; 4, L and G; 5, I and K; 6, M and N; 7, C and E**

Swanson, p. 4

Hunter, Mackin, Callahan, pp. 1428-1433

Dobyns in Mackin, Callahan, Skirven, et al, pp. 1899-1905

7. Which of the following means *webbed fingers*?

- **A.** Polydactyly
- **B.** Ectrodactyly
- **C.** Syndactyly
- **D.** Brachydactyly

Syndactyly means webbed fingers. The incidence of syndactyly and polydactyly is high among infants with congenital anomalies. Syndactyly is most commonly found in the third web space. The next most common area is the fourth web, followed by the second web and first web.

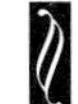

Answer: **C**

Green, p. 346

Dobyns in Mackin, Callahan, Skirven, et al, pp. 1899-1905

Refer to Fig. 20-3

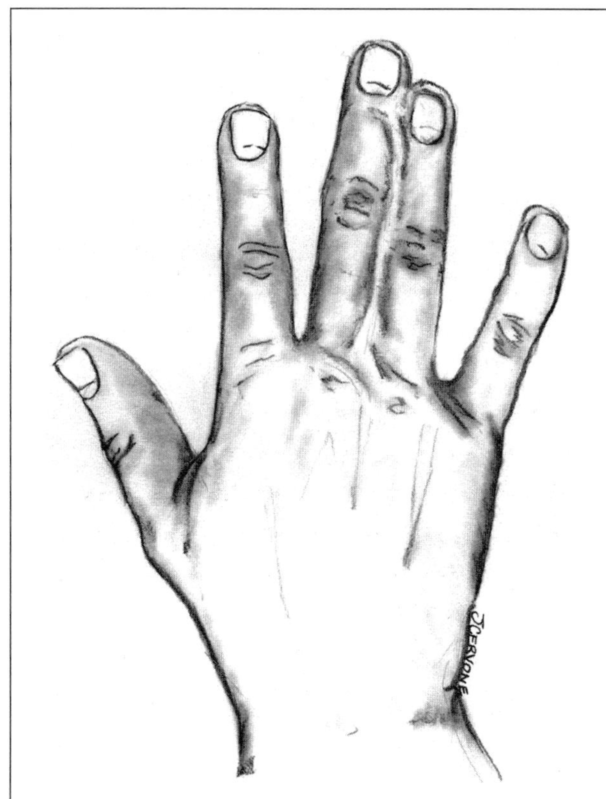

Fig. 20-3

8. Which disorder specifically affects the wrist?

A. Pterygium cubital contracture
B. Kirner's deformity
C. Phocomelia
D. Madelung's deformity

Madelung's deformity is a genetic disorder that, because of the limited distal radius development, does not become obvious until late childhood. Madelung's is more common in females. The classic deformity is a shortening of the radius at the wrist and is caused by inadequate development of the distal radius physis, thus resulting in an ulna that is longer than the radius; it appears as a subluxed wrist with a prominent ulnar head. The patient often has limited extension and supination. Madelung's deformity is most often seen bilaterally.

Function and appearance are rarely a problem until adolescence. Wrist pain may be noted with vigorous activities. Rest can be used when the pain is exacerbated. Surgical correction can be performed if needed.

Answer: **D**
Green, p. 515
Hunter, Mackin, Callahan, p. 1433
Dobyns in Mackin, Callahan, Skirven, et al, p. 1904
Smith, pp. 312-313

9. Which disorder involves the fifth digit but often is not obvious until the child reaches the age of 12?

A. Kirner's deformity
B. Hyperphalangism
C. Pterygium cubital contracture
D. Arthrogryposis

In 1927, Kirner described a condition of the fifth digit that was characterized by palmar and radial curving of the distal phalanx. This disorder is not considered strictly congenital because it often is not obvious until about age 12. It is more common in females and begins as a painless progressive curving of the distal phalanges of both hands, most commonly in the fifth digit.

Answer: **A**
Green, pp. 353-354
Dobyns in Mackin, Callahan, Skirven, et al, p. 1903
Refer to Fig. 20-4

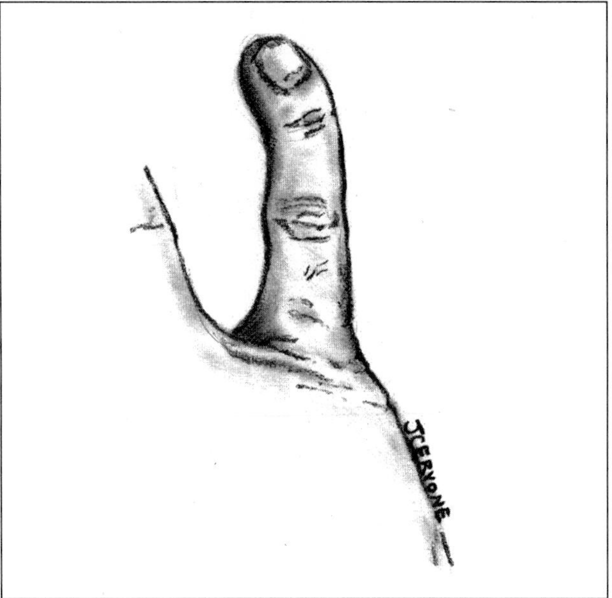

Fig. 20-4

10. Match each deformity with its definition.

Deformity

1. Pterygium cubital
2. Arthrogryposis
3. Polydactyly
4. Ectrodactyly

Definition

A. Persistent joint contracture
B. Congenital elbow webbing
C. Missing digits
D. Having more than the normal number of fingers and toes

Answers: **1, B; 2, A; 3, D; 4, C**
Green, pp. 304, 363, 370, 480-781

11. Which of the following terms means *seal limb*?

A. Ectrodactyly
B. Phocomelia
C. Clinodactyly
D. Syndactyly

The term *phocomelia* means seal limb. Patients with this failure of formation may produce an extreme shortening of the limb. The incidence of phocomelia is approximately 0.8% of all congenital upper limb anomalies. This deformity became notorious in the 1950s and early 1960s when pregnant women took thalidomide. There are few indications for surgery in patients with phocomelia, but prosthetics often are indicated, especially in individuals with bilateral phocomelia.

Answer: **B**
Green, p. 258
Swanson, p. 15
Dobyns in Mackin, Callahan, Skirven, et al, p. 1899
Refer to Fig. 20-5

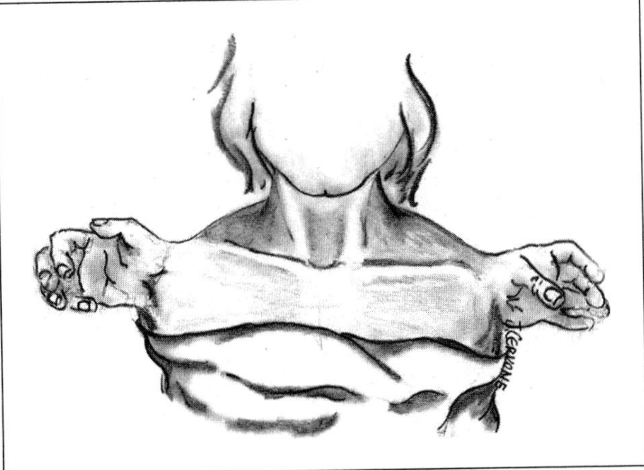

Fig. 20-5

12. True or False: Congenital ulnar drift of the fingers and congenital contracture of the digits also are referred to as *windblown hand.*

Windblown hand is a congenital deformity in the failure of differentiation category. It can be associated with whistling face syndrome and Freeman-Sheldon syndrome. Windblown hand also is known as *congenital ulnar drift fingers* and *congenital contracture of the digits.* This condition can be managed through therapy, adaptive equipment, or surgical correction. Surgical intervention is preferable at an early age.

Answer: **True**
Hunter, Mackin, Callahan, p. 1431
Dobyns in Mackin, Callahan, Skirven, et al, p. 1902
Refer to Fig. 20-6

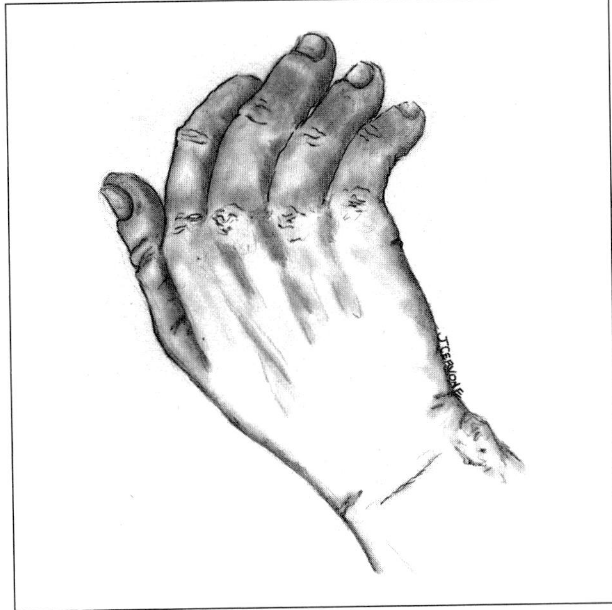

Fig. 20-6

13. Which term is commonly used to refer to a congenital flexion contracture of the PIP joint of the little finger in the sagittal plane?

A. Syndactyly
B. Kirner's deformity
C. Clinodactyly
D. Camptodactyly
E. Trigger digit

Camptodactyly classically presents with a flexion deformity of the PIP joint of the little finger in the sagittal plane (flexion/extension). However, a variety of presentations are noted in the literature. Camptodactyly often is hereditary and may present bilaterally. Often no treatment is necessary, unless it is disabling. Surgical treatment varies because of the multiplicity of structures. Conservative treatment consisting of static, dynamic, or serial casting/splinting has shown favorable results over a long period.

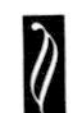

Answer: **D**
Swanson, p. 28
Hunter, Mackin, Callahan, p. 1430
Dobyns in Mackin, Callahan, Skirven, et al, p. 1902
Refer to Fig. 20-7

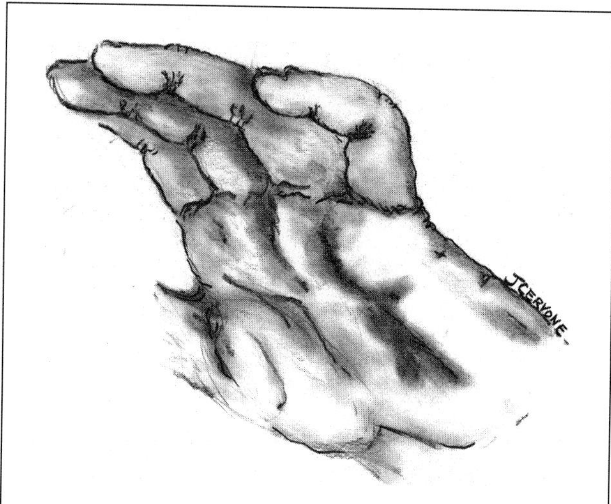

Fig. 20-7

14. An 11-year-old girl presents with a bent little finger and has no history of trauma. The patient's complaint is primarily cosmetic. Clinical examination and radiographs reveal middle phalanx involvement with curving in the coronal or radioulnar plane. What would you conclude?

A. The patient has a hypoplastic digit.
B. The patient hurt her finger but does not recall injury.
C. The patient has Maffucci's syndrome.
D. The patient has clinodactyly.

The patient's findings are classical indications of clinodactyly, which is a categorization of failure of differentiation. Clinodactyly is similar to camptodactyly; classically, both involve a bent finger in the fifth digit. In clinodactyly, the finger is bent in the coronal or radioulnar plane and most often affects the distal interphalangeal (DIP) joint; in camptodactyly the finger is bent in the sagittal or extension/flexion plane and most often affects the PIP joint. Often no intervention is needed for clinodactyly. Elective surgery may be indicated for cosmetic purposes.

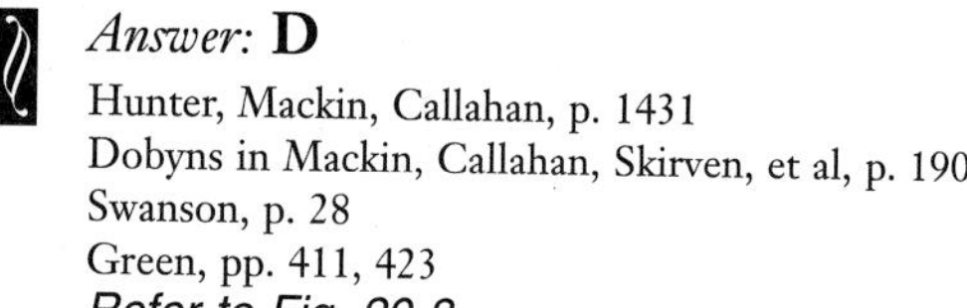

Answer: **D**

Hunter, Mackin, Callahan, p. 1431
Dobyns in Mackin, Callahan, Skirven, et al, p. 1902
Swanson, p. 28
Green, pp. 411, 423
Refer to Fig. 20-8

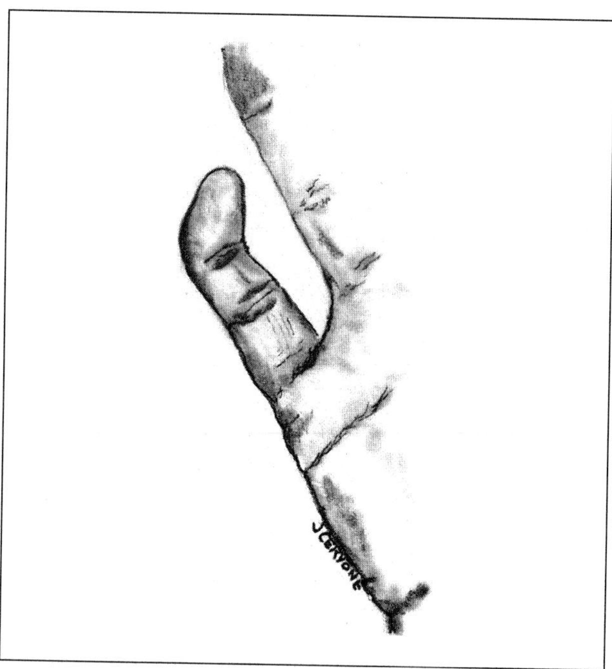

Fig. 20-8

15. Fig. 20-9 is an example of which of the following?

A. Apert's thumb
B. Congenital clasped thumb
C. Retroflexible thumb
D. Hypoplastic thumb

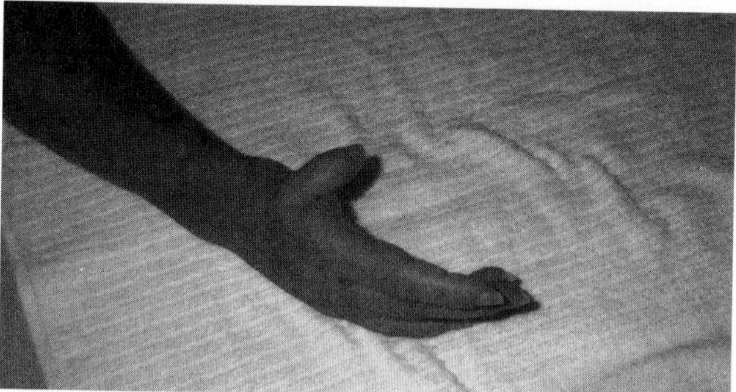

Fig. 20-9

The hypoplastic thumb is a defective digit that is incomplete in its development. The degree of hypoplasia ranges from minimal shortening to complete absence of the thumb. The remaining three answers are specific thumb disorders that are not applicable to the patient shown.

Apert's thumb is often short and angulated. The thumb and index webs are deficient, and the thumb must be separated early to allow for function. Congenital clasped thumb is characterized by a thumb that is flexed and adducted; this deformity sometimes is called *thumb-clutched hand*. The retroflexible thumb is a rare congenital anomaly; during physical examination, the metacarpophalangeal (MCP) joint is hyperextended, and the DIP joint is hyperflexed (resembling a type-III deformity of rheumatoid arthritis).

Answer: **D**
Green, pp. 385-409

16. Amputation at the shoulder level represents which percentage of impairment for the upper extremity?

A. 30%
B. 50%
C. 80%
D. 100%

An amputation of the arm at the shoulder level represents an impairment of 100% of the upper extremity. This corresponds to a 60% impairment of the whole person.

An amputation below the axilla and proximal to the biceps tendon is rated as a 95% to 100% impairment of the upper extremity and a 57% to 60% impairment of the whole person.

An amputation below the elbow and proximal to the MCP joints is rated as a 90% to 95% impairment of the upper extremity and a 54% to 57% impairment of the whole person.

An amputation of the fingers and thumb through the MCP joint is considered a 100% impairment of the hand, a 90% impairment of the upper extremity, and a 54% impairment of the whole person. Digit amputation is rated on a scale that is relative to the entire hand.

Answer: **D**
Hunter, Mackin, Callahan, pp. 1849, 1868
Schneider in Mackin, Callahan, Skirven, et al, pp. 300-301

17. Which technique is not appropriate for desensitization of the residual limb?

A. Tapping
B. Vibration
C. Use of graded textures
D. All of the above are appropriate desensitization techniques.

After the wound has healed, desensitization may be needed for a hypersensitive residual limb. The techniques cited as most appropriate include gentle massage, pressure, tapping, stroking, vibration, weight bearing, and the use of graded textures. Desensitization helps prepare the limb for application of the prosthetic socket.

Answer: **D**
Bowker, Michael, p. 279
Peimer, p. 2461
Hunter, Mackin, Callahan, pp. 614-615, 1229

18. Which of these phenomena is a normal response to an amputation that generally does not interfere with function or require any treatment?

A. Phantom limb sensation
B. Phantom limb pain
C. Residual limb pain
D. All of the above

Phantom limb sensation is the ability to perceive cortical images of the lost limb, and it occurs in almost every acquired amputee. Phantom limb sensation usually is no more than a minor annoyance and, on occasion, may even be useful during prosthetic training. New amputees should be educated that this is a normal phenomenon so that they do not think they are going crazy when they still “feel” the areas distal to the amputation. This sensation generally does not interfere with function or require any treatment.

Phantom limb pain can begin in the immediate postamputation phase and should diminish but can become a severe problem and result in chronic pain. If this pain interferes with normal activities of daily living and sleep patterns for more than 6 weeks after the amputation, it must be aggressively treated. Phantom pain is believed to occur because of deafferentation of the peripheral and central pain centers, especially the somatosensory cortex. Pain treatment modalities are used based on their mechanisms in modifying pain messages in these pathways. Many treatment techniques have been employed with varying success. Effective techniques include the use of drugs and conventional occupational/physical therapy modalities.

Residual limb pain is defined as pain in the residual limb that does not descend into the phantom. This pain may be related to neuroma formation or may be caused by physical changes in the residual limb. Another common cause is related to pressure from an ill-fitting prosthesis.

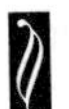

Answer: **A**

Hunter, Mackin, Callahan, p. 1229
Esquenazi, Meier, pp. 5-20
Peimer, p. 2465
Pillet, Mackin in Mackin, Callahan, Skirven, et al, pp. 1461-1472

CLINICAL GEM:
One way to treat phantom pain is by using a transcutaneous electrical nerve stimulation unit. One technique is electrode placement on the contralateral limb.

19. The "golden period" in prosthetic management denotes the most optimal time for the fitting of an upper extremity prosthesis to promote successful rehabilitation. This period occurs during which time after amputation?

A. The first 6 months
B. The first 60 days
C. The first 30 days
D. The first year

The first immediate-fit prosthesis was reported in 1958 and since then many studies have been conducted to show the effect of early-fit prosthetic fabrication on successful rehabilitation. The study conducted by Malone and others denoted a "golden period" of prosthetic fitting, which appeared to be within the first month after amputation. Early application of a prosthesis promotes the continuation of bilateral activities, better acceptance of the prosthesis, and better healing through edema and pain control. The success rate for patients fit within 1 month of amputation was 93%; the success rate for those fit after 1 month was only 42%.

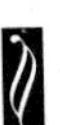

Answer: **C**

Malone, Fleming, Robertson, pp. 33-41
Hunter, Mackin, Callahan, p. 1211
Pillet, Mackin in Mackin, Callahan, Skirven, et al, pp. 1461-1472

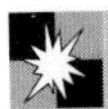

CLINICAL GEM:
An early-fit prosthesis may be fabricated within the first 2 weeks after surgery. In fact, an immediate fit can be fabricated in the operating room or shortly thereafter. This is called an *immediate postoperative prosthesis* (IPOP).

20. Which of the following is a developmental sign that indicates that a child is ready for the first fitting of an upper extremity prosthesis?

A. Child sits independently without support.
B. Child explores sound hand and residual limb while supine.
C. Child tries to hold object in elbow fold or against body.
D. Child responds to verbal instructions.
E. All of the above

A survey of child amputee clinics in North America done by Shaperman, Landsberger, and Setoguchi in 2003 indicated the top developmental signs as listed in choices A through D. Other indicators were child rolls over independently, parents request fitting and will support the program, child pulls to stand and cruises around furniture, child attempts to move from sitting to prone or prone to sitting, and child shifts weight from side to side in sitting.

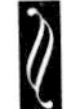

Answer: **E**

Shaperman, Landsberger, Setoguchi, p. 13

21. According to the leading pediatric amputee centers, the most appropriate time to fit a congenital unilateral transverse radioulnar limb–deficient child with his or her first prosthesis is which of the following?

A. Before 2 months of age, to aid in visually guided reaching
B. Birth to 3 months, to help promote incorporation of the prosthesis in the child's body image
C. Around 6 months, when the infant is achieving independent sitting balance
D. When the child is old enough to follow simple two-step commands

The appropriate time to fit a congenital amputee with his or her first prosthesis is probably one of the most controversial topics regarding the limb-deficient child. With recent technical advances and the availability of more types of prostheses, the controversy has become even more complicated because it involves the question of the most appropriate type of prosthesis. Hubbard documents many studies that support the belief that fitting a child as early as possible is important to facilitate the child's ability to become two-handed. She also references many articles that weigh the costs of early fitting against the benefits and questions the cost-benefit ratio. Review of the literature from many of the leading pediatric amputee centers seems to indicate a general agreement that the most appropriate time for fitting a first prosthesis on a congenital unilateral amputee is between 3 and 9 months of age, or at about 6 months, when the child is achieving sitting balance. Support for this idea follows.

The question of early fit to aid visually guided reaching was supported in a 1976 article by Fisher. She cited research that supports the belief that the development of visually guided reaching depends on the opportunity to see the limb moving in space. She questioned whether fitting the baby before 3 or 4 months of age would aid visually guided reaching and thus influence future prosthetic wearing and use patterns.

The Child Amputee Prosthetics Project (CAPP) at the University of California in Los Angeles has long been a proponent of early fitting and bases its criteria on developmental milestones. At the CAPP, the criterion for prescribing the first passive prosthesis for a baby with a below-elbow limb deficiency is the attainment of independent sitting balance. When the baby is sitting securely, has no need to use the arms for support, and has achieved some proficiency in creeping and pulling to a stand, a prosthesis can provide a functional advantage.

Wanner asserts that early fitting at 6 months of age enables the child to incorporate the prosthesis into his body image, which increases the likelihood of long-term prosthetic acceptance. At 6 months of age, most children begin to sit. The prosthesis enables the child to touch down on the limb-deficient side and thereby improves his sitting balance. It also helps the child to do bimanual activities at arm's length.

Hubbard's experience with myoprosthetics at the Hugh MacMillan Rehabilitation Center in Canada also supports this early fit. A passive, cosmetic prosthesis typically is provided to congenital amputees between 3 and 6 months of age to assist them in balance and gross motor activity and to condition them to wearing an artificial limb.

Shaperman, Landsberger, and Setoguchi also point out that "[t]he first actively operated terminal device is fitted when the child demonstrates awareness of cause and effect and tries to hold objects. Myoelectric hands are often fitted as early as 10 months and body-powered terminal devices between 18 and 24 months."

Finally, Jain has outlined in chart form the developmental milestones that are used to guide prescription of various prostheses and their components. He also states that "the initial prosthetic fitting . . . is done at age 3 to 9 months to assist in gross motor development tasks, allowing the use of both limbs for creeping, pulling to stand, and so on. Fitting at a later age (2 to 5 years) has been shown to result in greater rejection of the prosthesis because of the development of compensatory techniques."

Answer: **C**

Hunter, Mackin, Callahan, pp. 1205, 1242, 1246
Bowker, Michael, p. 779
Atkins, Meier, p. 138
Jain, p. 10
Shaperman, Landsberger, Setoguchi, p. 13

22. Congenital unilateral amputees can perform what percentage of activities of daily living without a prosthesis?

A. 10%
B. 30%
C. 50%
D. 100%

Congenital unilateral amputees manage all activities of daily living without a prosthesis. Therefore fitting a functional prosthesis for a patient with unilateral agenesis will often encumber the person.

Answer: **D**

Hunter, Mackin, Callahan, p. 1238
Beasley, p. 743
Pillet, Mackin in Mackin, Callahan, Skirven, et al, pp. 1461-1472

23. True or False: The Krukenberg procedure initially was indicated for blind, bilateral below-elbow amputees.

The Krukenberg procedure (Fig. 20-10, *A*) can be considered for treatment of mutilating upper-extremity injuries. Initially, the Krukenberg procedure was indicated for blind, bilateral below-elbow amputees. This procedure, however, has been used in children with absence of hands and is used in certain countries for unilateral amputees with normal sight. There is concern over the cosmesis of the stump, but the amount of function that is possible in these patients is astounding. There is not much enthusiasm for the Krukenberg procedure in the United States, probably because of a lack of experience and a poor understanding of both the procedure and of how functional (Fig. 20-10, *B*) the patient is afterward.

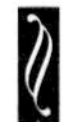

Answer: **True**

Hunter, Mackin, Callahan, p. 1055
Pillet, Mackin in Mackin, Callahan, Skirven, et al, pp. 1461-1472

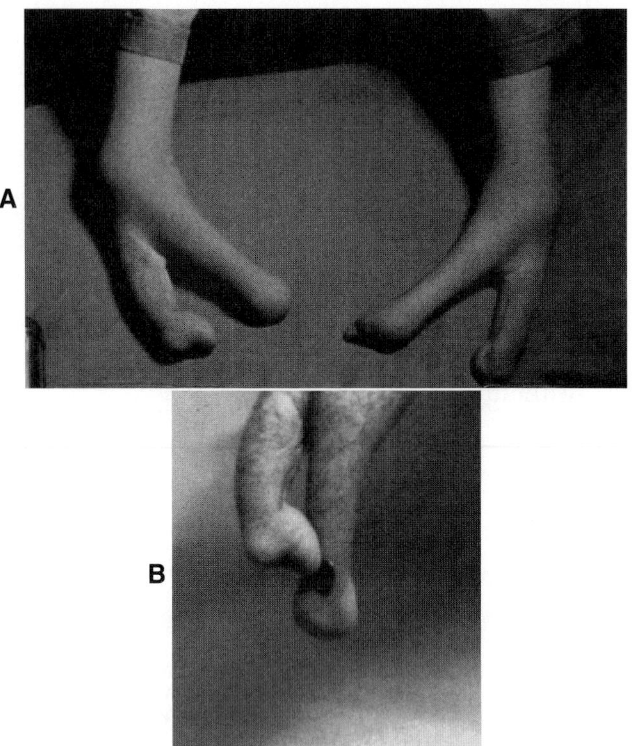

Fig. 20-10 ■ From Hunter JM, Mackin EJ, Callahan AD: *Rehabilitation of the hand: surgery and therapy,* ed 4, St Louis, 1995, Mosby.

24. True or False: A hybrid prosthesis combines body-powered control with myoelectric/external control.

A hybrid system can be an externally powered elbow and a body-powered TD or a body-powered elbow and an externally powered TD. Some advantages of a hybrid system include the following: greater functional envelope, reduced weight, reduced harness system, simultaneous use of the elbow and TD, and reduced cost.

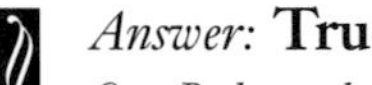

Answer: **True**

Otto Bock prosthetic compendium, upper extremity prostheses, p. 81

Refer to Fig. 20-11

25. True or False: A myoelectric TD is not an option for a unilateral transcarpal/transmetacarpal level amputee because it would make the limb much longer than the contralateral side.

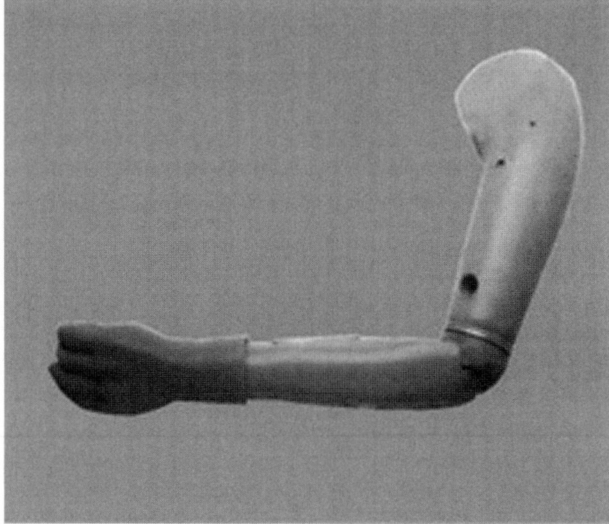

Fig. 20-11 ■ Hybrid prosthesis by Otto Bock Health Care: the ErgoArm (a body-powered elbow) and the Sensorhand (a myoelectric hand). (Courtesy Otto Bock Health Care, Minneapolis, MN.)

In the past, individuals with very long residual limbs had few fitting options for myoelectric hands. The transcarpal hand from Otto Bock Health Care is a microprocessor-controlled hand (Fig. 20-12) that has a grip force and speed force comparable to other adult hands, with one third less weight and one third less size. Now, the transcarpal/transmetacarpal-level amputee can have myoelectric grasp and release capability.

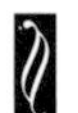

Answer: **False**

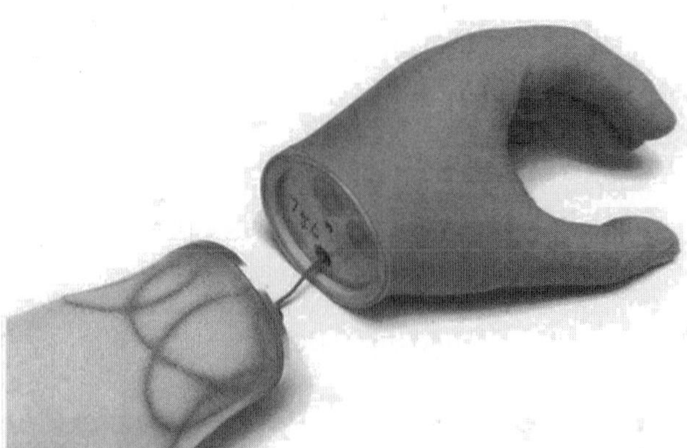

Fig. 20-12 ■ The transcarpal hand. (Courtesy Otto Bock Health Care, Minneapolis, MN.)

26. Which is the prehension pattern most commonly used by prosthetic hands?

A. Palmar
B. Hook
C. Lateral
D. Tip

Six different prehension patterns are used by the physiologic hand: palmar, hook, cylindrical, lateral, tip, and spherical. The most typical prehension pattern physiologically is palmar prehension, also known as "three-jaw Chuck" because the index and middle finger pads both make contact with the thumb. Mechanical and externally controlled prostheses all use this type of prehension, not only because it is the predominant prehension pattern, but it also provides both precision gripping at the fingertips and some power grasping within the palm of the hand.

Answer: **A**
Sarrafian, pp. 104-105
Light, pp. 133-136

27. Biscapular abduction in a transradial prosthesis is a control motion used for which of the following?

A. Activities at the midline
B. An assistive movement to glenohumeral flexion
C. Elbow unlock
D. A and B
E. All of the above

The primary work source for operating the transradial or transhumeral prosthesis is glenohumeral flexion, which can generate a fairly large amount of force and cable travel. For activities at midline, such as toileting, eating, or dressing, *biscapular abduction* is employed because the prosthesis must be used close to the body. *Glenohumeral flexion* can only be used for activities that are sufficiently away from the body. Biscapular abduction has excellent force characteristics but only a moderate amount of cable travel, which is adequate for small gripping tasks. The amount of biscapular abduction depends on the patient's posture and shoulder width.

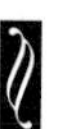
Answer: **D**
Fryer, pp. 104-105
Northwestern University upper extremity prosthetic manual, Sect. 4, pp. 1-6, Sect. 5, p. 8

28. The control mechanisms needed to lock or unlock a mechanical elbow in a conventional above-elbow prosthesis for a transhumeral amputee are which of the following?

A. Chest expansion and scapular abduction of the involved extremity
B. Shoulder depression, shoulder extension, and shoulder abduction of the involved extremity
C. Shoulder depression, shoulder flexion, and internal rotation of the involved extremity
D. Shoulder depression, shoulder extension, and external rotation of the uninvolved extremity

After the prosthesis fit, the first step in training is learning what body movements are needed to control the operation of the prosthetic devices. To operate the elbow lock on a conventional above-elbow prosthesis, the amputee needs shoulder depression, shoulder extension, and shoulder abduction of the involved extremity. The therapist must facilitate full ROM for these movements before acquisition of the prosthesis and should ensure that the amputee is proficient in these movements for control training before initiating functional use training. Recent improvements in products, such as the electric locking body-powered elbow and new three-point harnessing, will lead to new control mechanisms for the conventional user.

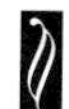
Answer: **B**
Bowker, Michael, p. 283
Atkins, Meier, p. 44
Pedretti, p. 430

29. To power a voluntary opening hook terminal device, a below-elbow (transradial) amputee would use which motion?

A. Humeral flexion
B. Humeral extension
C. Humeral abduction
D. Humeral adduction

A single-control system is used as a power source for a below-elbow (transradial) amputee to allow for prehension. Humeral flexion is used to operate the terminal device.

Answer: **A**
Hunter, Mackin, Callahan, p. 1234

30. What is the advantage of the canted hook over a mechanical hand?

A. Better sight lines for visual feedback
B. Grips cylindrical objects more easily
C. More cosmetically appealing
D. Uses a palmar three-jaw chuck prehension pattern

Because the prosthetic user does not have tactile sensation to determine gripping, he or she depends on visual feedback for grasping confirmation. It is interesting to note that a certain amount of tactile feeling may be perceived through the body-powered cable system to the harness. Prosthetic hands, while being cosmetically superior, block the line of sight to the object, thus making them less functional, especially for precision gripping. Canted hooks, designed to be rotated laterally for a side approach to the object, maximize the line of sight.

Answer: **A**
Fryer, pp. 104-105

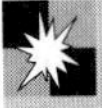
CLINICAL GEM:
The term *prosthetic hands* refers to a prosthesis that is designed with a functional hand, not a hook.

31. Which statement about a bilateral transhumeral patient is false?

A. Bilaterals benefit from different TDs on each side.
B. Bilaterals benefit from the use of wrist flexion devices.
C. Bilaterals should use external power for all components.
D. Bilaterals require push button rather than dial disconnect wrists.

Bilateral users benefit from the different prehension patterns offered by a canted hook on the dominant side and a lyre-shaped symmetric hook on the nondominant side. Hooks, as opposed to hands, are suggested because the great functional requirements of the bilateral patient offset the cosmetic needs. The canted hook permits a better line of sight on the dominant limb, and the lyre shape offers the alternative cylindrical prehension pattern on the nondominant side. Wrist flexion devices are a necessity for the bilateral patient to permit activities at the midline, which include eating, toileting, and dressing. Disconnect wrists are beneficial for switching to functional TDs or for locking pronation and supination. Push-button activation is best and can be activated by activating the push button to bump against a table, chair, or other prosthesis. *It is not advisable for a system to be all body or external power.* The dominant side typically is body powered because it usually has the required force and excursion requirements, and the nondominant side is often externally powered. This avoids interdependent controls, enhances function to the nondominant side, and ensures one device will always be operational.

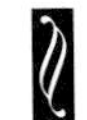
Answer: **C**
Lehneis, p. 316

32. True or False: A self-suspension socket design is preferred for fitting a transradial below-elbow amputee with external power.

One of the goals and benefits of providing a myoelectric prosthesis is the possibility for minimizing or eliminating any body harnessing. Self-suspension can come from many socket designs, all of which have their specific applications, depending on the residual limb presentation. Some of the different styles include the Muenster, Northwestern, Otto Bock, and a design called the *anatomically contoured controlled interface*, the newest design on the market for self-suspension (see Fig. 20-13). These designs depend on the anatomy of the residual limb to provide a bony lock that the socket can suspend over. In some situations it is not practical to suspend from the bony anatomy because it may limit anatomic movement of the residuum. In this case, using some sort of suspension liner may be best. Liners can come off the shelf with a generic shape or can be custom made to a cast of the individual's limb. Off-the-shelf liners are of lower cost and are easily formed with no unusual characteristics. Custom liners have a higher cost and make the fabrication process more time-consuming; however, they offer superior durability and can be fabricated to include any form of suspension modality. The socket style must be chosen with the thought of minimizing harnessing.

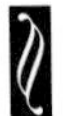
Answer: **True**
Hunter, Mackin, Callahan, pp. 1208, 1227

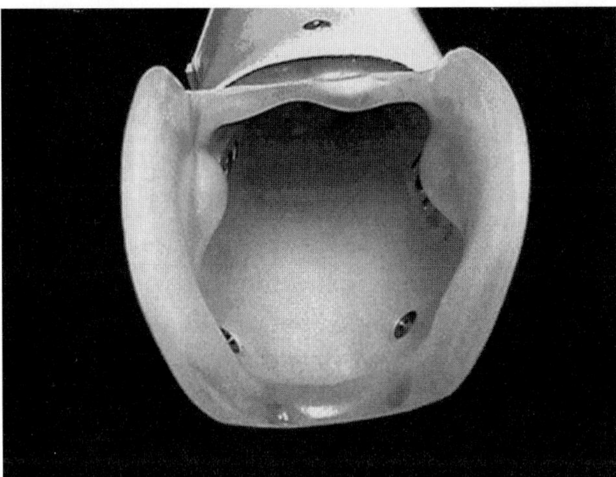

Fig. 20-13 ■ Courtesy Randall Alley BSc, CP, FAAOP, Head of Clinical Research and Business Development for the Hanger Prosthetics and Orthotics Upper Extremity Prosthetic Program.

33. Mr. X is an above-elbow (transhumeral) amputee with a conventional voluntary opening TD. How much should he be able to open his TD when the elbow is fully flexed or extended?

A. At least 50% of maximal available TD opening
B. 100% of maximal available TD opening
C. 15% to 35% of maximal available TD opening
D. It depends on the level of amputation.

A prosthetic checkout is the key to determining the proper fit, mechanical efficiency, and functioning of the control system. Many prosthetic evaluation checklists are available. Two suggested designs are those by New York University and Northwestern University. To evaluate TD opening as part of the full evaluation, the above-elbow amputee locks the elbow at 90 degrees. He or she then actively opens the TD fully. This opening is measured with a ruler and recorded. The same active opening of the TD is next measured with the elbow in full flexion and in full extension. The amputee should be able to open the TD at least 50% of the initial measurement when the elbow is at 90 degrees.

A below-elbow amputee should be able to open the TD to 70% to 100% of available TD opening in full elbow flexion and extension.

Answer: **A**
Hunter, Mackin, Callahan, p. 1233
Trombly, pp. 862-863
Atkins, Meier, p. 42

34. The pediatric "cookie-crusher" prosthesis uses which type of control system?

A. One-state/two-function (hand-opening/hand-closing)
B. Two-state/two-muscle
C. Two-state/two-muscle proportional
D. None of the above

The concept behind myoelectric prosthetics is that the contraction of a muscle can produce a strong enough electric signal to be detected at the surface of the skin. This electromyographic signal can be picked up by electrodes that control the flow of myoelectric energy from a battery to a motor. The motor can control a hand, elbow, or even a wrist unit. State-control systems function by turning the component either off or on (similar to the operation of a simple light switch). After the myoelectric system is activated by muscle contraction, the motor will operate at a constant speed until the muscle relaxes and the system is turned off.

Two-state control systems use a contraction of one muscle to activate a motor in one direction and a second (preferably antagonistic) muscle to operate the motor in another direction. Therefore two separate muscles are needed to operate a prosthesis. This two-state/two-muscle control system can operate many commercially available systems and is most commonly used to activate the following: 1) grasp/release in a hand unit using wrist flexors/extensors; and 2) elbow flexion/elbow extension using biceps/triceps. The Otto Block "digital two-site" electric hand system, the Otto Bock Greifer, and the New York Hosmer-Dorrance electric elbow are all examples of the two-state/two-muscle myoelectric system.

The Utah artificial arm system also is a two-state/two-muscle system with the addition of an internal electronic switch that is activated by cocontraction of the two muscles, alternating between elbow control and hand control. Spiegel describes the specific control technique in the Utah arm as two-state five-function myoelectric control. In proportional control systems, the speed or the prehensile force of the prosthesis is varied with the intensity of the electromyographic signal (similar to the effect of a dimmer switch). The Liberty Mutual Boston elbow is a proportional two-state/two-muscle system.

In some cases, controlling a prosthesis with just one muscle site is necessary. This may occur when only one muscle is available (e.g., after brachial plexus injury when only a few muscle sites are available and each is needed to control different movements). In this case, a one-state control system must be used. Rate-sensitive and level (amplitude)–sensitive control systems exist. In a rate-sensitive system, the speed at which the muscle is contracted determines the direction of movement. For example, a quick contraction may be used to open the hand, and a slow contraction may be used to close it. The hand continues to open or close as long as the muscle remains contracted. In a level-sensitive system, the strength of contraction determines the direction of movement. A hard contraction may be used to open the hand and a gentle contraction may be used to close it. The contractions also must be completed within a specified period. The pediatric "cookie-crusher" and the University New Brunswick System system are two examples.

Otto Bock's "double channel" electric hand system is a one-state, two-function myoswitch controller. So that the Otto Bock Greifer may be completely interchangeable with any of the electric hand systems, it also can be operated as a one-state/two-function system. Thus the Greifer can be made to be operated by both one-site or two-state control systems.

Answer: **A**

Hunter, Mackin, Callahan, pp. 1193, 1243
Atkins, Meier, p. 6
Spiegel, p. 62
Esquenazi, Meier, p. 12

35. The most commonly used body-powered TD is which of the following?

A. Voluntary opening hook
B. Voluntary opening hand
C. Voluntary closing hand and hook
D. Voluntary closing terminal device

The most distal part of an upper-limb prosthetic is the TD. Some authors have stated that this is the most important aspect of the prosthesis, just as the hand is the most important part of the arm. Certainly, a lot of attention has been generated toward the development of various types of TDs.

To date, the most common TD still operates in a gross grasp pattern of function. The mechanical and myoelectric hands function with a "three-jaw chuck" pinch pattern. Mechanical hooks generally have a stationary post with a movable "finger." All body-powered TDs are operated by a cable in one direction and a spring in the other direction.

Because most upper-limb amputees are unilateral, the residual limb functions as the dominant extremity, with the prosthetic limb operating as a functional assist. This is especially true because the science of prosthetic development has not progressed to isolated finger function in a prosthesis.

A "voluntary opening" indicates that the amputee must use his or her own body power to pull on the cable and *open* the TD; the spring automatically closes the device. The Hosmer-Dorrance hook TD is the device most commonly prescribed in North America. The pinch force of this TD is determined by the number of rubber bands or springs that are used. Each rubber band on the hook provides approximately 1 to 1½ pounds of pinch force.

Voluntary closing, conversely, uses the pulling action on the cable to *close* the TD. The advantages of the voluntary closing TD are that a greater maximal pinch strength is available and that graded prehension is allowed. The pinch force is as gentle or strong as the force generated by the amputee. Unfortunately, the mechanical complexity of this device makes it both expensive and prone to break down; for this reason, the voluntary closing TD is not popular.

Both voluntary closing and voluntary opening hands have the disadvantages of frictional losses in the mechanics, which are far greater than with either type of hook; restriction of movement by the cosmetic glove; and contours that block visualization of the fingertips. In addition to these disadvantages, some authors suggest that the practice of the hook-type TDs may have a high incidence of prosthetic rejection because psychosocial issues are not addressed.

Answer: **A**

Trombly, p. 854
Bowker, Michael, p. 107
Hunter, Mackin, Callahan, pp. 1193-1196
Esquenazi, Meier, p. 25

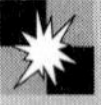

CLINICAL GEM:
Some authors believe that the TD is the most important component of the prosthesis; others believe the socket is the most important component.

Hunter, Mackin, Callahan, p. 1232

36. You are treating a patient, after an amputation, who wants a myoelectric prosthesis. Which testing device is used to assess the strength of a potential muscle group?

A. Nerve conduction velocity unit
B. Galvanic stimulation unit
C. Myotester
D. Direct current stimulation device

The myotester (Fig. 20-14) is useful in assessing the signal strength of potential muscle groups. A myotester also helps determine the best electrode placement. Visual feedback is provided on the unit with a meter or a light. The test is first performed on the sound side for training and then applied to the side with the amputation.

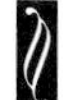

Answer: **C**
Hunter, Mackin, Callahan, p. 1248

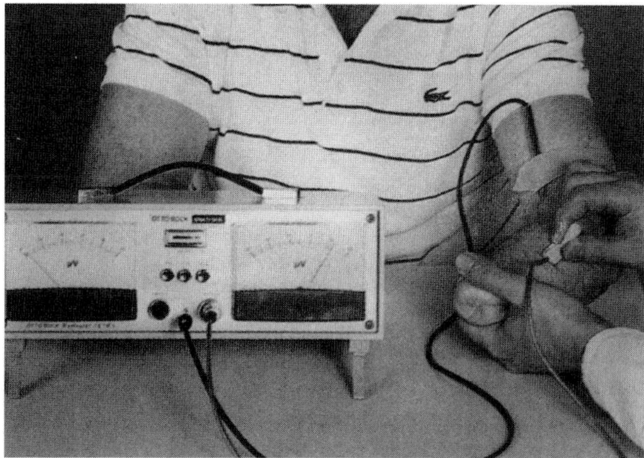

Fig. 20-14 ■ From Pedretti LW: *Occupational therapy: practice skills for physical dysfunction,* ed 4, St Louis, 1996, Mosby.

CLINICAL GEM:
Fig. 20-15 displays the Otto Bock MyoBoy, a muscle site–testing evaluation tool. This unique hardware and software product is used to evaluate muscle sites for a myoelectric prosthesis. The user can see the muscle signals and strength of those signals when hooked up to electrodes. A visual virtual hand and car game are two programs that can be used for training and muscle strengthening. This information can assist in the component selection process as well. All muscle-testing information gathered can be documented, saved, and printed (Fig. 20-15).

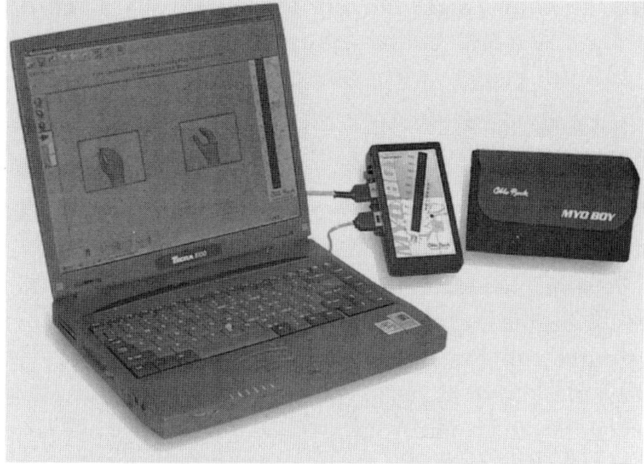

Fig. 20-15 ■ Courtesy Otto Bock, Minneapolis, MN.

37. A 36-year-old woman sustained a traumatic left transradial amputation. The perfect TD for maximizing her functional capabilities would be which of the following?

A. A myoelectric hand because of its cosmesis and functional abilities
B. A conventional body-powered voluntary opening hook because of the increased ability to visualize objects during functional use
C. A passive cosmetic hand because her nondominant extremity was amputated
D. None of the above

There are no absolutes in prosthetic prescription. Each individual must be evaluated individually for his or her own physiologic, anatomic, psychologic, activities of daily living, and lifestyle needs. A team-oriented approach is suggested for the prescriptive pattern. Sears has suggested a quantitative approach to prescriptions, but even he admits that this method has limitations because of the individual nature of this process. The "perfect" TD prescribed is determined by the patient's specific needs.

Answer: **D**
Sears, pp. 361-371
Meredith, p. 936
Spiegel, p. 61

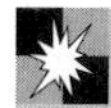

CLINICAL GEM:
Spiegel and Meredith describe the advantages and disadvantages of available components and believe that evaluating the pros and cons is vital to choosing a proper prosthesis.

38. True or False: During functional use training, a unilateral below-elbow amputee is taught to hold dishes with the prosthesis and use the sound extremity to hold the sponge or dishcloth when washing dishes.

Functional use training usually begins once the amputee has a beginning mastery of the controls. A unilateral amputee will generally find that the prosthesis becomes the nondominant, gross-assist extremity. Even with recent advances in myoelectrics and hybrid designs, the TD still functions in a gross grasp and release. For this reason, during dish washing, the prosthesis is used to grasp the sponge or dishcloth (with care taken to avoid immersing the prosthesis in water) while the sound extremity is used to hold the more fragile dish.

Answer: **False**

Atkins, Meier, p. 46
Bowker, Michael, p. 286

39. True or False: The two basic techniques for harnessing a transhumeral amputee are dual control and triple control.

Dual control is done through a Bowden cable with a split housing around the elbow. When the elbow is locked, the cable travels through the housing controlling the TD. When the elbow is unlocked, the cable acts to flex the elbow. The benefit of this control type is that the same movement for flexing the elbow is the movement that controls the TD. The problem is that it typically requires 4.5 inches of excursion to perform both functions and the elbow must be locked in order to operate the TD. When the elbow is being flexed and a heavier object is in the TD, the tension required to flex the elbow tends to open the hook and drops whatever is being held. Triple control allows for simultaneous and independent control over elbow flexion and TD activation. This control does not require that the elbow is locked to activate the TD. The difficulty of this control is that it requires separation between biscapular abduction and glenohumeral flexion. The benefit is that having separate controls allows the individual more freedom of movement and allows for positioning and grasping tasks to be performed quicker.

Answer: **True**

Bertels, pp. 1-5

Chapter 21

Hodge Podge of Treatment Techniques

1. True or False: Traditional athletic taping is the same as Kinesio taping.

Traditional taping encloses a joint to provide stability and restrict movement, whereas Kinesio taping focuses on the muscles that control movement.

Answer: **False**
Coopee in Mackin, Callahan, Skirven, et al, p. 1796

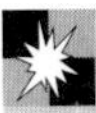
CLINICAL GEM:
Dr. Kenso Kase introduced his techniques of Kinesio taping in 1994 to a group of chiropractors in New Mexico. The technique has gained rapid popularity.

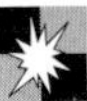
CLINICAL GEM:
The website www.kinesiotaping.com contains information about technique, instructional courses, and tape distributors.

2. Kinesio Taping is indicated for all except which of the following?

A. Relief of pain
B. Muscle support
C. Correction of joint misalignment by balancing muscles
D. All of the above are indications to use Kinesio taping.

Many conditions can be successfully treated with Kinesio taping. It is indicated for pain relief, muscle support, and correction of joint alignment.

Answer: **D**
Coopee in Mackin, Callahan, Skirven, et al, pp. 1805-1806

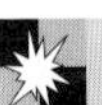
CLINICAL GEM:
Precautions/contraindications: Allergy to the adhesive or materials as well as improper tape tension can increase pain. Caution is advised with the elderly or patients with multiple health risks. During a patient's pregnancy, do not tape the neck, shoulder, and/or medial aspect of the lower leg because these are pressure points that induce labor. Additionally, avoid taping when a patient has malignancy, cellulitis, infection, fragile, or healing tissue.

3. Which of the following is not an indication for continuous passive motion (CPM) in the upper extremity?

A. Stable fractures after open reduction and internal fixation (ORIF)
B. Repaired tendons
C. Burns
D. All of the above are indications.

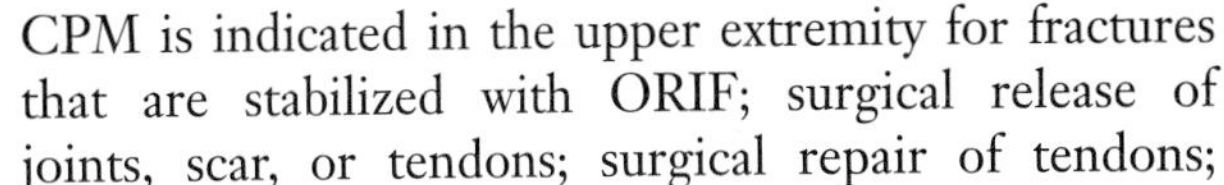

CPM is indicated in the upper extremity for fractures that are stabilized with ORIF; surgical release of joints, scar, or tendons; surgical repair of tendons;

reconstruction of ligaments; elimination of joint stiffness; inflammatory conditions; pain; burns; and total joint replacements.

Answer: **D**

LaStayo, Cass in Mackin, Callahan, Skirven, et al, p. 1768

4. According to Maitland, the shoulder quadrant technique, "rolling over the quadrant," is used to treat a patient whose disorder is described by which of the following?

A. Acute and irritable
B. Minor and chronic
C. Subacute and irritable
D. Subacute and improving

"Rolling over the quadrant" (Fig. 21-1, *A*) is used when the patient's disorder is minor and chronic. It is a painful procedure. The patient's arm is firstly held very firmly against the peak of the quadrant (Fig. 21-1, *B*) with his or her glenohumeral joint slightly medially rotated (Fig. 21-1, *C*); therefore you would not use this technique on an individual with an acute disorder or on one in whom you could easily convert a subacute condition into an acute condition with too vigorous a treatment.

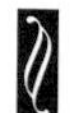

Answer: **B**

Maitland, pp. 135-136

5. True or False: When a concave surface is mobilized on a convex surface, the concave joint surface is glided in the same direction that the bone is moving.

The convex-concave rule denotes the mechanical relationship of the joint surfaces and is the basis for determining the direction of the mobilizing force when joint mobilization gliding techniques are used. When a concave surface is mobilized on a convex surface, the concave joint surface is glided in the same direction that the bone is moving (Fig. 21-2, *A*). If the convex surface is mobilized on a concave surface, bone movement and glide are in the opposite direction (Fig. 21-2, *B*).

Answer: **True**

Kisner, Colby, p. 153
Murphy, p. 2

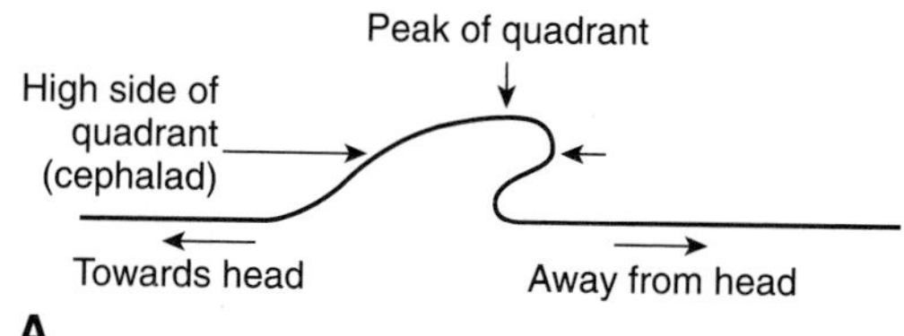

A

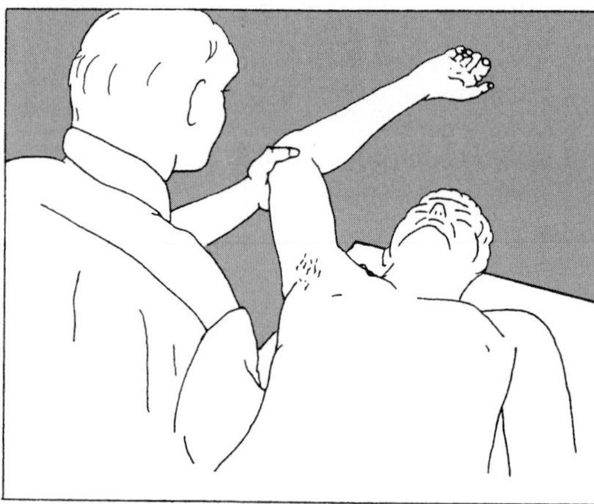

B

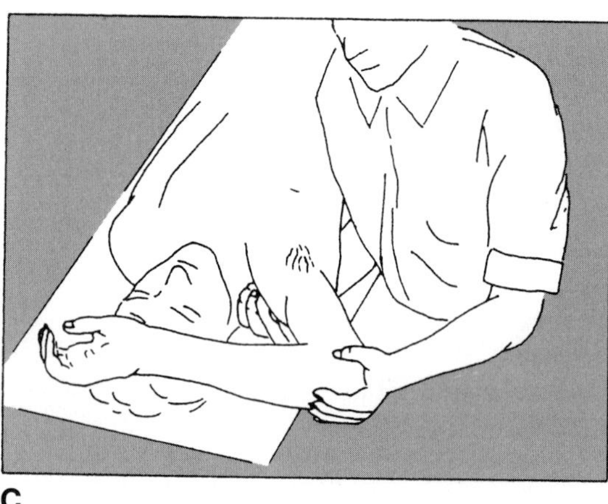

C

Fig. 21-1 ■ **A,** Peak of quadrant; **B,** viewed from caudad position; and **C,** viewed from cephalad position. (From Maitland GD: *Peripheral manipulation*, ed 3, Edinburgh, 1991, Butterworth Heinemann.)

Clinical Gem:
Controversy exists concerning the concave-convex theory of joint mobilization.

6. True or False: *Rolling, gliding,* and *spinning* are terms associated with the physiological movements of joint mobilization.

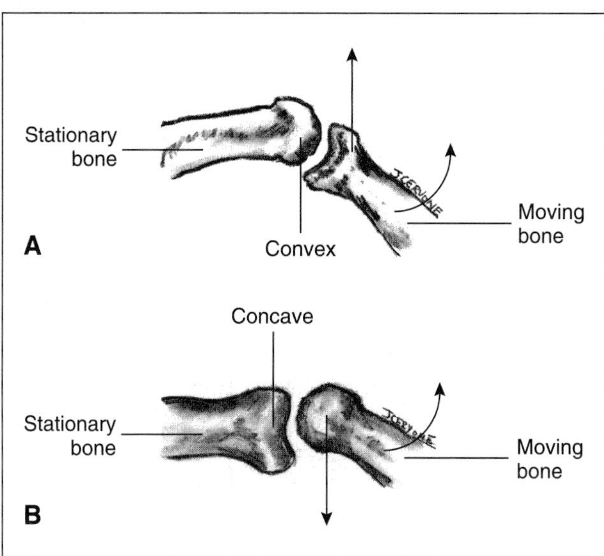

Fig. 21-2 ■ **A,** Moving bone is mobilized in the same direction as desired motion. **B,** Moving bone is mobilized in the direction opposite that of desired motion.

The techniques used in joint mobilization can be performed with physiological or accessory movements. Physiological movements are performed voluntarily by the patient (e.g., flexion, abduction, rotation). Accessory movements are those movements within the joint and surrounding tissues necessary for normal joint range of motion (ROM) that the patient cannot perform voluntarily (e.g., distraction, gliding, compression, rolling, spinning).

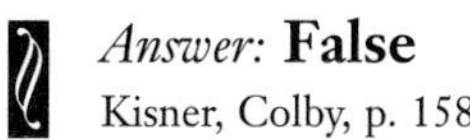

Answer: **False**
Kisner, Colby, p. 158

7. Which of the following is *not* a contraindication or precaution for joint mobilization?

A. Malignancy
B. Joint replacement arthroplasties
C. Pain
D. Infection

The reference sources cited give overlapping contraindications and precautions. It is important for the therapist to appropriately evaluate the patient and determine whether joint mobilization can be an effective adjunct to treatment. Grade I distraction and grade I oscillatory movements that do not stress or stretch the capsule help block the transmission of pain stimuli. Therefore pain is not a precaution or contraindication but may sometimes be a justification for joint mobilization. However, please note that caution must be taken in performing mobilization on a painful joint so as to not increase the pain. See the following Clinical Gem for precautions and contraindications to joint mobilization.

Answer: **C**
Kisner, Colby, pp. 156-158
Murphy, p. 1

CLINICAL GEM:
The following is a list of precautions and contraindications for joint mobilization.

Precautions: Osteoporosis, hypermobility, inability of patient to relax, and presence of protective muscle spasm

Contraindications: Joint replacement arthroplasty, unhealed fractures, acute arthritis, bone disease, infection, malignancy, and rheumatoid arthritis

8. Which of the following are benefits of joint mobilization?

A. Increased joint lubrication
B. Increased proprioceptive input
C. Temporary decrease in joint stiffness
D. Increased joint nutrition
E. All of the above

All of the above are benefits of joint mobilization. When joint mobilization is performed, synovial fluid production (joint lubrication) is stimulated, thus bringing nutrients to the cartilage of the joint surfaces. Old fibers are realigned and lengthened, and new collagen aligns in the direction of stress, thus decreasing joint stiffness. Joint mobilization assists in sending sensory information regarding pain, speed, and direction of movement and muscle tone to the brain.

Answer: **E**
Kisner, Colby, p. 156
Duda-Huys, pp. 7-12

9. A 42-year-old female typist presents with complaints of right shoulder pain. She is right hand–dominant. Before initiating treatment of her painful shoulder, you should first clear which area?

A. Fingers
B. Cervical spine
C. Thoracic spine
D. Wrist
E. All of the above

With all shoulder problems, excluding involvement of the cervical spine before commencing treatment at the shoulder is wise. Cervical problems can mimic shoulder lesions to the extent of painful and even restricted shoulder movements.

Answer: **B**
McKenzie, p. 193
Wells, p. 110

10. Which of the following causative factors is commonly said to be involved in rotator cuff tendonitis?

A. Vascular
B. Degenerative
C. Mechanical stress
D. Anatomy
E. All of the above

The consensus seems to be that the pathogenesis of rotator cuff tendonitis is multifactorial and thus may include relative contributions of vascular, degenerative, and mechanical stress and anatomical variations.

Answer: **E**
McKenzie, p. 194

11. A 16-year-old male presents with the chief complaint of neck and upper thoracic pain. His test movements are normal. He presents with normal ROM, and his pain cannot be reproduced by test movements. You send him out to the waiting area to evaluate your findings. After 30 minutes he complains to the receptionist about being uncomfortable. The cause of his symptoms is most likely which of the following?

A. Derangement
B. Postural
C. Dysfunction
D. All of the above

This is a typical clinical example of a patient with a postural syndrome. The patient has poor posture, and the pain cannot be reproduced by the test movements. To reproduce the appropriate postural stress, the patient must assume and maintain the position that is stated to cause pain. Only after the passage of sufficient time will the symptoms appear, and up to half an hour may be required before the pain is felt.

Answer: **B**
McKenzie, p. 153

12. True or False: According to Kaltenborn, joint play testing and mobilization must be done with the joint in a resting position.

Kaltenborn refers to bone and joint positions in terms of the maximum loose-packed position (MLPP—the resting position) and the close-packed position. In the MLPP, the greatest amount of joint play is possible; thus the assessment of joint play and treatment are performed in this position. In the close-packed position, there is maximum contact between the concave and convex articular surfaces; therefore the least amount of joint play is available.

Answer: **True**
Duda-Huys, pp. 7-8

13. True or False: According to Maitland, a grade IV joint mobilization movement is a large amplitude movement at end range.

A grade IV joint mobilization is a small-amplitude movement, performed at the limit of range. Maitland's treatment technique involves passive oscillatory movements and sustained stretches. He has defined four basic grades of movement, as described in Fig. 21-3.

Answer: **False**
Kisner, Colby, p. 160
Duda-Huys, p. 7-14

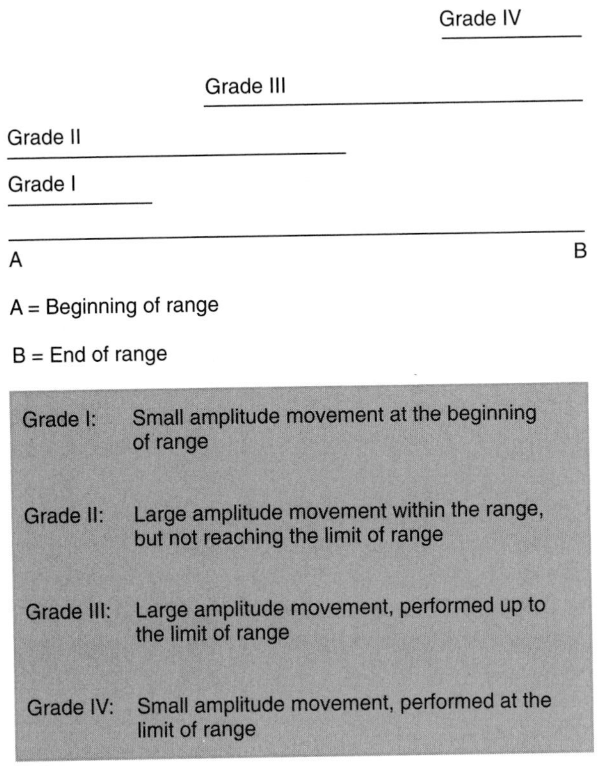

Grade IV

Grade III

Grade II

Grade I

A B

A = Beginning of range

B = End of range

Grade I:	Small amplitude movement at the beginning of range
Grade II:	Large amplitude movement within the range, but not reaching the limit of range
Grade III:	Large amplitude movement, performed up to the limit of range
Grade IV:	Small amplitude movement, performed at the limit of range

Fig. 21-3

14. A patient is 5 weeks status post repair of the flexor digitorum superficialis (FDS) and flexor digitorum profundus (FDP) for digits one through three. When he attempts to make a fist he can't make any gains into flexion, even with the uninjured digits. Application of which device will help determine whether the extensor digitorum communis (EDC) is firing higher than the flexors?

A. Electromyographic (EMG) biofeedback
B. High-voltage galvanic stimulation (HVGS)
C. Transcutaneous electrical nerve stimulation (TENS)
D. CPM

An EMG biofeedback device (Fig. 21-4) allows the therapist to see which muscles are contracting and helps the patient to retrain the proper muscles to work. In this case, the patient learns to perform place-and-hold techniques and light dowel squeezing to focus on FDS/FDP contraction while keeping EDC activity to a minimum. The patient has to learn control of the muscles before strengthening can be performed.

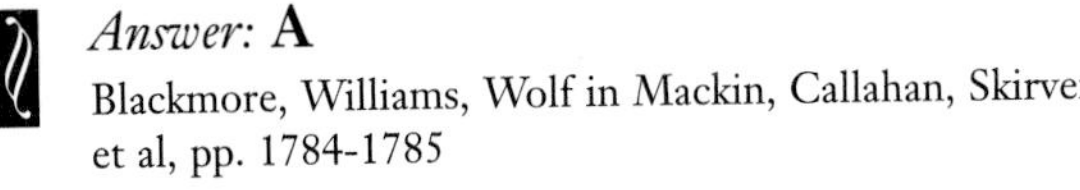

Answer: **A**
Blackmore, Williams, Wolf in Mackin, Callahan, Skirven, et al, pp. 1784-1785

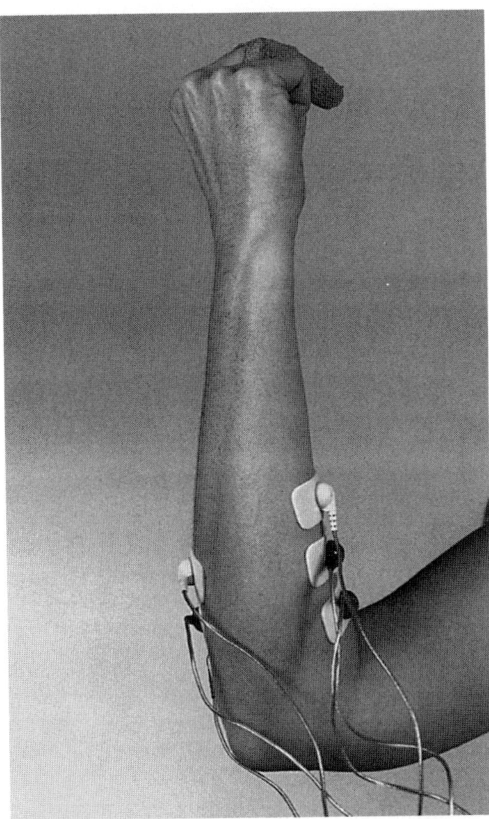

Fig. 21-4 ■ From Mackin EJ, Callahan AD, Skirven TM, et al: *Rehabilitation of the hand and upper extremity*, ed 5, St Louis, 2002, Mosby.

15. Match each practitioner with the associated treatment technique.

Practitioner

1. Mennel
2. Maitland
3. Kaltenborn
4. Cyriax

Techniques

A. Steroid injection, passive stretch, physiological movement in direction of limitation, deep friction massage
B. Glides, traction, "taking up the slack"
C. Quick-thrust mobilization followed by exercise to maintain range
D. Passive oscillatory movements, anteroposterior and posteroanterior glides, sustained stretch

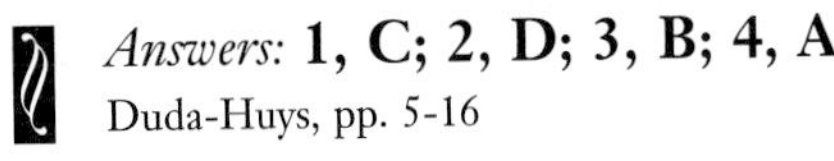

Answers: **1, C; 2, D; 3, B; 4, A**
Duda-Huys, pp. 5-16

16. The well-known acronym RICE stands for *r*est, *i*ce, *c*ompression, and *e*levation and is used as first-aid treatment for strains, sprains, and bruises. Other factors may or may not be as well known. Which of the following would you *not* do immediately after strains, sprains, and bruises?

A. Apply heat
B. Massage your injury
C. Drink alcohol
D. All of the above are inappropriate.

One should not apply heat, massage the injury, or drink alcohol immediately after an injury because these activities increase bleeding or swelling.

Answer: **D**
Lindsay, p. 110

17. Which of the following mobilization techniques may be beneficial for increasing shoulder external rotation?

A. Anterior glide
B. Posterior glide
C. Lateral glide
D. Inferior glide

The correct answer is A, anterior glide. External rotation of the humerus will stress the anterior aspect of the capsule, thus allowing further external rotation to occur. With mobilization, the head of the humerus moves anteriorly, thus helping to stretch the anterior portion of the shoulder capsule.

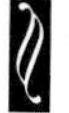

Answer: **A**
Donatelli, p. 247

18. A 28-year-old basketball player is referred to therapy 12 weeks after dorsal dislocation of the fifth proximal interphalangeal (PIP) joint. The patient presents with a 25-degree flexion contracture. One of your treatment techniques is joint mobilization. According to concave/convex theory, which glide is used to increase PIP joint extension?

A. Dorsal
B. Lateral
C. Radial
D. All of the above

According to the convex-concave rule, the digits are mobilized in the same direction as the desired motion. Therefore, in theory a dorsal glide is performed to achieve PIP joint extension. The restricting tissue, in all likelihood, is the volar plate and a dorsal glide will favorably mobilize the volar plate. In reality, a volar glide is also likely to mobilize the volar plate.

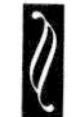

Answer: **A**
Malone, McPoil, Nitz, p. 373

CLINICAL GEM:
It often is helpful to distract a joint before mobilizing it.

19. According to Cyriax, a "springy" end feel is significant during evaluation of which condition?

A. Arthritis
B. Fracture
C. Internal derangement of the joint
D. Acute bursitis

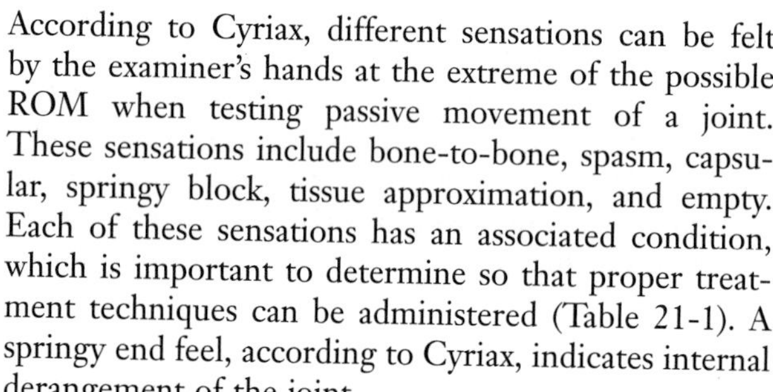

According to Cyriax, different sensations can be felt by the examiner's hands at the extreme of the possible ROM when testing passive movement of a joint. These sensations include bone-to-bone, spasm, capsular, springy block, tissue approximation, and empty. Each of these sensations has an associated condition, which is important to determine so that proper treatment techniques can be administered (Table 21-1). A springy end feel, according to Cyriax, indicates internal derangement of the joint.

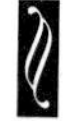

Answer: **C**
Cyriax, p. 53
Duda-Huys, pp. 7-16

20. All but which of the following are goals of shoulder taping?

A. Repositioning the humerus
B. Inhibiting the upper trapezius
C. Decreasing the patient's pain
D. Shortening the lower trapezius
E. All of the above are goals.

McConnell reports that shoulder taping repositions the humerus, inhibits activity of the upper trapezius,

Table 21-1

Cyriax's Description of End Feel

End feel	Description	Significance in evaluation
Bone-bone	Two hard surfaces meet—abrupt	Anatomic limit of joint
Spasm	Hardish feel; muscles reflexively stop movement	Acute and subacute arthritis; fracture
Capsular	Hardish feel; some give	Arthritis
Spring back	Rebound at end of movement	Internal derangement of joint
Tissue approximation	Soft-arrest movement	No mechanical block
Empty	Pain some distance from anatomic limit	Suspect acute bursitis, abscess, neoplasm

shortens the lower trapezius, and secondarily decreases pain. McConnell uses taping of the shoulder to treat impingement, simple tendonitis, anterior subluxation, frozen shoulder, and multidirectional instability.

Answer: **E**
Brecker, pp. 10-11

21. Deep friction is the most beneficial and, according to Cyriax, often the only beneficial treatment of strains at which location?

A. Muscle belly
B. Tendon
C. Ligament
D. Musculotendinous junction

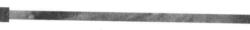

At the musculotendinous junction, the proximity of rigid tendon prevents the restoration of mobility except by manual means. Hence, according to Cyriax, the sort of strains that effect athletes and ballet dancers, especially at the leg, are often entirely incurable except by deep friction massage.

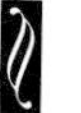
Answer: **D**
Cyriax, p. 19

22. Mr. B. is 23 years old and presents with a partial rupture of the triceps. Which of the following, according to Cyriax, would be an appropriate treatment technique?

A. Local anesthesia, followed by active off-weight exercise
B. Deep massage to torn fibers while the muscle is held in full relaxation, followed by active exercise without resistance
C. Avoidance of resisted exercise until recovery is well established
D. Stretch out if necessary
E. All of the above

According to Cyriax, rehabilitation for a partial rupture to a muscle would include Answers A through D after aspiration of the hematoma. Complete rupture would require operative suture.

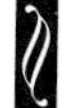
Answer: **E**
Cyriax, p. 34

23. True or False: Soft-tissue mobilization and myofascial release are both used to treat superficial tissues.

Soft-tissue mobilization is a gentle technique designed to loosen superficial cross-restrictions of fascia. Myofascial release is used to release the deeper layer of fascia.

Answer: **False**
Barnes, pp. 5-15

24. What diagnosis has held great promise in reference to treatment with thermal biofeedback?

A. Fractures
B. Reflex sympathetic dystrophy/complex regional pain syndrome (RSD/CRPS)
C. Tendon repair
D. All of the above will benefit greatly from thermal biofeedback.

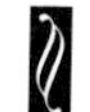

Studies have shown success in the treatment of RSD/CRPS with the use of adjunctive thermal biofeedback. This treatment technique allows patients to increase hand temperature and reduce pain intensity.

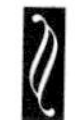
Answer: B
Blackmore, Williams, Wolf in Mackin, Callahan, Skirven, et al, p. 1787
Refer to Fig. 21-5

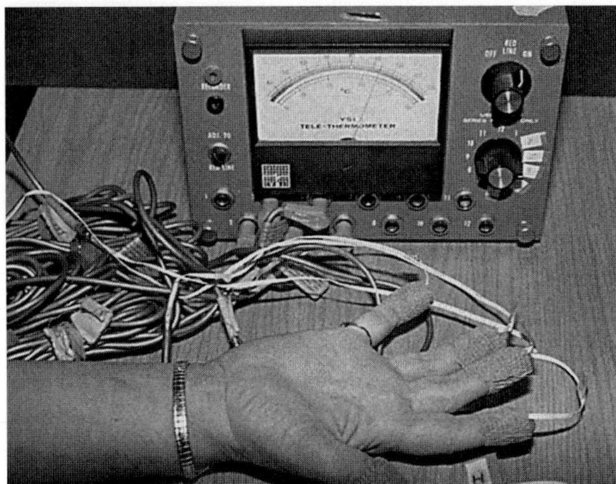

Fig. 21-5 ■ This thermal biofeedback unit is capable of monitoring 10 separate areas for skin temperature. The patient is attempting hand-warming techniques while monitoring the distal digit temperature. (From Mackin EJ, Callahan AD, Skirven TM, et al: *Rehabilitation of the hand and upper extremity*, ed 5, St Louis, 2002, Mosby.)

25. Which of the following might be a hyperirritable spot in a muscle or its fascia which is painful on compression and can give rise to referred pain?

A. Jump sign
B. Spasm
C. Bruxism
D. Trigger point

A trigger point is an area of hyperirritability in a tissue or muscle that, when compressed, is tender and hypersensitive and can give rise to referred pain. Types of trigger points include myofascial, cutaneous, fascial, ligamentous, and periosteal.

Answer: **D**
Travell, Simons, p. 4

26. True or False: Pressure to a trigger point can result in pilomotor activity.

Pilomotor activity (gooseflesh) can appear spontaneously with pressure application to active trigger points (see Fig. 4-14, Question 62).

Answer: **True**
Travell, Simons, p. 42

27. Which of the following is not helpful for treating a trigger point?

A. Light digital pressure
B. Deep stripping massage
C. Stretch and spray
D. Kneading massage

All of the above except light pressure are useful in helping to inactivate trigger points.

Answer: **A**
Travell, Simons, p. 25

28. According to Travell, what is the "workhorse" of myofascial therapy?

A. Manual pressure techniques
B. Moist heat treatment
C. Stretch and spray
D. Injection and stretch

Travell reports that stretch and spray is the "workhorse" of myofascial therapy because it quickly inactivates myofascial trigger points with less discomfort than with injection or ischemic compression (see Fig. 5-4, Question 18).

Answer: **C**
Travell, Simons, p. 63

29. Kinesio Tex Tape can be left on for how long?

A. 3 to 5 days
B. 5 to 7 days
C. 7 to 10 days
D. 3 to 4 weeks

Kinesio tape contains no latex or medicinal properties and can remain on the skin for 3 to 5 days. A patient can bathe without removing the tape. The tape is lightweight and barely perceptible to the wearer. It can stretch 30% to 40% of its resting length.

Answer: **A**
Mackin, Callahan, Skirven, et al, p. 1797

30. The upper limb tension test 1 (ULTT1) tests for the involvement of the median nerve. It is

a recommended test for patients with symptoms in which of the following?

A. Arm
B. Head
C. Neck
D. Thoracic spine
E. All of the above

With symptoms anywhere in the arm, head, neck, or thoracic spine, the ULTT1 should be included in the examination if a patient has neural complaints. It should be performed on the first examination if indications in the subjective and physical examination imply that impaired nervous system mechanics are a component of the patient's disorder.

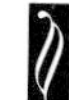

Answer: **E**
Butler, p. 150
Refer to Fig. 21-6

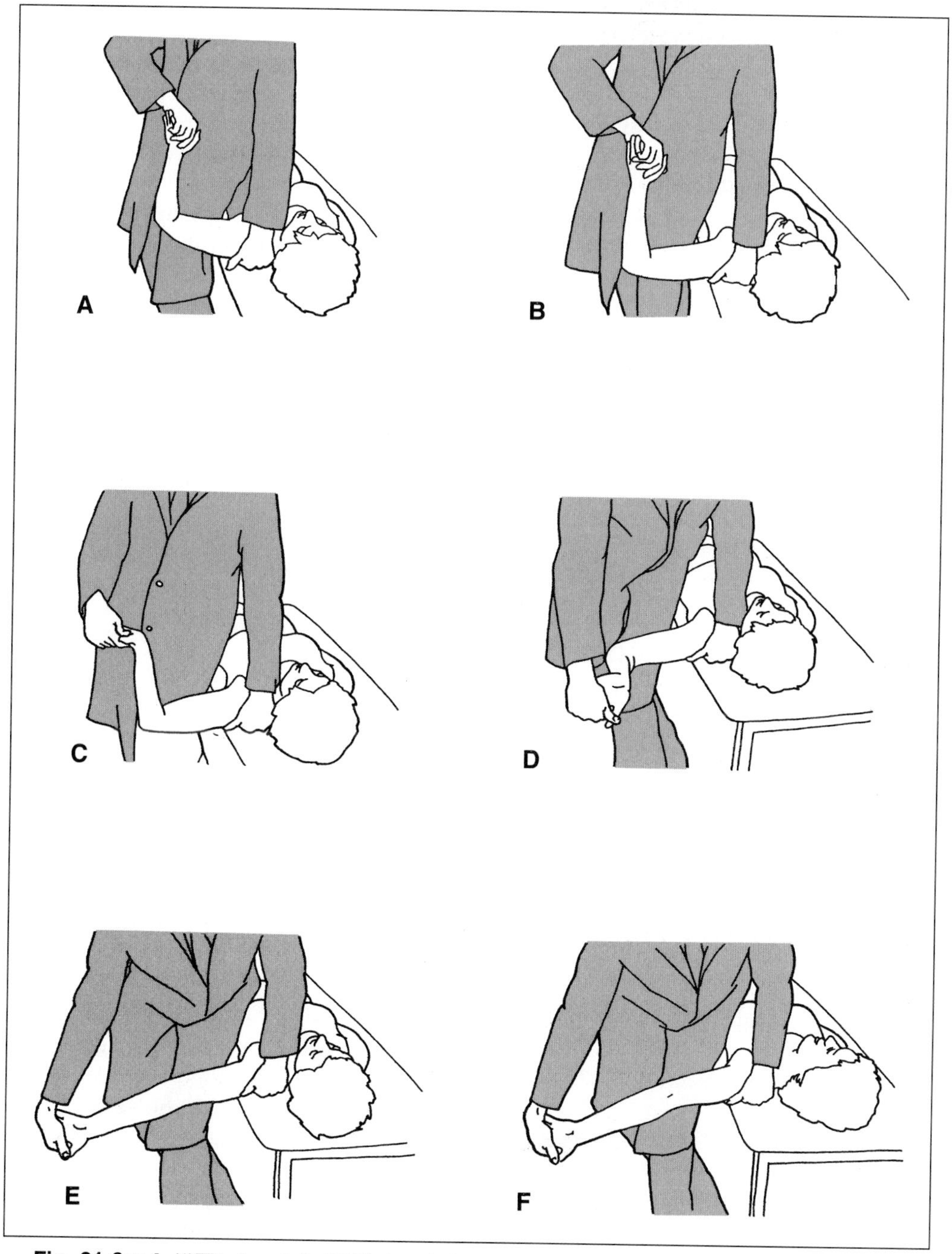

Fig. 21-6 ■ **A,** ULTT1 stage 1. **B,** ULTT1 stage 2. **C,** ULTT1 stage 3. **D,** ULTT1 stage 4. **E,** ULTT1 stage 5. **F,** ULTT1 stage 6. (From Butler D: *Mobilization of the nervous system*, New York, 1991, Churchill Livingstone.)

31. A normal response to the ULTT1 often will include which of the following?

A. Deep stretch or ache in the cubital fossa
B. Tingling sensation in the thumb and first three fingers
C. Stretch of the anterior shoulder area
D. All of the above

Kenneally et al (1988) listed the normal responses to the ULTT1 as seen in 400 "normal" volunteers as the following:

1. A deep stretch or ache in the cubital fossa (99% of volunteers) that extends down the anterior and radial aspects of the forearm and into the radial hand (80%)

2. A definite tingling sensation in the thumb and first three fingers

3. In a small percentage of subjects, a stretch in the anterior shoulder area

4. Cervical lateral flexion away from the side tested increased the response in approximately 90% of normal volunteers.

5. Cervical lateral flexion toward the tested side decreased the test response in 70% of normal volunteers.

Answer: **D**
Butler, p. 151

32. You are preparing a patient who sustained a distal tip amputation of his dominant index finger for discharge. What would be the most useful tool to help this patient return to his factory job?

A. Valpar work component number eight simulated assembly
B. McCarron-Dial System
C. Baltimore therapeutic equipment tool number (BTE) 162
D. Rolling putty in the clinic

Valpar work samples are used to help return injured industrial workers to gainful employment. Valpar number eight simulates assembly line work and would be useful to assist this patient in training to work on the assembly line at the factory. Valpar work samples are used for evaluation as well as treatment and are easy to administer and score.

The McCarron-Dial vocational rehabilitation system is used for the mentally challenged population. The exclusive use of BTE tool number 162 is insufficient for returning an employee to the assembly line. However, the BTE and BTE Primus are excellent modalities for evaluation, conditioning, functional capacity evaluations, and return to work rehabilitation.

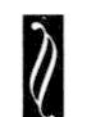

Answer: **A**
Hopkins, Smith, pp. 287-289

33. True or False: A concentric contraction is a form of isotonic exercise.

Isotonic exercise is a dynamic exercise that uses force with movement. An isotonic muscle contraction occurs when tension, usually with a constant resistive force, is developed in a muscle. The muscle length decreases or increases during the performance of work or exercise. All of the following are types of isotonic exercise: concentric contraction, eccentric contraction, constant loading, variable loading, and plyometric loading.

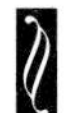

Answer: **True**
Hunter, Mackin, Callahan, p. 1733
Kasch in Mackin, Callahan, Skirven, et al, p. 1014
Taber's cyclopedic medical dictionary

34. Match each isotonic exercise with the correct definition.

Isotonic Exercise

1. Concentric contraction
2. Eccentric contraction
3. Constant loading
4. Variable loading
5. Plyometric loading

Definition

A. Occurs when muscles are loaded suddenly and forced to stretch before they can contract and elicit movement
B. Loading that remains the same
C. Contraction of muscle that results in shortening of muscle fibers
D. Imposing an increasing load throughout ROM so that a more constant stress is placed on muscles
E. Muscle contraction in a lengthened state

Answers: **1, C; 2, E; 3, B; 4, D; 5, A**
Hunter, Mackin, Callahan, p. 1733
Kasch in Mackin, Callahan, Skirven, et al, p. 1014
Weiss, LaStayo, Mills, pp. 218-219

35. A 58-year-old woman complains of bilateral pain in her carpometacarpal (CMC) joints of the thumbs. The patient does not want surgical intervention. She has difficulty peeling vegetables and is seeking help to ensure success in meal preparation. What can you do for this patient?

A. Refer her to durable medical equipment (DME) companies
B. Teach her pinching and grasping strengthening programs
C. Adapt or construct a peeling board
D. Fabricate a short opponens splint
E. C and D

Patients often experience limitations in functional tasks when osteoarthritis has affected the first CMC joint. Adaptive equipment may be used to help regain or maintain functional independence. A short opponens splint also is an excellent choice to include in your program. Splinting may help decrease inflammation, provide rest and support, position the joint, and minimize joint deformity. Splinting and adaptive equipment are excellent adjuncts that the skilled therapist can implement in a program to manage arthritis. Referral to a DME company is too vague and strength programs are inappropriate at this time.

Answer: **E**
Hunter, Mackin, Callahan, p. 1348
Kasch in Mackin, Callahan, Skirven, et al, pp. 1014-1020

36. True or False: Theoretically, Kinesio taping may stimulate the somatosensory system to reduce pain.

Theoretically, Kinesio taping may stimulate the somatosensory system to reduce pain. When properly applied, it increases sensory stimuli to mechanoreceptors, which activates the analgesic system. It may also activate the spinal inhibitory system through stimulation of touch receptors. It may activate the descending inhibitory system. In addition, taping decreases pain by reducing inflammation and decreasing pressure on nociceptors.

Answer: **True**
Coopee in Mackin, Callahan, Skirven, et al, p. 1799
Refer to Fig. 21-7

37. Which of the following statements is not true about Kinesio taping and supporting muscle function?

A. It enhances contraction of a weakened muscle by input through the somatosensory system.
B. It increases muscle fatigue by enhancing contraction.
C. It increases active ROM by assisting muscle function.
D. All of the above are false.

Answer B is incorrect because Kinesio taping will decrease muscle fatigue by enhancing contraction. The other statements are correct.

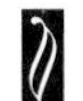
Answer: **B**
Coopee in Mackin, Callahan, Skirven, et al, p. 1802

38. According to Kaltenborn, what is the capsular pattern for the finger joints (dorsal interphalangeal [DIP] and PIP)?

A. Flexion followed by extension
B. Restricted in all directions with slightly more limitation in flexion
C. Extension followed by flexion
D. Flexion and rotation followed by extension

According to Kaltenborn, the capsular pattern for the digits is restricted in all directions with slightly more limitation in flexion.

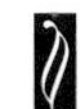
Answer: **B**
Kaltenborn, p. 52

39. A 62-year-old woman with a type I thumb deformity from rheumatoid arthritis is referred to you for evaluation and treatment. What is the best choice for intervention?

A. Refer her to a surgeon; there is nothing you can do.
B. Fabricate a dynamic interphalangeal (IP) joint extension splint
C. Educate your patient in joint protection and adaptive equipment principles
D. Begin an aggressive strengthening program

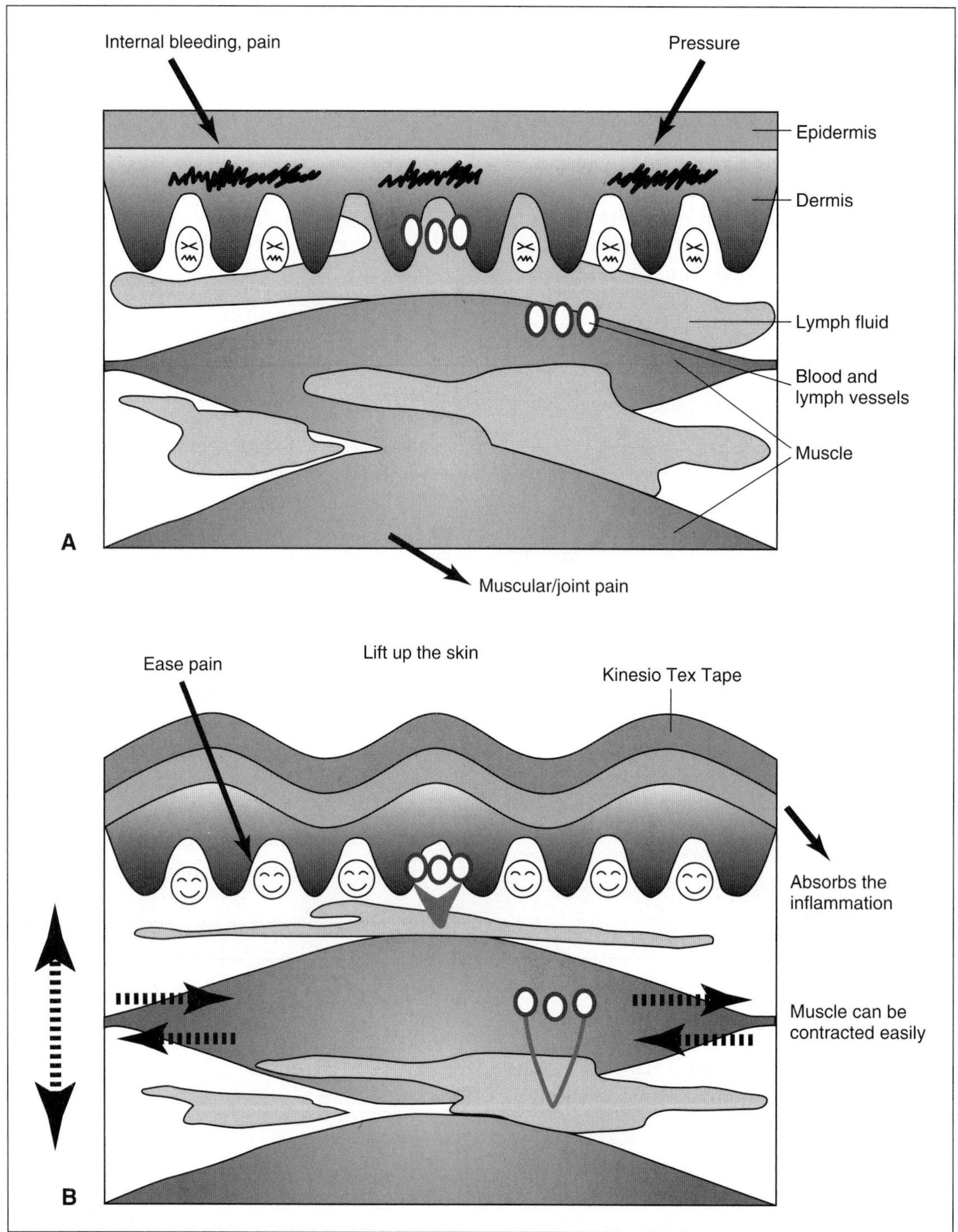

Fig. 21-7 ■ **A,** Traumatized fascia without Kinesio taping. **B,** Traumatized fascia with Kinesio taping. (Redrawn from Kase K, Kenishi Y: *Kinesio taping for the back and knee*, 1999, Kinesio Taping Association.)

A type I thumb deformity (see Fig. 13-4), which is similar to a boutonnière deformity, results in hyperextension of the IP joint secondary to flexion of the metacarpophalangeal (MCP) joint. Treatment goals are to decrease pain, decrease edema, maintain joint mobility, and prevent or minimize deformity. Teaching your patient joint-protection techniques and using adaptive equipment helps to minimize stress on the thumb.

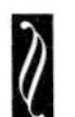
Answer: **C**
Hunter, Mackin, Callahan, p. 1348

40. Pushing a full cart of groceries from the store to the car is what kind of exercise?

A. Isokinetic exercise
B. Stretching
C. Closed-chain kinematics
D. Open-chain kinematics

Pushing a cart is an example of a closed-chain exercise. Closed-chain kinematics are load-bearing exercises used for stability. Closed-chain exercise transfers forces across more than one joint. Open-chain kinematics are exercises performed for mobility in which one joint or muscle group is isolated (e.g., isolated elbow flexion and extension).

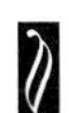
Answer: **C**
Hunter, Mackin, Callahan, p. 1734
Kasch in Mackin, Callahan, Skirven, et al, p. 1015

41. True or False: Isokinetic assessment is most often used to measure maximal strength.

Isokinetic assessment infrequently is used to measure maximal strength. Isokinetic exercise is contraction of a muscle, whereby speed is controlled and maximum exertion occurs through the full ROM. Isometric exercise is a static form of exercise that occurs when a muscle contracts against an immovable object. Isometric assessment is most often used for measuring maximal strength.

Answer: **False**
Hunter, Mackin, Callahan, p. 1733
Kasch in Mackin, Callahan, Skirven, et al, p. 1014
Taber's cyclopedic medical dictionary

42. Continuous pressure over a scar does all but which of the following?

A. Make it softer
B. Break up scar tissue
C. Improve cosmesis
D. It does all of the above.

Scar-management techniques such as continuous pressure soften tissues and improve cosmesis. Scar-management techniques do not break up scar tissue but are used to increase pliability and assist in tissue elongation.

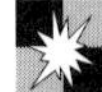
CLINICAL GEM:
Some physicians advocate application of otoform while sutures are intact. Others believe that application of otoform or other scar-remodeling techniques should be employed after suture removal.

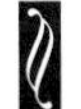
Answer: **B**
Hunter, Mackin, Callahan, p. 1062
Pettengill in Mackin, Callahan, Skirven, et al, p. 1416

43. You are treating a patient after carpal tunnel release. A silicone gel sheet and Tubigrip are applied 2 days after suture removal to soften scar tissue and decrease edema. During the patient's next visit, she reports increased numbness in the median nerve distribution and hypersensitivity over the incision. Which of the following would you do?

A. Continue silicone gel sheet and Tubigrip because hypersensitivity will decrease in a few days
B. Refer back to the physician to assess for infection
C. Remove silicone gel sheet and Tubigrip and reassess
D. Discontinue silicone gel sheet and commence ultrasound for scar management

Pressure application for scar management can result in skin maceration, allergies to products, decreased circulation, and nerve compression. This patient may have had an allergic reaction to the silicone gel sheet, or the

Tubigrip may have caused her hypersensitivity. The therapist should consider other scar-management techniques (e.g., otoform, silicone, elastomer). This patient's paresthesia may be related to a tight Tubigrip. The current Tubigrip should be removed, and a larger size should be applied. The therapist should consider discontinuing all scar products and compressive devices for a few days and then gradually reintroduce products and techniques.

Answer: **C**

Hunter, Mackin, Callahan, p. 1286
deLinde, Knotine in Mackin, Callahan, Skirven, et al, p. 1516

44. A patient is referred to you with bilateral symptoms of pain on the radial side of the forearm and hand. No objective sensory loss is noted. What is a possible diagnosis?

A. de Quervain's tenosynovitis (disease)
B. Intersection syndrome
C. Scalene trigger points
D. All of the above

If a patient experiences pain on the radial side of the forearm and hand without objective sensory loss, the patient could have a multitude of different diagnoses. Some of these diagnoses may include intersection syndrome, de Quervain's tenosynovitis, or scalene trigger points. The therapist must remember to look proximally when he or she is treating distal hand problems. It is easy to overlook proximal trigger points during treatment of hand patients; however, such oversight may lead to treating an incorrect diagnosis.

Answer: **D**

Travell, Simons, p. 350

45. In upper extremity neural tension testing, which of the following is the most relative comparative sign?

A. Overall ROM or flexibility
B. Manual muscle test results
C. Sensation mapping results
D. Opposite "normal' side comparisons

During the physical examination the therapist should test the sound limb first to have a better idea about what to expect from the affected limb.

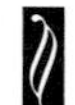
Answer: **D**

Butler, p. 169

46. Which of the following is not a joint-protection technique for patients with osteoarthritis?

A. Reduce excessive loading on the joints
B. Avoid pain in activities
C. Increase ROM of involved joints
D. Use built-up writing tools

Increasing ROM of involved joints is not a joint-protection technique. When treating patients with osteoarthritis with joint-protection techniques, the therapist tries to maintain ROM rather than increase ROM. You should increase muscle strength and physical fitness in the osteoarthritic hand because this will assist with maintaining ROM. Strengthening must be done in a pain-free fashion. Isometric exercise is often most beneficial with these patients. Aerobic activity is an excellent method for reducing pain with osteoarthritis because it increases stamina and decreases stress and depression while improving sleep patterns. Obviously, reduction of excessive loading on the joints, using adaptive equipment, and avoiding painful activities are protection techniques that should be employed.

Answer: **C**

Melvin in Mackin, Callahan, Skirven, et al, p. 1656

47. What is the best choice of the techniques listed below for prevention or reduction of subacute or chronic high-protein hand edema in patients who are postsurgical, posttraumatic, or postcerebrovascular accident (CVA)?

A. Manual edema mobilization
B. Kinesio taping
C. Joint mobilization
D. Thermal biofeedback

Manual edema mobilization (MEM) was developed by Sandra Artzberger in 1995 to prevent or reduce subacute or chronic high-protein hand edema in patients who are postsurgical, posttraumatic, or post-CVA. The role of the lymphatic system for edema reduction has not been readily addressed in American hand therapy literature but has been widely described in Europe since the 1930s. MEM is highly effective with cases of chronic edema, and it was designed to address lymphatic drainage principles to specific hand diagnoses.

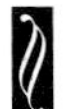

Answer: **A**

Artzberger in Mackin, Callahan, Skirven, et al, pp. 899-901

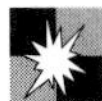

CLINICAL GEM:

The fifth edition of *Rehabilitation of the Hand* dedicates a chapter to MEM.

CLINICAL GEM:

MEM should not be performed in the following scenarios:

- Presence of infection—potential to spread the infection
- Over areas of inflammation—potential to increase inflammation and pain (Do MEM proximal to the inflammation to decrease congested fluid.)
- Blood clot or hematoma in the area—potential to activate (move) the clot
- Active cancer—controversial theory notes the potential to spread cancer. Absolutely never do MEM if the cancer is not being medically treated. Always seek a physician's advice.)
- Congestive heart failure, severe cardiac problems, or pulmonary problems—potential to overload the cardiac and pulmonary systems
- In the inflammation stage of acute wound healing—theoretical possibility of disrupting the clean-up process and the invasion of fibroblasts
- If renal failure or severe kidney disease problems exists—this is not a high-protein edema, and overloading the renal system and/or moving the fluid elsewhere is possible.
- If the patient has primary lymphedema or postmastectomy lymphedema—knowledge of how to reroute lymph to other parts of the body and of how to perform specific treatment techniques is necessary for successful treatment.

From Mackin EJ, Callahan AD, Skirven TM, et al: *Rehabilitation of the hand and upper extremity*, ed 5, St Louis, 2002, Mosby.

Chapter 22

Occupational Safety and Health Administration

1. True or False: Personal protection equipment is specialized clothing or equipment worn by an employee for protection against hazards.

General work clothes, uniforms, pants, and shirts or blouses are not intended to function as protection against hazards. Personal protective equipment includes gloves, masks, eye protection, and gowns and must be provided by the employer.

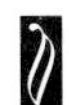

Answer: **True**
Federal Register

2. When prescription eyeglasses are used for eye protection, they must be equipped with which of the following?

A. Tint
B. Adjustable lenses
C. Protective side shields
D. All of the above

To be in compliance with Occupational Safety and Health Administration (OSHA) standards, eyeglasses must have protective side shields when being used as personal protective equipment.

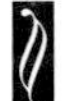

Answer: **C**
Florida Administrative Code

3. OSHA mandates the wearing of masks, eye wear, or face shields when one is exposed to which of the following potentially hazardous contents?

A. Splashes
B. Spray
C. Droplets
D. Aerosols
E. All of the above

OSHA mandates the use of personal protective equipment whenever an employee is at risk for exposure to any of the above.

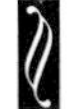

Answer: **E**
Florida Administrative Code

4. Universal Precautions is an employer's bloodborne exposure plan. This implies which of the following?

A. Treating 18- to 65-year-olds as if they were infected with a bloodborne infection
B. Defining certain patients as high-risk
C. Using precautions for all human blood fluids and certain human body fluids
D. Using precautions with selective body fluids and patients

According to Universal Precautions, all human blood fluids and certain human body fluids should be considered possibly infectious regardless of age or high-risk categorization.

Answer: **C**
Florida Administrative Code

5. All contaminated dressings are considered biomedical waste.

A. True
B. False
C. Maybe
D. Depends on state law

Contaminated dressings and gloves may be considered biomedical waste, depending on state law. For example, in Florida, dressings are biomedical waste only if they are supersaturated, with the potential to drip or splash body fluid. Gloves are considered biomedical waste if they are contaminated with blood or body fluid.

Answer: **D**
Federal Registry
Florida Administrative Code

6. For disposal of biomedical fluids in a rimmed clinical service sink, which type of personal protection should be used?

A. Gloves
B. Face shield
C. Both A and B
D. None of the above

Splashing from a clinical service sink can be of concern. A face shield and gloves should be used as minimum protection against body fluid splashing into the eyes, mouth, or hands.

Answer: **C**
Florida Administrative Code

7. True or False: Body excretions such as feces, nasal discharges, saliva, sputum, sweat, tears, urine, and vomitus must be treated as biomedical waste.

If there is no blood contamination, these body fluids are not considered biomedical waste.

Answer: **False**
Federal Register

8. True or False: Sharps should be packaged in impermeable red polyethylene or polyethylene plastic bags.

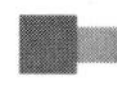

Sharps should not be packaged in red bags. They must be disposed of in a designated sharps container.

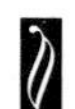

Answer: **False**
Federal Register

9. True or False: Surfaces contaminated with spilled or leaked biomedical waste should be cleaned with an approved disinfectant.

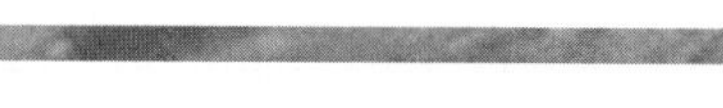

Any surface with visible soil must be disinfected with a chemical germicide that is registered by the U.S. Environmental Protection Agency.

Answer: **True**
Federal Register

10. At least 20 different pathogens have been transmitted by percutaneous exposure to blood. Which bloodborne diseases are of greatest concern in the healthcare setting?

A. Syphilis, Rocky Mountain spotted fever, malaria
B. Human immunodeficiency virus, hepatitis B, hepatitis C
C. *Staphylococcus aureus*, tuberculosis, *Streptococcus*
D. *Pseudomonas aeruginosa*, *Escherichia coli*, *Neisseria meningitidis*

The transmission of all organisms listed above is possible through blood exposure. However, the transmission of most of them is extremely rare compared with the transmission of human immunodeficiency virus, hepatitis B, and hepatitis C, which are the most common concerns of healthcare workers.

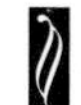

Answer: **B**
Centers for Disease Control and Prevention

11. A client has skin tears on the hands and arms. Which type of personal protection should you use?

A. Gloves
B. Gown
C. Face shield
D. Hair covering
E. All of the above

Personal protection should be selected according to the anticipated body fluid route of exposure. A skin tear could potentially bleed, thus contaminating through contact; therefore in this case, gloves are the protection of choice.

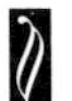

Answer: **A**
Florida Administrative Code

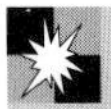

CLINICAL GEM:
It may be helpful to have gloves that extend up the length of the arms.

12. A client vomits in your work area. What should you do?

A. Clean the area with alcohol
B. Wear gloves to clean the area
C. Use a hospital-approved disinfectant to clean the area
D. B and C
E. A and B

According to the Standard Precautions, body fluids should be cleaned by a person wearing gloves and using a hospital-approved disinfectant. Alcohol is not an approved disinfectant. The disinfectant should be tuberculocidal for proper cleaning.

Answer: **D**
Florida Administrative Code

13. True or False: An individual receiving the hepatitis B vaccine cannot donate blood.

The hepatitis B vaccine should be offered to any healthcare worker, free of charge, who potentially could be exposed to the hepatitis B virus. The vaccine boosts the immune system to produce antibodies that will kill the virus if the vaccinated individual is exposed. Because this is a chemical vaccine and is not from serum, the vaccinated individual's blood is considered safe for donation.

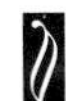

Answer: **False**
Centers for Disease Control and Prevention

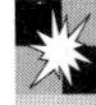

CLINICAL GEM:
The Centers for Disease Control and Prevention recommend that a person wait 2 weeks after immunization to give blood.

14. A therapist has been exposed to blood. A contaminated syringe with a needle was left in the patient area, and the therapist was stuck. According to OSHA standards, which of the following is true?

A. The therapist can report the exposure within 14 days.
B. The exposure must be reported immediately.
C. The therapist must report on the status of the exposure, in writing, within 6 months of exposure.
D. The therapist should ignore the exposure unless the patient is high-risk.

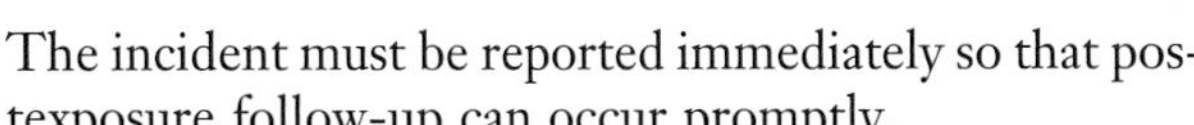

The incident must be reported immediately so that postexposure follow-up can occur promptly.

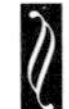

Answer: **B**
Federal Registry

Chapter 23

Research and Statistics

1. True or False: The research problem, statement of purpose, and statement of hypothesis all mean the same thing.

The research problem specifically defines the reason for the inquiries based on a framework of logical analysis of strengths and weaknesses of previous work. The problem should be stated clearly and concisely. This should precede the statement of purpose and the hypothesis.

The statement of purpose is drawn from the research problem and defines the parameters of the study. The statement of purpose is more detailed than the statement of the problem and gives the reader an insight into what and how things will be measured.

A hypothesis is a tentative idea or prediction about the potential direction or outcome of the study. It is more specific than the statement of purpose and often suggests a relationship between two or more test variables.

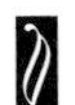

Answer: **False**
Mackin, Callahan, Skirven, et al, pp. 2106-2107

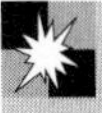

CLINICAL GEM:
We do not test the population as a whole. Rather, we use a sample drawn from the population in our studies and make inferences about the entire population. When a sample population is used, according to statistical theory, the hypothesis is stated as a null hypothesis. Additionally, an alternative hypothesis is formed as a statement complementary to the null hypothesis.

2. Literature reviews available on the Internet span how many previous years?

A. 10
B. 20
C. 30
D. 30 plus

The fact that literature reviews on the Internet span only the past 10 years is an important limitation of computer literature reviews. Reviewing *all* research related to the topic is crucial to give the current study significance. A literature review sets the stage for the study and provides motivation and insight for the reader into the direction, thoroughness, and integrity of the study.

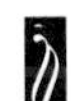

Answer: **A**
Fess in Mackin, Callahan, Skirven, et al, pp. 2106-2107

3. True or False: Inferential statistics can be divided into two categories: parametric and nonparametric.

Inferential statistical methods are classified as either parametric or nonparametric. Parametric statistical techniques are based on the assumption that population observations follow a known distribution, typically a normal distribution. In addition, most parametric tests require an interval scale of measurement. Nonparametric statistical techniques require few, if any, assumptions about the nature of the sampled population. Nonparametric tests can be used when the observations are measured on a nominal or ordinal scale.

Table 23-1

Data column #1	Data column #2	Data column #3	Data column #4
1. Marital Status	**2.** Satisfaction	**3.** Time in Treatment	**4.** Weight (pounds)
Married	Very satisfied	1 week	40
Single	Somewhat satisfied	2 weeks	50
Divorced	Somewhat dissatisfied	3 weeks	80
Widowed	Very dissatisfied	4 weeks	100

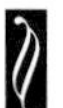

Answer: **True**

Knapp, pp. 28-30
Fess in Mackin, Callahan, Skirven, et al, pp. 2106-2108

4. Match the following columns of data in Table 23-1 with the correct scales of measurement (choices A through D).

A. Interval
B. Nominal
C. Ordinal
D. Ratio

Nominal: This is a variable such as marital status, in which the only distinction among "married," "single," "divorced," and "widowed" is that they are different categories (Data column #1).

Ordinal: There is a definite order to the measurements in column 2 because they can be ranked in terms of level of satisfaction. However, the distance between "very satisfied" and "somewhat satisfied" cannot be quantified (e.g., "very satisfied" is not a fixed amount better than "somewhat satisfied") (Data column #2).

Interval: Not only is there order to the measurements in column 3; the distance between any two numbers on the scale also is fixed and consistent (e.g., "4 weeks" minus "2 weeks" is the same as "3 weeks" minus "1 week") (Data column #3).

Ratio: The ratio scale is the same as the interval scale, except that it has a true zero, whether real or implied. Weight measurements in column 4 follow a ratio scale because there is a true zero (0 pounds) (Data column #4).

Answers: **1, B; 2, C; 3, A; 4, D**

Knapp, pp. 7-9
Portney, Watkins, pp. 44-48

CLINICAL GEM:

Here is a way to remember the differences among nominal, ordinal, and interval scales of measurement. **Nom**inal means that the measurements are ***names***, such as the names of categories (e.g., male/female, White/Black/Hispanic/Asian). **Ord**inal means that the measurements can be ***ordered*** (e.g., high/medium/low, excellent/good/average/poor). **Interval** means that the measurements are ***values*** on a well-defined scale, such as degrees Fahrenheit or degrees centigrade.

5. True or False: A histogram is a visual representation of data in which the data values are grouped into intervals and the relative frequency of values in each interval is plotted.

Individual data values collected in a study may be uninformative by themselves, but by organizing similar values together, trends can be seen. For example, the measured calcium values (mg/dl) for a group of 10 patients might be 8.6, 9.2, 8.0, 7.8, 9.7, 8.5, 10.4, 8.5, 9.3, and 10.1. By grouping these values into four intervals of equal width, the raw data can be summarized as follows:

Interval	Count (frequency)	Relative frequency
7.0 to 7.9	1	0.1
8.0 to 8.9	4	0.4
9.0 to 9.9	3	0.3
10.0 to 10.9	2	0.2
Total	10	1.0

Created by Doug Shier

The last column of this table (the relative frequency) can be plotted with the intervals on the horizontal axis and the relative frequency on the vertical axis, as in Fig. 23-1.

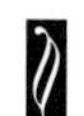

Answer: **True**

Knapp, pp. 28-30

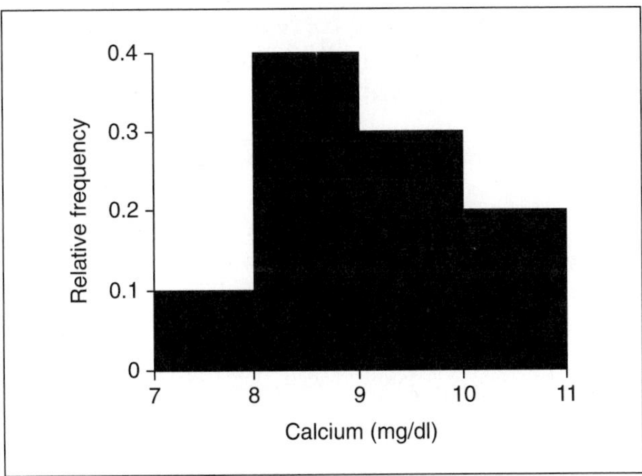

Fig. 23-1 ■ Created by Doug Shier.

6. Match each measure of central tendency with the correct definition.

Measure of Central Tendency

1. Mean
2. Median
3. Mode

Definition

A. The most frequent score in a distribution
B. The average score in a distribution
C. The score at the midpoint of the distribution

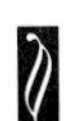

Answers: **1, B; 2, C; 3, A**
Portney, Watkins, p. 323
Refer to Fig. 23-2

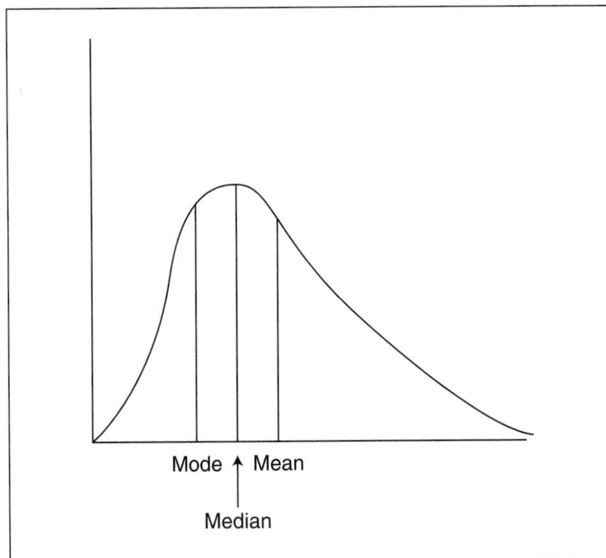

Fig. 23-2

7. What do you call a distribution in which the mean, mode, and median scores are all the same?

A. Gaussian distribution
B. Normal distribution
C. Bell curve
D. All of the above

In a bell curve—which also is known as a *gaussian distribution* or *normal distribution*—the mean, mode, and median scores are all the same.

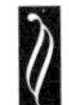

Answer: **D**
Portney, Watkins, p. 323
Refer to Fig. 23-3

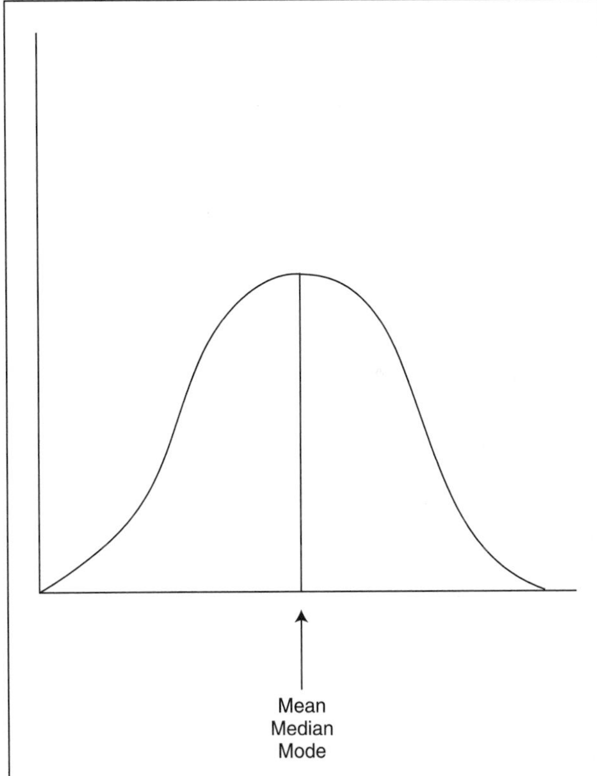

Fig. 23-3

8. True or False: The range (high score minus low score) by itself is a useful measure of variability.

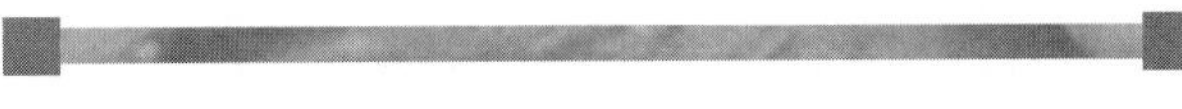

The range is the difference between the highest and lowest value in a set of variables. A few deviant scores would mislead an observer as to the variability in a distribution. The range by itself is not useful but can be useful in combination with measures of central tendency.

Answer: **False**
Portney, Watkins, p. 323

9. True or False: The standard deviation is the square root of the variance in a distribution.

Variance is a measure of variability in a distribution and is equal to the square of the standard deviation. The standard deviation is a descriptive statistic that reflects the variability or dispersion of scores around the mean. The standard deviation (which has the same measurement units as the original observations) is often used as a basis for comparing samples.

Answer: **True**
Knapp, pp. 44-56
Portney, Watkins, pp. 326-327

10. In a screening program for hypertension, the average systolic blood pressure for males in a certain population is 140 mm Hg, and the standard deviation is 8 mm Hg. One particular individual has a reading of 165 mm Hg. Does this person have a significantly elevated blood pressure?

It is reasonable to assume that this population of individuals has systolic blood pressure values that are normally distributed. In a normal distribution, approximately 68% of the observations fall within (plus or minus) one standard deviation of the mean; 95% fall within two standard deviations of the mean; and 99% fall within three standard deviations of the mean. The individual reading of 165 is 25 units (165-140) greater than the mean, and this translates into 3.125 (25/8 = 3.125) standard deviations greater than the mean. This puts the individual over three standard deviations from the mean. Therefore, a blood pressure as high as this occurs in less than 1% of the population. This individual has a blood pressure reading that is statistically significant.

Answer: **Yes**
Knapp, pp. 62-66

11. True or False: The correlation coefficient indicates the extent of a linear relationship between two measurements.

When two measurements, such as Scholastic Aptitude Testing (SAT) scores or grade point averages (GPAs), co-vary systematically, the relationship can be graphed as points in a two-dimensional scatter plot, which create a more or less straight line. In a significant correlation, the scores may be related *directly* (i.e., as one increases so does the other) or *inversely* (i.e., as one increases the other decreases). Fig. 23-4, *A* shows a direct relationship.

Fig. 23-4, *B* illustrates an inverse relationship between age and joint flexibility. This relationship shows that as age increases, flexibility decreases.

The degree of linear relationship ranges from −1 (exact inverse relation) to +1 (direct relationship). A correlation coefficient of 0 indicates no linear relationship between the variables.

Answer: **True**
Knapp, pp. 217-218

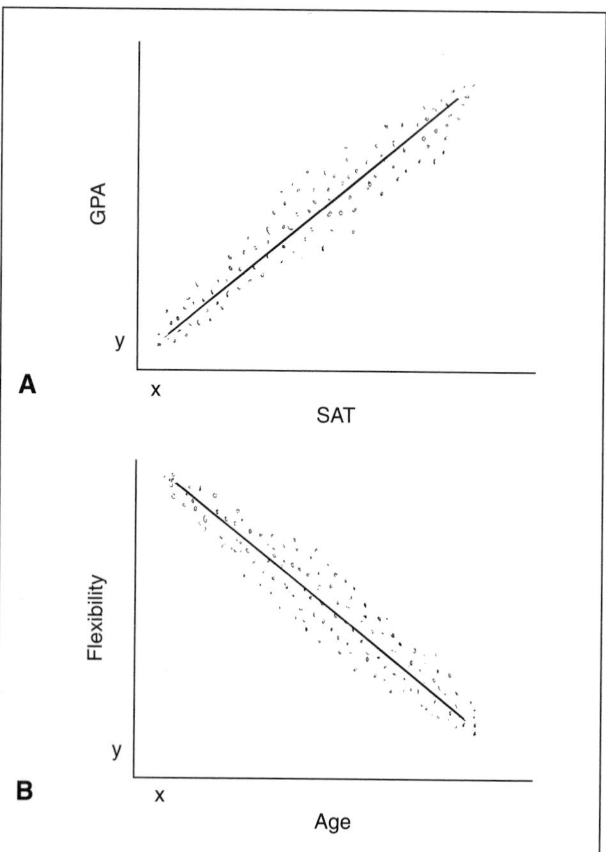

Fig. 23-4

12. True or False: In Fig. 23-4, GPAs and flexibility are the dependent variables, and SAT scores and age are the independent variables.

GPA and flexibility are dependent variables. SAT scores and age are independent variables. Dependent variables are outcomes or results. Independent variables are presumed to cause or determine outcomes; often these variables are manipulated or controlled by the researcher, who sets their "values," or levels. It should be noted, however, that correlations do not indicate cause and effect. Age, *per se*, does not cause loss of flexibility. SAT scores do not cause GPAs, although they are clearly a predictor.

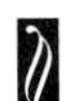

Answer: **True**

Portney, Watkins, pp. 90-93, 684
Knapp, pp. 6-7

13. True or False: Dependent variables tend to be placed on the Y axis of a graph.

Researchers tend to place independent variables along the horizontal axis of a graph, which is called the *X axis*. The results, or dependent variables, appear on the vertical, or ordinate axis (Y axis). In Fig. 23-4, *A*, the independent variable, SAT, is plotted along the horizontal (X) axis and the dependent variable, GPA, is plotted along the vertical axis (Y).

Answer: **True**

Portney, Watkins, pp. 90-94

14. Which of the following statements describes the difference between statistics and parameters?

A. Statistics are used only in research; parameters can be used in real life.
B. Parameters always are expressed in whole numbers; statistics are expressed in decimals.
C. A statistic is a descriptive measure based on a sample. When an entire population is measured, it is called a *parameter*.
D. All of the above are true.

This question has to do with how researchers can look at a segment of a population and make inferences about the whole population. This process is called *sampling*. The researcher determines the population, which is the entire set of individuals or units about which data will be generalized. However, if the researcher samples randomly from that population and measures that sample, the results can be generalized to the entire population. A sample is a subset of a population chosen for study. The results obtained from the sample are called *statistics*.

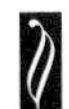

Answer: **C**

Portney, Watkins, pp. 111-124

CLINICAL GEM:
To remember the concept "populations," think of a large group of individuals, such as those who make up the U.S. population. In contrast, a "sample" consists of a small group of individuals, such as 100 patients participating in clinical research. Samples are the basis for making inferences about an entire population.

15. True or False: The null hypothesis states that the differences found among samples are caused by an experimental intervention.

The statement above characterizes the experimental (alternative) hypothesis, not the null hypothesis. The null hypothesis states that differences found among samples are caused by sampling error. Typically, the null hypothesis is a hypothesis of no difference. Experiments can never prove or disprove either hypothesis; rather, they report the probability that one or the other is true.

Answer: **False**

Portney, Watkins, p. 346
Knapp, pp. 108-109
Fess in Mackin, Callahan, Skirven, et al, p. 2106

16. Match each statistical term with the correct definition.

Statistical Term

1. T Test
2. β Level
3. Parameter
4. Type II error
5. *p* Value
6. Independent variable
7. α Level
8. Type I error

Definition

A. The probability that the observed difference is caused by sampling error
B. A parametric test for comparing two means
C. The percent set by the experimenter at which she/he will reject the null hypothesis when it is true
D. An incorrect decision to reject the null hypothesis
E. An incorrect decision to accept the null hypothesis
F. A descriptive measurement of a population
G. The characteristic of experimental units that is expected to influence an outcome
H. The percent set by the experimenter at which she/he will accept the null hypothesis when it is false

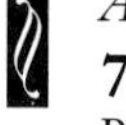

Answers: **1, B; 2, H; 3, F; 4, E; 5, A; 6, G; 7, C; 8, D**
Portney, Watkins, pp. 677-694

CLINICAL GEM:
Here is a way to remember type I and type II errors. In Western justice systems, a person is presumed innocent until proven guilty beyond a reasonable doubt. In this case, the null hypothesis is that the defendant is innocent (the presumption), and the experimental hypothesis is that the defendant is guilty. A type I error is rejecting the null hypothesis when it is true (i.e., convicting an innocent person). Use the mnemonic **ONE: One is Needlessly Executed.** A type II error is not rejecting the null hypothesis when it is false (i.e., letting a guilty person go free). Use the mnemonic **TWO: The Wicked get Out.**

17. True or False: Clinical services continue to be offered without an established base of experimental data.

With increasing economic challenges in healthcare, practitioners must justify clinical decisions with an identified body of knowledge. Unfortunately, many health professionals share the dilemma that clinical services continue to be offered without a base of experimental data. A scientific rationale does exist for practice, but often it comes from other disciplines such as anatomy, physiology, or psychology. Healthcare professionals must establish their own special professional knowledge base to effectively change or develop practice techniques.

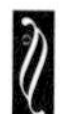

Answer: **True**
Portney, Watkins, p. 3

18. True or False: Intrarater reliability refers to the variation between two or more raters who measure the same group of subjects.

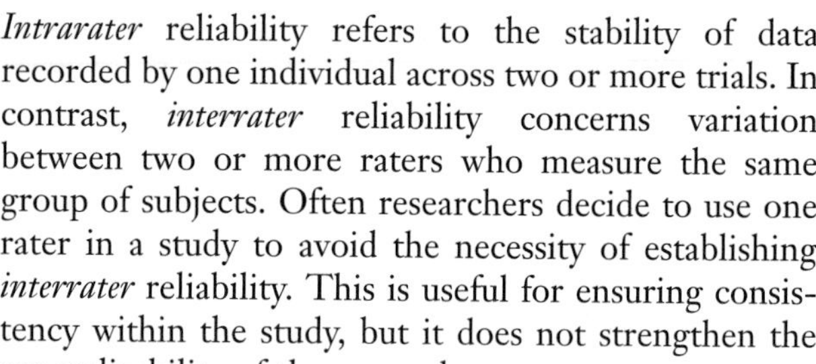

Intrarater reliability refers to the stability of data recorded by one individual across two or more trials. In contrast, *interrater* reliability concerns variation between two or more raters who measure the same group of subjects. Often researchers decide to use one rater in a study to avoid the necessity of establishing *interrater* reliability. This is useful for ensuring consistency within the study, but it does not strengthen the generalizability of the research outcomes.

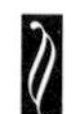

Answer: **False**
Portney, Watkins, pp. 60-61

19. True or False: Validity is the degree of consistency with which an instrument or rater measures a variable.

Reliability is the degree of consistency with which an instrument or rater measures a variable. Validity is the degree to which an instrument measures what it is intended to measure.

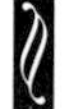

Answer: **False**
Portney, Watkins, pp. 690, 694

20. True or False: The goal of the researcher is to reject the null hypothesis.

The null hypothesis, H_0, states that any observed differences between the means are caused by chance. The goal always is to statistically test the null hypothesis, usually with the intent of rejecting it. This concept is similar to a legal assumption that a person is innocent until proven guilty. The null hypothesis suggests we assume that no relationship exists between variables until significant evidence is accumulated to convince us otherwise. The goal is not to "prove" the null hypothesis but to give the data a chance to disprove the null hypothesis.

The alternative hypothesis, H_1, is what the researcher hopes the data will support; the alternative hypothesis indicates that the observed difference is "real."

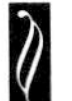
Answer: **True**
Portney, Watkins, p. 346
Fess in Mackin, Callahan, Skirven, et al, p. 2106

21. While establishing a research study, you decide that the level of significance in your study will be 0.05. To improve your confidence level, what would you do to the *p* value?

A. Lower it to 0.025
B. Increase it to 0.10
C. Increase it to 0.50
D. None of the above

The traditional designation of 0.05 is an arbitrary standard. When this standard is used, it means that we are willing to accept a 5% chance of incorrectly rejecting the null hypothesis. To improve our confidence level, we can minimize the risk of statistical error by lowering the level of significance in the study to 0.025 or 0.01. In other words, rejection of the null hypothesis at the 0.01 level is stronger or more believable than is rejection at the 0.05 level because the odds of an event happening by chance is 1 time in 100 compared with 5 times in 100.

Answer: **A**
Portney, Watkins, p. 349
Fess in Mackin, Callahan, Skirven, et al, p. 2106

Appendix 1

Hand Enthusiasts Vendor and Website List

This appendix provides a sampling of companies, professional organizations, and Internet sites related to hand therapy that will be beneficial to the hand enthusiast. This is not an all-inclusive listing and is not intended to endorse any specific company, product, or website. This information is also included on your CD-ROM so that you can click on the websites and access the information. Have fun!

Exploring Hand Therapy
Founded by Susan Weiss and Nancy Falkenstein.
http://www.exploringhandtherapy.com
8318 40th Place North
St. Petersburg, FL 33709
(727) 341-1674
Exploring Hand Therapy (EHT) is an organization dedicated to providing "Excellence In Education" for occupational therapists, physical therapists, certified hand therapists, and other medical professionals.
Earn all your CEUs.
AOTA-approved provider for CEUs.

Live Conferences
http://www.liveconferences.com
7991 9th Avenue South
St. Petersburg, FL 33707
(727) 341-1823
This is the best way to earn CEUs from the comfort of your own home!

Treatment 2 Go
Founded by Susan Weiss and Nancy Falkenstein.
http://www.treatment2go.com
7991 9th Avenue South
St. Petersburg, FL 33707
(727) 341-1823
Order a DVD, CD-ROM, or VHS, and earn CEUs.

INFORMATIONAL WEBSITES

American Association for Hand Surgery
http://www.handsurgery.org

American Association of Surgery of the Hand
http://www.hand-surg.org/

American Hand Therapy Foundation
http://www.ahtf.org

American Occupational Therapy Association
http://www.aota.org

American Physical Therapy Association
http://www.apta.org

American Society of Hand Therapists
http://www.asht.org

American Society of Plastic and Reconstructive Surgeons
http://www.plasticsurgery.org

Arthritis Foundation
http://www.arthritis.org

Biometrics
http://www.biometricsltd.com

Common Hand Problems
http://ozarkortho.com/patiented/hands.htm

Common Orthopedic Conditions of the Hand
http://www.med.und.nodak.edu/users/jwhiting/hand.html

CTD News
http://www.ctdnews.com

Dynamic Learning Online
http://www.dynamic-online.com

Eaton's Hand Surgery Links
http://www.eatonhand.com

Elsevier (Mosby)
http://www.us.elsevierhealth.com/

ERGOPRO
http://www.ergopro.com

Hand Therapy Certification Commission
http://www.htcc.org

Indiana Hand Center
http://www.indianahandcenter.com

International Federation of Societies for Hand Therapy
http://www.ifsht.org

Journal of Hand Therapy
http://www.jhandtherapy.org

Journal of American Society for Surgery of the Hand
http://www.clinicalhandjournal.org

National Board for Certification in Occupational Therapy
http://www.nbcot.org

OrbiTouch Keyless Keyboard
http://www.keybowl.com

Wheeless' Textbook of Orthopedics
http://www.ortho-u.net/med.htm

Working Well Ergonomics
http://www.working-well.org

World Wide Wounds
http://www.worldwidewounds.com

Worldortho
http://www.worldortho.com

VENDOR LIST

Advanced Therapy Products
PO Box 3420
Glen Allen, VA 23058
(800) 548-4550
(804) 747-0676 (fax)
http://www.atpwork.com

Alimed
297 High Street
Dedham, MA 02026
(800) 225-2610
(800) 437-2966 (fax)
http://www.alimed.com

Armaid: the new solution to repetitive strain
(800) 549-3904
http://www.armaid.com

Austin Medical Equipment
1900 South Mannheim Road
Westchester, IL 60154
(800) 382-0300
800-422-0515 (fax)
http://www.austinmedical.com

Bailey Manufacturing Company
PO Box 130
Lodi, OH 44254
(800) 321-8372
(800) 224-5390 (fax)
http://www.baileymfg.com

Baltimore Therapeutic Equipment
7455 L New Ridge Road
Hanover, MD 21076
(800) 331-8845
(410) 850-5244 (fax)
http://www.bteco.com

Better Hand Glove Products
Sof*Brace and thermal glove products
PO Box 21641
Concord, CA 94521
(800) 242-2850
(800) 97 HANDS (974-2637)
(209) 755-5746 (fax)
http://betterhands.com

Bio-Concepts, Inc.
2424 East University
Phoenix, AZ 85034-6911
(800) 421-5647
(602) 273-6931 (fax)
http://www.bio-con.com

Biodex Medical Systems
Brookhaven R&D Plaza
20 Ramsay Rd, Box 702
Shirley, NY 11967-0702
(800) 224-6339
(516) 924-9338 (fax)
http://www.biodex.com

Bio Med Sciences, Inc.
1111 Hamilton Street
Allentown, PA 18101
(800) 257-4566
(610) 974-8831 (fax)
http://www.silon.com

Bio Technologies
2160 North Central Road, Suite 204
Fort Lee, NJ 07024
(800) 971-2468
(201) 947-4495 (fax)

Carolon Hot Mitt
601 Forum Parkway
Rural Hall, NC 27045
(800) 334-0414
http://www.carolon.com

Chattanooga Group
4717 Adams Road
Hixson, TN 37343
(800) 592-7329
(800) 242-8329 (fax)
http://www.chattgroup.com

ClikStrips
WFR Corporation
30 Lawlins Park
Wyckoff, NJ 07446
(800) 526-5247
http://www.reveals.com/clikstrips.htm

Cold Laser Products
674 Ponce De Leon Drive
Tierra Verde, FL 33715
(727) 804-7754
(727) 865-2040 (fax)
sales@laserhealthproducts.com
http://laserhealthproducts.com

CP Motion
7211 S.W. 62nd Avenue, Suite 120
South Miami, FL 33143
(305) 668-7858
(305) 740-3390 (fax)
http://www.cpmotion.net

DeRoyal/LMB
200 DeBusk Lane
Powell, TN 37849
(888) 938-7828
(800) 938-7828 (fax)
http://www.deroyal.com

Dynasplint
770 Ritchie Highway, Suite W 21
Severna Park, MD 21146-3937
(800) 638-6771
http://www.dynasplint.com

Dynatronics Corporation
7030 Park Centre Drive
Salt Lake City, UT 84121
(800) 874-6251
(800) 221-1919 (fax)
http://www.dynatron.com

Empi
599 Cardigan Road
St. Paul, MN 55126-4099
(800) 328-2536, extension 1773
http://www.empi.com

Enablemart
400 Columbia Street, Suite 100
Vancouver, WA 98660
(888) 640-1999
(360) 695-4133 (fax)
http://www.enablemart.com

Ergodyne
1410 Energy Park Drive, Suite One
St. Paul, MN 55108
(800) 225-8238
(651) 642-1882 (fax)
http://www.ergodyne.com

Ergoscience, Inc.
15 Office Park Circle, Suite 214
Birmingham, AL 35223
(866) 779-6447
(205) 879-6397 (fax)
http://www.ergoscience.com

Fiskars, Inc.
780 Carolina Street
Sauk City, WI 53583
(800) 500-4849
(608) 643-4908 (fax)
http://www.fiskars.com

Four Hands
Accessories and jewelry for health professionals
(866) 678-9145
http://www.fourhandsonline.com

The Healthy Back Store
8245 Backlick Rd, Suite D
Lorton, VA 22079
(888) 469-2225
703-339-0671 (fax)
http://www.healthyback.com

Hoggan Health Industries, Inc.
(800) 678-7888
http://www.hogganhealth.com

Iomed
2441 South 3850 West, Suite A
Salt Lake City, UT 84120
(800) 621-3347
(801)972-9072 (fax)
http://www.iomed.com

Jobst
5825 Carnegie Building
Charlotte, NC 28209
(800) 537-1063
(800) 228-2736 (in Ohio)
(419) 691-4511 (fax)
http://www.jobst-usa.com

Joint Active Systems
2600 South Raney Street
Effingham, IL 62401
(800) 879-0117
(217) 347-3384 (fax)
http://www.jointactivesystems.com

Joint Jack Company
108 Britt Road
East Hartford, CT 06118
(860) 568-7338
(860) 568-9588 (fax)
http://www.jointjackcompany.com

Jtech Medical Industries
4314 Zevex Park Lane
Salt Lake City, UT 84123
(800) 970-2337
http://www.zevex.com

Kinesis Corporation
22121 17th Avenue SE, Suite 112
Bothell, WA 98021
(800) 454-6374
(425) 402-8181 (fax)
http://www.kinesis-ergo.com

Lafayette Instruments
PO Box 5729
Lafayette, IN 47903
(800) 428-7545
(765) 423-1505 (fax)
http://www.licmef.com

Medical Specialties, Inc.
4600 Lebanon Road
Charlotte, NC 28227
(800) 582-4040
http://www.medspec.com

Mettler Electronics Corporation
1333 S. Claudina Street
Anaheim, CA 92805
(800) 854-9305
(714) 635-7539 (fax)
http://www.mettlerelec.com

Northcoast Medical
18305 Sutter Boulevard
Morgan Hill, CA 95037
(800) 821-9319
(877) 213-9300 (fax)
http://www.ncmedical.com

Orfit Industries America
165 EAB Plaza
West Tower
6th Floor
Uniondale, NY 11556
(516) 522-2662
E-mail: martinj.ratner@orfit.com

Orfit Industries: Thermoplastics for Medical Industries
Vosveld 9A
B-2110 Wijnegem
BELGIUM
Phone 32 (0)3 326 20 26
Fax 32 (0)3 326 14 15
http://orfit.com/en/index.html

OrthoLogic/Sutter Corporation
1275 West Washington Street
Tempe, AZ 85281
(800) 286-5520
http://www.orthologic.com

Otto Bock USA
North American Headquarters
Two Carlson Parkway North, Suite 100
Minneapolis, MN 55447-4467
http://www.ottobockus.com

Physicians Sales and Service/World Medical, Inc.
4345 Southpoint Boulevard
Jacksonville, FL 32216
(904) 380-5900
(904) 281-0752 (fax)
http://www.pssd.com

Primal Pictures—Interactive Hand CD-ROM
AIDC, PO BOX 2246
Williston, VT 05495
(800) 716 2475
http://www.anatomy.tv
http://www.primalpictures.com

Quest Medical Group, Inc.
248 Pom Hill Senior Boulevard, Suite 219
Macon, GA 31210
(800) 248-8846
(801) 572-6514 (fax)
http://www.hoganhealth.com

RCAI—Restorative Care of America
12221 33rd Street North
St. Petersburg, Florida 33716
(800) 627-1595
http://www.rcai.com

Rehabilicare
PO Box 30244
Tampa, FL 33633
(800) 343-0488
(800) 272-6458 (fax)
http://www.rehabilicare.com

RS Medical
14401 Southeast First Street
Vancouver, WA 98684
(800) 935-7763
(800) 929-1930 (fax)
http://www.rsmedical.com

Sammons Preston Rolyan
4 Sammons Court
Bolingbrook, IL 60440
(800) 323-5547
(800) 547-4333 (fax)
http://www.sammonspreston.com

Silver Ring Splint Company
PO Box 2856
Charlottesville, VA 22902
(800) 311-7028
(888) 456-8828 (fax)
http://www.silverringsplint.com

Smith & Nephew
PO Box 1005
Germantown, WI 53022
(800) 228-3693
(414) 251-7758 (fax)
http://www.smith-nephew.com

Soft FLEX computer gloves—Four Points Products, Inc.
4230 Winding Willow Drive
Tampa, FL 33618
(800) 216-8415
http://www.softflex.com

Specialty Therapy Equipment, Inc.
8209 Rider Ave.
Townson, MD 21204
(800) 999-7839
(410) 821-8429 (fax)
gkrame@compcast.net

Tetra Medical Supply Corporation
6364 West Gross Point Road
Niles, IL 60714-3916
(800) 621-4041
(847) 647-9034 (fax)
http://www.tetramed.com

Therakinetics
55 Carnegie Plaza
Cherry Hill, NJ 08003-1020
(800) 800-4276
(800) 701-9964 (fax)

UE Tech
PO Box 2145
Edwards, CO 81632
(800) 736-1894
(970) 926-8870 (fax)
http://www.uetech.com

Valpar
PO Box 5767
Tucson, AZ 85703-5767
(800) 528-7070
(520) 292-9755 (fax)
http://www.valparint.com

Appendix 2

Drugs Commonly Encountered in Hand Therapy

Introduction

One of the areas of upper extremity rehabilitation seldom addressed in the occupational and physical therapy literature is prescription and nonprescription drugs and their effects on wound care, healing, and rehabilitation. The goal of this appendix is to introduce the hand therapist to some of the most common medications prescribed by hand surgeons and often encountered in a rehabilitation setting. Additionally, the commonly used or abused nonprescription drugs nicotine, alcohol, and caffeine are also presented. Finally, an alphabetical list of the drugs discussed in the chapter and the classification of each is provided for quick reference. Addressing all classes of medications, their indications, side effects, and interactions is beyond the scope of this chapter (please refer to the *Physicians' Desk Reference* and other pharmacology reference books).

Common Medications Prescribed by Hand Surgeons

Narcotic analgesics

Narcotic pain medicines are among the most common drugs that hand therapists encounter daily. They are most often prescribed to reduce pain after surgery or trauma. Narcotics may be useful—especially in the early postoperative period—to allow the patient to comply with the treatment regimen without undue discomfort, so that therapeutic progression may be achieved. Narcotics, however, can be associated with a number of common side effects that may interfere with treatment sessions and compliance with exercises at home. These include sedation, drowsiness, and other symptoms associated with central nervous system (CNS) depression (see Alcohol); nausea and vomiting; rash; and pruritus (itching). Additionally, abuse could occur. If you feel that your patient exhibits these symptoms, notify the referring physician, who may change the medication or place the patient on a structured pain medication protocol. Remember that because the therapist typically spends more one-on-one time with the patient than the physician does, therapists are more often in a position to identify these problems, and physicians generally appreciate these observations and input.

Common narcotic analgesics (or drugs containing a narcotic analgesic) include the following: butorphanol (Stadol), codeine, dolophine (Methadone), hydrocodone (Lorcet, Lortab, Vicodin), hydromorphone (Dilaudid), meperidine (Demerol), morphine (MS Contin, Roxanol), nalbuphine (Nubain), oxycodone (Percocet, Percodan, Tylox), pentazocine (Talwin), and propoxyphene (Darvocet-N, Darvon). One other drug, tramadol (Ultram), is commonly prescribed for pain and related to the opiates but is not considered a narcotic. It acts on the CNS and should not be given in conjunction with the narcotics or to patients who are addicted to narcotics.

Nonsteroidal antiinflammatory drugs

Nonsteroidal antiinflammatory drugs (NSAIDs) are an ever-expanding class of drugs useful in the treatment of arthritis, musculoskeletal disorders and injuries, and postoperative patients because of their analgesic, antipyretic, and antiinflammatory properties. Their mechanism of action is through the inhibition of prostaglandin synthesis. Prostaglandins are reported to cause pain, redness, fever, and edema in various musculoskeletal conditions, including osteoarthritis, rheumatoid arthritis, and related disorders. NSAIDs avoid the CNS side effects associated with narcotics and many of the adverse reactions associated with steroids; however, they commonly cause gastrointestinal (GI) side effects that may be serious. These can be displayed as abdominal pain, indigestion, nausea, diarrhea, constipation, or even GI bleeding (typically dark tarry stools) from gastritis or peptic ulcer disease. The NSAIDs that have a salicylate (aspirin) component may cause oozing, bleeding, and bruising postoperatively because of their anticoagulant (blood-thinning) properties. Other common side effects of NSAIDs include rash, pruritus, headache, and dizziness. Examples of commonly prescribed and over-the-counter NSAIDs are aspirin, celecoxib (Celebrex), diclofenac (Cataflam, Voltaren), diflunisal (Dolobid), etadolac (Lodine), fenoprofen (Nalfon), flurbiprofen (Ansaid), ketorolac (Toradol), ibuprofen (Advil, Motrin, Nuprin), indomethacin (Indocin), ketoprofen (Orudis, Oruvail), meloxicam (Mobic), nabumetone (Relafen), naproxen (Aleve, Anaprox, Naprosyn), oxaprozin (Daypro), piroxicam (Feldene), rofecoxib (Vioxx), salicylate (Trilisate), salsalate (Disalcid), sulindac (Clinoril), and valdecoxib (Bextra).

Corticosteroids

Corticosteroid drugs are used principally as antiinflammatory agents in most patients encountered in a hand therapy setting. Oral steroids are used to treat medical conditions such as asthma, chronic obstructive pulmonary disease (COPD), dermatologic conditions, and rheumatic or autoimmune disorders. In hand surgery, however, they are mainly used to decrease edema and inflammation. Side effects of oral steroids may be serious in conditions that require high doses and/or prolonged treatment and may include GI ulcers, osteoporosis, hip necrosis, diabetes, insomnia, irritability, weight gain, Cushingoid features, impaired wound healing, and susceptibility to infections. In hand conditions, however, steroids are more commonly used in an injectable form, which allows localization of their effects and fewer systemic side effects. Depending on the condition and location, the steroid may be combined with a local anesthetic such as Xylocaine (lidocaine) or Marcaine (bupivicaine). Injections should not be given into a previously infected or unstable joint because they may interfere with the body's wound-healing responsiveness and ability to fight infection. Local injections, especially if repeated, can cause thinning of overlying skin, a discolored and shiny appearance, and atrophy of subcutaneous tissues. Examples of oral corticosteroid preparations include cortisone, dexamethasone (Decadron), methylprednisolone (Medrol, Medrol Dosepak), and prednisone (Deltasone). Injectable steroids include betamethasone (Celestone), dexamethasone (Decadron), methylprednisolone (Depo-Medrol), and triamcinolone (Aristocort, Kenalog).

Disease-modifying antirheumatic drugs

Disease-modifying antirheumatic drugs (DMARDs) are an inhomogeneous class of drugs used predominantly by rheumatologists to treat rheumatoid arthritis (RA) and other inflammatory or autoimmune arthritides (e.g., lupus, psoriatic arthritis). Original treatments for rheumatoid arthritis included the gold salts auranofin (Ridaura), and aurothioglucose (Lomosol, Solganal), and penicillamine (Cuprimine); these still may be infrequently encountered today by the hand therapist. These drugs have been supplanted mostly by hydroxychloroquine (Plaquenil), sulfasalazine (Azulfidine) and the more traditional immunosuppressive agents such as methotrexate (Rheumatrex), cyclosporine (Neoral), and azathioprine (Imuran), which are used to suppress the body's immune-mediated joint destruction. Newer immunomodulating agents include the tumor necrosis factor blockers infliximab (Remicade) and etanercept (Enbrel), the interleukin-1 receptor antagonist anakinra (Kineret), and the pyrimidine synthesis inhibitor leflunomide (Arava). Many of these agents may suppress the immune system and make patients susceptible to infection, and the therapist should be alert to signs of infection, especially in the postoperative period.

Antibiotics and antimicrobial drugs

Antimicrobial drugs are commonly employed postoperatively in hand-surgery patients, topically or orally, and in severe infections, intramuscularly or intravenously. Depending on the type of surgery, conditions of the injury, and preference of the surgeon, oral antibiotics may be given prophylactically in the early postoperative period. However, because of the increasing emergence of resistant strains of bacteria, these medications should not be given casually for "possible" infection and should ideally have a culture taken before initiating treatment. Once the patient is on an antibiotic, the full prescription should be completed, even if the infection visually appears resolved. The most common side effects are gastrointestinal and may present as abdominal pain, indigestion, nausea, vomiting, diarrhea, or constipation. Rash, pruritus, photosensitivity, headache, and dizziness are also common. Some examples of antibiotics likely to be encountered in a hand setting include the following: amoxicillin/clavulanate (Augmentin), ampicillin/sulbactam IM/IV (Unasyn), azithromycin (Zithromax), clarithromycin (Biaxin), cefaclor (Ceclor), cefadroxil (Duricef), cefazolin IM/IV (Ancef, Kefzol), cefotaxime IM/IV (Claforan), ceftazidime IM/IV (Fortaz), ceftriaxone IM/IV (Rocephin), cefuroxime (Ceftin), cephalexin (Keflex), ciprofloxacin (Cipro), clindamycin (Cleocin), doxycycline (Vibramycin), erythromycin (EES, Ery-Tab), gatifloxacin (Tequin), levofloxacin (Levaquin), metronidazole (Flagyl), moxifloxacin (Avelox), nafcillin (Unipen), ofloxacin (Floxin), penicillin V (Pen-Vee K), and vancomycin (Vancocin, Vancor).

Anticoagulants and antithrombotics

Patients who undergo microvascular surgery or are predisposed to thromboembolic complications (history of deep venous thrombosis, pulmonary embolism, peripheral vascular disease, cardiac arrhythmias, or other cardiac diseases or stroke) are often placed on blood-thinning or anticoagulant medications. In hand surgery these drugs are used to prevent arterial (and venous) occlusions, especially after soft tissue flaps or replants. Arterial thrombosis or embolism may otherwise lead to necrosis or death of the flap, digit, or the entire extremity. In some cases, hand surgeons may use medicinal leeches to decrease venous engorgement of skin flaps postoperatively. The leeches suck out the blood and fall off when they are full. Bleeding is, of course, the most common complication of anticoagulant therapy, and patients on these medications typically have repeated blood testing to maintain the equilibrium between the desired effect and frank bleeding. On these drugs, patients will typically have more oozing, drainage, and prolonged wound healing times. Numerous prescription and over-the-counter medications may affect the blood levels of these drugs or intensify the anticoagulant effect; therefore a patient who experiences increased or continued problems with bleeding should list all medications so that the referring physician can be contacted. As patients progress postoperatively, the physician may change from one of the more potent anticoagulants to aspirin products (Bayer, Bufferin, or Ecotrin). Some of the more potent anticoagulant drugs are the following: ardeparin (Normiflo), dipyridamole (Persantine), enoxaparin (Lovenox), heparin, danaparoid (Orgaran), ticlopidine (Ticlid), and warfarin (Coumadin).

Sympatholytic or antiadrenergic drugs

These medications work by interfering with the sympathetic nervous system's constriction of peripheral blood vessels in the skin and subcutaneous tissues of the upper extremity in conditions such as Raynaud's syndrome and reflex sympathetic dystrophy (RSD). They do not significantly increase skeletal muscle blood flow and therefore do not have much use in the treatment of other types of peripheral vascular disease. They can, however, dilate blood vessels in the superficial tissues and skin. The most common side effect of these agents is orthostatic hypotension (dizziness or lightheadedness on standing or changing body position). To date, the most effective alpha-blocking agent with the least undesirable side effects is phenoxybenzamine (Dibenzyline). Some other agents are guanethidine (Ismelin), methyldopa (Aldomet), phentolamine (Regitine), prazosin (Minipress), reserpine (Serpasil), and tolazoline (Priscoline).

Miscellaneous drugs used in hand conditions

Nifedipine (Adalat, Procardia) is a calcium channel blocker commonly employed in the treatment of hypertension and other cardiovascular diseases. Nifedipine works on the vascular smooth muscle to cause dilation of blood vessels and increased peripheral blood flow. It may also reverse the signs of vasomotor instability, and for these reasons may be useful in the treatment of Raynaud's syndrome and RSD. It is also sometimes used postoperatively after microvascular surgery. Nifedipine has been shown to decrease vasospasm and may decrease the frequency and severity of attacks in Raynaud's syndrome.

Amitriptyline (Elavil) is a tricyclic antidepressant used in the treatment of RSD, neuralgias, and other chronic pain disorders of the upper extremity. Elavil is of benefit in RSD patients because many of them have some degree of clinical depression, but it also produces some vasodilation and has analgesic action. Elavil commonly causes drowsiness, orthostatic hypotension, and marked anticholinergic side effects, including dry mouth, blurred vision, tachycardia, urinary retention, and slowed gastric emptying. It can be very dangerous in overdoses—a fact that should be remembered in patients with severe depression or suicidal tendencies.

Capsaicin (Zostrix) is a topical ointment derived from the red capsicum pepper, which has shown promise in the local relief of hyperalgesia and hypersensitivity of the skin and pain associated with various neuropathies as well as some arthritic conditions. Topical application may be helpful in some patients with RSD.

Gabapentin (Neurontin) is an anticonvulsant drug that is used to treat some forms of epilepsy. Some hand surgeons also use it in the treatment of RSD and neuropathic pain or phantom pain after peripheral nerve injuries. Its mechanism of action in these conditions is unclear.

Drugs of Abuse and Their Roles in Hand Rehabilitation

Nicotine

Nicotine—found in cigarettes, cigars, chewing tobacco, snuff, and pipe tobacco—causes peripheral vasoconstriction along with increased heart rate and blood pressure. Nicotine has an adverse effect on wound healing in the hand therapy patient. Vasoconstriction decreases the blood supply to bone, muscle, and soft tissue, thus delaying overall healing, especially in those who have undergone microvascular procedures such as flaps or replants, after which smoking is definitely contraindicated. These effects are often more pronounced in the elderly or debilitated patient who may already have conditions that adversely affect healing and circulation. Nicotine can also alter the activity of other concomitant prescription and over-the-counter medications.

Remember also that drugs used to help with smoking cessation typically contain nicotine, and if patients smoke while taking these medications, the level of nicotine in the bloodstream increases dramatically and may be dangerous. Some examples of these drugs include Habitrol, Nicoderm CQ, Nicorette gum, Nicotrol, and Prostep.

Alcohol

Because alcohol is water-soluble, it affects every living cell in the body. In contrast to nicotine, moderate doses of alcohol can cause vasodilation, especially in cutaneous vessels. Alcohol is also a CNS depressant that not only affects reasoning but also memory and coordination. This commonly has a profound effect on therapy because it may influence understanding and compliance with wound care as well as clinic and home exercise programs. Chronic alcohol abuse may cause GI distress and interfere with normal digestion and may be accompanied by poor nutrition, often leading to impaired wound healing. When alcohol is combined with other prescription or nonprescription drugs such as pain medications or sedatives, it may cause overdose, liver failure, or death.

Caffeine

Caffeine is a drug that few people consider when taking a medical history. In addition to coffee, caffeine is found in many beverages, foods, and medications and may cause vasoconstriction in the hand therapy patient, thus resulting in numbness and pain in the extremities. Caffeine may also exacerbate previous medical problems such as hypertension, tachycardia, cardiac arrhythmias, and coronary artery disease. Because of their altered work and activity schedules, many hand patients substantially increase their intake of coffee and caffeine. Some common medications that contain caffeine are butalbital (Esgic, Fioricet, Fiorinal), ergotamine (Cafergot, Wigraine), Excedrin, and orphenadrine (Norgesic).

References

American Medical Association: *Drug evaluations annual 1992*, Chicago, 1991, American Medical Association.

Gellman H, Nichols D: Reflex sympathetic dystrophy in the upper extremity, *J Am Acad Orthop Surg* 5:313-22, 1997.

Green DP, Hotchkiss RN, Pederson WC: *Green's Operative hand surgery*, ed 4, New York, 1999, Churchill Livingstone.

Mosby's Drug consult 2003, St Louis, 2003, Mosby.

Physician assistants' prescribing reference, Spring 2003, New York, 2003, Prescribing Reference.

Physicians' desk reference, ed 57, Montvale, NJ, 2003, Medical Economics Company, Inc.

List of Drugs Commonly Encountered in Hand Therapy

Drug name (common trade names are capitalized; generic names are lowercase)	Indication/drug category
Adalat (nifedipine)	hypertension, Raynaud's syndrome
Advil (ibuprofen)	NSAID
alcohol	CNS depressant
Aldomet (methyldopa)	hypertension/sympatholytic
Aleve (naproxen)	NSAID
amitriptyline (Elavil)	depression, neuropathic pain
amoxicillin/clavulanate (Augmentin)	antibiotic
ampicillin/sulbactam (Unasyn)	antibiotic
Anacin (aspirin)	NSAID, anticoagulant
anakinra (Kineret)	DMARD
Anaprox (naproxen sodium)	NSAID
Ancef (cefazolin IV)	antibiotic
Ansaid (flurbiprofen)	NSAID
Arava (leflunomide)	DMARD
ardeparin (Normiflo)	anticoagulant
Aristocort (triamcinolone)	corticosteroid
aspirin	NSAID, anticoagulant
Augmentin (amoxicillin/ clavulanate)	antibiotic
auranofin (Ridaura)	DMARD
aurothioglucose (Lomosol, Solganal)	DMARD
Avelox (moxifloxacin)	antibiotic
azathioprine (Imuran)	DMARD
azithromycin (Zithromax)	antibiotic
Azulfidine (sulfasalazine)	DMARD
Bayer (aspirin)	NSAID, anticoagulant
betamethasone (Celestone)	corticosteroid
Bextra (valdecoxib)	NSAID
Biaxin (clarithromycin)	antibiotic
Bufferin (aspirin)	NSAID, anticoagulant
butalbital (Esgic, Fioricet, Fiorinal)	migraine headache, caffeine
butorphanol (Stadol)	narcotic analgesic
Cafergot (ergotamine)	migraine headache, caffeine
caffeine	stimulant
capsaicin (Zostrix)	neuropathic pain
Cataflam (Voltaren)	NSAID
Ceclor (cefaclor)	antibiotic
cefaclor (Ceclor)	antibiotic
cefadroxil (Duricef)	antibiotic
cefazolin (Kefzol, Ancef)	antibiotic
Cefotan (cefotetan)	antibiotic
cefotaxime (Claforan)	antibiotic
cefotetan (Cefotan)	antibiotic
cefprozil (Cefzil)	antibiotic
ceftazidime (Fortaz)	antibiotic
Ceftin (cefuroxime)	antibiotic
ceftriaxone (Rocephin)	antibiotic
cefuroxime (Ceftin)	antibiotic
Cefzil (cefprozil)	antibiotic
Celebrex (celecoxib)	NSAID
celecoxib (Celebrex)	NSAID
Celestone (betamethasone)	corticosteroid
cephalexin (Keflex)	antibiotic
Cipro (ciprofloxacin)	antibiotic
ciprofloxacin (Cipro)	antibiotic
Claforan (cefotaxime)	antibiotic

Drug name (common trade names are capitalized; generic names are lowercase)	Indication/drug category
clarithromycin (Biaxin)	antibiotic
Cleocin (clindamycin)	antibiotic
clindamycin (Cleocin)	antibiotic
Clinoril (sulindac)	NSAID
codeine	narcotic analgesic
cortisone	corticosteroid
Coumadin (warfarin)	anticoagulant
Cuprimine (penicillamine)	DMARD
cyclosporine (Neoral)	DMARD
danaparoid (Orgaran)	anticoagulant
Darvocet-N (propoxyphene)	narcotic analgesic
Darvon (propoxyphene)	narcotic analgesic
Daypro (oxaprozin)	NSAID
Decadron (dexamethasone)	corticosteroid
Deltasone (prednisone)	corticosteroid
Demerol (meperidine)	narcotic analgesic
Depo-Medrol (methylprednisolone)	corticosteroid
dexamethasone (Decadron)	corticosteroid
Dibenzyline (phenoxybenzamine)	hypertension/sympatholytic
diclofenac (Cataflam, Voltaren)	NSAID
diflunisal (Dolobid)	NSAID
Dilaudid (hydromorphone)	narcotic analgesic
dipyridamole (Persantine)	anticoagulant
Disalcid (salsalate)	DMARD
Dolobid (diflunisal)	NSAID
dolophine (Methadone)	narcotic analgesic
doxycycline (Vibramycin)	antibiotic
Duricef (cefadroxil)	antibiotic
E-mycin (erythromycin)	antibiotic
EES (erythromycin)	antibiotic
Ecotrin (aspirin)	NSAID, anticoagulant
Elavil (amitriptyline)	depression, neuropathic pain
Enbrel (etanercept)	DMARD
enoxaparin (Lovenox)	anticoagulant
ergotamine (Cafergot, Wigraine)	migraine headache, caffeine
erythromycin (E-mycin, EES)	antibiotic
Esgic (butalbital)	migraine headache, caffeine
etadolac (Lodine)	NSAID
etanercept (Enbrel)	DMARD
Excedrin (aspirin, caffeine)	NSAID, anticoagulant, caffeine
Feldene (piroxicam)	NSAID
fenoprofen (Nalfon)	NSAID
Fioricet (butalbital)	migraine headache, caffeine
Fiorinal (butalbital)	migraine headache, caffeine
Flagyl (metronidazole)	antibiotic
Floxin (ofloxacin)	antibiotic
flurbiprofen (Ansaid)	NSAID
Fortaz (ceftazidime)	antibiotic
gabapentin (Neurontin)	seizures, RSD/neuropathic pain
gatifloxacin (Tequin)	antibiotic
guanethidine (Ismelin)	hypertension/sympatholytic
Habitrol (nicotine)	smoking cessation
heparin	anticoagulant
hydrocodone (Lorcet, Lortab, Vicodin)	narcotic analgesic
hydromorphone (Dilaudid)	narcotic analgesic
hydroxychloroquine (Plaquenil)	DMARD
ibuprofen (Advil, Motrin, Nuprin)	NSAID
Imuran (azathioprine)	DMARD
Indocin (indomethacin)	NSAID
indomethacin (Indocin)	NSAID
infliximab (Remicade)	DMARD

Drug name (common trade names are capitalized; generic names are lowercase)	Indication/drug category
Ismelin (guanethidine)	hypertension/sympatholytic
Keflex (cephalexin)	antibiotic
Kefzol (cefazolin)	antibiotic
Kenalog (triamcinolone)	corticosteroid
ketoprofen (Orudis)	NSAID
ketorolac (Toradol)	NSAID
Kineret (anakinra)	DMARD
leflunomide (Arava)	DMARD
Levaquin (levofloxacin)	antibiotic
levofloxacin (Levaquin)	antibiotic
Lodine (etadolac)	NSAID
Lomosol (aurothioglucose)	DMARD
Lorcet (hydrocodone)	narcotic analgesic
Lortab (hydrocodone)	narcotic analgesic
Lovenox (enoxaparin)	anticoagulant
Medrol (methylprednisolone)	corticosteroid
meperidine (Demerol)	narcotic analgesic
Methadone (dolophine)	narcotic analgesic
methotrexate (Rheumatrex)	DMARD
methyldopa (Aldomet)	hypertension/sympatholytic
methylprednisolone (Depo-Medrol, Medrol)	corticosteroid
metronidazole (Flagyl)	antibiotic
Minipress (prazosin)	hypertension/sympatholytic
morphine (MS Contin, Roxanol)	narcotic analgesic
Motrin (ibuprofen)	NSAID
moxifloxacin (Avelox)	antibiotic
MS Contin (morhpine)	narcotic analgesic
nabumetone (Relafen)	NSAID
nafcillin (Unipen)	antibiotic
nalbuphine (Nubain)	narcotic analgesic
Nalfon (fenoprofen)	NSAID
Naprosyn (naproxen)	NSAID
naproxen (Aleve, Anaprox, Naprosyn)	NSAID
Neoral (cyclosporine)	DMARD
Neurontin (gabapentin)	seizures, RSD/neuropathic pain
Nicoderm CQ (nicotine)	smoking cessation
Nicorette gum (nicotine)	smoking cessation
nicotine	stimulant
Nicotrol	smoking cessation
nifedipine (Adalat, Procardia)	hypertension, Raynaud's
Norgesic (orphenadrine)	muscle relaxant, caffeine
Normiflo (ardeparin)	anticoagulant
Nubain (nalbuphine)	narcotic analgesic
Nuprin (ibuprofen)	NSAID
ofloxacin (Floxin)	antibiotic
Organan (danaparoid)	anticoagulant
orphenadrine (Norgesic)	muscle relaxant,caffeine
Orudis (ketoprofen)	NSAID
oxaprozin (Daypro)	NSAID
oxycodone (Percocet, Percodan, Tylox)	narcotic analgesic
Pen-Vee K (penicillin V)	antibiotic
penicillamine (Cuprimine)	DMARD
penicillinV (Pen-VeeK)	antibiotic
pentazocine (Talwin)	narcotic analgesic
Percocet (oxycodone)	narcotic analgesic
Percodan (oxycodone)	narcotic analgesic
Persantine (dipyridamole)	anticoagulant
phenoxybenzamine (Dibenzyline)	hypertension/sympatholytic

Drug name (common trade names are capitalized; generic names are lowercase)	Indication/drug category
phentolamine (Regitine)	hypertension/sympatholytic
piroxicam (Feldene)	NSAID
Plaquenil (hydroxychloroquine)	DMARD
prazosin (Minipress)	hypertension/sympatholytic
prednisone (Deltasone)	corticosteroid
Priscoline (tolazoline)	hypertension/sympatholytic
Procardia (nifedipine)	hypertension, Raynaud's
propoxyphene (Darvocet-N, Darvon)	narcotic analgesic
Prostep (nicotine)	smoking cessation
Regitine (phentolamine)	hypertension/sympatholytic
Relafen (nabumetone)	NSAID
Remicade (infliximab)	DMARD
reserpine (Serpasil)	hypertension/sympatholytic
Rheumatrex (methotrexate)	DMARD
Ridaura (auranofin)	DMARD
Rocephin (ceftriaxone IV)	antibiotic
rofecoxib (Vioxx)	NSAID
Roxanol (morphine)	narcotic analgesic
salicylate (Trilisate)	DMARD
salsalate (Disalcid)	DMARD
Serpasil (reserpine)	hypertension/sympatholytic
Solganal (aurothioglucose)	DMARD
Stadol (butorphanol)	narcotic analgesic
sulfasalazine (Azulfidine)	DMARD
sulindac (Clinoril)	NSAID
Talwin (pentazocine)	narcotic analgesic
Tequin (gatifloxacin)	antibiotic
Ticlid (ticlopidine)	anticoagulant
ticlopidine (Ticlid)	anticoagulant
tolazoline (Priscoline)	hypertension/sympatholytic
Toradol (ketorolac)	NSAID
tramadol (Ultram)	nonnarcotic analgesic
triamcinolone (Aristocort)	corticosteroid
triamcinolone (Kenalog)	corticosteroid
Trilisate (salicylate)	DMARD
Tylox (oxycodone)	narcotic analgesic
Ultram (tramadol)	nonnarcotic analgesic
Unasyn (ampicillin/sulbactam)	antibiotic
Unipen (nafcillin)	antibiotic
valdecoxib (Bextra)	NSAID
Vancocin (vancomycin)	antibiotic
Vancor (vancomycin)	antibiotic
vancomycin (Vancocin, Vancor)	antibiotic
Vibramycin (doxycycline)	antibiotic
Vicodin (hydrocodone)	narcotic analgesic
Vioxx (rofecoxib)	NSAID
Voltaren (diclofenac)	NSAID
warfarin (Coumadin)	anticoagulant
Wigraine (ergotamine)	migraine headache, caffeine
Zithromax (azithromycin)	antibiotic
Zostrix (capsaicin)	neuropathic pain

NOTE: Common trade names are capitalized; generic names are in lowercase.

DMARD, Disease-modifying antirheumatic drug; NSAID, nonsteroidal antiinflammatory drug.

Appendix 3

Nutrition

The following is a quick nutritional reference for therapists. This appendix will assist therapists in discussing optimal nutrition with their patients. While compiling information for this section, the contributors selected vitamins, minerals, and food supplements—as well as their benefits and cautions—with the hand therapy patient in mind. Further study is recommended for an in-depth evaluation of this subject. Vitamins, minerals, or supplements that contain extensive precautions or are controversial are omitted from this section.

Vitamins

Vitamin	Benefits*	Cautions†
Vitamin A	Assists in the development and maintenance of epithelial tissue; improves immune function	
Vitamin B_1 (Thiamine)	Enhances circulation; assists blood formation; optimizes brain and nerve cell function	
Vitamin B_2 (Riboflavin)	Assists red blood cell formation, antibody production, and cell respiration and growth; people with carpal tunnel syndrome may benefit from use of this vitamin in combination with vitamin B_6	
Vitamin B_3 (Niacin)	Assists nervous system function and circulation; a particular form of niacin, inositol hexaniacinate, has been shown to increase circulation to the extremities	A flush, usually harmless, may occur after ingestion of niacin supplements; those who are pregnant, diabetic, or have glaucoma, gout, liver disease, or peptic ulcers should use cautiously because amounts over 500 mg daily may cause liver damage if taken for prolonged periods
Vitamin B_5 (Pantothenic acid)	Assists stress reduction and production of neurotransmitters; decreases morning stiffness and pain; assists in red blood cell formation	
Vitamin B_6 (Pyridoxine)	Assists sodium and potassium balance; required by nervous system; maintains healthy nerve tissue; assists immune system function; decreases water retention; decreases inflammation; increases circulation; increases gamma-aminobutyric acid (GABA) to help control pain perception; thought to be helpful for treatment of carpal tunnel syndrome and other common peripheral nerve pathologies; has a vital role in the multiplication of all cells	Doses greater than 2000 mg/day can produce symptoms of nerve toxicity

Vitamins—cont'd

Vitamin	Benefits*	Cautions†
Vitamin B_{12} (Cyanocobalamin)	Helps prevent nerve damage; maintains fatty sheaths that cover and protect nerve endings	
Folic acid	Needed for red blood cell formation; aids in proper functioning of white blood cells, thereby strengthening immunity	Those with a hormone-related cancer or convulsive disorder must not take high doses of folic acid for extended periods
Vitamin C (Ascorbic acid)	Assists tissue growth and repair; enhances immunity; guards against infection; increases bone mass; promotes healing of wounds and burns through improved function of collagen; helps with nerve transmission	Pregnant women should not take more than 5000 mg daily because infants may become dependent on this supplement and develop scurvy when deprived of the accustomed megadoses after birth; if aspirin and vitamin C are taken together, stomach irritation may occur
Vitamin D	Especially important for normal growth and development of bones and teeth in children; benefits immune system; assists blood clotting; stimulates absorption of calcium	Should not be taken without calcium; toxicity may result from taking more than 65,000 international units over a period of years; excessive amounts may cause vomiting, diarrhea, weight loss, and kidney damage
Vitamin E	Improves circulation; necessary for tissue repair; assists blood clotting/healing; reduces scarring in some wounds; synergistic relationship with Vitamin C (effectiveness enhanced when taken together); may soften abnormal connective tissue in Dupuytren's disease	Those taking a blood thinner should not take more than 1200 international units of vitamin E daily; those with diabetes, rheumatic heart disease, or overactive thyroid should not take more than the recommended dosage; if patient is hypertensive, start with small amounts such as 200 mg daily and gradually increase dosage
Vitamin K	Necessary for blood clotting; aids in bone formation and repair	Large doses of synthetic vitamin K should not be taken during the last few weeks of pregnancy because it can be toxic for newborns; megadoses can cause flushing and sweating; excessive amounts of the synthetic vitamin may cause jaundice
Vitamin P (Bioflavonoids)	Used extensively in athletic injuries for relieving pain and bruises; has an antibacterial effect; promotes circulation; decreases edema	Very high doses may cause diarrhea

*The benefits listed in this table have been indicated to be effective according to the cited references.

†Blank spaces indicate no significant cautions associated with use according to the cited references.

Minerals

Mineral	Benefits*	Cautions†
Boron	Small amount needed for healthy bones and metabolism of calcium	No more than 3 mg should be taken daily
Calcium	Vital for strong bones; aids in transmission of nerve impulses	Calcium supplements should not be taken by those with history of kidney stones or kidney disease; doses of 2000 mg/day may increase risk for kidney stones as well as heterotopic ossification; may interfere with effects of verapamil (Calan, Isoptin, Verelan); a calcium channel blocker sometimes is prescribed for hypertension or cardiac problems
Copper	Aids in formation of bone, hemoglobin, and red blood cells; works in balance with zinc and vitamin C to form elastin; necessary for healing; promotes healthy nerves and joints; essential for collagen formation; has antiinflammatory effects	High doses may result in a rare metabolic condition (Wilson's disease)
Germanium	Improves cellular oxygenation; helps fight pain; keeps immune system functioning	
Iron	Oxygenates red blood cells; aids immune system function	Iron supplements should not be taken if active infection is present because extra iron can increase bacterial growth in the body; high doses can lead to cirrhosis of the liver
Magnesium	Helps prevent calcification of soft tissue; aids in bone formation; maintains body pH balance; increases energy; aids in muscle relaxation and blood vessel relaxation	Diarrhea may result if large doses are consumed
Manganese	Required for normal bone growth and reproduction and formation of cartilage and synovial fluid	
Phosphorus	Aids in bone formation; promotes normal cell function	
Potassium	Promotes healthy nervous and muscular function; helps control water retention with sodium	Excess can result in muscular weakness or death
Silicon	Aids in formation of collagen for bones and connective tissue; aids in calcium absorption in early stages of bone formation	Inhalation of small silicon particles into the lungs may lead to silicosis
Sodium	Helps maintain proper water balance; helps control blood pH	Large doses can cause high blood pressure
Sulfur	Necessary for collagen synthesis	
Vanadium	Needed for cellular metabolism; aids in production of bone	High doses may cause lung irritation
Zinc	Required for protein synthesis; aids in collagen formation; promotes healthy immune system function; assists in wound healing	More than 100 mg daily can depress the immune system; excess amounts may lead to vomiting, nausea, fever, and diarrhea

*The benefits listed in this table have been proven effective according to the cited references.

†Blank spaces indicate no significant cautions associated with use.

Natural Food Supplements

Natural food supplement	Benefits*	Cautions†
Alfalfa	Good for arthritis pain; contains chlorophyll, which aids in healing of infections and burns	May reactivate symptoms in people with quiescent systemic lupus
Aloe vera	Skin healer and moisturizer; good for treatment of burns and cuts	Should be used only topically for therapeutic purposes described here
Barley grass	Acts as an antiinflammatory	
Boswellia	May inhibit inflammation; builds cartilage	
Bovine cartilage	Accelerates wound healing; reduces inflammation; helpful in treatment of rheumatoid arthritis	
Bromelain	Antiinflammatory enzyme particularly helpful in reducing postsurgical edema; decreases pain; decreases healing time of wounds and soft-tissue injuries; works best in combination with vitamin B_6	
Cayenne	Relieves pain when applied topically through inhibition of substance P	
Comdalis	Has potent pain-relieving properties; reduces neuralgia	
Echinacea	Boosts immune response; repairs skin and tissues; prevents scarring	
Evening primrose oil	Controls inflammation	
Fish oil	Relieves arthritis/combats stiffness	Not for diabetic patients because of the high fat content of this oil (but people with diabetes should consume fish for essential fatty acids)
Flaxseed oil or flaxseed	Decreases pain, inflammation, and edema associated with arthritis	
Garlic	Stimulates immune system; acts as a natural antibiotic	
Ginger	Has antiinflammatory and pain-relieving properties	
Ginkgo biloba	Increases circulation to the extremities	Not to be taken by those who routinely take aspirin or blood thinners
Glucosamine	Involved in formation of tendons, skin, bones, and ligaments; can be helpful for tendonitis and bursitis	
Gotukola	Stimulates growth of connective tissue; helps with wound healing; decreases joint pain and immobility of fingers	
Grapeseed extract	Inhibits edema	
Hawthorn	Increases circulation to the extremities	
Honey	Promotes healing; natural antiseptic; good salve for burns and wounds	Not to be taken by babies under 1 year of age, or those with diabetes
Horsetail	Helps produce calcium and strengthen bones	
Kelp	Beneficial for sensory nerves and spinal cord	
Lactobacillus bifidus	Helps maintain healthy intestinal flora when antibiotics are taken	
Sea cucumber	Relieves arthritis; reduces pain and stiffness; has been shown to boost grip strength in the arthritic hand	
Sea mussel	Helps relieve pain and stiffness associated with arthritis	
Shark cartilage	Relieves arthritis; promotes healthy immune system	Should not be taken by pregnant women, children, or those who have had recent heart attacks or surgery

*The benefits listed in this table have been proven to be effective according to the cited references.

†Blank spaces indicate no significant cautions associated with use.

References

Balch JF, Balch PA: *Prescription for nutritional healing: a practical A-Z reference to drug-free remedies using vitamins, minerals, herbs, and food supplements*, ed 2, Garden City Park, New York, 1997, Avery Publishing Group.

Kalyn W: *The healing power of vitamins, minerals, and herbs*, Pleasantville, New York, 1999, Reader's Digest.

Linnger J: *The natural pharmacy: complete home reference to natural medicine*, ed 2, 1999, Prima Publishing.

Peterson MS: *Eat to compete: a guide to sports nutrition*, ed 2, St Louis, 1996, Mosby.

White LB: *The herbal drugstore*, 2000, Rodale, Inc.

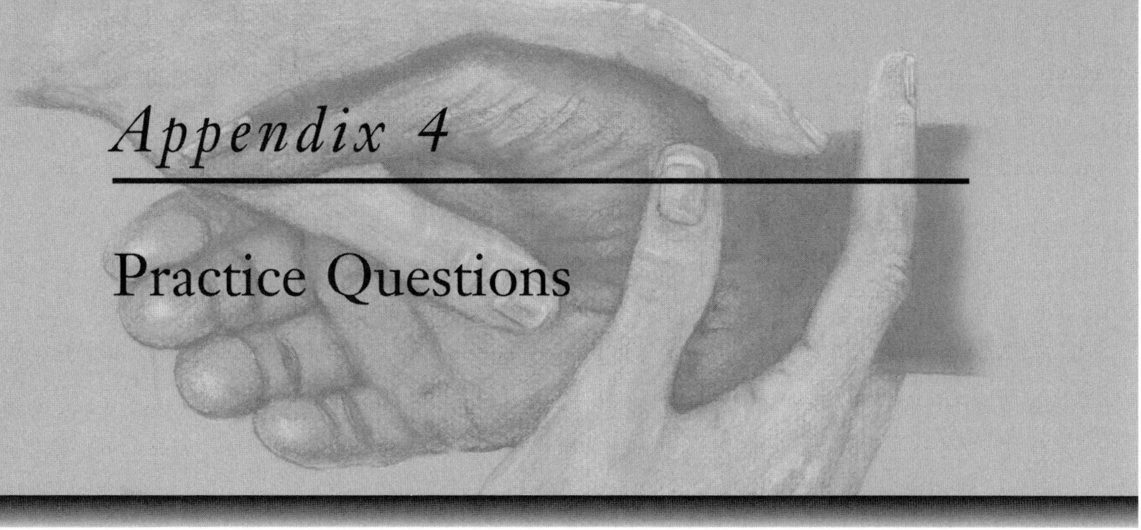

Appendix 4

Practice Questions

The following are more than 200 questions for you to answer as a self-review of the material you have learned in this text.

1. The articular disc of the wrist is also known as which of the following?

A. The triangular fibrocartilage (TFC)
B. Space of Poirier
C. Arcade of Struthers
D. Distal radioulnar (DRU) joint

2. What procedure provides fusion at the distal radial joint with the creation of a pseudoarthrosis proximal to the fusion to allow for forearm rotation?

A. Darrach procedure
B. Sauve-Kapandji
C. Four-corner fusion
D. None of the above

3. A fracture of the radial styloid is termed which of the following?

A. Smith's fracture
B. Die punch fracture
C. Chauffeur's fracture
D. Colles fracture

4. The Frykman's classification system classifies fractures of which of the following?

A. Elbow
B. DRU joint
C. Proximal interphalangeal (PIP) joint
D. Thumb

5. Which portion of the triangular fibrocartilage complex (TFCC) is avascular?

A. Peripheral
B. External
C. Central
D. None of the above

6. What does CIND stand for?

A. Carpal instability nondissociative
B. Carpal icebreakers normal distance
C. Carpal independence not disoriented
D. None of the above

7. Four-bone fusion includes which of the following four bones?

A. Scaphoid, lunate, capitate, hamate
B. Capitate, scaphoid, lunate, triquetrum
C. Trapezium, trapezoid, capitate, hamate
D. Lunate, capitate, hamate, triquetrum

8. Speed's test is used to assess which of the following?

A. Tennis elbow
B. Trigger finger
C. Biceps tendonitis
D. Rotator cuff pathology

9. What type of scar is considered an extreme variant of hypertrophic scars?

A. Carloid
B. Fire
C. Swollen
D. Keloid

10. During the initial stage of a burn (first 24 to 72 hours), the hand should be elevated to what level?

A. Above the heart
B. To heart level but not above
C. Below the heart
D. All of the above are appropriate.

11. What finger is *most* often affected by tendon ruptures in rheumatoid arthritis (RA) patients?

A. Small
B. Ring
C. Middle
D. Index

12. What deformity presents with hyperextension of the PIP joint and flexion of the distal interphalangeal (DIP) joint?

A. Boutonnière
B. Mallet
C. Pseudo-boutonnière
D. Swan-neck

13. When treating scleroderma, what is/are the primary hand motions that need to be maintained?

A. Metacarpophalangeal (MCP) joint flexion
B. PIP joint extension
C. Thumb abduction
D. All of the above are primary motions.

14. What is a way to determine if a reflex sympathetic dystrophy/complex regional pain syndrome (RSD/CRPS) patient has sympathetic maintained pain (SMP) or sympathetic independent pain (SIP)?

A. X-ray
B. Magnetic resonance imaging (MRI)
C. Triple-phase bone scan
D. Diagnostic blockade

15. True or False: Conventional transcutaneous electrical nerve stimulation (TENS) is theorized to modulate pain via the gate-control theory of Melzack and Wall.

16. What technique is proposed via Watson and Carlson to treat RSD/CRPS?

A. Stress loading
B. Nerve blocks
C. Active range of motion (AROM)
D. Passive range of motion (PROM)

17. Ultrasound at 1 MHz may have an effect on tissue up to what depth?

A. 5 cm
B. 7 cm
C. 9 cm
D. 10 cm

18. Ultrasound at 3 MHz affects tissues up to what depth?

A. 6 cm
B. 5 cm
C. 4 cm
D. 2 cm

19. What modality uses the induction of topically applied ions into the tissue by application of a low-voltage direct current (DC)?

A. Phonophoresis
B. Iontophoresis
C. Ultrasound
D. Functional electrical stimulation

20. True or False: Primary healing occurs in rigidly immobilized bones.

21. What type of healing occurs when there is motion at the fracture site?

A. Primary
B. Secondary
C. Tertiary
D. Healing cannot occur with motion at the fracture site.

22. Webbed fingers are termed which of the following?

A. Polydactyly
B. Clinodactyly
C. Syndactyly
D. Kirners

23. True or False: A torn radial collateral ligament that becomes trapped superficially to the proximal edge of the adductor aponeurosis is termed a *Stener's lesion.*

24. A rupture of the extensor mechanism of the terminal phalanx is termed which of the following?

A. Jersey finger
B. Mallet finger
C. Flexor digitorum profundus (FDP) rupture
D. Bowler's digit

25. Ruptures of the extensor mechanism of the PIP result in what deformity?

A. Boutonnière
B. Swan-neck
C. Mallet
D. None of the above

26. Avulsion of the FDP is termed which of the following?

A. Mallet finger
B. Jersey finger
C. Baseball finger
D. Bowler's digit

27. What bone ties the axial skeleton to the upper limb?

A. Ribs
B. Collar bone (clavicle)
C. Humerus
D. Sternum

28. What is the only joint that attaches the upper limb directly to the axial skeleton?

A. Sternoclavicular joint
B. Acromioclavicular (AC) joint
C. Glenohumeral joint
D. None of the above

29. Weak or absent adductor function of the thumb results in flexion of the interphalangeal (IP) joint during pinch and is termed which of the following?

A. Stenner's lesion
B. Wartenburg's sign
C. Froment's sign
D. None of the above

30. The abductor pollicis brevis (APB) is innervated by what nerve?

A. Median
B. Ulnar
C. Radial
D. Posterior interosseous nerve (PIN)

31. The flexor pollicis brevis (FPB) deep head is innervated by what nerve?

A. Anterior interosseous nerve (AIN)
B. Median
C. PIN
D. Ulnar

32. CMMS stands for which of the following?

A. Casting minimal motion splints
B. Casting motion to mobilize stiffness
C. Casting mainly to manage stiffness
D. Casting to maintain motion from splinting

33. The brachioradialis (BR) is innervated by what nerve?

A. Median
B. Radial
C. Ulnar
D. Long thoracic

34. What test is used with a mild axial compression of the thumb to assess for first carpometacarpal (CMC) joint osteoarthritis (OA)?

A. Finkelstein's
B. Watson's
C. Grind
D. Ballottement

35. The wrist flexion test for carpal tunnel is termed which of the following?

A. Tinel's
B. Finkelstein's
C. Phalen's test
D. All of the above could be correct.

36. What is the term for avascular necrosis of the lunate?

A. Kienbock's disease
B. Preiser's disease
C. Huntington's disease
D. Parkinson's disease

37. What is the term for avascular necrosis of the scaphoid?

A. Kienbock's disease
B. Preiser's disease
C. Huntington's disease
D. Parkinson's disease

38. What does SLAC stand for?

A. Stagnate lunate and capitate
B. Scaphoid lunate access celebrities
C. Scapholunate advanced collapse
D. Scaphoid- and lunate-accelerated coordination

39. True or False: Edema is an accumulation of excessive fluid in the intercellular spaces.

40. How much volume is increased in the interstitial fluids before edema is visible?

A. 30%, as much as 50 ml of edema can go without notice
B. 40%, as much as 65 ml of edema can go without notice
C. 50%, as much as 75 ml of edema can go without notice
D. 60%, as much as 90 ml of edema can go without notice

41. 3.61 on the Semmes Weinstein monofilament test is considered which of the following?

A. Normal
B. Diminished light touch
C. Decreased protective sensation
D. Asensate

42. 4.31 on the Semmes Weinstein monofilament test is considered which of the following?

A. Normal
B. Diminished light touch
C. Diminished protective sensation
D. Asensate

43. True or False: *Creep* is the term that is used when the skin undergoes plastic deformation. The skin becomes tense and begins to fatigue (break down) and is unable to return to normal resting length.

44. What is desiccation in regards to wound healing?

A. Keeping it moist
B. Drying out
C. Keeping it clean
D. Strong odors

45. What is the term for a skin graft that uses the entire epidermis and a portion of the dermis?

A. Split-thickness graft
B. Full-thickness graft
C. Pedicled graft
D. Pedicled flap

46. True or False: A paronychia is a bacterial infection of the nail fold and/or nail plate and is one of the most common infections of the hand.

47. What is the term for a deep infection of the pad of the finger?

A. Glomus tumor
B. Splinter
C. Felon
D. Herpetic whitlow

48. Most animal bites are from which of the following animals?

A. Cats
B. Dogs
C. Bees
D. Rats

49. A superficial viral infection that appears as one or more vesicles on or near the finger pad and is often seen in medical and dental personnel and caregivers is which of the following?

A. Glomus tumor
B. Paronychia
C. Herpetic whitlow
D. Enchondroma

50. What is a growth of granulation tissue above the skin that is caused by a chronic low-grade infection or foreign body called?

A. Pyogenic granuloma
B. Enchondroma
C. Ganglion cyst
D. Herpetic whitlow

51. With what is a pyogenic granuloma best treated?

A. Mitraflex
B. Dry sterile gauze
C. Adaptic
D. Silver nitrate

52. After a dorsal dislocation of the PIP joint, how should the patient be positioned?

A. Dorsal extension block splint with the amount of flexion required to keep the finger reduced (25 degrees or less)
B. Dorsal extension block splint with full extension allowed at the PIP joint
C. Volar splint with the PIP joint at 10 degrees of flexion
D. Volar splint holding the PIP joint at 0 for 6 weeks

53. The flexor digitorum superficialis (FDS) is absent in what percentage of patients?

A. 21%
B. 31%
C. 41%
D. 51%

54. How many pulleys are on the thumb?

A. One
B. Two
C. Three
D. Four

55. What are the most important finger pulleys?

A. A1 and A3
B. A2 and A4
C. A1, A2, and A3
D. All pulleys are equally important.

56. What position provides maximum FDS glide?

A. Hook fist
B. Full fist
C. Straight fist
D. Full extension

57. What disease has been considered synonymous with factitious edema?

A. Secretan's
B. Faker's
C. Madelung's
D. Longerberger's

58. What is the most disabling impairment after rupture of the extensor pollicis longus (EPL)?

A. Loss of MCP joint extension
B. Loss of IP joint flexion
C. Loss of IP extension
D. Loss of CMC joint extension

59. What is the biggest impairment after a boutonnière deformity?

A. MCP extension contracture
B. Lack of DIP joint flexion
C. PIP joint stiffness
D. Lack of PIP joint extension

60. What zone is over the MCP joint?

A. Zone 1
B. Zone 3
C. Zone 4
D. Zone 5

61. Carpal tunnel syndrome (CTS) patients should be splinted with the wrist in what position?

A. Wrist at 20 degrees of extension
B. Wrist at 20 degrees of flexion
C. Neutral
D. Splinting is contraindicated.

62. True or False: The ulnar nerve arises from the medial cord of the brachial plexus.

63. True or False: The elbow should be splinted in 70 degrees at night for cubital tunnel syndrome.

64. Which is *not* one of the four *Ps* with compartment syndrome?

A. Pain with passive muscle stretch
B. Paresthesias
C. Pallor
D. All of the above are correct.

65. What two tendons pass through the first dorsal compartment?

A. EPL and extensor pollicis brevis (EPB)
B. Abductor pollicis longus (APL) and EPB
C. Abductor pollicis brevis (APB) and EPB
D. Extensor digitorum communis (EDC) and EPB

66. What tendons are involved with intersection syndrome?

A. Extensor carpi radialis longus (ECRL), EDC, APL, and EPB
B. ECRL, extensor carpi radialis brevis (ECRB), extensor indicis proprius (EIP), and EPB
C. ECRL, ECRB, APL, and EPB
D. ECRL, ECRB, APL, and APB

67. What is the most common soft-tissue tumor of the hand and wrist?

A. Ganglion cysts
B. Lipoma
C. Enchondroma
D. Glomus tumor

68. True or False: A Z-plasty procedure to release a Dupuytren's contracture is termed a *McCash procedure*.

69. What artery provides the primary blood supply to the hand?

A. Radial
B. Median
C. Ulnar
D. All of the above provide equal contribution.

70. What is the recommended Jamar Dynamometer handle position by the American Society of Surgery of the Hand (ASSH)?

A. First
B. Second
C. Third
D. Fourth

71. What is the normal carrying angle of the elbow in males?

A. 5 degrees
B. 15 degrees
C. 25 degrees
D. 35 degrees

72. True or False: The interosseous membrane is a structure that binds the radius and ulna together.

73. True or False: The MCP collateral ligament is taut in extension.

74. True or False: Systemic lupus erythematosus is a disease that affects the major body organs.

75. A wheelbarrow is an example of what type of lever?

A. First class
B. Second class
C. Third class
D. It is not a lever.

76. The retrovascular cord in Dupuytren's disease is responsible for contracture at which joint level?

A. DIP
B. PIP
C. MCP
D. CMC

77. A patient with RA is unable to flex the thumb at the IP joint after working in the garden. What might she be diagnosed with?

A. Madelung's
B. Scapholunate (SL) ligament tear
C. Mannerfelt
D. Preiser's

78. How should a patient be positioned after a boxer's fracture?

A. MCP flexed with IPs extended
B. MCPs extended with IPs flexed
C. MCP flexed with IPs flexed to 30 degrees
D. MCPs extended and IPs extended

79. A boxer's fracture occurs in what part of the metacarpal?

A. Base
B. Shaft
C. Neck
D. It does not occur in the metacarpal.

80. What is the most commonly injured carpal bone?

A. Scaphoid
B. Lunate
C. Capitate
D. Triquetrum

81. What is the Watson's test used to diagnose?

A. Lunotriquetral (LT) injuries
B. SL injuries
C. Interosseous injuries
D. TFCC tears

82. A disruption of the radioulnar joint displaced radial head fracture and proximal migration of the radius describes what injury?

A. Galezzi
B. Essex-Lopresti injury
C. TFCC tears
D. Monteggia

83. What structure in Dupuytren's disease is solely responsible for the development of contractures involving the MCP joint?

A. Palmer nodules
B. Pretendinous band
C. Grayson's ligament
D. Cleland's ligament

84. True or False: Lister's tubercle is a useful anatomic landmark on the dorsal distal ulna.

85. Which of the following muscles is *not* innervated by the AIN?

A. Flexor pollicis longus (FPL)
B. FDP
C. Pronator quadratus (PQ)
D. All of the above are innervated by the AIN.

86. The coracobrachialis muscle is innervated by what nerve?

A. Muscolocutaneous
B. Radial
C. PIN
D. AIN

87. Ten to what power is considered bacterial infection?

A. 10 to the second
B. 10 to the third
C. 10 to the fourth
D. 10 to the fifth

88. What nerve passes through the quadrangular space?

A. Long thoracic
B. Dorsal scapular
C. Axillary
D. No nerve is in this space.

89. What type of suture is used around a core suture in flexor tendon repairs?

A. Two-strand
B. Four-strand
C. Six-strand
D. Epitendinous

90. What nerve is entrapped in Wartenberg's syndrome?

A. Dorsal branch of the ulnar nerve
B. AIN
C. PIN
D. Radial sensory

91. What is the term for a nontraumatic flexion deformity of the PIP joint of the small finger?

A. Camptodactyly
B. Clinodactyly
C. Syndactyly
D. Kirners

92. True or False: A Martin-Gruber connection is an anatomic communication between the median and the ulnar nerves in the forearm.

93. Winging of the scapula occurs when what nerve is damaged?

A. Dorsal scapular
B. Radial
C. Long thoracic
D. It does not occur from nerve damage.

94. Which of the following is *not* part of the contents of the carpal tunnel?

A. Median nerve
B. Palmaris longus
C. FDS
D. FDP

95. What position provides the maximum glide to the FDP?

A. Hook fist
B. Straight fist
C. Full fist
D. All of the above provide equal glide.

96. True or False: Allen's test is the best clinical test for evaluating the arterial blood supply to the hand.

97. What is the most common joint disease in the upper extremity?

A. RA
B. OA
C. Psoriatic arthritis
D. All of the above are equally common.

98. What percentage of people over 65 has OA on x-rays?

A. 30%
B. 50%
C. 70%
D. 90%

99. True or False: Bouchard's is the node on the dorsal aspect of the DIP joint in OA.

100. True or False: Heberden's is the node at the PIP joint in OA.

101. What is the syndrome that occurs in the extensors with OA and begins with the small fingers and moves down the line?

A. Vaughn-Jackson syndrome
B. Caput ulnae syndrome
C. Preiser's disease
D. Psoriatic arthritis

102. Which of the following muscle(s) extends the IP joints of the digits?

A. Interossei
B. Lumbricals
C. EDC
D. All of the above can contribute to extension.

103. True or False: The lumbricals are weak MCP flexors.

104. Which muscle resembles an earthworm?

A. Interossei
B. Lumbricals
C. Adductor pollicis
D. FPB

105. True or False: Manual edema mobilization (MEM) is acceptable when infection is present.

106. True or False: CRPS type two presents with a corresponding peripheral nerve or nerve branch injury.

107. Which of the following is not a criterion of the International Association Pain Society (IAPS) for a diagnosis of CRPS?

A. An inciting noxious event or immobilization
B. Continuing pain that is disproportionate to the event
C. Evidence of edema at some time, changes in skin blood flow, or abnormal sudomotor activity
D. Limited range of motion (ROM)

108. Which neural tension test puts the patients arm into the pronated position along with wrist flexion?

A. Median nerve
B. Ulnar nerve
C. Radial nerve
D. All of the above

109. Which of the following is *not* a contraindication to neural tension as a treatment technique?

A. Recently repaired peripheral nerve
B. Malignancy
C. Active inflammatory conditions
D. All of the above are contraindications.

110. Which of the following is *not* a contraindication to MEM?

A. If the patient has congestive heart failure
B. Over areas of inflammation
C. Blood clot or hematoma
D. All of the above are contraindications.

111. True or False: MEM is especially effective for treating the chronically edematous hand.

112. True or False: MEM should begin in the inflammatory stage of wound healing.

113. True or False: Trigger fingers can be released with open percutaneous methods.

114. True or False: The MCP joint collateral ligaments are taught in extension.

115. Which of the following is a superficial infection of the skin?

A. Cellulitis
B. Mycobacteria
C. Pyogenic granuloma
D. Felon

116. True or False: The pedicle is the part of the flap that provides the skin coverage.

117. What is a new surgical device that is used for tendon repairs that allows therapists to being early motion?

A. Teno-fix
B. Collagenase
C. Mitek anchors
D. Button pull-out

118. Which of the following is the excursion distance for the digital flexors?

A. 2 to 3 cm
B. 3 to 4 cm
C. 4 to 5 cm
D. 6 to 7 cm

119. Which tendon transfer for median nerve palsy uses the palmaris longus?

A. Huber
B. Stiles Bunnell
C. Camitz
D. Rolye-Thompson

120. Which is the most common primary bone tumor in the hand?

A. Enchondroma
B. Glomerulus tumor
C. Volar wrist ganglion
D. Lipoma

121. A patient presents to your clinic with complaints of persistent numbness in the index and long fingers. She reports that the numbness increases when she drives or does needlepoint. She also reports often waking up at night with pain in her hand. Which is the most likely diagnosis?

A. Compression of the ulnar nerve at Guyon's canal
B. Compression of the ulnar nerve at the cubital tunnel
C. Compression of the median nerve at the wrist
D. Compression of the radial nerve at the arcade of Frohse

122. You are treating a patient with a diagnosis of pronator syndrome. Which of the following is not a potential site of compression in pronator syndrome?

A. The arcade of Struthers
B. The lacertus fibrosus
C. The pronator teres
D. The arch of the FDS

123. You are treating a patient who complains of pain in the forearm as well as weakness that affects the thumb and index fingers. Evaluation reveals minimal function of the FDP to the index and long fingers and decreased function of the FPL. Sensation is normal. Which syndrome might this patient have?

A. CTS
B. AIN syndrome
C. Radial nerve palsy
D. PIN syndrome

124. Which of the following is not a site of compression in radial tunnel syndrome?

A. Fibrous bands anterior to radial head
B. Recurrent radial vessels
C. Tendinous margin of the ECRB
D. The arcade of Frohse
E. All of the above are sites of compression.

125. You are treating a patient who complains of dorsal wrist pain and numbness affecting the thumb, index, and long fingers. The patient has severe shooting pain with thumb and wrist motion. Which diagnosis might be appropriate for this patient?

A. Radial tunnel syndrome
B. CTS
C. Wartenberg's syndrome
D. Pronator syndrome

126. You are treating a patient who complains of intermittent pain along the medial proximal forearm and numbness in the small and ring fingers. He reports waking at night with numbness in the hand and pain in his arm. The patient also has a positive Tinel's sign at the medial epicondyle. Which diagnosis might be appropriate for this patient?

A. CTS
B. Cubital tunnel syndrome
C. Pronator syndrome
D. AIN syndrome

127. Which of the following is not a compression site of the ulnar nerve in cubital tunnel syndrome?

A. Medial head of the triceps
B. Aponeurosis of the flexor carpi ulnaris (FCU)
C. Ligament of Struthers
D. All of the above are compression sites for the ulnar nerve.

128. Which of the following is a contraindication for replantation of digits?

A. Proximal phalanx level amputation of the thumb in a 40-year-old man
B. Multiple digit amputation in a 65-year-old woman
C. Distal fingertip amputation in a 35-year-old man
D. Distal tip amputation in a 7-year-old child

129. You are treating a patient after his replant. Venous outflow appears to be a problem. What should you do?

A. Lower the limb
B. Elevate the limb
C. Tighten the dressing
D. Make the limb colder

130. What is the maximal warm ischemic time that will not produce deleterious effects for digit replantation?

A. 2 hours
B. 6 hours
C. 12 hours
D. 24 hours

131. Pinch strength is achieved primarily by muscular innervation supplied by which of the following?

A. The deep branch of the ulnar nerve
B. The AIN
C. The PIN
D. The deep branch of the median nerve

132. Perception of touch in the fingertips is mediated by which of the following?

A. Nonmyelinated C fibers
B. Large, myelinated group A–beta fibers
C. Small, myelinated free nerve endings
D. Myelinated C fibers

133. The deep motor branch of the ulnar nerve enters the hand through which of the following?

A. Carpal tunnel
B. Cubital tunnel
C. Guyon's canal
D. Hunter's canal

134. An advancing Tinel's sign along the course of a repaired nerve is which of the following?

A. Indicative of the number of regenerating axons progressing down the nerve
B. The only way to predict return of nerve function
C. An indication of the presence of both sensory and motor axons distal to the repair site
D. An indication of nerve regeneration but not a predictive value

135. By week 3, a sutured wound has which percentage of its tensile strength?

A. 15%
B. 35%
C. 50%
D. 75%

136. A pathologic process similar to Dupuytren's disease occurs in which of the following?

A. Albright's disease
B. Ledderhose's disease
C. Dercum's disease
D. Paschen's disease

137. A patient exhibits tenderness in the snuffbox. Which bone might be fractured?

A. Lunate
B. Triquetrum
C. Scaphoid
D. Trapezium

138. What is stenosing tenosynovitis involving the APL and the EPB called?

A. de Quervain's disease
B. Preiser's disease
C. Intersection syndrome
D. Wartenberg's syndrome

139. Which of the following muscles abducts the fingers?

A. Volar interossei
B. Dorsal interossei
C. Lumbricals
D. FPL

140. As the median nerve courses through the carpal tunnel, it innervates which muscle first after crossing the wrist?

A. Pronator quadratus
B. Opponens pollicis
C. APB
D. FPB

141. When manual muscle testing (MMT) the supinator, you are evaluating which nerve?

A. Radial nerve
B. Musculocutaneous nerve
C. Ulnar nerve
D. Median nerve

142. The resisted middle finger test is used to evaluate irritation of which nerve?

A. Median
B. Radial
C. Ulnar
D. Musculocutaneous

143. Which muscle is found in extensor compartment five?

A. EPB
B. Extensor carpi ulnaris (ECU)
C. EDC
D. Extensor digiti minimi (EDM)

144. Which dermatome provides sensory innervation to the middle finger?

A. C5
B. C6
C. C7
D. C8

145. A distal radius fracture presenting with volar displacement of the distal fragment is called which of the following?

A. Colles' fracture
B. Essex-Lopresti fracture
C. Smith's fracture
D. Galeazzi fracture

146. Which of the following is not an intraarticular fracture?

A. Bennett's
B. Barton's
C. Monteggia
D. All of the above are intraarticular fractures.

147. Ganglion cysts occur commonly and are most often present where?

A. At the dorsal SL interval
B. At the volar SL interval
C. At the volar LT interval
D. At the dorsal LT interval

148. Stress loading is a treatment used for RSD. Lois Carlson recommends how many minutes of scrubbing for the initial treatment?

A. 3 minutes
B. 6 minutes
C. 9 minutes
D. 15 minutes

149. Which of the following is the most common rheumatoid thumb deformity?

A. Swan-neck deformity
B. Lateral instability of the IP joint
C. Boutonnière deformity
D. None of the above

150. Which of the following thumb muscles is innervated by two nerves?

A. Opponens pollicis
B. FPL
C. APB
D. FPB

151. Which of the following muscles should be the first to be reinnervated after a laceration of the median nerve above the elbow?

A. Pronator teres
B. Supinator
C. Palmaris longus
D. Flexor carpi radialis (FCR)

152. Which structure centralizes the tendons of the EDC over the MCP joints?

A. Transverse fibers
B. Collateral ligaments
C. Sagittal bands
D. Oblique retinacular ligament (ORL)

153. Which of the following is the anatomic term for the communications between the extensor tendons on the dorsum of the hand?

A. Sagittal bands
B. Lateral bands
C. Juncturae tendinea
D. Interosseous membrane

154. Which of the following are the primary receptors for tactile gnosis?

A. Merkel cells
B. Meissner cells
C. Pacinian corpuscles
D. Ruffini end organ

155. Which is the first sensation to return after nerve repair?

A. Light touch
B. Pain and temperature
C. Deep pressure
D. Moving two-point discrimination

156. Which of the following is the classification for the least complicated nerve injury?

A. Neuronotmesis
B. Neuralgia
C. Neuropraxia
D. Neuroma

157. Which percentage of ROM is lost with a radiocarpal fusion?

A. 12%
B. 27%
C. 55%
D. 80%

158. Which muscle is most commonly involved in a rotator cuff repair?

A. Subscapularis
B. Infraspinatus
C. Supraspinatus
D. Teres major

159. You are treating a patient with ulnar nerve problems. You notice a positive Froment's sign. Which muscle is atrophied?

A. APB
B. Adductor pollicis
C. Opponens pollicis
D. FPB

160. Which of the following carpal bones does not articulate with the lunate?

A. Trapezium
B. Triquetrum
C. Hamate
D. Capitate
E. Scaphoid

161. Which of the following tendons does not originate off of the ulna?

A. EIP
B. EPL
C. FPL
D. APL

162. Gamekeeper's thumb refers to which of the following?

A. Radial collateral ligament injury of the thumb at the MCP joint
B. Fracture at the base of the thumb
C. Ulnar collateral ligament injury of the thumb at the MCP joint
D. Fracture at the radial styloid

163. A positive Terry Thomas sign on a radiograph indicates which of the following?

A. SL dissociation
B. Scaphoid fracture
C. LT tear
D. TFCC tear

164. What is the name of a test that Dellon developed?

A. Two-point discrimination
B. Semmes-Weinstein
C. Moving two-point discrimination
D. Ninhydrin

165. A patient presents with hyperextension of the thumb MCP joint with lateral pinch after an

ulnar nerve lesion. What is the term for this hand posture?

A. Froment's sign
B. Duchenne's sign
C. Jeanne's sign
D. Wartenberg's sign

166. The patient described in the previous question presents with a flattened metacarpal arch. What is the name for this clinical presentation?

A. Froment's sign
B. Masse's sign
C. Duchenne's sign
D. Wartenberg's sign

167. Paraffin should be applied at which temperature?

A. 160° to 170° F
B. 125° to 135° F
C. 102° to 104° F
D. 80° to 90° F

168. Which type of prosthesis is a Pillet prosthesis?

A. Myoelectric hand
B. Above-elbow prosthesis
C. Prosthesis for shoulder disarticulation
D. Aesthetic prosthesis

169. You are performing MMT on a patient's biceps. The patient is able to achieve full ROM against gravity. He is not able to tolerate any resistance. Which muscle grade is he?

A. Trace
B. Poor
C. Fair
D. Good
E. Normal

170. Which structures pass through the quadrangular space?

A. Median nerve and brachial artery
B. Ulnar nerve and brachial artery
C. Axillary nerve and posterior circumflex artery
D. Axillary nerve and anterior circumflex humeral artery

171. The rotator cuff comprises which muscles?

A. Supraspinatus, infraspinatus, subscapularis, and teres minor
B. Supraspinatus, subscapularis, teres major, and infraspinatus
C. Supraspinatus, infraspinatus, teres major, and latissimus dorsi
D. Teres minor, infraspinatus, subscapularis, and coracobrachialis

172. All but which of the following muscles insert into the greater tuberosity?

A. Supraspinatus
B. Infraspinatus
C. Teres minor
D. Subscapularis

173. The mobile wad of Henry is composed of all but which of the following muscles?

A. BR
B. ECRL
C. EDC
D. ECRB

174. What is the normal "carrying angle" of the elbow in females?

A. 50 degrees valgus
B. 15 to 20 degrees valgus
C. 50 degrees varus
D. 10 degrees varus

175. You are treating a patient with a radial head fracture and a disruption of the DRU joint. What is this injury called?

A. Chauffeur's fracture
B. Monteggia's fracture
C. Bennett's fracture
D. Essex-Lopresti injury

176. After elbow dislocation, what nerve is most commonly injured from valgus stress at the time of the dislocation?

A. Radial nerve
B. Median nerve
C. Ulnar nerve
D. None of the above

177. The tendon most commonly involved in lateral epicondylitis is which of the following?

A. ECRL
B. ECRB
C. EDC
D. ECU

178. A patient has sustained a severe injury to the elbow, and the surgeon has determined that fusion is the only option. In which position is the elbow usually fused to maximize function?

A. Flexed at 130 degrees
B. Flexed at 90 degrees
C. Flexed at 60 degrees
D. Flexed at 30 degrees

179. You are treating a patient who reports that he felt a "pop" in his shoulder while attempting to lift a bag of heavy groceries. You note a bulge in the anterior aspect of his right arm. What might have happened to this patient?

A. Rupture of the long head of the biceps
B. Rupture of the triceps
C. Distal humerus fracture
D. Proximal humerus fracture

180. Which of the following is *not* a provocative test for thoracic outlet syndrome?

A. Adson's test
B. Allen's test
C. Wright's hyperabduction test
D. Costoclavicular maneuver

181. Which ligament holds the skin in place on the digit?

A. The ORL
B. The transverse retinacular ligament
C. Cleland ligament
D. The collateral ligaments

182. Which of the following may be recommended for treatment of acute lateral epicondylitis?

A. Wrist splint at 30 to 40 degrees of extension
B. Wrist splint with wrist at neutral
C. Wrist splint with wrist in slight flexion
D. No splint is indicated.

183. In relation to sympathetic function, *vasomotor* refers to which of the following?

A. Skin color
B. Sweat
C. Gooseflesh response
D. Trophic nail changes

184. In reference to the Semmes-Weinstein monofilaments, monofilament number 3.22 correlates with which of the following?

A. Normal sensation
B. Diminished light touch
C. Diminished protective sensation
D. Loss of protective sensation

185. When fabricating a splint for a patient with ulnar nerve palsy, the therapist must take into consideration which of the following goals of the splint?

A. Assist function of the thumb for tip prehension
B. Assist grasp by providing a stable wrist in extension
C. Prevent clawing and assist in grasp and release
D. Prevent overstretch of the wrist extensors

186. When performing MMT for the EDC, the therapist must do which of the following?

A. Position the forearm in pronation with the wrist stabilized and ask the patient to extend the MCP joints with the IP joints flexed
B. Have the forearm supinated and the wrist stabilized and ask the patient to extend the MCP joints with the IP joints extended
C. Have the forearm in neutral and the wrist stabilized and ask the patient to extend the MCP joints with the IP joints extended
D. Have the forearm pronated and the wrist stabilized and ask the patient to extend the index finger while all other fingers are flexed

187. In reference to functional electrical stimulation, amplitude refers to which of the following?

A. Duration of treatment
B. Intensity
C. Duty cycle
D. Frequency

188. In relation to the muscle and nerve fibers in the strength duration curve, which of the following is true?

A. Muscle fibers require low-intensity, short-duration current, and nerve fibers require long-duration, high-intensity current before response.
B. Nerve fibers require low-intensity, short-duration current, and muscle fibers require long-duration, high-intensity current before response.
C. Nerve fibers require long-duration, low-intensity current, and muscle fibers require short-duration, high-intensity current before response.
D. Nerve and muscle tissues respond in an equal manner to elicit a response.

189. During treatment of a patient who has a proximal phalanx fracture with stable internal fixation, when can AROM and PROM exercises be initiated?

A. Between 1 and 3 days after surgery
B. 1 week after surgery
C. 3 to 4 weeks after surgery
D. 6 weeks after surgery

190. A 26-year-old male sustained a crush injury to the DIP joint 3 months ago. The patient has difficulty performing prehension tasks primarily because of hypersensitivity. However, his occupation requires prehension tasks. The patient's insurance allows only one visit for hand rehabilitation. What should be done?

A. A Stax splint should be provided to protect the DIP joint
B. The patient should be instructed to wear latex gloves to decrease the irritation of the DIP joint
C. The patient should be given a TENS unit
D. The patient should be taught desensitization techniques

191. According to Gelberman, which amount of tendon glide is needed to stimulate intrinsic healing at the repair site without creating significant gap formation?

A. 1 to 2 mm
B. 3 to 4 mm
C. 4 to 6 mm
D. 8 to 10 mm

192. In relation to ergonomic management, the recommended handle length for a hand-held tool is which of the following?

A. 4 cm
B. 9 cm
C. 11 cm
D. 15 cm

193. A complication that may occur after a distal radius fracture is which of the following?

A. EPL rupture
B. Radial nerve compression
C. Median nerve compression
D. A and C are correct.
E. B and C are correct.

194. What is the most common carpal coalition?

A. Scaphoid-triquetrum
B. Lunate-triquetrum
C. Hamate-triquetrum
D. Scaphoid-hamate

195. Which of the following does not serve as a border for the anatomic snuffbox?

A. APL
B. EPB
C. EPL
D. APB

196. Which of the following is not true about a myoelectric prosthesis?

A. It is considered a body-powered prosthesis.
B. It does not require a body harness.
C. It is powered by the amplified action potentials of underlying muscles.
D. It has no sensory feedback.

197. A patient presents to the clinic with a zone IV flexor tendon laceration. Where is this zone?

A. Within the carpal tunnel
B. Proximal to the carpal tunnel
C. Within the fibroosseous canal
D. At the level of palm

198. You are treating a patient in the clinic who has greater passive DIP joint flexion with the PIP joint flexed than with it extended. Which structure is involved?

A. Sagittal band
B. Lateral band
C. ORL
D. FDP

199. Which of the following is considered the most severe form of nerve injury?

A. Neuropraxia
B. Neurotmesis
C. Axonotmesis
D. Wallerian degeneration

200. Which of the following is the most common ganglion to develop in the hand and the wrist?

A. Volar wrist ganglion
B. Mucus cyst
C. Dorsal wrist ganglion
D. Squamous-cell carcinoma

201. Which of the following is not true about the management of a patient with frostbite?

A. The frozen extremity should be allowed to rewarm at room temperature.
B. The patient's core body temperature should be restored with external warming and ingestion of warm fluids by mouth.
C. The frozen extremity should be rewarmed rapidly at 40° to 44°C.
D. All of the above are true.

202. Which angle of pull is recommended when using dynamic splinting?

A. 30-degree angle
B. 60-degree angle
C. 90-degree angle
D. 120-degree angle

203. Which grade of movement is used to perform a small amplitude of movement at the beginning of the ROM to treat a painful joint?

A. Grade I
B. Grade II
C. Grade III
D. Grade IV

Answer Key

1. A, **2.** B, **3.** C, **4.** B, **5.** C, **6.** A, **7.** D, **8.** C, **9.** D, **10.** B, **11.** A, **12.** D, **13.** D, **14.** D, **15.** True, **16.** A, **17.** A, **18.** D, **19.** B, **20.** True, **21.** B, **22.** C, **23.** False, **24.** B, **25.** A, **26.** B, **27.** B, **28.** A, **29.** C, **30.** A, **31.** D, **32.** B, **33.** B, **34.** C, **35.** C, **36.** A, **37.** B, **38.** C, **39.** True, **40.** A, **41.** B, **42.** C, **43.** True, **44.** B, **45.** A, **46.** True, **47.** C, **48.** B, **49.** C, **50.** A, **51.** D, **52.** A, **53.** A, **54.** C, **55.** B, **56.** C, **57.** A, **58.** A, **59.** B, **60.** D, **61.** C, **62.** True, **63.** False, **64.** D, **65.** B, **66.** C, **67.** A, **68.** False, **69.** C, **70.** B, **71.** A, **72.** True, **73.** False, **74.** True, **75.** B, **76.** A, **77.** C, **78.** A, **79.** C, **80.** A, **81.** B, **82.** B, **83.** B, **84.** False, **85.** D, **86.** A, **87.** D, **88.** C, **89.** D, **90.** D, **91.** A, **92.** True, **93.** C, **94.** B, **95.** C, **96.** True, **97.** B, **98.** C, **99.** False, **100.** False, **101.** A, **102.** D, **103.** True, **104.** B, **105.** False, **106.** True, **107.** D, **108.** C, **109.** D, **110.** D, **111.** True, **112.** False, **113.** True, **114.** False, **115.** A, **116.** False, **117.** A, **118.** D, **119.** C, **120.** A, **121.** C, **122.** A, **123.** B, **124.** E, **125.** C, **126.** B, **127.** C, **128.** C, **129.** B, **130.** C, **131.** A, **132.** B, **133.** C, **134.** D, **135.** A, **136.** B, **137.** C, **138.** A, **139.** B, **140.** C, **141.** A, **142.** B, **143.** D, **144.** C, **145.** C, **146.** C, **147.** A, **148.** A, **149.** C, **150.** D, **151.** A, **152.** C, **153.** C, **154.** A, **155.** B, **156.** C, **157.** C, **158.** C, **159.** B, **160.** A, **161.** C, **162.** C, **163.** A, **164.** C, **165.** C. **166.** B, **167.** B, **168.** D, **169.** C, **170.** C, **171.** A, **172.** D, **173.** C, **174.** B, **175.** D, **176.** C, **177.** B, **178.** B, **179.** A, **180.** B, **181.** C, **182.** A, **183.** A, **184.** B, **185.** C, **186.** A, **187.** B, **188.** B, **189.** A, **190.** D, **191.** B, **192.** B, **193.** D, **194.** B, **195.** D, **196.** A, **197.** A, **198.** C, **199.** B, **200.** C, **201.** A, **202.** C, **203.** A.

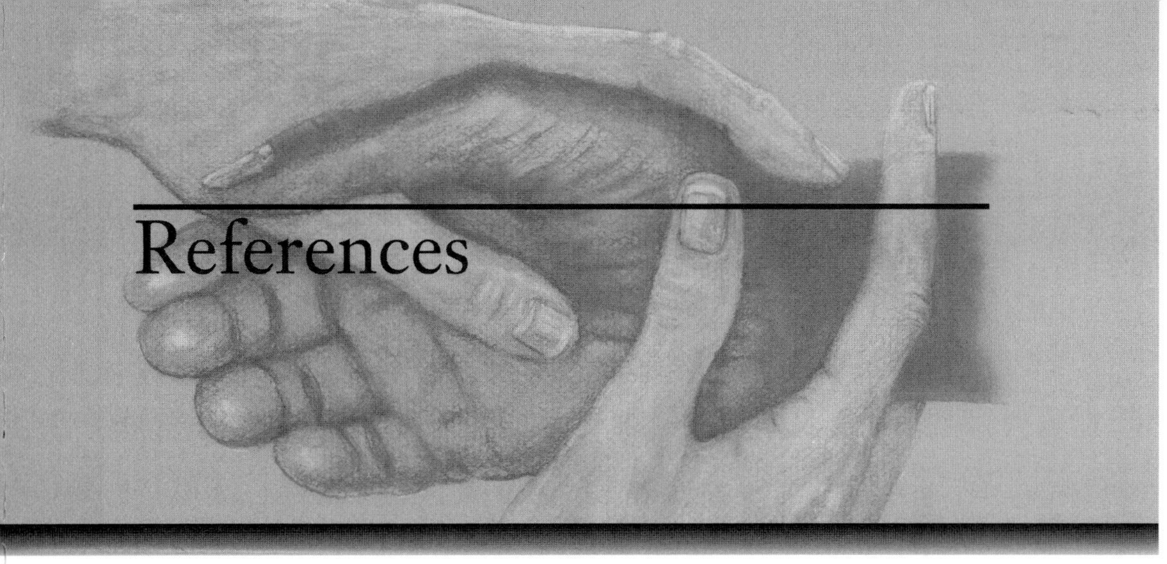

References

Ablove RH, Howell RM: The physiology and technique of skin grafting, *Hand Clin* 13:2, 1997.

Abram SE, Haddox JD: *The pain clinic manual*, ed 2, Baltimore, 2000, Lippincott Williams & Wilkins.

Achauer BM: The burned hand. In Green DR, Hotchkiss RN, Pederson WC, eds: *Green's Operative hand surgery*, ed 4, pp. 2045-2060, Philadelphia, 1999, Churchill Livingstone.

Adams BD, Samani JE, Holley KA: Triangular fibrocartilage injury: a laboratory model, *J Hand Surg* [Am] 21(2): 189-193, 1996.

Adams LS, Greene LW, Topoozian E: Range of motion. In *ASHT clinical assessment recommendations*, ed 2, Chicago, 1992, American Society of Hand Therapists.

Allan CH, Joshi A, Lichtman DM: Kienbock's disease: diagnosis and treatment, *J Am Acad Orthop Surg* 9(2):128-136, 2001.

Almquist EE: Kienbock's disease, *Hand Clin* 3(1):141-148, 1987.

Alter S, Feldon P, Terrono AL: Pathomechanics of deformities in the arthritic hand and wrist. In Mackin EJ, Callahan AD, Skirven TM, et al, eds: *Rehabilitation of the hand and upper extremity*, ed 5, pp. 1545-1555, St Louis, 2002, Mosby.

Alverez O, Rozint J, Wiseman D: Moist environment for healing: matching the dressing to the wound, *Wound* 1:35, 1989.

American Society for Surgery of the Hand: *Hand surgery update*, Rosemont, IL, 1996, American Academy of Orthopaedic Surgeons.

Anderson JE: *Grant's Atlas of anatomy*, ed 8, Baltimore, 1983, Williams & Wilkins.

Anderson, Good, Kerr, et al: *Low level laser therapy in the treatment of carpal tunnel syndrome*, Automotive Safety and Health Research, Detroit, 1995, NAO Research and Development Center.

Andrew JR, Jelsma RD, Joyce ME, et al: Open surgical procedures for injuries to the elbow in throwers. In Drez D, Jr, DeLee JC, Miller MD, eds: *Operative techniques in sports medicine*, pp. 109-113, Philadelphia, 1996, WB Saunders.

Angelides AC: Ganglions of the hand and wrist. In Green DR, Hotchkiss RN, Pederson WC, eds: *Green's Operative hand surgery*, ed 4, pp. 2171-2183, Philadelphia, 1999, Churchill Livingstone.

Arnheim DD, Prentice W: *Principles of athletic training*, ed 8, St Louis, 1993, Mosby.

Aszmann OC, Kress K, Dellon AL: Results of decompression of peripheral nerves in diabetics: a prospective, blinded study, *Plast Reconstr Surg* 106(4):816-822, 2000.

Athanasian EA: Bone and soft tissue tumors. In Green DP, Hotchkiss RN, Pederson WC, eds: *Green's Operative hand surgery*, ed 4, pp. 2223-2253, Philadelphia, 1999, Churchill Livingstone.

Atkins DJ: Adult upper limb prosthetic training. In Bowker JH, Michael JW, eds: *Atlas of limb prosthetics*, ed 2, St Louis, 1992, Mosby.

Atkins DJ, Alley RD: Upper-extremity prosthetics, an emerging specialization in a technologically advanced field, *AOTA Continuing Educ Article*, *OT Practice*, February, 2003.

Atkins DJ, Meier RH: *Comprehensive management of the upper-limb amputee*, New York, 1989, Springer-Verlag.

Aulicino PL: Clinical examination of the hand. In Mackin EJ, Callahan AD, Skirven TM, et al, eds: *Rehabilitation of the hand and upper extremity*, ed 5, pp. 120-142, St. Louis, 2002, Mosby.

Aulicino PL: Neurovascular injuries in the hands of athletes, *Hand Clin* 6(3):455-466, 1990.

Baker LL, Wederich CL, McNeal DR, et al: *Neuromuscular electrical stimulation: a practical guide*, ed 4, Downey, CA, 2000, Los Amigos Research and Education Institute, Inc.

Baltimore Therapeutic Equipment Company user's guide, Hanover, MD.

Baratz ME, Divelbiss B: Fixation of phalangeal fractures, *Hand Clin* 13(4):541-555, 1997.

Barnes DA, Tullos HS: An analysis of 100 symptomatic baseball players, *Am J Sports Med* 6:62-67, 1978.

Barnes J: *Myofascial release* I, Presented Clearwater, FL, January, 1996.

Basti J, Dionysian E, Sherman PW, et al: Management of proximal humeral fractures, *J Hand Ther* 7(2):111-121, 2003.

Beasley RW: General considerations in managing upper-limb amputations, *Orthop Clin North Am* 12(4):743-749, 1981.

Bednar JM, Lersner-Beson, CV: Wrist reconstruction: salvage procedures. In Mackin EJ, Callahan AD, Skirven TM, et al, eds: *Rehabilitation of the hand and upper extremity*, ed 5, pp. 1195-1202, St Louis, 2002, Mosby.

Bednar JM, Osterman L: Carpal instability: evaluation and treatment, *J Am Acad Orthop Surg* 1(1):10-17, 1993.

Belanger AY: *Evidence-based guide to therapeutic physical agents*, Philadelphia, 2002, Lippincott, Williams & Wilkins.

Bell-Krotoski JA: A study of peripheral nerve involvement underlying physical disability of the hand in Hansen's disease, *J Hand Ther* 5:3, 1992.

Bell-Krotoski JA: Preoperative and postoperative management of tendon transfers after median-and ulnar-nerve injury. In Mackin EJ, Callahan AD, Skirven TM, et al, eds: *Rehabilitation of the hand and upper extremity*, ed 5, pp. 799-820, St Louis, 2002, Mosby.

Bell-Krotoski JA: Sensibility testing with the Semmes-Weinstein monofilaments. In Mackin EJ, Callahan AD, Skirven TM, et al, eds: *Rehabilitation of the hand and upper extremity*, ed 5, St Louis, 2002, Mosby.

Berger RA: The anatomy of the ligaments of the wrist and distal radioulnar joints, *Clin Orthop* Feb (383):32-40, 2001.

Berger RA: The anatomy and basic biomechanics of the wrist joint, *J Hand Ther* 9(2):84-93, 1996.

Bertels TH: *Functions of the body harness for upper extremity prosthesis*, Minneapolis, 2003, Otto Bock Health Care.

Biese J: Therapist's evaluation and conservative management of rheumatoid arthritis in the hand and wrist. In Mackin EJ, Callahan AD, Skirven TM, et al, eds: *Rehabilitation of the hand and upper extremity*, ed 5, pp. 1569-1582, St Louis, 2002, Mosby.

Blackmore SM: Therapist's management of ulnar nerve neuropathy at the elbow. In Mackin EJ, Callahan AD, Skirven TM, et al, eds: *Rehabilitation of the hand and upper extremity*, ed 5, pp. 2076-2104, St Louis, 2002, Mosby.

Blackmore SM, Williams DA, Wolf SL: The use of biofeedback in hand rehabilitation. In Mackin EJ, Callahan AD, Skirven TM, et al, eds: *Rehabilitation of the hand and upper extremity*, ed 5, pp. 1779-1795, St Louis, 2002, Mosby.

Blair WF: *Techniques in hand surgery*, Baltimore, 1996, Williams & Wilkins.

Bley L, Seitz WH, Jr: Injuries about the distal ulna in children, *Hand Clin* 14(2):231-237, 1998.

Bogumill G: Functional anatomy of the shoulder. In Hunter JM, Mackin EJ, Callahan AD, eds: *Rehabilitation of the hand: surgery and therapy*, ed 4, St Louis, 1995, Mosby.

Bonatz E, Kramer TD, Masear VR: Rupture of the extensor pollicis longus tendon, *Am J Orthop* 25(2):118-122, 1996.

Bond JR, Berquist TH: Radiologic evaluation of hand and wrist motion, *Hand Clin* 7(1):113-123, 1991.

Boscheinen-Morrin J, Conolly WB: *The hand: fundamentals of therapy*, ed 3, Boston, 2001, Butterworth-Heinemann.

Boyer MI, Strickland JW, Engles DR, et al: Flexor tendon repair and rehabilitation: state of the art in 2002, *J Bone Joint Surg* [Am] 84(9):1684-1706, 2002.

Bowker JH, Michael JW: *Atlas of limb prosthetics: surgical, prosthetic, and rehabilitation principles*, ed 2, St Louis, 1992, Mosby.

Boyes JH: Tendon transfers for radial nerve palsy, *Bull Hosp Joint Dis* 21:97-105, 1960.

Bozentka DJ: Pathogenesis of osteoarthritis. In Mackin EJ, Callahan AD, Skirven TM, et al, eds: *Rehabilitation of the hand and upper extremity*, ed 5, pp. 1637-1645, St Louis, 2002, Mosby.

Brach P, Goitz R: An update on the management of carpal fractures, *J Hand Ther* 16(2):152-160, 2003.

Brand PW, Hollister A: *Clinical mechanics of the hand*, ed 2, St Louis, 1993, Mosby.

Brandsma W: Secondary defects of the hand with intrinsic paralysis: prevention, assessment and treatment, *J Hand Ther* 3(1):14-17, 1990.

Brandt KD: *Diagnosis and nonsurgical management of osteoarthritis*, 1996, Professional Communications, Inc.

Brandt KD: In Kelley W, Harris ED, Jr, Ruddy S, et al, eds: *Textbook of rheumatology*, ed 5, Philadelphia, 1997, WB Saunders.

Brecker L: Jenny McConnell offers new techniques for problem shoulders, *Advance for Physical Therapists* December, 1993.

Brotzman SB: *Clinical orthopaedic rehabilitation*, St Louis, 1996, Mosby.

Brown FE, Hamlet MP, Feehan L: Acute care and rehabilitation of the hand after cold injury. In Mackin EJ, Callahan AD, Skirven TM, et al, eds: *Rehabilitation of the hand and upper extremity*, ed 5, pp. 1527-1539, St Louis, 2002, Mosby.

Brown PW: Reconstruction for pinch in ulnar intrinsic palsy, *Orthop Clin North Am* 5:323-342, 1974.

Browne EZ: Skin grafts. In Green DR, Hotchkiss RN, Pederson WC, eds: *Green's Operative hand surgery*, ed 4, pp. 1759-1782, Philadelphia, 1999, Churchill Livingstone.

Browner BD, Jupiter J, Levine A, et al: *Skeletal trauma: fractures, dislocations, and ligamentous injuries*, Philadelphia, 1992, WB Saunders.

Brushart TM: Nerve repair and grafting. In Mackin EJ, Callahan AD, Skirven TM, et al, eds: *Rehabilitation of the hand and upper extremity*, ed 5, pp. 1381-1403, St Louis, 2002, Mosby.

Bryant RA, Rolstad BS: *Autolysis: a clinical approach to selective debridement*, Minneapolis, 1999, Bryant Rolstad Consultants LLC.

Burkhart SS, Morgan CD, Kibler WB: The disabled throwing shoulder: spectrum of pathology. Part I: Pathoanatomy and biomechanics, *Arthroscopy* 19(4):404-420, 2003.

Burkhead WZ, Jr, Rockwood CA, Jr: Treatment of instability of the shoulder with and exercise program, *J Bone Joint Surg* [Am] 74(6):890-896, 1992.

Burton RI, Melchior JA: Extensor tendons—late reconstruction. In Green DP, Hotchkiss RN, Pederson WC, eds: *Green's Operative hand surgery*, ed 4, pp. 1988-2021, Philadelphia, 1999, Churchill Livingstone.

Burton R, Pellegrini V: Surgical management of basal joint arthritis of the thumb. Part II. Ligament reconstruction with tendon interposition arthroplasty, *J Hand Surg* [Am] 11(3):324-332, 1986.

Bush DC: Soft tissue tumors of the forearm and hand. In Mackin EJ, Callahan AD, Skirven TM, et al, eds: *Rehabilitation of the hand and upper extremity*, ed 5, pp. 954-970, St Louis, 2002, Mosby.

Butler DS: *Mobilization of the nervous system*, New York, 1991, Churchill Livingstone.

Byl NN, Merzenich MM: Focal hand dystonia. In Mackin EJ, Callahan AD, Skirven TM, et al, eds: *Rehabilitation of the hand and upper extremity*, ed 5, pp. 2053-2075, St Louis, 2002, Mosby.

Cailliet R: *Shoulder pain*, Philadelphia, 1975, FA Davis.

Cambridge-Keeling CA: Range-of-motion measurement of the mind. In Mackin EJ, Callahan AD, Skirven TM, et al, eds: *Rehabilitation of the hand and upper extremity*, ed 5, pp. 169-182, St Louis, 2002, Mosby.

Campbell PJ, Wilson RL: Management of joint injuries and intraarticular fractures. In Mackin EJ, Callahan AD, Skirven TM, et al, eds: *Rehabilitation of the hand and upper extremity*, ed 5, pp. 396-411, St Louis, 2002, Mosby.

Canale TS: *Campbell's Operative orthopaedics*, ed 10, St Louis, 2003, Mosby.

Cannon NM: Postoperative management of metacarpophalangeal joint capsulectomies. In Mackin EJ, Callahan AD, Skirven TM, et al, eds: *Rehabilitation of the hand and upper extremity*, ed 5, pp. 1060-1074, St Louis, 2002, Mosby.

Cannon NM: Rehabilitation approaches for distal and middle phalanx fractures of the hand, *J Hand Ther* 16(2):105-116, 2003.

Carlson L, Watson K: Treatment of reflex sympathetic dystrophy using the stress-loading program, *J Hand Ther* 1:149-154, 1988.

Carroll R: Acute calcium deposits in the hand, *JAMA* 273(5):422-426, 1995.

Casanova JS: *Clinical assessment recommendations*, ed 2, Chicago, 1992, American Society of Hand Therapists.

Chang LD, Buncke G, Slezak S, et al: Cigarette smoking, plastic surgery and microsurgery, *J Reconstr Microsurg* 12(7):467-474, 1996.

Chase RA: Anatomy and kinesiology of the hand. In Mackin EJ, Callahan AD, Skirven TM, et al, eds: *Rehabilitation of the hand and upper extremity*, ed 5, pp. 61-76, St Louis, 2002, Mosby.

Chinchalkar SJ, Gan BS: Management of proximal interphalangeal joint fractures and dislocations, *J Hand Ther* 16(2):117-128, 2003.

Chung KC, Spilson MS, Kim MH: Is negative ulnar variance a risk factor for Kienbock's disease? A meta-analysis, *Ann Plast Surg* 47(5):494-499, 2001.

Clark GC, Wilgis EFS, Aiello B, et al: *Hand rehabilitation: a practical guide*, ed 2, New York, 1996, Churchill Livingstone.

Coe M, Trumble T: Biomechanical comparison of methods used to treat Kienbock's disease, *Hand Clin* 9(3):417-429, 1993.

Cohen MS: Fractures of the carpal bones, *Hand Clin* 13(4):587-599, 1997.

Cohen MD, Dellon AL: Computer-assisted sensorimotor testing documents neural regeneration after ulnar nerve repair at the wrist, *Plast Reconstr Surg* 107(2):501-505, 2001.

Colditz JC: Functional fracture bracing. In Mackin EJ, Callahan AD, Skirven TM, et al, eds: *Rehabilitation of the hand and upper extremity*, ed 5, pp. 1875-1886, St Louis, 2002, Mosby.

Colditz JC: Splinting the hand with a peripheral-nerve injury. In Mackin EJ, Callahan AD, Skirven TM, et al, eds: *Rehabilitation of the hand and upper extremity*, ed 5, pp. 622-634, St Louis, 2002, Mosby.

Colditz JC: Therapist's management of the stiff hand. In Mackin EJ, Callahan AD, Skirven TM, et al, eds: *Rehabilitation of the hand and upper extremity*, ed 5, pp. 1021-1049, St Louis, 2002, Mosby.

Conrad EU III, Enneking WF: *Clinical symposia: common soft tissue tumors*, 42, #1, New York, 1990, Ciba-Geigy.

Cooney WP: Contractures and burns. In Morrey BF, ed: *The elbow and its disorders*, ed 3, pp. 433-451, Philadelphia, 2000, WB Saunders.

Cooney WP, Linscheid RL, An KN: Opposition of the thumb: an anatomic and biomechanical study of tendon transfers, *J Hand Surg* [Am] 9(6):777-786, 1984.

Cooney WP, Linscheid RL, Dobyns JH: *The wrist: diagnosis and operative treatment*, St Louis, 1998, Mosby.

Coons MS, Green SM: Boutonniere deformity, *Hand Clin* 11:387-402, 1995.

Coopee RA: Kinesio Taping. In Mackin EJ, Callahan AD, Skirven TM, et al, eds: *Rehabilitation of the hand and upper extremity*, ed 5, pp. 1796-1807, St Louis, 2002, Mosby.

Coppard BM, Lohman H: *Introduction to splinting: a clinical-reasoning and problem-solving approach*, ed 2, St Louis, 2001, Mosby.

Culp RW, Taras JS: Primary care of flexor tendon injuries. In Mackin EJ, Callahan AD, Skirven TM, et al, eds: *Rehabilitation of the hand and upper extremity*, ed 5, pp. 415-430, St Louis, 2002, Mosby.

Curtis RM: Fundamental principles of tendon transfer, *Orthop Clin North Am* 5(2):231-242, 1974.

Cyriax J: Diagnosis of soft tissue lesions. In *Textbook of orthopedic medicine*, ed 8, London, 1982, Bailliere Tindall.

Davidson PA, Pink M, Perry J: Functional anatomy of the flexor-pronator muscle group in relation to the medial collateral ligament of the elbow, *Am J Sports Med* 23:245-250, 1995.

Dávila SA: Therapist's management of fractures and dislocations of the elbow. In Mackin EJ, Callahan AD, Skirven TM, et al, eds: *Rehabilitation of the hand and upper extremity*, ed 5, pp. 1171-1184, St Louis, 2002, Mosby.

Davis TR, Barton NJ: Median nerve palsy. In Green DR, Hotchkiss RN, Pederson WC, eds: *Green's Operative hand surgery*, ed 4, pp. 1497-1525, Philadelphia, 1999, Churchill Livingstone.

DeHaven KE, Linter DM: Athletic injuries: comparison by age, sport and gender, *Am J Sports Med* 14:218-224, 1986.

DeLee JC: *Orthopaedic sports medicine*, Philadelphia, 1994, WB Saunders.

DeLee JC, Drez D, Miller MD: *DeLee & Drez's Orthopaedic sports medicine*, ed 2, Philadelphia, 2003, WB Saunders.

deLinde GL, Knothe B: Therapists management of the burned hand. In Mackin EJ, Callahan AD, Skirven TM, et al, eds: *Rehabilitation of the hand and upper extremity*, ed 5, pp. 1492-1526, St Louis, 2002, Mosby.

Dell PC, Dell RB: Management of carpal fractures and dislocations. In Mackin EJ, Callahan AD, Skirven TM, et al, eds: *Rehabilitation of the hand and upper extremity*, ed 5, pp. 1171-1184, St Louis, 2002, Mosby.

Dellon AL: Clinical grading of peripheral nerve problems, *Neurosurg Clin N Am* 12(2):229-240, 2001.

Dellon AL: Diagnosis and treatment of ulnar nerve compression at the elbow, *Tech Hand Upper Extremity Surg* 4:127-136, 2000.

Dellon AL: Discussion of "Surgical treatment of painful neuromas of the medial antebrachial cutaneous nerve" by Stahl and Rosenberg, *Ann Plast Surg* 48(2):158-160, 2002.

Dellon AL: *Evaluation of sensibility and re-education of sensation in the hand*, Baltimore, 1981, Williams & Wilkins.

Dellon AL: Management of peripheral nerve problems in the upper and lower extremity using quantitative sensory testing, *Hand Clin* 15(4):697-715, 1999.

Dellon AL: *Somatosensory testing and rehabilitation*, Bethesda, MD, 1997, American Occupational Therapy Association, Inc.

Dellon AL: Use of a silicon tube for the reconstruction of a nerve injury, *J Hand Surg* [Br] 19(3):271-272, 1994.

Dellon AL, Aszmann OC, Muse V: Evidence in support of collateral sprouting after sensory nerve resection, *Ann Plast Surg* 37(5):520-525, 1996.

Dellon AL, Hament W, Gittelsohn A: Non-operative management of cubital tunnel syndrome; results of eight year prospective study, *Neurol* 43:1673-1677, 1993.

Dellon AL, Mackinnon SE: Radial sensory nerve entrapment in the forearm, *J Hand Surg* [Am] 11(2):199-205, 1986.

Dellon AL, Mackinnon SE, Brandt KE: The markings of the Semmes-Weinstein nylon monofilaments, *J Hand Surg* [Am] 18(4):756-757, 1993.

Department of Health and Human Services, FDA Re: K010175.

De Smet L, Fabry G: Grip force reduction in patients with tennis elbow: influence of elbow position, *JHT* 10(31):229, 1997.

Diao E: Metacarpal fixation, *Hand Clin* 13(4):555-571, 1997.

Dictionary of titles, ed 4, revised 1991, U.S. Government Printing Office.

Disa JJ, Wang B, Dellon AL: Correction of scapular winging by supraclavicular neurolysis of the long thoracic nerve, *J Reconstr Microsurg* 17(2):79-84, 2001.

Dobyns JH: Management of congenital hand anomalies. In Mackin EJ, Callahan AD, Skirven TM, et al, eds: *Rehabilitation of the hand and upper extremity*, ed 5, pp. 1889-1906, St Louis, 2002, Mosby.

Donatelli R: Clinics in physical therapy. In Donatelli R, ed: *Physical therapy of the shoulder*, ed 3, New York, 1997, Churchill Livingstone.

Doran MF, Pond GR, Crowson, et al: Trends in incidence and mortality in rheumatoid arthritis in Rochester, Minnesota, over a forty-year period, *Arthritis Rheum* 46(3):625-631, 2002.

Dorland's Illustrated medical dictionary, ed 30, Philadelphia, 2003, WB Saunders.

Doyle JR: Extensor tendons—acute injuries. In Green DP, Hotchkiss RN, Pederson WC, eds: *Green's Operative hand surgery*, ed 4, pp. 1950-1987, Philadelphia, 1999, Churchill Livingstone.

Duda-Huys S: *Joint mobilization: hand therapy course review-study guide*, Atlanta, 1990.

Dumitru D: Reflex sympathetic dystrophy. Rehabilitation of chronic pain, *Phys Med Rehabil State of the Art Rev* 5(1):89-101, 1991.

Earle AS, Vlastou C: Crossed fingers and other tests of ulnar nerve motor function, *J Hand Surg* [Am] 5(6):560-565, 1980.

Eaton R, Malerich M: The volar plate arthroplasty in the proximal phalangeal joint: a review of ten years' experience, *J Hand Surg* [Am] 5(3):260-268, 1980.

Ejeskar A: Finger flexion force and hand grip strength after tendon repair, *J Hand Surg* 9:4, 1982.

Engkvist O, Lundburg G: Rupture of the extensor pollicis longus tendon after fracture of the lower end of the radius: a clinical and microangiographic study, *Hand Clin* 11(1): 76-86, 1979.

Esquenazi A, Meier RH: Rehabilitation in limb deficiency. 4. Limb amputation, *Arch Phys Med Rehabil* 77(3 Suppl): S18-S28, 1996.

Evans GRD, Dellon AL: Implantation of the palmar cutaneous branch of the median nerve into the pronator quadratus for treatment of painful neuroma, *J Hand Surg* [Am] 19(2):203-206, 1994.

Evans RB: Clinical management of extensor tendon injuries. In Mackin EJ, Callahan AD, Skirven TM, et al, eds: *Rehabilitation of the hand and upper extremity*, ed 5, pp. 542-579, St Louis, 2002, Mosby.

Evans RB: Eleventh Natalie Barr lecture. The source of our strength, *J Hand Ther* 10(1)14-23, 1997.

Evans RB: Therapist's management of carpal tunnel syndrome. In Mackin EJ, Callahan AD, Skirven TM, et al, eds: *Rehabilitation of the hand and upper extremity*, ed 5, pp. 660-671, St Louis, 2002, Mosby.

Evans RB, McAuliffe JA: Wound classification and management. In Mackin EJ, Callahan AD, Skirven TM, et al, eds: *Rehabilitation of the hand and upper extremity*, ed 5, pp. 311-330, St Louis, 2002, Mosby.

Evans RB, Thompson DE: The application of force to the healing tendon, *J Hand Ther* 6(4):266-284, 1993.

Eversmann WW: Compression and entrapment neuropathies of the upper extremity, *J Hand Surg* [Am] 8:759-766, 1983.

Falkenburg SA, Schultz DJ: Ergonomics for the upper extremity: occupational diseases of the hand, *Hand Clin* 9(2):263-271, 1993.

Federal register, Department of Labor, Part II, Occupational Safety and Health Administration, December, 1991.

Fedorczyk JM: Therapist's management of elbow tendonitis. In Mackin EJ, Callahan AD, Skirven TM, et al, eds: *Rehabilitation of the hand and upper extremity*, ed 5, pp. 1271-1281, St Louis, 2002, Mosby.

Fedorczyk JM, Barbe MF: Pain management: principles of therapists' intervention. In Mackin EJ, Callahan AD, Skirven TM, et al, eds: *Rehabilitation of the hand and upper extremity*, ed 5, pp. 1725-1741, St Louis, 2002, Mosby.

Fernandez DL, Palmer AK: Fractures of the distal radius. In Green DP, Hotchkiss RN, Pederson WC, eds: *Green's Operative hand surgery*, ed 4, pp 929-985, Philadelphia, 1999, Churchill Livingstone.

Fess EE: Clinical validation of hand rehabilitation: evaluating published research. In Mackin EJ, Callahan AD, Skirven TM, et al, eds: *Rehabilitation of the hand and upper extremity*, ed 5, pp. 2105-2109, St Louis, 2002, Mosby.

Fess EE: Principles and methods of splinting for mobilization of joints. In Mackin EJ, Callahan AD, Skirven TM, et al, eds: *Rehabilitation of the hand and upper extremity*, ed 5, pp. 1818-1827, St Louis, 2002, Mosby.

Fess EE, Philips CA: *Hand splinting: principles and methods*, ed 2, St Louis, 1987, Mosby.

Fess EE, Gettle K, Philips CA, et al: *Hand and upper extremity splinting: principles and methods*, ed 3, St Louis, 2004, Mosby.

Flatow EL, editor: *Orthop Clin North Am* 28(2), 1997.

Fleegler EJ: Skin tumors. In Green DP, Hotchkiss RN, Pederson WC, eds: *Green's Operative hand surgery*, ed 4, pp. 2184-2205, Philadelphia, 1999, Churchill Livingstone.

Fleisig GS, Dillman CJ, Andrews JR: Proper mechanics for baseball pitching, *Clin Sports Med* 1:151-170, 1989.

Florida administrative code biomedical waste, Chapter 64, June 1997.

Floyd W, Troom J: Tumors of the hand and forearm, *Hand Clin* 11(2):127, 1995.

Freeland AE: *Hand fractures*, New York, 2000, Churchill Livingstone.

Freeland AE, Hardy MA, Singletary S: Rehabilitation for proximal phalangeal fractures, *J Hand Ther* 16(2):129-142, 2003.

Freeland AE, Jabaley ME, Hughes JL: *Stable fixation of the hand and wrist*, New York, 1986, Springer-Verlag.

Fryer C: Harnessing and controls for body-powered devices. In Bowker JH, Michael JW, eds: *Atlas of limb prosthetics*, ed 2, St Louis, 1992, Mosby.

Frykman GK, Watkins BE: The distal radioulnar joint. In Mackin EJ, Callahan AD, Skirven TM, et al, eds: *Rehabilitation of the hand and upper extremity*, ed 5, pp. 1124-1135, St Louis, 2002, Mosby.

Frymoyer KW: *Orthopedic knowledge update 4: home study syllabus*, Rosemont, IL, 1993, American Academy of Orthopaedic Surgeons.

Fu FH, Ticker JB, Imhoff AB: *An atlas of shoulder surgery*, New York, 1998, McGraw-Hill.

Garrison SL: *Handbook of physical medicine and rehabilitation basics*, Philadelphia, 1995, JB Lippincott.

Geissler WB: Carpal fractures in athletes, *Clin Sports Med* 20(1):167-188, 2001.

Gelb RI: Tendon transfer for rupture of the extensor pollicis longus tendon, *Hand Clin* 11(3):411-422, 1995.

Gelberman RH, Woo SL: The physiological basis for application of controlled stress in the rehabilitation of flexor tendon injuries, *J Hand Ther* 2(2):66-83, 1989.

Gellman H, Buch K: Acute compartment syndrome of the arm, *Hand Clin* 14(3):385.

Gerber C, Hersche O, Farron A: Isolated rupture of the subscapularis tendon, *J Bone Joint Surg* [Am] 78(7):1015-1023, 1996.

Giannakopoulos PN, Sotereanos DG, Tomaino MM, et al: Benign and malignant muscle tumors in the hand and forearm, *Hand Clin* 11(2):191-201, 1995.

Gilberman KH: *Operative nerve repair and reconstruction*, Philadelphia, 1991, JB Lippincott.

Giurintano DJ: Basic biomechanics, *J Hand Ther* 8(2)79-84, 1995.

Green DP: *Operative hand surgery*, ed 3, New York, 1993, Churchill Livingstone.

Green DP: Radial nerve palsy. In Green DP, Hotchkiss RN, Pederson WC, eds: *Green's Operative hand surgery*, ed 4, pp. 1481-1496, Philadelphia, 1999, Churchill Livingstone.

Green DP, Hotchkiss RN, Pederson WC, eds: *Green's Operative hand surgery*, ed 4, Philadelphia, 1999, Churchill Livingstone.

Greenfield B, Syen D: Brachial plexus lesions: physical therapy of the shoulder. In *Clinics in physical therapy*, ed 2, New York, 1991, Churchill Livingstone.

Griffith AJ: Therapist's management of the stiff elbow. In Mackin EJ, Callahan AD, Skirven TM, et al, eds: *Rehabilitation of the hand and upper extremity*, ed 5, pp. 1245-1261, St Louis, 2002, Mosby.

Gupta R, Allaire RB, Fornalski S, et al: Kinematic analysis of the distal radioulnar joint after a simulated progressive ulnar-sided wrist injury, *J Hand Surg* [Am] 27(5):854-862, 2002.

Hahn DH: In Kelley WN, Harris ED, Ruddy S, et al, eds: *Textbook of rheumatology*, ed 5, Philadelphia, 1997, Saunders, pp. 1015–1054.

Hardy MA, Hardy SG: Reflex sympathetic dystrophy: the clinician's perspective, *J Hand Ther* 10(2):137-150, 1997.

Hareau J: What makes treatment for reflex sympathetic dystrophy successful? *J Hand Ther* 9(4):367-370, 1996.

Harris C Jr, Rutledge GL, Jr: The functional anatomy of the extensor mechanism of the finger, *J Bone Joint Surg* [Am] 54(4):713-726, 1972.

Hastings H, Davidson S: Tendon transfers for ulnar nerve palsy, *Hand Clin* 4(2):167-178, 1988.

Hastings H II, Ernst JM: Dynamic external fixation for fractures of the proximal interphalangeal joint, *Hand Clin* 9(4):659-674, 1993.

Hastings H II, Graham TJ: The classification and treatment of heterotopic ossification about the elbow and forearm, *Hand Clin* 10(3):417-437, 1994.

Hawkins R, Bell R, Lippitt S: *Atlas of shoulder surgery*, St Louis, 1996, Mosby.

Hayes EP, Carney K, Wolf J, et al: Carpal tunnel syndrome. In Mackin EJ, Callahan AD, Skirven TM, et al, eds: *Rehabilitation of the hand and upper extremity*, ed 5, pp. 643-659, St Louis, 2002, Mosby.

Hayes K: *Manual for physical agents*, ed 4, Stanford, CT, 1993, Appleton & Lange.

Hecox B, Mehreteab TA, Weisberg J: *Physical agents: a comprehensive text for physical therapists*, Stanford, CT, 1994, Appleton & Lange.

Heggers JP: Assessing and controlling wound infection, *Clin Plast Surg* 30(1):25-35, 2003.

Herndon DN: *Total burn care*, Philadelphia, 1996, WB Saunders.

Herndon JH: Neuromas. In Green DR, Hotchkiss RN, Pederson WC, eds: *Green's Operative hand surgery*, ed 4, pp. 1469-1480, Philadelphia, 1999, Churchill Livingstone.

Hess CT: *Clinical guide to wound care*, ed 4, Philadelphia, 2002, Lippincott, Williams & Wilkins.

Hodges PL: *Surgical flaps*. In *Selected readings in plastic surgery*, Waco, TX, 1992, Baylor University Medical Center.

Hopkins H, Smith H, eds: *Willard and Spackman's Occupational therapy*, ed 7, Philadelphia, 1988, JB Lippincott.

Hoppenfeld S: *Physical examination of the spine and extremities*, Norwalk, CT, 1976, Appleton-Century-Crofts.

Hoppenfeld S, de Boer P: *Surgical exposures in orthopedics, the anatomic approach*, Philadelphia, 1994, JB Lippincott.

Hornbach EE, Culp RW: Radial tunnel syndrome. In Mackin EJ, Callahan AD, Skirven TM, et al, eds: *Rehabilitation of the hand and upper extremity*, ed 5, St Louis, 2002, Mosby.

House HJ, Fidler MO: Frostbite of the hand. In Green DR, Hotchkiss RN, Pederson WC, eds: *Green's Operative hand surgery*, ed 4, pp. 2061-2067, Philadelphia, 1999, Churchill Livingstone.

Hunter JM: Atlas on regional anatomy of the neck, axilla, and upper extremity. In Mackin EJ, Callahan AD, Skirven TM, et al, eds: *Rehabilitation of the hand and upper extremity*, ed 5, pp. 3-49, St Louis, 2002, Mosby.

Hunter JM, Mackin EJ, Callahan AD, eds: *Rehabilitation of the hand: surgery and therapy*, ed 4, St Louis, 1995, Mosby.

Hunter JM, Schneider LH, Mackin EJ, eds: *Tendon and nerve surgery in the hand: a third decade*, St Louis, 1997, Mosby.

Hurst LC, Badalamente MA: Nonoperative treatment of Dupuytren's disease, *Hand Clin* 15(1):97-107, 1999.

Idler RS: General principles of patient evaluation in nonoperative management of cubital syndrome, *Hand Clin* 12(2):397-403, 1996.

Imatami J, Hashizume H, Wake H, et al: The central slip attachment fracture, *J Hand Surg* [Br] 22:107-109, 1997.

Innis PC: Surgical management of the stiff hand. In Mackin EJ, Callahan AD, Skirven TM, et al, eds: *Rehabilitation of the hand and upper extremity*, ed 5, pp. 1050-1059, St Louis, 2002, Mosby.

Jabaley ME, Wegener EE: Principles of internal fixation as applied to the hand and wrist, *J Hand Ther* 16(2):95-104, 2003.

Jacobs M, Austin N: *Splinting the hand and upper extremity*, Philadelphia, 2003, Lippincott, Williams & Wilkins.

Jaffe R, Chidgey LK, LaStayo PC: The distal radioulnar joint: anatomy and management of disorders, *J Hand Ther* 9(2):129-138, 1996.

Jain S: Rehabilitation in limb deficiency. 2: The pediatric amputee, *Arch Phys Med Rehabil* 77(3 Suppl):S9-S13, 1996.

Jarvis C: *Wound management in the elderly*, course 907, Las Vegas, p. 39.

Jebson PJL, Kasdan ML: *Hand secrets*, ed 2, Philadelphia, 2001, Hanley & Belfus.

Jensen JA, Goodson WH, Hopf HW, et al: Cigarette smoking decreases tissue oxygen, *Arch Surg* 126(9):1131-1134, 1991.

Jobe FW: *Operative techniques in upper extremity sports injuries*, St Louis, 1996, Mosby.

Johnson SL: Ergonomic hand tool design, *Hand Clin* 9(2):299-311, 1993.

Jones B, Stern P: Interphalangeal joint arthrodesis, *Hand Clin* 10(2):267-275, 1994.

Jones NF, Chang J, Kashani P: The surgical and rehabilitative aspects of replantation and revascularization of the hand. In Mackin EJ, Callahan AD, Skirven TM, et al, eds: *Rehabilitation of the hand and upper extremity*, ed 5, pp. 1428-1449, St Louis, 2002, Mosby.

Jorgensen LN, Kallehave F, Christensen E, et al: Less collagen production in smokers, *Surg* 123(4):450-455, 1998.

Jupiter JB, Fernandez DL: Complications following distal radial fractures, *Instr Course Lect* 51:203-219, 2002.

Kader P: Therapist's management of the replanted hand, *Hand Clin* 2(1):179-191, 1986.

Kaempffe FA: External fixation for distal radius fractures: adverse effects of excess distraction, *Am J Orthop* 25(3):205-209, 1996.

Kaltenborn FM: *Manual mobilization of the extremity joints*, Bokrardel, Sweden, 1989, Olaf Norlis.

Kandel ER, Schwartz JH: *Principles of neuroscience*, ed 2, New York, 1985, Elsevier.

Kasch MC: Therapist's evaluation and treatment of upper extremity cumulative trauma disorder. In Mackin EJ, Callahan AD, Skirven TM, et al, eds: *Rehabilitation of the hand and upper extremity*, ed 5, pp. 1005-1018, St Louis, 2002, Mosby.

Kasdan ML: Occupational hand injuries. In *Occupational medicine: state-of-the-art reviews*, Philadelphia, 1989, Hanley & Belfus.

Kasdan ML, Amadio PC, Bowers WH: *Technical tips for hand surgery*, Philadelphia, 1994, Hanley & Belfus.

Kelley WN, Wortmann RL: In Kelley WN, Harris ED, Ruddy S, et al, eds: *Textbook of rheumatology*, ed 5, Philadelphia, 1997, WB Saunders.

Khandwala AR, Webb J, Harris SB, et al: A comparison of dynamic extension splinting and controlled active mobilization of complete divisions of extensor tendons in zones 5 and 6, *J Hand Surg* [Br] 25(2):140-146, 2000.

Kibler WB: Biomechanical analysis of the shoulder during tennis activities, *Clin Sports Med* 14:79-85, 1995.

Kimura J: Principles and pitfalls of nerve conduction studies, *Ann Neurol* 16:418, 1984.

Kindwall EP, Gottlieb LJ, Larson DL: Hyperbaric oxygen therapy in plastic surgery: a review article, *Plast Reconstr Surg* 88(5):898-908, 1991.

King GJ, Morrey BF, An KN: Stabilizers of the elbow, *J Shoulder Elbow Surg* 2:165-174, 1993.

King II T: The effect of water temperature on hand volume during volumetric measurement using the water displacement method, *J Hand Ther* 6(3):202-204, 1993.

Kirkpatrick A, ed: *Clinical practice guidelines*, ed 3, Milford, CT, November 25, 2003, International Research Foundation for RSD/CPRS.

Kisner C, Colby L: *Therapeutic exercise: peripheral joint mobilization*, Philadelphia, 1985, FA Davis.

Kloth L, McCulloch JM: *Wound healing: alternatives in management*, ed 3, Philadelphia, 2002, FA Davis.

Knapp RG: *Basic statistics for nurses*, ed 2, New York, 1985, John Wiley & Sons.

Koman LA, Poehling GG, Smith TL: Complex regional pain syndrome: reflex sympathetic dystrophy and causalgia. In Green DR, Hotchkiss RN, Pederson WC, eds: *Green's Operative hand surgery*, ed 4, pp. 636-666, Philadelphia, 1999, Churchill Livingstone.

Koman LA, Ruch DS, Smith BP, et al: Vascular disorders. In Green DP, Hotchkiss RN, Pederson WC, eds: *Green's Operative hand surgery*, ed 4, pp 2254-2302, Philadelphia, 1999, Churchill Livingstone.

Koman LA, Smith BP, Smith TL: Reflex sympathetic dystrophy (complex regional pain syndromes-types 1 and 2). In Mackin EJ, Callahan AD, Skirven TM, et al, eds: *Rehabilitation of the hand and upper extremity*, ed 5, pp. 1695-1706, St Louis, 2002, Mosby.

Kornberg M, Aulicino PL, Du Puy TE: Ulnar arterial aneurysms and thromboses in the hand and forearm, *Orthop Rev* 12:25-33, 1983.

Kostopoulos D, Rizopoulos R: *Trigger point and myofascial therapy*, Thorofare, NJ, 2001, Slack.

Kottke FJ, Stillwell GK, Lehmann JF: Reconstructive surgery of extremities. In Kottke FJ, Lehmann JF, eds: *Krusen's Handbook of physical medicine and rehabilitation*, ed 3, Philadelphia, 1982, WB Saunders.

Kozin SH: Incidence, mechanism, and natural history of scaphoid fractures, *Hand Clin* 17(4):515-524, 2001.

Kozin SH: Perilunate injuries: diagnosis and treatment, *J Am Acad Orthop Surg* 6(2):114-120, 1998.

Krop PN: Fractures: general principles of surgical management. In Mackin EJ, Callahan AD, Skirven TM, et al, eds: *Rehabilitation of the hand and upper extremity*, ed 5, pp. 371-381, St. Louis, 2002, Mosby.

Kwiatkowski TC, Hanley EN, Jr, Ramp WK: Cigarette smoking and its orthopedic consequences, *Am J Orthop* 25(9):590-597, 1996.

van der Laan L, Goris RJ: Reflex sympathetic dystrophy. An exaggerated regional inflammatory response? *Hand Clin* 13(3):373-385, 1997.

Laseter GF: Therapist's management of distal radius fractures. In Mackin EJ, Callahan AD, Skirven TM, et al, eds: *Rehabilitation of the hand and upper extremity*, ed 5, pp. 1136-1155, St Louis, 2002, Mosby.

Laseter GF, Carter PR: Management of distal radius fractures, *J Hand Ther* 9(2):114-128, 1996.

LaStayo PC: Ulnar wrist pain and impairment: a therapist's algorithmic approach to the triangular fibrocartilage complex. In Mackin EJ, Callahan AD, Skirven TM, et al, eds: *Rehabilitation of the hand and upper extremity*, ed 5, pp. 1156-1170, St Louis, 2002, Mosby.

LaStayo PC, Cass R: Continuous passive motion for the upper extremity: why, when, and how. In Mackin EJ, Callahan AD, Skirven TM, et al, eds: *Rehabilitation of the hand and upper extremity*, ed 5, pp. 1745-1763, St Louis, 2002, Mosby.

LaStayo PC, Howell J: Clinical provocative tests used in evaluating wrist pain: a descriptive study, *J Hand Ther* 8(1): 10-17, 1995.

LaStayo PC, Michlovitz SL: The wrist and hand. In Kolt GS, Snyder-Mackler L, eds: *Physical therapies in sport and exercise*, Edinburgh, UK, 2003, Churchill Livingstone.

LaStayo PC, Weiss S: The GRIT: a quantitative measure of ulnar impaction syndrome, *J Hand Ther* 14(3):173-179, 2001.

LaStayo PC, Wheeler DL: Reliability of passive wrist flexion and extension goniometric measurements: a multicenter study, *Phys Ther* 74(2):162-174, 1994.

LaStayo PC, Winters KM, Hardy M: Fracture healing: bone healing, fracture management, and current concepts related to the hand, *J Hand Ther* 16(2):81-93, 2003.

Lazarus MD, Sidles JA, Harryman DT II, et al: Effect of chondral-labral defect on glenoid concavity and glenohumeral stability: a cadaveric model, *J Bone Joint Surg* [Am] 78:94-102, 1996.

Leclercq C: Compression of the ulnar nerve in the wrist and hand. In Tubiana R, ed: *The hand*, vol 4, Philadelphia, 1993, Saunders.

Leddy JP, Packer JW: Avulsion of the profundus tendon insertion in athletes, *J Hand Surg* [Am] 2:66-69, 1977.

van Lede P: Minimalistic splint design: a rationale told in a personal style, *J Hand Ther* 15(2):192-201, 2002.

van Lede P, van Veldhoven G: *Therapeutic hand splints: a rationale approach*, Antwerp, Belgium, 1998, Provan.

Lee MP, Nasser-Sharif S, Zelouf DS: Surgeon's and therapist's management of tendonopathies in the hand and wrist. In Mackin EJ, Callahan AD, Skirven TM, et al, eds: *Rehabilitation of the hand and upper extremity*, ed 5, pp. 931-953, St Louis, 2002, Mosby.

Lee MP, Susan MS, David SZ: Surgeon's and therapist's management of tendonopathies in the hand and wrist. In Mackin EJ, Callahan AD, Skirven TM, et al, eds: *Rehabilitation of the hand and upper extremity*, ed 5, pp. 931-953, St Louis, 2002, Mosby.

Lehneis R: Fitting and training the bilateral upper-limb amputee. In Bowker JH, Michael JW, eds: *Atlas of limb prosthetics*, ed 2, St Louis, 1992, Mosby.

Leibovic SJ: Internal fixation for small joint arthrodesis in the hand and the interphalangeal joints, *Hand Clin* 13(4): 601-613, 1997.

Lennard T: *Physiatric procedures in clinical practice*, Philadelphia, 1995, Hanley & Belfus.

Levin LS, Moorman GJ, Heller L: Management of skin grafts and flaps. In Mackin EJ, Callahan AD, Skirven TM, et al, eds: *Rehabilitation of the hand and upper extremity*, ed 5, pp. 344-356, St Louis, 2002, Mosby.

Light T: Kinesiology of the upper limb. In Bowker JH, Michael JW, eds: *Atlas of limb prosthetics*, ed 2, St Louis, 1992, Mosby.

Light T, Bednar M: Management of intra-articular fractures of the metacarpophalangeal joint, *Hand Clin* 10(2):303-314, 1994.

Lillegard WA, Butcher JD, Rucker KS: *Handbook of sports medicine: a symptom-oriented approach*, ed 2, Boston, 1998, Butterworth-Heinemann.

Lindenfeld TN: Medial approach in elbow arthroscopy, *Am J Sports Med* 18:413-417, 1990.

Lindsay R, Watson G, et al: *Treat your own strains, sprains, and bruises*, New Zealand, 1994, Spinal Publications, Ltd.

Linscheid R: Historical perspective of finger joint motion: the hand-me-downs of our predecessors. The Richard J. Smith Memorial Lecture, *J Hand Surg* [Am] 27(1):1-25, 2002.

Lippitt SB, Vanderhooft JE, Harris SL, et al: Glenohumeral stability from concavity-compression: a quantitative analysis, *J Shoulder Elbow Surg* 2:27-35, 1993.

Lister DG, Pederson CW: Skin Flaps. In Green DR, Hotchkiss RN, Pederson WC, eds: *Green's Operative hand surgery*, ed 4, pp. 1783-1850, Philadelphia, 1999, Churchill Livingstone.

Loth T, Wadsworth C: *Orthopaedic review for physical therapists*, St Louis, 1998, Mosby.

Louis DS, Jebson PJL, Graham TJ: Amputations. In Green DP, Hotchkiss RN, Pederson WC, eds: *Green's Operative hand surgery*, ed 4, pp. 48-94, Philadelphia, 1999, Churchill Livingstone.

Lubahn JD: Open-palm technique and soft-tissue coverage in Dupuytren's disease, *Hand Clin* 15(1):127-136, 1999.

Lubahn JD, Wolfe TL: Surgical treatment and rehabilitation of tendon ruptures in the rheumatoid hand. In Mackin EJ, Callahan AD, Skirven TM, et al, eds: *Rehabilitation of the hand and upper extremity*, ed 5, pp. 1598-1607, St Louis, 2002, Mosby.

Ludlow KS, Merla JL, Cox JA, et al: Pillar pain as a postoperative complication of carpal tunnel release: a review of the literature, *J Hand Ther* 10(4):277-282, 1997.

Mackin EJ, Callahan AD, Skirven TM, et al, eds: *Hunter, Mackin, & Callahan's Rehabilitation of the hand and upper extremity*, ed 5, St Louis, 2002, Mosby.

Mackinnon SE, Dellon AL: *Surgery of the peripheral nerve*, New York, 1988, Thieme.

Maddy L, Meyerdierks E: Dynamic extension assist splints of acute central slip lacerations, *J Hand Ther* 10(3):206-212, 1997.

Magee D: *Orthopedic physical assessment*, ed 2, Philadelphia, 1992, WB Saunders.

Maitland GD: *Peripheral manipulation*, ed 3, Boston, 1991, Butterworth-Heinemann.

Malick MH: *Manual on static splinting*, ed 3, Pittsburgh, 1985, AREN Publishing.

Malick MH, Kasch M: *Manual of management of specific hand problems*, Pittsburgh, 1984, AREN Publishing.

Malone JM, Fleming LL, Robertson J, et al: Immediate, early, and late postsurgical management of upper-limb amputation, *J Rehabil Res Dev* 21(1):33-41, 1984.

Malone TR, McPoil TG, Nitz AJ: *Orthopaedics and sports physical therapy*, ed 3, St. Louis, 1997, Mosby.

Manktelow RT, Anastakis DJ: Functioning free muscle transfers. In Green DR, Hotchkiss RN, Pederson WC, eds: *Green's Operative hand surgery*, ed 4, pp. 1201-1219, Philadelphia, 1999, Churchill Livingstone.

Marks PH, Warner JJ, Irrgang JJ: Rotator cuff disorders of the shoulder, *J Hand Ther* 7(2):90-98, 1994.

Marshall RW, Williams DH, Birch R, et al: Operations to restore elbow flexion after brachial plexus injuries, *J Bone Joint Surg* [Br] 70(4):577-582, 1988.

Martin DS, Collins ED: *Manual of acute hand injuries*, St Louis, 1998, Mosby.

Matloub HS, Yousef NJ: Peripheral nerve anatomy and innervation patterns, *Hand Clin* 8:201, 1992.

Matsen FA III, Lippitt SB, Sidles JA, et al: *Practical evaluation and management of the shoulder*, Philadelphia, 1994, WB Saunders.

May MM, Lawton JN, Blazar PE: Ulnar styloid fractures associated with distal radius fractures: incidence and implications for distal radioulnar joint instability, *J Hand Surg* [Am] 27(6):965-971, 2002.

McAuliffe JA: Clinical and radiographic evaluation of the elbow. In Mackin EJ, Callahan AD, Skirven TM, et al, eds: *Rehabilitation of the hand and upper extremity*, ed 5, St Louis, 2002, Mosby.

McCollister EC: *Surgery of the musculoskeletal system*, ed 2, New York, 1990, Churchill Livingstone.

McCulloch JM, Kloth L, Feedar J: *Wound healing alternatives in management*, ed 2, Philadelphia, 1995, FA Davis.

McDowell CL, House JH: Tetraplegia. In Green DR, Hotchkiss RN, Pederson WC, eds: *Green's Operative hand surgery*, ed 4, pp. 1588-1606, Philadelphia, 1999, Churchill Livingstone.

McFarlane R: Dupuytren's disease, invitational lecture, ASHT 19th annual meeting, *J Hand Ther* 10(1):8-13, 1997.

McFarlane RM, MacDermid JC: Dupuytren's disease. In Mackin EJ, Callahan AD, Skirven TM, et al, eds: *Rehabilitation of the hand and upper extremity*, ed 5, pp. 971-988, St Louis, 2002, Mosby.

McGrouther DA: Dupuytren's contracture. In Green DR, Hotchkiss RN, Pederson WC, eds: *Green's Operative hand surgery*, ed 4, pp. 563-591, Philadelphia, 1999, Churchill Livingstone.

McKee P, Morgan L: *Orthotics in rehabilitation: splinting the hand and body*, Philadelphia, 1998, FA Davis.

McKenzie RA: *Lumbar spine—mechanical diagnosis and therapy*, New Zealand, 1981, Spinal Publications, Ltd.

McKenzie RA: *The human extremities—mechanical diagnosis and therapy*, New Zealand, 2000, Spinal Publications, Ltd.

McLaughlin HL: Complex "locked" dislocation of the metacarpophalangeal joints, *J Trauma* 5:683-688, 1965.

McNemar TB, Howell JW, Chang E: Management of metacarpal fractures, *J Hand Ther* 16(2):143-151, 2003.

Medicare coverage issues manual, transmittal 166, 2003, Department of Health & Human Services (DHHS), Coverage Issues Manual, Centers for Medicare & Medicaid Services (CMS). Accessed at http://www.cms.hhs.gov/manuals/pm_trans/R166CIM.pdf.

Mehlhoff TL, Noble PC, Bennett JB, et al: Simple dislocation of the elbow in the adult: Results after closed treatment, *J Bone Joint Surg* [Am] 70(2):244-249, 1998.

Mehta AJ: *Common musculoskeletal problems*, Philadelphia, 1997, Hanley & Belfus.

Melvin JL: Scleroderma (systemic sclerosis): treatment of the hand. In Mackin EJ, Callahan AD, Skirven TM, et al, eds: *Rehabilitation of the hand and upper extremity*, ed 5, pp. 1677-1691, St Louis, 2002, Mosby.

Melvin JL: Systemic lupus erythematosus of the hand. In Mackin EJ, Callahan AD, Skirven TM, et al, eds: *Rehabilitation of the hand and upper extremity*, ed 5, pp. 1667-1676, St Louis, 2002, Mosby.

Melvin JL: Therapist's management of osteoarthritis in the hand. In Mackin EJ, Callahan AD, Skirven TM, et al, eds: *Rehabilitation of the hand and upper extremity*, ed 5, pp. 1646-1663, St Louis, 2002, Mosby.

Melzak R, Stillwell DM, Fox EJ: Trigger points and acupuncture points for pain: correlations and implications, *Pain* 3: 3-23, 1977.

Mendez-Eastman S: When wounds won't heal, *RN* 61(1): 20-24, 1998.

Meredith JM: Comparison of three myoelectrically controlled prehensors and the voluntary-opening split hook, *Am J Occup Ther* 48(10):932-937, 1994.

Meyer T: *Review book for physical therapy licensing exam*, vol 1 & 2, 1997, Midwest Hi-Tech Publishers.

Meyerdierks E, Werner F: Limited wrist arthrodesis: a laboratory study article, *J Hand Surg* [Am] 12(4):526-529, 1987.

Michlovitz SL: *Thermal agents in rehabilitation*, ed 3, Philadelphia, 1996, FA Davis.

Michlovitz SL: Ultrasound and selected physical agent modalities in upper extremity rehabilitation. In Mackin EJ, Callahan AD, Skirven TM, et al, eds: *Rehabilitation of the hand and upper extremity*, ed 5, pp. 1745-1763, St Louis, 2002, Mosby.

Mih AD: Limited wrist fusion, *Hand Clin* 13(4):615-625, 1997.

Milford L: Tumors and tumorous conditions of the hand. In *The hand*, St Louis, 1988, Mosby.

Millender LH, Louis DS, Simmons BP: *Occupational disorders of the upper extremity*, New York, 1992, Churchill Livingstone.

Miller MD: *Review of orthopaedics*, ed 3, Philadelphia, 2000, Saunders.

Moojen TM, Snel JG, Ritt MJ, et al: In vivo analysis of carpal kinematics and comparative review of the literature, *J Hand Surg* [Am] 28(1):81-87, 2003.

Morrey BF: *Master techniques in orthopaedic surgery: the elbow*, Baltimore, 1994, Raven Press.

Morrey BF: *The elbow and its disorders*, ed 3, Philadelphia, 2000, WB Saunders.

Mosby's Medical, nursing & allied health dictionary, ed 6, St Louis, 2002, Mosby.

Mulligan BR: *Manual therapy "nags, snags, MWM's, etc."* 1995, Plane View Services, Ltd.

Mullins PA: Postsurgical rehabilitation of Dupuytren's disease, *Hand Clin* 15(1):167-174, 1999.

Murphy LD: *Joint mobilization: a comprehensive review of hand therapy*, ASHT, June, 1995.

Naidu SH, Heppenstall RB: Compartment syndrome of the forearm and hand, *Hand Clin* 10(1):13-27, 1994.

Nathan R, Taras JS: Common infections in the hand. In Mackin EJ, Callahan AD, Skirven TM, et al, eds: *Rehabilitation of the hand and upper extremity*, ed 5, pp. 359-368, St Louis, 2002, Mosby.

National Collegiate Athletic Association: Illegal equipment. In Nelson DM, ed: *1988 NCAA football rules and interpretations*. Mission, KS, 1988, National Collegiate Athletic Association.

National Federation Football Rules Committee: Player equipment. In Schindler D, ed: *1988 official high school football rules*. Kansas City, 1988, National Federation of State High School Associations.

Nelson C, Sawmiller S, Phalen G: Ganglions of the wrist and hand, *J Bone Joint Surg* [Am] 54(7):1459-1464, 1972.

Netter FH: Anatomy, physiology, and metabolic disorders. In *The Ciba collection of medical illustration*, vol 8, Musculoskeletal System, West Caldwell, NJ, 1987-1991, Ciba-Geigy Corp.

Nirschl R: Sports and overuse injuries to the elbow. In Morrey BF, ed: *The elbow and its disorders*, ed 2, Philadelphia, 1993, Saunders.

Norkin CC, Levangie PK: *Joint structure and function: a comprehensive analysis*, ed 3, Philadelphia, 2001, FA Davis.

Norkin CC, White DJ: *Measurement of joint motion: a guide to goniometry*, Philadelphia, 1995, FA Davis.

Norris C: *Sports injuries: diagnosis and management for physiotherapists*, Oxford, UK, 1993, Butterworth-Heinemann.

Norris TR: *Orthopedic knowledge update: shoulder and elbow*, Rosemont, IL, 1997, American Academy of Orthopaedic Surgeons.

Northwestern University upper extremity prosthetic manual, Chicago, IL, 2002, Northwestern University Prosthetic-Orthotic Center.

Oates SD, Daley, RA: Thoracic outlet syndrome, *Hand Clin* 12(4):705-728, 1996.

Olave E, Prates JC, Del Sol M, et al: Distribution patterns of the muscular branch of the median nerve in the thenar region, *J Anat* 186(Pt 2):441-446, 1995.

Omer GE: Diagnosis and management of cubital tunnel syndrome. In Mackin EJ, Callahan AD, Skirven TM, et al: *Rehabilitation of the hand and upper extremity*, ed 5, pp. 672-678, St Louis, 2002, Mosby.

Omer GE: Ulnar nerve palsy. In Green DR, Hotchkiss RN, Pederson WC, eds: *Green's Operative hand surgery*, ed 4, pp. 1526-1541, Philadelphia, 1999, Churchill Livingstone.

Omer GE, Spinner M, Van Beek AL: *Management of peripheral nerve problems*, ed 2, Philadelphia, 1998, WB Saunders.

Orenstein HH: Hand I: fingernails and soft tissue trauma: infections, tumors and reconstruction. In *Selected reading in plastic surgery*, vol 6, Waco, TX, 1992, Baylor University Medical Center.

Orwoll ES, Bliziotes M: *Osteoporosis: pathophysiology and clinical management*, Totowa, NJ, 2003, Humana Press.

Osterman AL: Wrist arthroscopy: operative procedures. In Green DP, Hotchkiss RN, Pederson WC, eds: *Green's Operative hand surgery*, ed 4, pp 207-222, Philadelphia, 1999, Churchill Livingstone.

Otto Bock prosthetic compendium, upper extremity prostheses, Germany, 1990, Schiele & Schon.

Owen D: In Kelley W, Harris ED, Jr, Ruddy S, et al, eds: *Textbook of rheumatology*, ed 5, Philadelphia, 1997, Saunders.

O'Young BJ, Young MA, Stiens SA: *Physical medicine and rehabilitation secrets*, ed 2, Philadelphia, 2002, Hanley & Belfus.

Ozkaya N, Nordin M: *Fundamentals of biomechanics: equilibrium, motion, and deformation*, New York, 1991, Van Nostrand Reinhold.

Palmer AK: Fractures of the distal radius. In Green DP, ed: *Operative hand surgery*, ed 3, pp. 929-971, New York, 1993, Churchill Livingstone.

Pascarelli E, Quilter D: *Repetitive strain injury: a computer user's guide*, New York, 1994, John Wiley & Sons.

Pedretti LW: *Occupational therapy practice skills for physical dysfunction*, ed 4, St Louis, 1996, Mosby.

Peimer CA: *Surgery of the hand and upper extremity*, New York, 1996, McGraw-Hill.

Pettengill KM, Strien VG: Postoperative management of flexor tendon injuries. In Mackin EJ, Callahan AD, Skirven TM, et al, eds: *Rehabilitation of the hand and upper extremity*, ed 5, pp. 431-456, St Louis, 2002, Mosby.

Pettengill KS: Therapist's management of the complex injury. In Mackin EJ, Callahan AD, Skirven TM, et al, eds: *Rehabilitation of the hand and upper extremity*, ed 5, pp. 1411-1427, St Louis, 2002, Mosby.

Pettrone FA: *Athletic injuries of the shoulder*, New York, 1995, McGraw-Hill.

Pillet J, Mackin EJ: Aesthetic hand prosthesis: its psychologic and functional potential. In Mackin EJ, Callahan AD, Skirven TM, et al, eds: *Rehabilitation of the hand and upper extremity*, ed 5, pp. 1461-1472, St Louis, 2002, Mosby.

Pink MM, Screnar PM, Tollefson KD, et al: Injury prevention and rehabilitation in the upper extremity. In Jobe FW, ed: *Operative techniques in upper extremity in sports injuries*, pp. 3-15, St Louis, 1996, Mosby.

Pollack FH, Drake D, Bovill EG, et al: Treatment of radial neuropathy associated with fractures of the humerus, *J Bone Joint Surg* [Am] 63(2):239-243, 1981.

Portney LG, Watkins MP: *Foundations of clinical research: applications to practice*, Stanford, CT, 1993, Appleton & Lange.

Prasartritha T, Liupolvanish P, Rojanakit A: A study of the posterior interosseous nerve and the radial tunnel in thirty Thai cadavers, *J Hand Surg* 18(1):107-112, 1993.

Pratt AL, Burr N, Grobbelaar AO: A prospective review of open central slip laceration repair and rehabilitation, *J Hand Surg* [Br] 27(6):530-534, 2002.

Pratt NE: Anatomy and biomechanics of the shoulder, *J Hand Ther* 7(2):65-76, 1994.

Prentice WE: *Therapeutic modalities for physical therapists*, ed 2, New York, 2002, McGraw Hill.

Pritchard CH, Sripada P, Bankes, PF, et al: A retrospective comparison of the efficacy and tolerability of sodium hyaluronate and hylan G-F20 in the treatment of osteoarthritis in the knee, *J Musculoskel Res* 6(3-4):197-205, 2002.

Prosser R, Conolly WB: Complication following surgical treatment for Dupuytren's contracture, *J Hand Ther* 9(4):344-348, 1996.

Prosser R, Herbert T: The management of carpal fractures and dislocations, *J Hand Ther* 9(2):139-147, 1996.

Purdy BA, Wilson RL: Management of nonarticular fractures of the hand. In Mackin EJ, Callahan AD, Skirven TM, et al, eds: *Rehabilitation of the hand and upper extremity*, ed 5, pp. 382-395, St Louis, 2002, Mosby.

Putz-Anderson V: *Cumulative trauma disorders: a manual for musculoskeletal disease of the upper extremity*, New York, 1988, Taylor & Francis.

Ranney D: *Chronic musculoskeletal injuries in the workplace*, Philadelphia, 1977, WB Saunders.

Raj PP: *Pain medicine: a comprehensive review*, St Louis, 1996, Mosby.

Rajon: *Hand Clin*, 1999.

Rayhack JM: The history and evolution of percutaneous pinning of displaced distal radius fractures, *Orthop Clin North Am* 24(2):287-300, 1993.

Reginato AJ, Hoffman GS: In Fauci AS, Braunwald E, Isselbacher KJ, et al, eds: *Harrison's Principles of internal medicine*, New York, 1998, McGraw-Hill.

Reid DC: *Sports injury assessment and rehabilitation*, ed 2, Philadelphia, 2002, WB Saunders.

Reiner M, Lohman W: *Medical management program for cumulative trauma disorders of the upper-extremity*, St Paul, MN, 1992, Hand Rehab, Inc.

Rettig AC, Ryan RO, Stone JA: Epidemiology of hand injuries in sports. In Strickland JW, Retting AC, eds: *Hand injuries in athletes*, pp. 37-48, Philadelphia, 1992, WB Saunders.

Reynolds CC: Preoperative and postoperative management of tendon transfers after radial nerve injury. In Mackin EJ, Callahan AD, Skirven TM, et al, eds: *Rehabilitation of the hand and upper extremity*, ed 5, pp. 821-831, St Louis, 2002, Mosby.

Richards RS, Bennett JD, Roth JH, et al: Arthroscopic diagnosis of intra-articular soft tissue injuries associated with distal radial fractures, *J Hand Surg* [Am] 22(5):772-776, 1997.

Richards R, Staley M: *Burn care and rehabilitation principles and practice*, Philadelphia, 1994, FA Davis.

Rockwood C, Matsen F: *The shoulder*, vols 1 and 2, Philadelphia, 1990, WB Saunders.

Rosenberg D, Conolley J, Dellon AL: Thenar eminence quantitative sensory testing in the diagnosis of proximal median nerve compression, *J Hand Ther* 14(4):258-265, 2001.

Rosenthal EA: The extensor tendons: anatomy and management. In Mackin EJ, Callahan AD, Skirven TM, et al, eds: *Rehabilitation of the hand and upper extremity*, ed 5, pp. 498-541, St Louis, 2002, Mosby.

Rowe CR, Zarins B: Recurrent transient subluxation of the shoulder, *J Bone Joint Surg* [Am] 63(6):863-872, 1981.

Rowland SA: Fasciotomy: the treatment of compartment syndrome. In Green DP, Hotchkiss RN, Pederson WC, eds: *Green's Operative hand surgery*, ed 4, pp. 689-710, Philadelphia, 1999, Churchill Livingstone.

Ruby LK, Cooney WP, An KN, et al: Relative motion of selected carpal bones: a kinematic analysis of the normal wrist, *J Hand Surg* [Am] 13(1):1-10, 1988.

Ruch DS, Poehling GS: Arthroscopic treatment of Panner's disease, *Clin Sports Med* 10:629-636, 1991.

Ryu JY, Cooney WP III, Askew LJ, et al: Functional ranges of motion of the wrist joint, *J Hand Surg* [Am] 16(3):409-419, 1991.

Sailer SM: The role of splints in rehabilitation in the treatment of carpal and cubital syndrome, *Hand Clin* 12(2): 223-241, 1996.

Sarrafian S: Kinesiology and functional characteristics of the upper limb. In Bowker JH, Michael JW, eds: *Atlas of limb prosthetics*, ed 2, St Louis, 1992, Mosby.

Saunders HD: *Evaluation, treatment and prevention of musculoskeletal disorders*, 1985, Viking Press.

Scheker LR, Hodges A: Brace and rehabilitation after replantation and revascularization, *Hand Clin* 17(3):473-480, 2001.

Schenck R: Intraarticular fractures of the phalanges, *Hand Clin* 10(2), 1994.

Schneider LH: Fractures of the distal interphalangeal joint, *Hand Clin* 10(2): 1994.

Schneider LH: Flexor tendons-late reconstruction. In Green DR, Hotchkiss RN, Pederson WC, eds: *Green's Operative hand surgery*, ed 4, pp. 1898-1949, Philadelphia, 1999, Churchill Livingstone.

Schneider LH: Fractures of the distal interphalangeal joint, *Hand Clin* 10(2):277-285, 1994.

Schneider LH: Impairment evaluation. In Mackin EJ, Callahan AD, Skirven TM, et al, eds: *Rehabilitation of the hand and upper extremity*, ed 5, St Louis, 2002, Mosby.

Schneider LH, Feldscher SB: Tenolysis: dynamic approach to surgery and therapy. In Mackin EJ, Callahan AD, Skirven TM, et al, eds: *Rehabilitation of the hand and upper extremity*, ed 5, pp. 457-468, St Louis, 2002, Mosby.

Schreuders TAR, Stam HJ: Strength measurements of lumbrical muscles, *J Hand Ther* 9:4, 1996.

Schultz-Johnson K: Upper extremity functional capacity. In Mackin EJ, Callahan AD, Skirven TM, et al, eds: *Rehabilitation of the hand and upper extremity*, ed 5, St Louis, 2002, Mosby.

Schwartz E, Warren RF, O'Brien SJ: Posterior shoulder instability, *Orthop Clin North Am* 18:409-419, 1987.

Sears HH: Approaches to prescription of bodypowered and myoelectric prosthesis, *Phys Med Rehabil Clin North Am* 2(2):361-371, 1991.

Seibold JR: In Kelley WN, Harris ED, Ruddy S, et al, eds: *Textbook of rheumatology*, ed 5, Philadelphia, 1997, WB Saunders.

Shaperman J, Landsberger SE, Setoguchi Y: Early upper limb prosthesis fitting: when and what do we fit, *J Prosthet Orthot Prosthet Orthot Sci* 15(1):13, 2003.

Sieg K, Adams SP: *Illustrated essentials of musculoskeletal anatomy*, ed 2, Gainesville, FL, 1985, Megabooks.

Silver Ring Splint Company catalog, Charlottesville, VA, 1994.

Simmons BP, McKenzie WD: Symptomatic carpal coalition, *J Hand Surg* [Am] 10(2):190-193, 1985.

Simonich SD, Wright TW: Terrible triad of the shoulder, *J Shoulder Elbow Surg* 6:566-568, 2003.

Simpson RL, Gartner MC: Management of burns of the upper extremity. In Mackin EJ, Callahan AD, Skirven TM, et al, eds: *Rehabilitation of the hand and upper extremity*, ed 5, pp. 1475-1491, St Louis, 2002, Mosby.

Singletary S, Freeland AE, Jarrett CA: Metacarpal fractures in athletes: treatment, rehabilitation, and safe early return to play, *J Hand Ther* 16(2):171-179, 2003.

Skirven TM: *Therapy post wrist arthroscopy: a comprehensive approach to challenging wrist problems*, Chicago, 1995, American Society of Hand Therapists.

Skirven TM, Callahan AD: Tenolysis: dynamic approach to surgery and therapy. In Mackin EJ, Callahan AD, Skirven TM, et al, eds: *Rehabilitation of the hand and upper extremity*, ed 5, pp. 599-621, St Louis, 2002, Mosby.

Skirven TM, Callahan AD: Therapist's management of peripheral-nerve injuries. In Mackin EJ, Callahan AD, Skirven TM, et al, eds: *Rehabilitation of the hand and upper extremity*, ed 5, pp. 599-621, St Louis, 2002, Mosby.

Skirven TM, Osterman AL: Clinical examination of the wrist. In Mackin EJ, Callahan AD, Skirven TM, et al, eds: *Rehabilitation of the hand and upper extremity*, ed 5, pp. 1099-1116, St Louis, 2002, Mosby.

Smith JR: *Modern treatment for lymphedema*, ed 5, Australia, 1997, Bowden.

Smith JW, Aston SJ: *Grabb and Smith's Plastic surgery*, ed 4, Boston, 1991, Little, Brown and Company.

Smith KL, Price JL: Care of the hand wound. In Mackin EJ, Callahan AD, Skirven TM, et al, eds: *Rehabilitation of the hand and upper extremity*, ed 5, pp. 331-343, St Louis, 2002, Mosby.

Smith MA, Muehlberger T, Dellon AL: Peripheral nerve compression associated with low-voltage electrical injury without associated significant cutaneous burn, *Plast Reconstr Surg* 109(1):137-144, 2002.

Smith P: *Lister's The hand: diagnosis and indications*, ed 4, London, 2003, Churchill Livingstone.

Smith RJ: Intrinsic Contracture. In Green DR, Hotchkiss RN, Pederson WC, eds: *Green's Operative hand surgery*, ed 4, pp. 604-618, Philadelphia, 1999, Churchill Livingstone.

Snyder SJ, Karzel R: Evaluation and treatment of the rotator cuff, *Orthop Clin North Am* 24(1), 1993.

Spiegel SR: Adult myoelectric upper-limb prosthetic training. In Atkins DJ, Meier RH, eds: *Comprehensive management of the upper-limb amputee*, New York, 1989, Springer-Verlag.

Spinner M: *Kaplan's Functional and surgical anatomy of the hand*, ed 3, Philadelphia, 1984, JB Lippincott.

Stabile KJ, Pfaeffle HJ, Tomaino MM: The Essex-Lopresti fracture-dislocation factors in early management and salvage alternatives, *Hand Clin* 18(1):195-204, 2002.

Stanley B, Tribuzi S: *Concepts in hand rehabilitation*, Philadelphia, 1992, FA Davis.

Steindler A: Reconstruction work on hand and forearm, *NY State Med J* 108:117-119, 1918.

Stener B: Displacement of the ruptured ulnar collateral ligament of the metacarpophalangeal joint of the thumb, *J Bone Joint Surg* [Br] 44:869-879, 1962.

Stern PJ: Fractures of the metacarpals and phalanges. In Green DP, Hotchkiss RN, Pederson WC, eds: *Green's Operative hand surgery*, ed 4, pp. 711-771, Philadelphia, 1999, Churchill Livingstone.

Stern PJ: Tendonitis, overuse syndromes, and tendon injuries, *Hand Clin* 6(3): 467, 1990.

Stirrat CR: Metacarpophalangeal joints in rheumatoid arthritis of the hand, *Hand Clin* 12(3):515-529, 1996.

Stokes LO, Stokes M: *Neurological physiotherapy*, St Louis, 1998, Mosby.

Strickland JW: Biologic rationale, clinical application, and results of early motion following flexor tendon repair, *J Hand Ther* pp. 30-41, 1989.

Strickland JW: Flexor tendons—acute injuries. In Green DP, Hotchkiss RN, Pederson WC, eds: *Green's Operative hand surgery*, ed 4, pp. 1851-1897, Philadelphia, 1999, Churchill Livingstone.

Sussman C, Bates-Jensen BM: *Wound care: a collaborative practice manual for physical therapists and nurses*, ed 2, New York, 2001, Aspen.

Swanson AB: Congenital limb defects classification and treatment, *Clin Symp* 33(3):1-32, 1981.

Szabo RM: Entrapment and compression neuropathies. In Green DR, Hotchkiss RN, Pederson WC, eds: *Green's Operative hand surgery*, ed 4, pp. 1404-1447, Philadelphia, 1999, Churchill Livingstone.

Taleisnik J: *The wrist*, New York, 1985, Churchill Livingstone.

Tan JC: *Practical manual of physical medicine and rehabilitation*, St Louis, 1998, Mosby.

Tan V, Rothenfluh DA, Beredjiklian PK, et al: Interosseous-lumbrical adhesions of the hand: contribution of magnetic resonance imaging to diagnosis and treatment planning, *J Hand Surg* [Am] 27(4):639-643, 2002.

Taras JS, Lemel MS, Nathan R: Vascular disorders of the upper extremity. In Mackin EJ, Callahan AD, Skirven TM, et al, eds: *Rehabilitation of the hand and upper extremity*, ed 5, pp. 879-898, St Louis, 2002, Mosby.

Terrono AL, Nalebuff EA, Philips CA: The rheumatoid thumb. In Mackin EJ, Callahan AD, Skirven TM, et al, eds: *Rehabilitation of the hand and upper extremity*, ed 5, pp. 1555-1568, St Louis, 2002, Mosby.

Thomas D, Moutet F, Guinard D: Postoperative management of extensor tendon repairs in zones V, VI, and VII, *J Hand Ther* 9(4):309-314, 1996.

Thomes L, Thomes B: Early mobilization method of surgically repaired Zone III extensor tendons, *J Hand Ther* 8(3):195-198, 1995.

Thorson EP, Szabo R: Tendonitis of the wrist and elbow in occupational hand injuries. In Kosdan M, ed: *Occupational medicine*, vol 4, Philadelphia, 1989, Hanley & Belfus.

Topper SM: Hand and microsurgery. In *Miller's Review of orthopaedics*, ed 3, Philadelphia, 2000, WB Saunders.

Topical wound care algorithms, ed 3, Humlebaek, Denmark, Coloplast.

Travell JG, Simons DG: *Myofascial pain and dysfunction: the trigger point manual*, Baltimore, 1983, Williams & Wilkins.

Tribuzi SM: Serial plaster splinting. In Mackin EJ, Callahan AD, Skirven TM, et al, eds: *Rehabilitation of the hand and upper extremity*, ed 5, pp. 1828-1838, St Louis, 2002, Mosby.

Trombly CA: *Occupational therapy for physical dysfunction*, ed 4, Baltimore, 1995, Williams & Wilkins.

Trombly CA, Scott: *Occupational therapy for physical dysfunction*, ed 4, Baltimore, 1995, Williams and Wilkins.

Tubiana R, Thomine JM, Mackin E: *Examination of the hand and wrist*, London, 1996, Martin Dunitz.

Varitimidis SE, Plakseychuk AY, Sotereanos DG: Reconstruction of the elbow: surgeon's perspective, *JHT* pp. 66, 1996.

Vasudevan SV, Melvin JL: Upper-extremity edema control: rationale of the techniques, *Am J Occup Ther* 33(8):520-523, 1979.

Venes D, Thomas CL: *Taber's Cyclopedic medical dictionary*, ed 19, Philadelphia, 2001, FA Davis.

Vicar A: Proximal interphalangeal joint dislocations without fractures, *Hand Clin* 4(1):5-13, 1988.

Villeco JP, Mackin EJ, Hunter JM: Edema: therapist's management. In Mackin EJ, Callahan AD, Skirven TM, et al, eds: *Rehabilitation of the hand and upper extremity*, ed 5, St Louis, 2002, Mosby.

Wadsworth TG: Elbow tendonitis. In Mackin EJ, Callahan AD, Skirven TM, et al, eds: *Rehabilitation of the hand and upper extremity*, ed 5, pp. 1263-1270, St Louis, 2002, Mosby.

Walch G, Boileau P, Noel E, et al: Impingement of the deep surface of the supraspinatus tendon on the posterosuperior glenoid: an arthroscopic study, *J Shoulder Elbow Surg* 1:238-245, 1992.

Walsh MT: Rationale and indications for the use of nerve mobilization and nerve gliding as a treatment approach. In Mackin EJ, Callahan AD, Skirven TM, et al, eds: *Rehabilitation of the hand and upper extremity*, ed 5, pp. 762-775, St Louis, 2002, Mosby.

Walsh MT, Muntzer E: Therapist's management of complex regional pain syndrome (reflex sympathetic dystrophy). In Mackin EJ, Callahan AD, Skirven TM, et al, eds: *Rehabilitation of the hand and upper extremity*, ed 5, pp. 1707-1724, St Louis, 2002, Mosby.

Walters KJ: *Understanding intrinsic and extrinsic tendon tightness and how to correct the problem.* Presented at Indiana Hand Care, Indianapolis, 1996.

Warmer Dam AD: *Manual therapy: improve muscle and joint function*, 1999, p. 261.

Warner JJ: Frozen shoulder: diagnosis and management, *J Am Acad Orthop Surg* 5(3):130-140, 1997.

Warwick L, Seradge H: Early versus later range of motion following cubital tunnel surgery, *J Hand Ther*, 8(4):245-248, 1995.

Watson HK, Weinzweig J: Intercarpal arthrodesis. In Green DP, Hotchkiss RN, Pederson WC, eds: *Green's Operative hand surgery*, ed 4, pp. 108-130, Philadelphia, 1999, Churchill Livingstone.

Watson HK, Weinzweig J, Guidera PM, et al: One thousand intercarpal arthrodeses, *J Hand Surg* [Br] 24(3):307-315, 1999.

Watson HK, Weinzweig J, Zeppieri J: The natural progression of scaphoid instability, *Hand Clin* 13(1):39-49, 1997.

Wehbe MA: Tendon gliding exercises, *Am J Occup Ther* 41(3):164-167, 1987.

Weinblatt ME, Keystone EC, Furst DE, et al: Adalimumab, a fully human anti-tumor necrosis factor alpha monoclonal antibody, for the treatment of rheumatoid arthritis in patients taking concomitant methotrexate: the ARMADA trial, *Arthritis Rheum* 48(1):35-45, 2003.

Weinzweig J: *Hand and wrist surgery secrets*, Philadelphia, 2000, Hanley & Belfus.

Weiss S, LaStayo P, Mills A, et al: Prospective analysis of splinting the first carpometacarpal joint: an objective, subjective, and radiographic assessment, *J Hand Ther* 13(3):218-226, 2000.

Werner FW, An KN: Biomechanics of the elbow and forearm, *Hand Clin* 10(3):357-373, 1994.

Whintraur M: Chapter 21 p. 268-277.

Wilder RT, Berde CB, Wolohan M, et al: Reflex sympathetic dystrophy in children: clinical characteristics and follow-up of seventy patients, *J Bone Joint Surg* [Am] 74(6):910-919, 1992.

Wilk KE, Voight ML, Keirns MA: Stretch-shortening drills for the upper extremities: theory and clinical application, *J Orthop Sports Phys Ther* 17:225-239, 1993.

Wilton JC, Dival TA: *Hand splinting: principles of design and fabrication*, Philadelphia, 1997, WB Saunders.

Wong GY, Wilson PR: Classification of complex and regional pain syndrome: new concepts, *Hand Clin* 13(3):319-325, 1997.

Wong L, Dellon AL: Brachial neuritis presenting as anterior interosseous nerve compression—implications for diagnosis and treatment: a case report, *J Hand Surg* [Am] 22(3):536-539, 1997.

Wright H: The hand in sports, *J Hand Ther* 4(2):49, 1991.

Wright HH, Rettig AC: Management of common sports injuries. In Mackin EJ, Callahan AD, Skirven TM, et al, eds: *Rehabilitation of the hand and upper extremity*, ed 5, pp. 2076-2104, St Louis, 2002, Mosby.

Wright TW, Dobyns JH: Carpal instability nondissociative. In Cooney WP, Linscheid RL, Dobyns JH, eds: *The wrist: diagnosis and operative treatment*, pp. 550-568, St Louis, 1998, Mosby.

Wright TW, Michlovitz SL: Management of carpal instabilities, *J Hand Ther* 9(2):148-156, 1996.

Wounds: a compendium of clinical research and practice, 13(2):suppl B, 2001.

Wynn Parry CB: *Rehabilitation of the hand*, ed 3, London, 1978, Butterworth-Heinemann.

Yamaguchi S, Viegas SF, Patterson RM: Anatomic study of the pisotriquetral joint: ligament anatomy and cartilaginous change, *J Hand Surg* [Am] 23(4):600-606, 1998.

Yaremchuk MJ: Plastic surgery inservice exam: hand and extremities.

Zyto K, Kronberg M, Brostrom LA: Shoulder function after displaced fractures of the proximal humerus, *J Shoulder Elbow Surg* 4(5):331-336, 1995.